Lung Transplantation: Principles and Practice

Lung Transplantation: Principles and Practice

Edited by Dylan Long

hayle medical

New York

Hayle Medical,
750 Third Avenue, 9th Floor,
New York, NY 10017, USA

Visit us on the World Wide Web at:
www.haylemedical.com

ISBN: 978-1-63241-433-5

Cataloging-in-Publication Data

Lung transplantation : principles and practice / edited by Dylan Long.
    p. cm.
Includes bibliographical references and index.
ISBN 978-1-63241-433-5
1. Lungs--Transplantation. 2. Transplantation of organs, tissues, etc. I. Long, Dylan.
RD539 .L86 2017
617.542--dc23

Table of Contents

Table of Contents

Preface

It is often said that books are a boon to mankind. They document every progress and pass on the knowledge from one generation to the other. They play a crucial role in our lives. Thus I was both excited and nervous while editing this book. I was pleased by the thought of being able to make a mark but I was also nervous to do it right because the future of students depends upon it. Hence, I took a few months to research further into the discipline, revise my knowledge and also explore some more aspects. Post this process, I began with the editing of this book.

This book discusses the fundamentals as well as modern approaches of lung transplantation. It unfolds the innovative aspects of this subject which will be crucial for the progress of this field in the future. Lung transplantation is an extensive surgical procedure in which the diseased lung is partially or fully replaced by a healthy lung. The various types of lung transplants are lobe transplant, heart-lung transplant, double-lung transplant, etc. This text aims at providing readers the most important concepts, theories and applications related to this field. It studies, analyses and upholds pillars of lung transplantation and its utmost significance in modern times. This book consists of contributions made by international experts. It will prove to be a beneficial resource guide for readers.

I thank my publisher with all my heart for considering me worthy of this unparalleled opportunity and for showing unwavering faith in my skills. I would also like to thank the editorial team who worked closely with me at every step and contributed immensely towards the successful completion of this book. Last but not the least, I wish to thank my friends and colleagues for their support.

Editor

Preface

It is often said that books are a boon to mankind. They document every progress and pass on the knowledge from one generation to the other. They play a crucial role in our lives. Thus I was both excited and nervous while editing this book. I was pleased by the thought of being able to make a mark but I was also nervous to do it right because the future of students depends upon it. Hence, I took a few months to research further into the discipline, revise my knowledge and also explore some more aspects. Post this process, I began with the editing of this book.

This book discusses the fundamentals as well as modern approaches of lung transplantation. It unfolds the innovative aspects of this subject which will be crucial for the progress of this field in the future. Lung transplantation is an extensive surgical procedure in which the diseased lung is partially or fully replaced by a healthy lung. The various types of lung transplants are lobe transplant, heart-lung transplant, double-lung transplant, etc. This text aims at providing readers the most important concepts, theories and applications related to this field. It studies, analyses and upholds pillars of lung transplantation and its utmost significance in modern times. This book consists of contributions made by international experts. It will prove to be a beneficial resource guide for readers.

I thank my publisher with all my heart for considering me worthy of this unparalleled opportunity and for showing unwavering faith in my skills. I would also like to thank the editorial team who worked closely with me at every step and contributed immensely towards the successful completion of this book. Last but not the least, I wish to thank my friends and colleagues for their support.

Editor

Changes in the Lung Microbiome following Lung Transplantation Include the Emergence of Two Distinct Pseudomonas Species with Distinct Clinical Associations

Robert P. Dickson[1], John R. Erb-Downward[1], Christine M. Freeman[1,2], Natalie Walker[1], Brittan S. Scales[1,3], James M. Beck[4], Fernando J. Martinez[1], Jeffrey L. Curtis[1,5], Vibha N. Lama[1], Gary B. Huffnagle[1,3]*

1 Division of Pulmonary and Critical Care Medicine, Department of Internal Medicine, University of Michigan Medical School, Ann Arbor, Michigan, United States of America, 2 Research Service, Department of Veterans Affairs Health Care System, Ann Arbor, Michigan, United States of America, 3 Department of Microbiology and Immunology, University of Michigan Medical School, Ann Arbor, Michigan, United States of America, 4 Department of Medicine, University of Colorado Denver, Aurora, Colorado and Medicine Service, Veterans Affairs Eastern Colorado Health Care System, Denver, Colorado, United States of America, 5 Pulmonary & Critical Care Medicine Section, Medical Service, VA Ann Arbor Healthcare System, Ann Arbor, Michigan, United States of America

Abstract

Background: Multiple independent culture-based studies have identified the presence of *Pseudomonas aeruginosa* in respiratory samples as a positive risk factor for bronchiolitis obliterans syndrome (BOS). Yet, culture-independent microbiological techniques have identified a negative association between *Pseudomonas* species and BOS. Our objective was to investigate whether there may be a unifying explanation for these apparently dichotomous results.

Methods: We performed bronchoscopies with bronchoalveolar lavage (BAL) on lung transplant recipients (46 procedures in 33 patients) and 26 non-transplant control subjects. We analyzed bacterial communities in the BAL fluid using qPCR and pyrosequencing of 16S rRNA gene amplicons and compared the culture-independent data with the clinical metadata and culture results from these subjects.

Findings: Route of bronchoscopy (via nose or via mouth) was not associated with changes in BAL microbiota (p = 0.90). Among the subjects with positive *Pseudomonas* bacterial culture, *P. aeruginosa* was also identified by culture-independent methods. In contrast, a distinct *Pseudomonas* species, *P. fluorescens*, was often identified in asymptomatic transplant subjects by pyrosequencing but not detected via standard bacterial culture. The subject populations harboring these two distinct pseudomonads differed significantly with respect to associated symptoms, BAL neutrophilia, bacterial DNA burden and microbial diversity. Despite notable differences in culturability, a global database search of UM Hospital Clinical Microbiology Laboratory records indicated that *P. fluorescens* is commonly isolated from respiratory specimens.

Interpretation: We have reported for the first time that two prominent and distinct *Pseudomonas* species (*P. fluorescens* and *P. aeruginosa*) exist within the post-transplant lung microbiome, each with unique genomic and microbiologic features and widely divergent clinical associations, including presence during acute infection.

Editor: Ian C. Davis, The Ohio State University, United States of America

Funding: Funding provided by National Institutes of Health grants T32HL00774921 (RPD), U01HL098961 (JMB, JLC, GBH), R01HL094622 (VNL), R01HL114447 (GBH, FJM), T32AI007528 (BSS) and the Biomedical Laboratory and Clinical Science Research & Development Services, Department of Veterans Affairs (CMF, JMB, JLC). The funders had no role in study design, data collection and analysis, decision to publish, or preparation of the manuscript.

Competing Interests: The authors have declared that no competing interests exist.

* E-mail: ghuff@umich.edu

Introduction

In recent years, novel culture-independent techniques of microbial identification have permitted analysis of entire bacterial communities within the airways of patients with various diseases [1–4]. Lung transplantation is the only therapeutic option for many end-stage lung diseases [5]. Microbial infection and colonization have been associated with increased morbidity and mortality among lung transplant recipients, due to pneumonia or bronchiolitis obliterans syndrome (BOS) [5–8]. Lung transplantation and the immunosuppressive therapies it requires result in numerous changes to host defenses that may alter the microbiota

of the respiratory tract [9,10]. In a recent study of lung transplant recipients using culture-independent techniques, Willner et. al observed a negative association between the abundance of *Pseudomonas* species (spp). and the diagnosis of BOS [11], a surprising result given the numerous independent studies demonstrating that the detection of *P. aeruginosa* in respiratory cultures is a positive risk factor for the subsequent development of BOS [6,12,13]. Additionally, studies of the post-transplant lung microbiome have conflicted regarding the impact of transplantation on microbial diversity, with one report finding increased diversity compared to controls [14] and another reporting decreased diversity [15]. The source of these conflicting findings, as well as the clinical significance and associated clinical factors of post-transplant microbial diversity, remain undetermined.

In this study, we aimed to address these conflicting findings via culture-independent identification of microbial communities in BAL samples obtained from lung transplant recipients, stratified by clinical parameters, and non-transplant control subjects. We hypothesized that the post-transplant lung microbiome would be distinct from that of non-transplant controls, and, consistent with the dichotomous reports, would contain more than one prominent species of *Pseudomonas* that would correlate with transplant health. We also hypothesized that the diversity of post-transplant lung microbiota would not be uniform among transplant recipients and would correlate with clinically significant parameters.

Methods

Ethics Statement

All clinical investigations were conducted according to the principles expressed in the Declaration of Helsinki. The study protocol was approved by the institutional review boards of the University of Michigan Healthcare System and the Ann Arbor Veterans Affairs Healthcare System. All patients provided written informed consent. The institutional review boards have examined the protocols and certified that "The risks are reasonable in relation to benefits to subjects and the knowledge to be gained. The risks of the study have been minimized to the extent possible."

Subject enrollment

Lung transplant recipients. BAL samples were obtained from lung transplant recipients undergoing bronchoscopy at the University of Michigan. All lung transplant recipients at the University of Michigan were eligible for enrollment in the study. Specimens were collected consecutively between 11/1/2011 and 8/1/2012.

Non-transplant control subjects. Specimens were obtained from volunteers enrolled in the Lung HIV Microbiome Project who underwent research bronchoscopy at the VA Ann Arbor Healthcare System [16,17]. All subjects were HIV-negative.

Clinical data

Clinical data regarding lung transplant recipients was abstracted from the electronic medical record of the University of Michigan and from the Organ Transplant Information System (OTIS). BOS was defined by physiologic testing according to the International Society of Heart and Lung Transplantation guidelines [18].

Sample acquisition and processing

Patients received conscious sedation and nebulized lidocaine. The bronchoscope was advanced via the mouth or nose and through the vocal cords. After a brief airway exam, the bronchoscope was wedged in the right middle lobe or lingula of the allograft (for surveillance bronchoscopies) or, in the case of symptomatic patients with available imaging, in the segment with the most evidence of radiographic abnormality. In non-transplant control subjects, the bronchoscope was wedged in the right middle lobe and lingula. BAL was performed with instillation of between 120 and 300 ml of sterile isotonic saline. Samples were stored on ice, centrifuged at 13,000 RPM for 30 minutes (Hermle Z 231 M microcentrifuge) in dolphin-nosed Eppendorf tubes and stored at $-80°C$ until the time of DNA extraction. All samples obtained from transplant subjects were processed by the University of Michigan Microbiology Laboratory for routine microbial analysis (bacterial, fungal and AFB culture). For bacterial culture, BAL fluid was plated on chocolate, sheep blood and MacConkey agar

plates and incubated for ≥ 72 hours. Bacteria were identified and reported if they grew more than 10^4 colony forming units (CFU) per mL, or if under 10^4 CFU/mL but were a single gram negative bacillus species and the only reportable pathogen.

DNA isolation

Genomic DNA was extracted from BAL pellets resuspended in 360 µl ATL buffer (Qiagen DNeasy Blood & Tissue kit) and homogenized in UltraClean fecal DNA bead tubes (MO-BIO, Carlsbad, CA) using a modified protocol previously demonstrated to isolate bacterial DNA [19].

Quantitative Polymerase Chain Reaction (qPCR)

Quantification of bacterial 16S rDNA was performed by real-time PCR utilizing TaqMan hydrolysis probes on a Roche 480 LightCycler. Degenerate bacterial 16S rDNA specific primers were targeted to the V1-V2 regions of the 16S rDNA gene using the following sequences: 5'-AGAGTTTGATCCTGGCTCAG-3' (forward); 5'-CTGCTGCCTYCCGTA-3' (reverse); (5'-FAM-TA+ACA+CATG+CA+AGTC+GA- BHQ1-3' (probe). [20–22]. The probe was developed for the primer BSR65/17 landing site using the following sequence: 5'-TCGACTTGCATGTRTTA-3'. 16S clones derived from a *Haemophilus* species were used for generation of a standard curve. After an initial denaturation of five minutes at 95°C, 40 cycles of amplification were performed: 30 seconds at 94°C, 30 seconds at 50°C and 30 seconds at 72°C. A final elongation step was performed at 72°C.

454 Pyrosequencing

The V3–V5 hypervariable regions of the bacterial 16S rRNA gene were sequenced in the V5–V3 direction using barcoded primer sets corresponding to 357F and 926R [23]. These barcoded primers were originally developed by the Broad Institute. Primary PCR cycling conditions were 95°C for two minutes, followed by 20 cycles of touchdown PCR (95°C 20 seconds, followed by an annealing for 30 seconds beginning at 60°C and decreasing one degree every two cycles until 50°C, and an elongation of 72°C 45 seconds), then 20 cycles of standard PCR (95°C for 20 seconds, 50°C for 30 seconds, and 72°C for 45 seconds), and finished with 72°C for 5 minutes. Quality control and sequencing was carried out at the University of Michigan, using the Roche 454 GS Junior according to established protocols [24]. Pre-procedure bronchoscope rinse controls, reagent water controls and mock community standards were analyzed with each sequencing run as quality controls.

Data analysis

Sequence data were processed and analyzed using the software mothur v.1.27.0 according to the Standard Operating Procedure for 454 sequence data (http://www.mothur.org) using a minimum sequence length of 250 basepairs [25]. A shared community file and a phylotyped (genus-level grouping) file were generated using operational taxonomic units (OTUs) binned at 97% identity generated using the dist.seqs, cluster, make.shared and classify.otu commands in mothur. No subsampling was performed and all subsequent phylogenetic analysis was performed in R. Amounts of bacterial DNA detected in reagent water controls were small relative to BAL and mock community specimens (discussed in results below). OTUs detected in reagent water controls were removed from all BAL specimens prior to analysis. OTU numbers were arbitrarily assigned in the binning process and are referred to throughout the manuscript in association with their most specified level of taxonomy.

Changes in the Lung Microbiome following Lung Transplantation Include the Emergence of Two Distinct...   3

These files, along with the files containing the taxonomic information for the OTUs, were imported and further analyzed in R using the R-package vegan 2.0–4 for diversity analyses and ordinations, and a custom R script for sorting classification results into tables. Classification of OTUs was carried out using the mothur implementation of the Ribosomal Database Project (RDP) Classifier and the RDP taxonomy training set 9 (fasta reference = trainset9_032012.pds.fasta, taxonomy reference = train-set9_032012.pds.tax), available on the mothur website. A mean of 1476±703 high-quality reads were obtained per BAL specimen. 1109 unique OTUs were identified across all the specimens. For relative abundance and ordination analysis, samples were normalized to the percent of total reads and we restricted analysis to OTUs that were present at greater than 1% of the sample population; all OTUs were included in diversity analysis. Sequences are available online at the NIH Sequence Read Archive (http://www.ncbi.nlm.nih.gov/sra, accession numbers 2419687–2419764).

Microbe-Specific PCR

Select BAL specimens were analyzed via PCR using microbe-specific primers. *Pseudomonas aeruginosa*-targeted primers used were PA-SS-F (5′-GGG GGA TCT TCG GAC CTC A-3′, location: 189-206) and PA-SS-R (5′-TCC TTA GAG TGC CCA CCC G-3′, location: 1124-1144) [26]. These primers were targeted at species-specific signature sequences in the 16S rDNA variable regions 2 and 8 and validated in our laboratory against numerous *Pseudomonas* species. For these primers, the initial denaturization step was at 95 C for 10 minutes, followed by 25 cycles of 94 C for 20 seconds, 58 C for 20 seconds and 72 C for 40 seconds with a final extension step of one minute at at 72 C. *Pseudomonas fluorescens*-targeted primers used were 16SPSEfluF (5′-TGC ATT CAA AAC TGA CTG-3′, location: 493-510) and 16SPSER (5′-AAT CAC ACC GTG GTA ACC G-3′, location: 1323–1338) [27]. For these primers, the initial denaturization step was at 95 C for 10 minutes, followed by 5 cycles of 94 C for 45 seconds, 55 C for 1 minute and 72 C for 2 minutes. This was followed by 35 cycles of 92 C for 45 seconds, 60 C for 45 seconds, 72 C for 2 minutes and a final extension step of 72 C for 2 minutes. Final cooling was performed at 4 C.

Phylogenetic Tree Generation

Bacterial genomes were uploaded into DNASTAR SeqBuilder (Lasergene). Sequences corresponding to the V3–V5 region of the 16S rRNA gene were aligned to each genome. A fasta-format document containing V3–V5 sequences was uploaded into MAFFT v.7, an online multiple sequence alignment program (http://mafft.cbrc.jp/alignment/server/) [28]. Details regarding the tree-building algorithm can be found at http://mafft.cbrc.jp/alignment/software/algorithms/algorithms.html. After sequence alignment, bootstrapping was performed and 1000 re-sample iterations were executed before generation of the final phylogenetic tree.

Statistical analysis

Statistical analyses were performed using Prism 5 (GraphPad Software) for ANOVA, t-test and regression analysis, and vegan and R for all diversity, rank abundance and ordination analyses. ANOVA-like permutation testing of constrained ordinations, both redundancy analysis (RDA) and by canonical correspondence analysis (CCA), was performed using the anova.cca function in the R package vegan. Significant differences in community membership identified via constrained ordination were confirmed using PERMANOVA (permutational multivariate analysis of variance) via the *adonis* function in vegan.

Study population

46 bronchoscopies were performed on 33 lung transplant recipients (**Table 1**). Six patients underwent two bronchoscopies, two underwent three and one patient underwent four; the remaining 24 patients underwent one bronchoscopy. Of the 46 specimens, two had minimal 16S bacterial DNA signal and were excluded from subsequent diversity, ordination, and rank-abundance analysis, but were included in relative 16S rDNA qPCR comparisons.

26 bronchoscopies were performed on 26 non-transplant control subjects, all lacking known history of lung disease (**Table 2**). All 26 specimens were included in all analyses.

For the purposes of analysis, transplant recipients were considered asymptomatic if the bronchoscopy was performed as a scheduled surveillance bronchoscopy (performed routinely at the University of Michigan following transplantation at six weeks, three months, six months and 12 months) and the patient had no acute complaints of cough, dyspnea, fever or increased sputum production and was not undergoing bronchoscopy for a newly appreciated radiographic infiltrate or decrease in lung function.

Patient Demographics

Most transplant recipients were male and had undergone bilateral lung transplantation (**1**). The most common pre-transplant diagnosis was pulmonary fibrosis, followed by cystic fibrosis (CF) and chronic obstructive pulmonary disease (COPD). Most bronchoscopies (67%) were performed within one year of transplantation.

When compared to patients who were asymptomatic at the time of bronchoscopy, symptomatic patients were more likely to be female and to have a history of BOS ($p < 0.05$, **Table 1**). Symptomatic and asymptomatic patients did not differ significantly with regard to time since transplant or pre-transplant diagnosis ($p > 0.05$, **Table 1**). A higher fraction of symptomatic subjects had recent antibiotic exposure and positive BAL bacterial culture (both *Pseudomonas* and otherwise), though these did not meet statistical significance ($p > 0.05$, **Table 1**, **Table 3**). The most commonly prescribed classes of antibiotics were fluoroquinolones, tetracyclines and macrolides. Only three subjects received nebulized tobramycin in the time prior to BAL. There were no significant differences in immunosuppression between the symptomatic and asymptomatic subjects.

Results

BAL from Lung Transplant Recipients Contains Distinct Bacterial Microbiota from that of Non-transplant Control Subjects

Bacteria levels in the samples from the various groups were determined by quantifying 16S rRNA gene copy numbers in 5 ml of unfractionated BAL. The amount of bacterial DNA detected in the pre-procedure bronchoscope rinse was at or near the limit of detection (**Figure 1**). In healthy, non-smoking individuals (non-transplant controls), the amount of bacteria in the BAL was significantly higher than in the pre-procedure control samples. Most importantly, the bacteria levels in the BAL specimens from lung transplant recipients were significantly higher than those in the healthy controls (**Figure 1**). On average, there was 15-fold more bacterial in the BAL specimens from transplant recipients than in those from non-transplant controls, with some samples 1000 fold higher (**Figure 1**). There was no significant difference

Table 1. Patient and Bronchoscopy Characteristics.

Patient characteristics

		Total (33)	Asymptomatic (17)	Symptomatic (16)	p
Patient demographics:	Male	29 (79%)	16 (94%)	10 (62%)	*0.04*
	Age	20–66 (49.9±15.8)	22–66 (52.6±17.2)	20–62 (47.0±14.4)	0.32
	Age at transplant	19–65 (48.7±15.5)	22–65 (51.6±16.6)	20–61 (45.7±14.2)	0.29
	Days post-transplant	26–2626 (431.7±575)	26–2626 (407.4±661.8)	58–1827 (457.6±487.5)	0.81
Type of transplant:	Bilateral lung	26 (79%)	11 (65%)	15 (94%)	0.08
	Single lung	13 (21%)	6 (35%)	1 (6%)	0.08
Pre-transplant diagnosis:	Pulmonary fibrosis	13 (39%)	6 (35%)	7 (44%)	0.73
	Cystic fibrosis	8 (24%)	4 (24%)	4 (25%)	1
	COPD	5 (15%)	4 (24%)	2 (12%)	0.65
	Other	7 (21%)	3 (18%)	3 (19%)	1
BOS:	BOS (ever)	7 (21%)	1 (6%)	6 (38%)	*0.04*
	BOS (at time of bronchoscopy)	4 (12%)	0 (0%)	4 (25%)	*0.04*

Bronchoscopy characteristics

		Total (44)	Asymptomatic (23)	Symptomatic (21)	p
Antibiotics:	Antibiotics within one month	28 (64%)	12 (52%)	16 (76%)	0.13
	Antibiotics within one week	19 (43%)	8 (35%)	11 (52%)	0.36
	Antibiotics at bronchoscopy	16 (36%)	6 (26%)	10 (48%)	0.21
Pathology:	Acute cellular rejection (A-grade)	5 (11%)	2 (9%)	3 (14%)	0.66
	Acute airway inflammation (B-grade)	2 (4%)	2 (9%)	0 (0%)	0.49
	Organizing pneumonia	6 (14%)	3 (13%)	3 (14%)	1

Depending on variable type, data are presented as either *N (% of group)* or as *range (mean ± standard deviation)*.

in bacterial 16S rRNA gene levels between symptomatic and asymptomatic transplant recipients. Thus, the BAL from lung transplant recipients contained significantly more bacteria than that from non-transplant control subjects.

Because bronchoscopies of transplant subjects were performed both via the nose and mouth, which contain distinct microbiota, and given the possibility of upper respiratory tract contamination of BAL specimens, we asked whether route of bronchoscope insertion was associated with differences in BAL microbiota. The majority (61%) of bronchoscopies performed on transplant subjects were performed via nasal insertion of the bronchoscope; the remainder were performed via an oral route. We employed the data visualization technique of Principal Components Analysis (PCA) to compare the bacterial communities in these specimen groups. We detected no spatial separation of BAL specimens obtained via the nose and those obtained via the mouth

(**Figure 2**). The two specimen groups were not statistically distinct when tested either via ANOVA-like permutation testing of constrained ordination (both redundancy analysis [RDA] and canonical correspondence analysis [CCA]) or via the *adonis* (PERMANOVA) function in vegan (p = 0.90). Thus route of bronchoscope insertion had no appreciable effect on BAL microbiota, arguing against significant contamination via upper respiratory tract microbiota.

Our next objective was to compare the composition of the BAL microbiota between transplant subjects and non-transplant controls, as well as between symptomatic and asymptomatic recipients. Using an unconstrained PCA of all samples (**Figure 3A**), we observed spatial separation of the three pre-specified subject groups (non-transplant controls, asymptomatic transplant recipients and symptomatic transplant recipients), though location of each group's members within the ordination

Table 2. Non-transplant Control Subject Characteristics (n = 26).

Male	8 (31%)
Age	18–75 (40.2±16.6)
Current Smoker	5 (19%)
Former Smoker	4 (15%)
FEV1% predicted	59–150 (103.2±16.9)

Table 3. Culture Results of Lung Transplant BAL Specimens.

	Total (44)	Asymptomatic (23)	Symptomatic (21)	p
Positive bacterial growth (any)	35 (80%)	19 (83%)	16 (76%)	0.72
Positive bacterial growth (>10K CFU/mL)	18 (41%)	7 (30%)	11 (52%)	0.22
Positive *Pseudomonas aeruginosa* growth	9 (20%)	2 (9%)	7 (33%)	0.06

was heterogenous. This separation of specimens by subject group was apparent when each group's centroid was plotted (**Figure 3B**), implying differences in the collective microbiota of each group when compared to the others. To test for statistical significance of these findings, we performed ANOVA-like permutation testing of constrained ordination, both by RDA and CCA. RDA demonstrated that significantly different microbial communities were associated with each of the subject groups (control, symptomatic recipients or asymptomatic recipients) (p<0.005, **Figure 3C**). This significance persisted when controlled for pretransplant diagnosis, time since transplant and FEV1 at the time of bronchoscopy (p<0.005 for all), and was confirmed using *adonis* (PERMANOVA) function in vegan (p<0.005) and corresponding multivariable analyses. When constrained by clinical parameters, only the presence of BOS at the time of bronchoscopy (p = 0.01) or of BOS at any point (p = 0.02) were associated with significant differences in BAL microbiota composition by ordination (**Table 4**). The significance of the distinct microbiota detected in subjects with BOS persisted when tested using adonis (p = 0.03) and when controlled for FEV1 at the time of bronchoscopy (p = 0.02) but not when controlled for time since transplant (p = 0.06). No significant differences were found when ordination

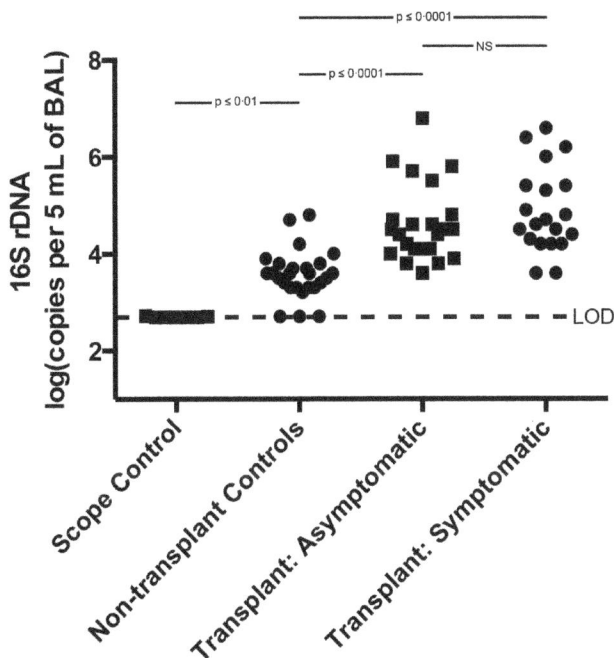

Figure 1. 16S rRNA gene qPCR of DNA prepared from unfractionated BAL samples. The number of copies of bacterial 16S rRNA genes per 5 mL of BAL was measured using qPCR as described in the methods. Specimen groups were compared using ANOVA and Tukey's multiple comparisons test.

was constrained by any other clinical parameter (p>0.05 for all) (**Table 4**). These analyses demonstrated that significant differences in the BAL bacterial communities could be identified between non-transplant, asymptomatic and symptomatic subjects, with BOS associated with significant differences in BAL microbiota among lung transplant recipients.

Decreased Bacterial Diversity is Associated with Evidence of Acute Bacterial Infection

We also investigated microbial diversity in the BAL from transplant recipients. The overall microbial diversity, as measured by the Shannon diversity index, was decreased among lung transplant recipients as compared to non-transplant controls (p = 0.001, **Figure 4A**). The distribution of diversity among transplant subjects was not uniform on inspection of this figure, with most subjects comparable to nontransplant control subjects but with 12 (27.2%) exhibiting markedly decreased bacterial diversity. When specimens were analyzed according to bronchoscopy indication, diversity among non-transplant control subjects was significantly higher than that of symptomatic transplant recipients (p ≤ 0.001) but not that of asymptomatic transplant recipients (p>0.05) (**Figure 4B**). Microbial diversity was not associated with exposure to antibiotics at the time of BAL or within seven days or 30 days of BAL (p>0.05 for all) (**Figure 4C**). Microbial diversity was significantly and negatively associated with the presence of BAL neutrophilia (p = 0.017) (**Figure 4D**), bacterial DNA burden (p≤0.0001) (**Figure 4E**) and positive bacterial culture (p≤0.001) (**Figure 4F**). Microbial diversity was not associated with any other tested clinical parameters, including pre-transplant diagnosis (**Table 4**). Thus, microbial diversity is not uniform in the lungs of transplant recipients and is negatively associated with other culture-independent indices of acute bacterial respiratory infection.

BAL from Lung Transplant Recipients Contain Increased levels of Pseudomonadaceae, Enterobacteriaceae and Staphylococcaceae and Decreased Levels of Prevotellaceae, Veillonellaceae, and Streptococcaceae

Despite the statistically significant differences in the PCA clusters between subject groups (**Figure 3**), some overlap existed between 1) the non-transplant controls and asymptomatic transplant recipients as well as between 2) asymptomatic and symptomatic transplant recipients. To explore whether we could determine the microbial constituents that were responsible for clustering of specimens in the PCA, we utilized a biplot analysis of the PCA (**Figure 3D**). This revealed that one of the major factors accounting for the difference in the non-transplant control subjects and many asymptomatic transplant subjects compared to other subjects was the abundance of OTU 1054 (**Figure 3D, x**). This OTU was classified as a *Prevotella* sp.. The major factor accounting for the difference in the heterogenous symptomatic transplant recipient group was the abundance of a single OTU (1065) in five

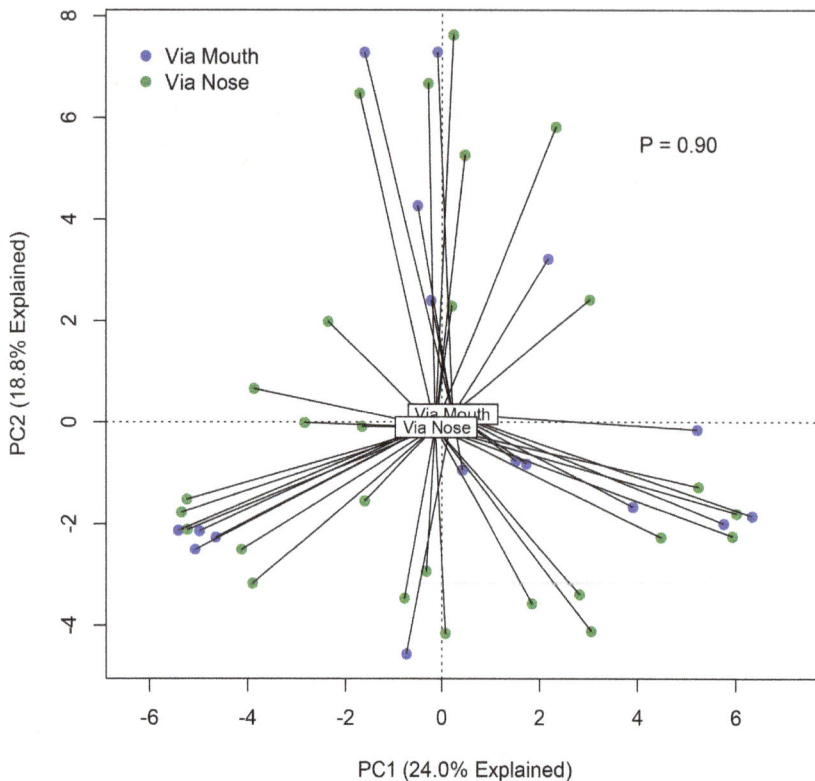

Figure 2. Comparison of transplant BAL specimens obtained via nasal and oral routes of bronchoscopy. Unsupervised principal component analysis (PCA) labeled by route of bronchoscope insertion. Group dissimilarity tested using ANOVA permutation test of ordination constrained by route of insertion.

of the subjects. This OTU was classified as a *Pseudomonas* sp. (**Figure 3D, y**). Finally, the PCA region that included most asymptomatic and some symptomatic transplant recipients (**Figure 3D, z**) was largely defined by the presence of two other OTUs (1025 and 1080). OTU 1080 was classified as an *Escherichia* sp., while OTU 1025 was classified as a *Pseudomonas* sp., distinct from the other *Pseudomonas* OTU (1065). Thus, the bacteria identified in the collection of lung transplant recipient BALs in our study included at least two distinct *Pseudomonas* spp. that appeared to be differentially represented in asymptomatic vs. symptomatic subjects.

We next analyzed the differences in the BAL microbiota among our subject groups at a taxonomic level. At the levels of phylum and family taxonomic classification, symptomatic and asymptomatic transplant recipients were markedly distinct from non-transplant controls but indistinguishable from each other (**Figure 5A**). Among non-transplant control subjects, the most commonly observed phyla (in descending order) were *Bacteroidetes*, *Firmicutes*, and *Proteobacteria*. These three phyla were also those most commonly observed among lung transplant recipients, though their relative frequency of detection was reversed, with *Proteobacteria* most commonly observed phylum. The most common bacterial families detected among non-transplant control subjects were *Prevotellaceae*, *Veillonellaceae*, and *Streptococcaceae*, while the most frequently detected families in BAL from transplant recipients were *Pseudomonadaceae*, *Enterobacteriaceae* and *Staphylococcaceae* (**Figure 5A**). There was minimal difference at a family level of taxonomy between symptomatic and asymptomatic transplant recipients. The presence of *Pseudomonadaceae* in the lung transplant recipients, which was rare in control subjects, was reflected in the

biplot PCA (**Figure 3D**). Overall, the majority of nontransplant control subjects had greater than 10% of their BAL microbiota consisting of *Prevotella* spp. and *Veillonella* spp., while this was infrequent among transplant subjects (**Table 5**). In contrast, the majority of transplant subjects had greater than 10% *Pseudomonas* spp. and *Escherichia* spp., which was infrequent among nontransplant control subjects (**Table 5**).

Two Distinct Pseudomonas Species Can Be Identified in the BAL from Lung Transplant Recipients

The most abundant OTU among symptomatic transplant recipients was a *Pseudomonas* sp. (OTU 1065) that, when present, was found in very high relative abundance (**Table 6, Figure 5B, y; Figure S1**). This OTU was the same that defined the cluster of symptomatic transplant subjects in PCA analysis (**Figure 3B, y**). In contrast, the most commonly detected OTU among asymptomatic transplant recipients (OTU 1025) was separately classified also as a *Pseudomonas* sp. (**Table 6, Figure 5B, z**) and was the same OTU that was the major factor that accounted for the clustering of asymptomatic transplant subjects in the PCA analysis (**Figure 3B, z**). A third OTU (OTU 1024) was also classified as a *Pseudomonas* sp. but was relatively infrequent and was detected in low abundance compared to the other *Pseudomonas* OTUs (**Table 6, Figure S1**). A fourth *Pseudomonas*-classified OTU (OTU 955) was detected in only one specimen, for which it comprised only 0.19% of total reads; it was excluded from subsequent analysis. **Figure S2** shows the representative sequences for the three most abundant *Pseudomonas* OTUs as well as their phylogenetic relationships. As OTU 1024 was not a significant factor in the clustering of the samples by PCA, we focused our

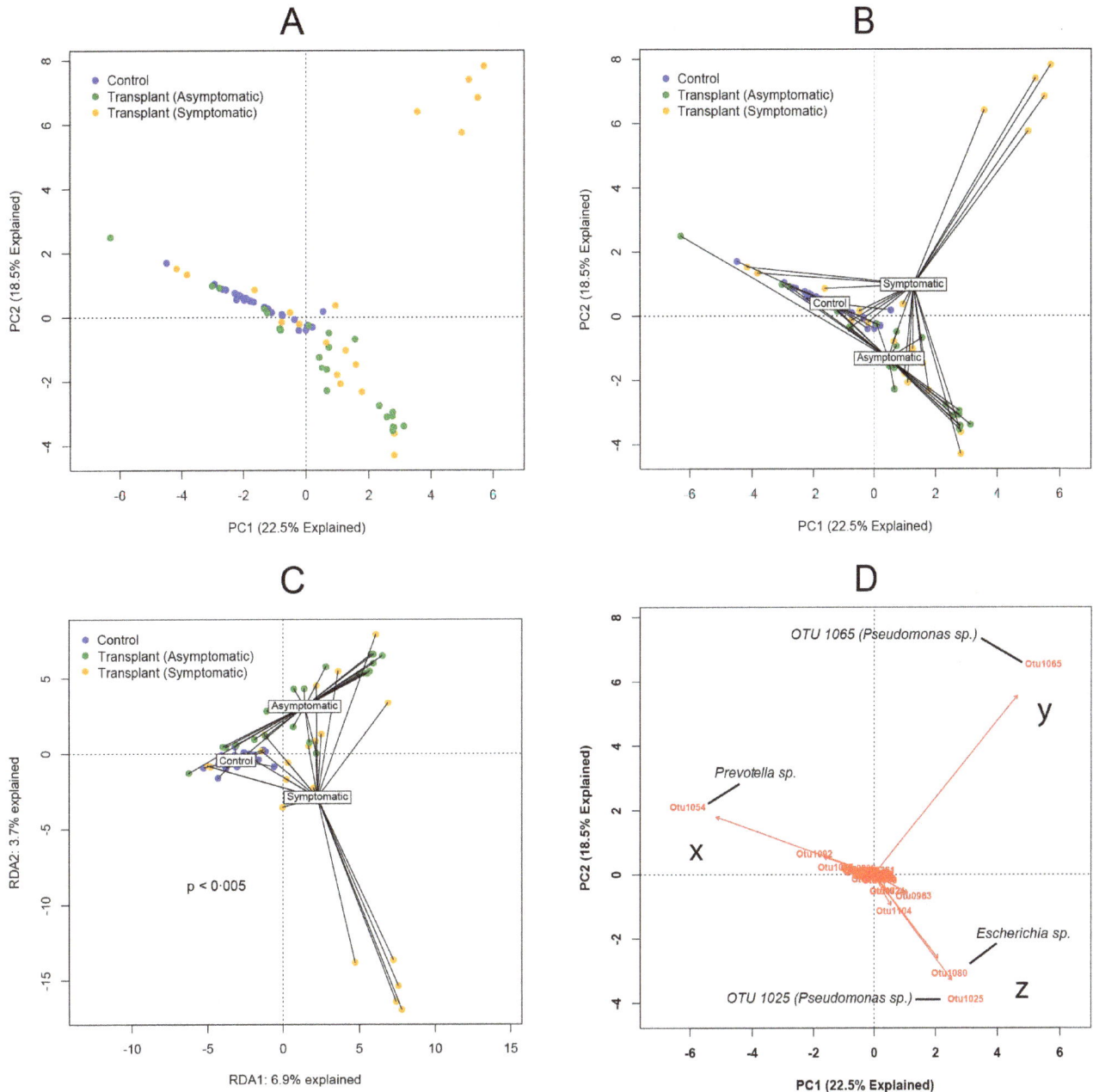

Figure 3. Ordination analyses of bacterial communities detected in BAL samples. Unsupervised principal component analysis (PCA): labeled by specimen group (A) and with specimen group centroids labeled (B) C: Ordination constrained by specimen group (RDA). Group dissimilarity tested using ANOVA permutation test. D: Biplot analysis of PCA plot with prominent OTUs labeled.

subsequent analysis on the two most common and significant *Pseudomonas* OTUs, 1025 and 1065.

In order to more thoroughly characterize the *Pseudomonas* OTUs, we utilized the National Center for Biotechnology Information Basic Local Alignment Search Tool (BLAST) (http://blast.ncbi.nlm.nih.gov/Blast.cgi). We screened all fully sequenced microbial genomes within the NCBI database using the *Pseudomonas* OTUs' 97% homologous representative nucleotide sequences. Of the 10 speciated bacterial strains in the NCBI database sharing 100% coverage and homology with the representative sequence of the *P. aeruginosa* OTU (OTU 1065), nine were identified as *P. aeruginosa* (**Table 7**, **Table S1**). In

contrast, the speciated bacterial strains sharing 100% coverage and homology with the other prominent *Pseudomonas* OTU (OTU 1025) were exclusively members of the *P. fluorescens* group (**Table 7**, **Table S1**, http://www.uniprot.org/taxonomy/200451).

Given the potential limitations of BLAST analysis in determining species-level taxonomic designations using 16S sequences, we designed a phylogenetic analysis utilizing existing sequences of clinically-obtained and reference genomes of 42 various *Pseudomonas* species as well as five non-*Pseudomonas* species. Using ten different housekeeping genes, we built MLST phylogeny trees (**Figure S3**) and compared them to trees generated using only 16S

Table 4. Significance of Comparisons of Lung Transplant Recipients by Diversity Analysis and Constrained Ordination.

Clinical Characteristic		Constrained Ordination Significance (p)	Shannon Diversity Index Significance (p)
Transplant/ Patient Factors	Pre-transplant diagnosis	>0.05	>0.05
	Type of transplant (single/bilateral)	>0.05	>0.05
	Sex	>0.05	>0.05
	Age	>0.05	>0.05
	Time over one year	>0.05	>0.05
	Antibiotics within 30 days	>0.05	>0.05
	Antibiotics within 7 days	>0.05	>0.05
	Antibiotics at time of BAL	>0.05	>0.05
	Pneumocystis prophylaxis agent	>0.05	>0.05
BAL Results	Bacterial DNA (16S qPCR)	>0.05	**p≤0.001**
	BAL neutrophilia	>0.05	**p = 0.017**
	Bacterial growth (>10^4 CFU/mL)	>0.05	**p≤0.001**
	Bacterial growth (any)	>0.05	>0.05
	Fungal growth	>0.05	>0.05
	Acute cellular rejection	>0.05	>0.05
Airway Factors	FEV1 under 70% predicted	>0.05	>0.05
	BOS (ever)	0.0225	>0.05
	BOS (at bronchoscopy)	0.01	>0.05

Statistical significance of comparisons of Shannon Diversity Indices was determined using Student's t-test and ANOVA for categorical variables and linear regression analysis for continuous variables. Constrained ordination was performed using Canonical Correspondance Analysis, and significance was determined using ANOVA-like permutation testing.

representative sequences (**Figure S2**). These trees illustrate that with these *Pseudomonas* species, MLST- and 16S-generated phylogenetic trees are similar. *P. aeruginosa* consistently separates from members of the *P. fluorescens* group in both, implying that enough genomic divergence is present in the 16S region to distinguish the two species. From our specimens, the *P. aeruginosa* OTU (OTU 1065) clustered exclusively with previously sequenced *P. aeruginosa* species. The other prominent *Pseudomonas* OTU (OTU 1025) clustered tightly and exclusively with members of the *P. fluorescens* group.

We also analyzed a number of the BAL samples with *P. aeruginosa* and *P. fluorescens*-specific PCR primers [26,27]. Three BAL specimens from subjects with high abundance of OTU 1065 (and low OTU 1025) and five BAL specimens with high abundance of OTU 1025 (and low 1065) were analyzed. The specimens with high abundance of OTU 1065 were PCR-positive for *P. aeruginosa* while those with a high abundance of OTU 1025 were PCR-positive for *P. fluorescens*. All patients who had OTU 1065 as the singular dominant OTU in their BAL microbiota also grew *P. aeruginosa* from their BAL (using conventional clinical microbiology techniques). In contrast, *P. aeruginosa* was not grown from any of the 11 BALs for which OTU 1025 was the most abundant OTU. Thus, when considered in aggregate, the pyrosequencing, BLAST, phylogenetic-tree analysis, microbe-specific PCR and culture data all support the conclusion that OTU 1065 represents *P. aeruginosa* and OTU 1025 represents *P. fluorescens*.

The Presence of P. aeruginosa and P. fluorescens in the BAL of Lung Transplant Recipients are Associated with Distinct Clinical Features

In order to assess potential differences in clinical significance associated with the presence of these two pseudomonads, we directly compared all subjects who had greater than 10% relative abundance of either prominent *Pseudomonas* OTU (**Figure 6**). No subjects had greater than 10% of both OTU (**Figure 6A**). When compared to subjects with greater than 10% *P. fluorescens*, subjects with *P. aeruginosa* had higher levels of BAL neutrophilia (**Figure 6B, p = 0.003**), bacterial DNA (**Figure 6C, p = 0.001**), and lower bacterial diversity (**Figure 6D, p<0.001**). All of the subjects with greater than 10% *P. aeruginosa* also had positive bacterial culture identified as *Pseudomonas*, while this was true of only one of the 15 subjects with greater than 10% *P. fluorescens* (**Figure 6E, p = 0.001**). Pre-transplant *Pseudomonas* infection was not more common among specimens with greater than 10% *P. aeruginosa* (2/6, 33%) than among other specimens (13/38, 34% (p>0.05). The most striking observation was that all of the subjects with greater than 10% *P. aeruginosa* were symptomatic at the time of bronchoscopy (**Table 6**), while most of the subjects with greater then 10% *P. fluorescens* were asymptomatic (**Figure 6F**).

Pseudomonas fluorescens has Strong Positive and Negative Correlations with Prominent Lung Microbes

Given the known ability of *P. fluorescens* to produce numerous antimicrobial molecules, we investigated the presence of correlations between its relative abundance and that of other prominent lung microbes. Significant positive and linear associations were

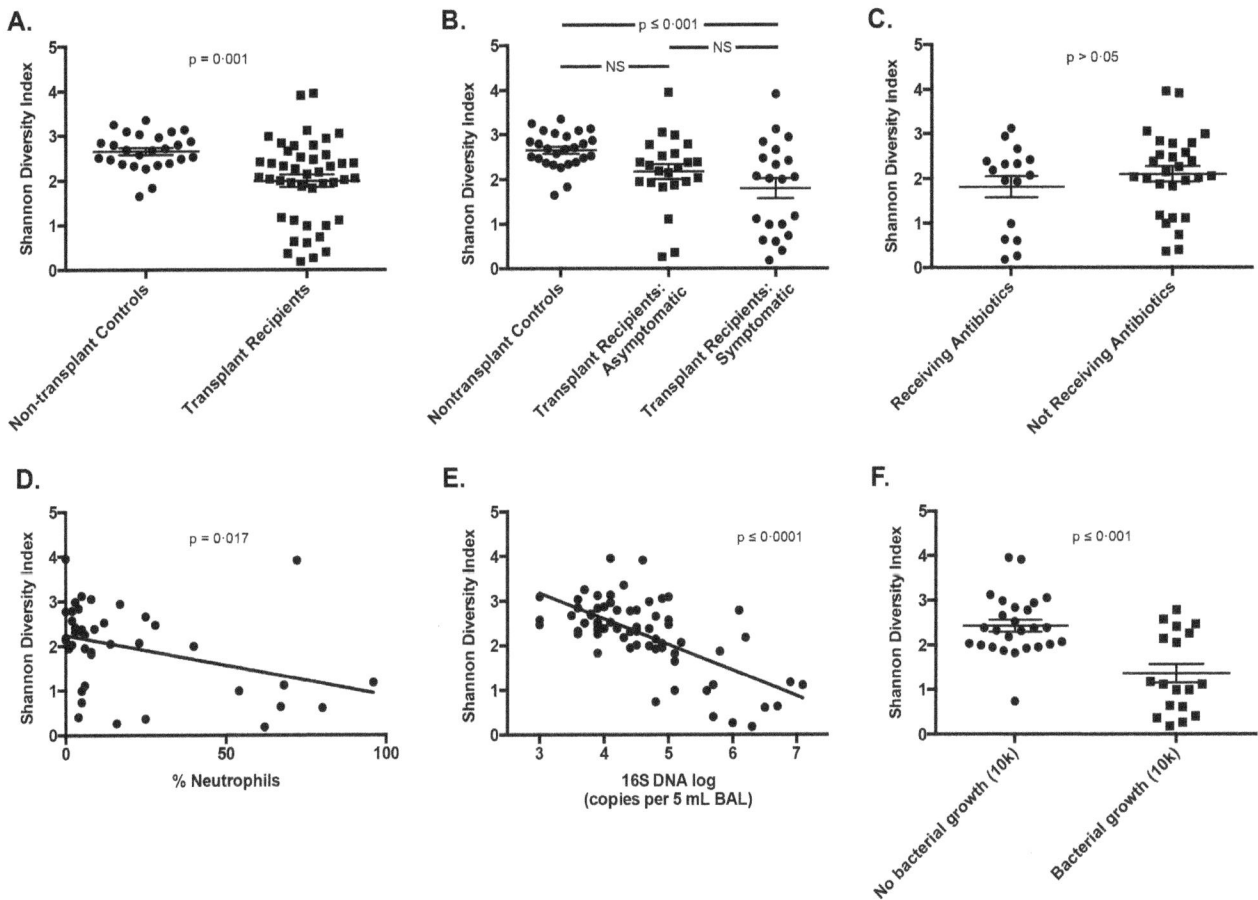

Figure 4. Shannon Diversity Indices of bacterial communities in BAL samples from lung transplant recipients. A-C: Comparison of bacterial community diversity by transplant status (A), specimen group (symptomatic/transplant status) (B) and antibiotic exposure (C). D-E: Bacterial community diversity correlated with BAL neutrophilia (D) and 16S DNA (E). F: Comparison of bacterial community diversity among transplant subjects by culture results. Comparison of group means performed with unpaired t-test and ANOVA with Tukey's multiple comparisons test. Continuous variables assessed for correlation with linear regression.

found between *P. fluorescens* and a common *Escherichia* OTU (OTU 1080) (p<0.0001, $R^2 = 0.37$), and significant negative nonlinear associations were found between *P. fluorescens* and OTUs of *Prevotella* and *Veillonella* (p = 0.003 and 0.01, respectively) **(Figure 7)**. Among transplant subjects, *P. fluorescens* also had a significant, negative and nonlinear association with the presence of *P. aeruginosa* (p = 0.05, unpaired t test).

Pseudomonas fluorescens is Commonly Isolated from the Airways of Lung Transplant Recipients and Patients with Other Chronic Lung Diseases

Given the prominence of *P. fluorescens* in the respiratory microbiota of our lung transplant recipients, we searched the database of bacterial culture isolates from the University of Michigan Clinical Microbiology Laboratory to determine how frequently it is cultured from respiratory specimens. Between January 1, 2002 and December 31, 2012, *P. fluorescens* was cultured from 242 distinct respiratory specimens, roughly 2 specimens per month. Of these, 59.9% were cultured using routine laboratory protocols for respiratory specimens; the remainder were cultured using a modified protocol adapted for specimens collected from patients with cystic fibrosis (CF). The majority (53.7%) were cultured from sputum specimens; 21.1% were cultured from

throat swabs, and 13.2% were cultured from bronchoscopically-obtained specimens (BAL or brushings). The most common underlying condition was CF (38.8% of all isolates), followed by other chronic airway disease (COPD, asthma and non-CF bronchiectasis: 16.1%) and lung transplantation (7.4%, 18 specimens). 10.7% (26) of the specimens were obtained from patients with suspected acute pneumonia, and in all but four of these instances the patient was either chronically immunosuppressed or had recent healthcare exposures meeting criteria for healthcare-associated pneumonia. In most isolates (85.1%), *P. fluorescens* was co-isolated with species classified by the laboratory as "oral flora." Other species commonly co-isolated were *P. aeruginosa* (25.6%), *Staphylococcus aureus* (15.7%) and *Stenotrophomonas maltophilia* (11.6%). Thus despite the notable differences observed in the culturability of pseudomonads in our study, a global database search of UM Hospital Clinical Microbiology Laboratory records indicated that *P. fluorescens* is commonly isolated from respiratory specimens.

Discussion

Using culture-independent techniques and BAL specimens from 59 total subjects, we identified that two distinct *Pseudomonas* species dominate the BAL microbiota of some transplant recipients.

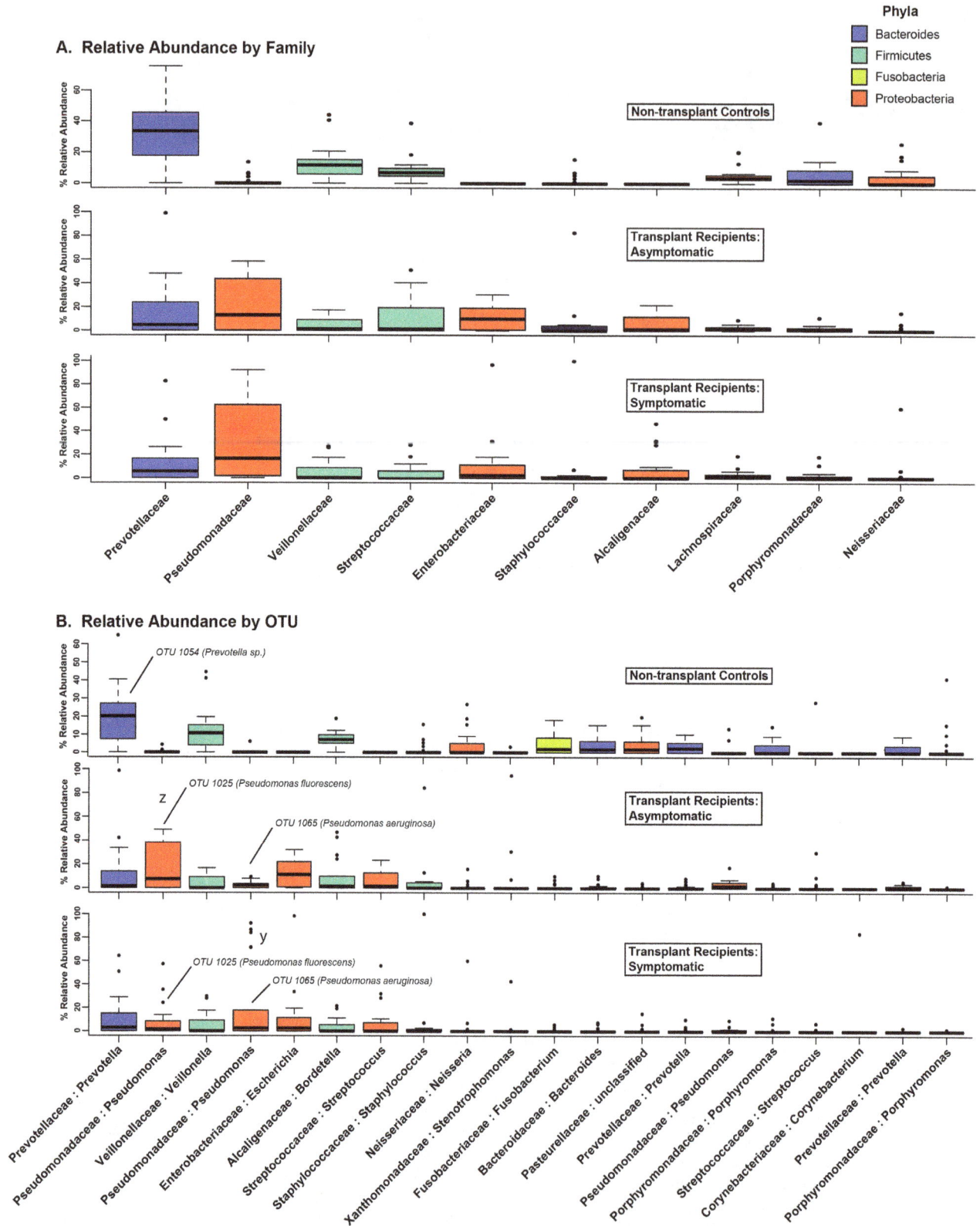

Figure 5. Taxonomic classification of the bacterial OTUs detected in BAL samples. Families and OTUs are ranked in descending order of mean relative abundance among all subjects. Box plots are colored according to phylum (see Phyla legend). Outliers are plotted as circles. A: Relative abundance of the 10 most abundant bacterial families. B: Relative abundance of 20 most abundant bacterial OTUs.

Table 5. Percentage of Subjects with >10% Relative Abundance of Prominent Genera.

Subject Group	Prevotella	Veillonella	Streptococcus	Pseudomonas	Escherichia
Nontransplant Control Subjects (26)	65.4%	53.8%	23.1%	3.8%	0.0%
Asymptomatic Transplant Subjects (23)	8.7%	17.4%	30.4%	52.2%	52.2%
Symptomatic Transplant Subjects (21)	4.8%	23.8%	14.3%	57.1%	28.6%

Whereas *P. aeruginosa*, when present, is detected in high abundance and is associated with clinical evidence of acute infection, *P. fluorescens* is commonly detected in moderate abundance and is rarely associated with parameters of acute infection. We observed that the decreased diversity of post-transplant lung microbiota is correlated with features of acute infection and is not uniform among transplant recipients.

Our results reveal that among post-transplant microbiota, at least two distinct *Pseudomonas* species are prominent and have widely divergent clinical associations, which provides a potential unifying explanation for the apparently dichotomous reports of the association between *Pseudomonas* and the development of BOS. Multiple independent studies have identified the presence of *P. aeruginosa* in respiratory cultures as a positive risk factor for the subsequent development of BOS [6,12,13]. Yet in the largest published study to date of lung transplant subjects utilizing culture-independent techniques of microbial identification, Willner et. al. observed a negative association between *Pseudomonas* spp. and the diagnosis of BOS [11]. While the subjects in our study with abundant *P. aeruginosa* exhibited evidence consistent with acute infection (symptoms of acute infection, BAL neutrophilia, increased bacterial burden, decreased bacterial diversity), the many subjects with abundant *P. fluorescens* exhibited little evidence of acute infection (**Figure 6B-6E**). The stark difference in culture positivity between these pseudomonads (**Figure 6E**) may explain the differences between prior culture-based studies and the culture-independent study by Willner et. al.. The distinctions between these two *Pseudomonas* species, while of clear clinical and biological significance, are unappreciated when analysis is limited to the family level of taxonomic designation (**Figure 5A**). Our results highlight the discriminatory power of incorporating additional techniques of microbial identification (e.g. culture, BLAST, phylogenetic tree generation, microbe-specific PCR) to complement the level of taxonomy provided by pyrosequencing and other culture-independent techniques.

The lack of detection of *P. fluorescens* via culture among our specimens was stark and surprising, especially given the relative frequency with which it is isolated in our clinical microbiology laboratory. Multiple explanations are possible. *P.fluorescens* is well-described to exist in a viable but not-culturable state in the environment[22,23]. All clinical respiratory specimens at our institution are incubated at 37°C, while the optimal growth temperature of P. fluorescens is below 32°C (a temperature range that is found in the airways [29]). *P. fluorescens* produces numerous antimicrobial metabolites and inhibits *in vitro* growth of other organisms[20,21], and in a one report could only be cultured after the fluid containing it was dialyzed [30]. Thus its culture-negativity may reflect production of active culture inhibitors.

Our study is the first to describe the widespread abundance of *P. fluorescens* in the BAL of lung transplant recipients. We are aware of only one published report of the detection of *P. fluorescens* in BAL fluid (a single patient with ventilator-associated pneumonia, detected using 16S analysis and not via BAL culture) [31]. The *Pseudomonas* genus is large and contains an extremely diverse group of bacteria at the genomic level. Much work has been done on the phylogeny of this genus, and recent studies have demonstrated that *P. fluorescens* and *P. aeruginosa* characterize very distinct genomic groups [32]. *P. aeruginosa* strains, when analyzed using either multi-locus sequence typing (MLST) or 16S rRNA gene sequence comparisons, cluster tightly within a single related group, while analysis of *P. fluorescens* strains has identified three distinct genetic clades [33]. For this reason, *P. fluorescens* bacteria have been suggested to belong in a species-complex rather than a single species [34]. Members of this *P. fluorescens* species complex include all sequenced *P. fluorescens* genomes, along with numerous other speciated pseudomonads [33]. *P. poae*, encountered during our BLAST analysis (**Table S1**), is a fluorescent pseudomonad that is genetically included within the *P. fluorescens* group [32] and phylogenetic analysis within our laboratory using MLST of nine selected housekeeping genes also clusters it within the *P. fluorescens* species-complex (manuscript in preparation). Taken together, analysis using culture, 16S analysis, MLST and PCR all indicate that the two prominent *Pseudomonas* OTUs in lung transplant BAL represent two distinct pseudomonads: *P. aeruginosa* and *P. fluorescens*. Indeed, our review of *P. fluorescens* isolates from our own clinical microbiology laboratory found that the organism is cultured from respiratory specimens of patients with lung transplantation and other chronic lung diseases with relative frequency.

Other recent culture-independent studies have located *P. fluorescens* elsewhere in the aerodigestive tract. A recent culture-independent analysis of the human salivary microbiome found increased prevalence of *P. fluorescens* among solid organ transplant

Table 6. Percentage of Subjects with >10% Relative Abundance of Prominent Pseudomonas OTUs.

Subject Group	OTU 1065: P. aeruginosa	OTU 1025: P. fluorescens	OTU 1024
Nontransplant Control Subjects (26)	0.0%	0.0%	3.8%
Asymptomatic Transplant Subjects (23)	0.0%	47.8%	4.3%
Symptomatic Transplant Subjects (21)	28.6%	23.8%	0.0%

Table 7. Abundance and Identification of Prominent Pseudomonas OTUs in Lung Transplant BALs.

OTU	% of BALs containing OTU	Mean abundance (SD)	Culture Results[1]	BLAST identification (100% coverage, 100% identity)
1065	66%	11.6% (25.6)	P. aeruginosa	P. aeruginosa[2]
1025	61%	13.5% (18.0)	No growth	P. fluorescens group[3]
1024	43%	1.9% (3.4)	No growth	None[4]

1: All BALs with OTU 1065 as the most abundant OTU grew P. aeruginosa. No BALs with either other OTU as the most abundant had positive cultures; 2: Of the 10 completed genomes in the database with 100% homology and 100% identity, nine were P. aeruginosa. 3: Of the two completed genomes in the database with 100% homology and 100% identity, one was P. fluorescens and one was P. poae, a recently described member of the P. fluorescens group (http://www.uniprot.org/taxonomy/200451); 4: No BLAST matches met 100% identity and homology. The genomes with the highest identity and homology were exclusively members of the P. fluorescens group.

recipients, [35] and a separate study found *P. fluorescens* in the vast majority (93%) of gastric antrum biopsies taken from patients with acid-related gastrointestinal disorders [36]. Members of the *P.*

fluorescens species-complex are obligate aerobic Gram-negative bacilli that are ubiquitous in plant, soil and water environments [37]; they are prominent plant commensals and are very rarely

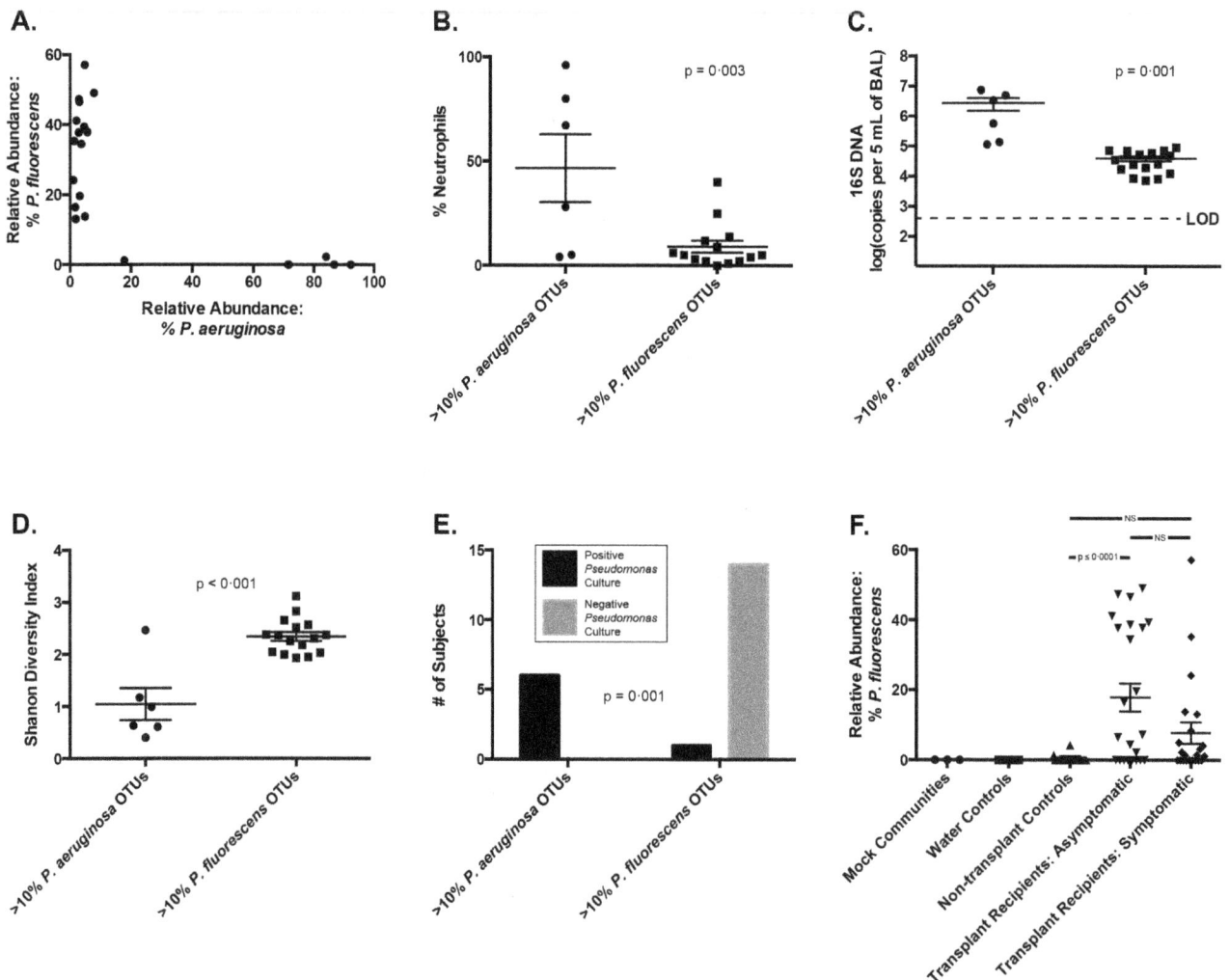

Figure 6. Clinical comparison among lung transplant recipients in relationship to two distinct *Pseudomonas* OTUs in BAL fluid. *P. aeruginosa* refers to OTU 1065, and *P. fluorescens* refers to OTU 1025 (see text). A: Relative abundance of each OTU in transplant recipients with greater than 10% of either. B-E: Comparison of *P. aeruginosa*-prominent and *P. fluorescens*-prominent BAL specimens by BAL neutrophilia (B), bacterial DNA burden (C), bacterial community diversity (D) and culture results (E). F: Relative abundance of *P. fluorescens* among pre-defined subject groups. Comparison of group means performed using unpaired t-test and ANOVA with Tukey's multiple comparisons test. Contingency testing performed using Fisher's exact test.

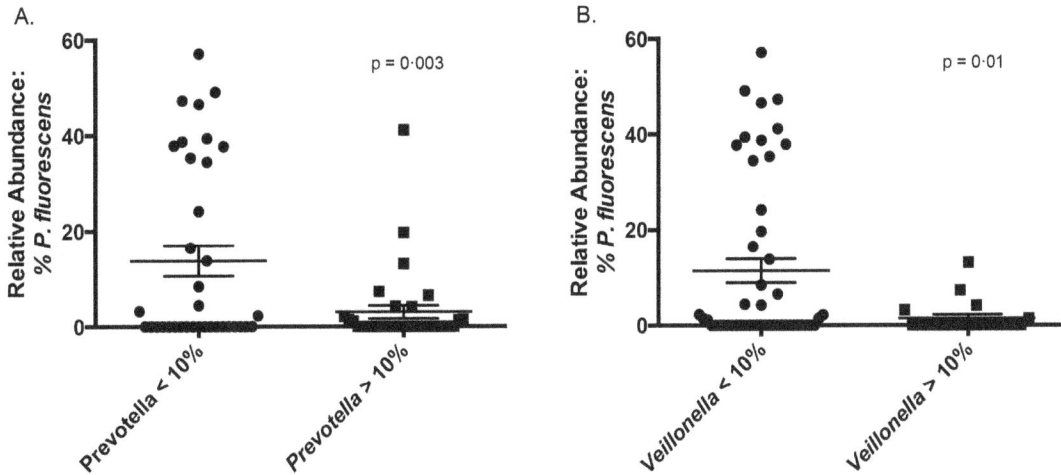

Figure 7. *In vivo* associations between *P. fluorescens* (OTU 1025) and other prominent bacteria: *Prevotella* (A) and *Veillonella* (B). Group means compared using unpaired t-test.

described as pathogenic in humans [38]. They have been commonly detected in the home environments of patients with respiratory disease [39]. Increased abundance of *P. fluorescens* has been observed in the oropharyngeal microbiota of patients infected with the H1N1 influenza virus [40]. Antibodies against *P. fluorescens* are common among patients with Crohn's disease [41,42], though whether it is a marker or mediator of human disease remains undetermined.

The significant associations (both positive and negative) between abundance of *P. fluorescens* and that of other prominent bacteria has several possible interpretations. *P. fluorescens* actively inhibits in vitro growth of other bacteria [43]. It produces numerous antibiotics (including mupirocin [44]) and is used in agriculture as a biological control organism [37]. Hence, although the observed associations may be secondary to the presence of conditions that are jointly favorable to *P. fluorescens* and *Escherichia* sp. and unfavorable to *Prevotella* and *Veillonella* spp., an important research direction will be to determine whether *P. fluorescens* exhibits in vivo pro- and anti-biotic effects in the respiratory tract.

We observed decreased bacterial diversity in the BAL of transplant recipients when compared to controls and identified negative associations between BAL diversity and multiple clinical features associated with acute infection. Recent studies are divergent regarding changes in BAL microbiota diversity among lung transplant recipients when compared to non-transplant controls. Borewicz et al. observed increased BAL microbiota diversity among transplant recipients [15], while two other published reports reported decreased diversity [11,14]. In COPD and asthma, the relationship between disease severity and lung microbial diversity has been similarly conflicting [1]. Most BAL microbiota studies to date have either excluded patients with active infection or have made no distinction in analysis between symptomatic and asymptomatic subjects (as in the above-cited lung transplant studies). Our findings are consistent with observations from the CF literature indicating that decreased diversity is not a direct consequence of duration of illness or impaired lung function but is instead driven by other factors [4].

To our knowledge, ours is the first report observing significant associations between BAL microbiota diversity and other BAL indices of acute infection. In our population, this decreased diversity did not appear to be secondary to recent exposure to

antibiotics, as patients who had received antibiotics other than their *Pneumocystis* prophylaxis agent in the preceding 30 days, seven days and at the time of BAL did not have decreased BAL bacterial diversity indices. These results are surprising and divergent from the cystic fibrosis literature [4]. The fact that all transplant subjects are at baseline on antibiotics for *Pneumocystis* prophylaxis (unlike subjects with other lung pathologies such as CF) may be relevant to this difference. While decreased bacterial diversity in the gut has been associated with obesity and geography [45,46], its significance in the lung apart from as a marker of acute infection is uncertain.

A potential limitation of this study is the absence of concurrent oral and nasal sampling for identification of "lung-specific" bacteria. There has been discussion in the literature about the extent to which microbiota detected in BAL reflect lung-resident organisms as opposed to oral-derived microbes picked up during sedation-related aspiration or broncho-scopic carryover. One study of six healthy subjects observed a similar constitution in the bacterial communities of the lower and upper respiratory tracts [20]; however, subsequent published studies from the NIH-funded LHMP consortium have identified bacterial species by BAL with significantly disproportionate representation in lower respiratory tract samples [16,17]. These newer, larger studies suggest that some bacteria might replicate in or colonize the lower respiratory tract, with specific selective pressures favoring some species over others. Such preferential accumulation of certain OTUs supports the existence of lung-specific microbiota. An important contribution of the current study is the observation that route of bronchoscopy insertion (nasal or oral) has no appreciable effect on BAL microbiota (**Figure 2**) despite the markedly divergent microbial communities detected in the human mouth and nose [47]. This finding suggests that passage of the bronchoscope through these spaces has little impact on detected BAL microbiota, and bronchoscopic carryover of upper respiratory tract microbiota in BAL fluid is minimal. Further, the strong and significant associations we found between BAL bacterial community diversity and composition on one hand, and clinically and biologically significant parameters on the other, is relevant to ongoing discussions about the diagnostic implications of sampling lung microbiota via BAL [48]. We believe that the associations we report between BAL microbiota communities and significant clinical parameters indicate that the microorganisms detected in BAL specimens have clinical and biological significance, regardless of their derivation.

Another limitation of this study, common to all studies utilizing BAL, is the potentially variable effect of dilution on BAL assays. Despite efforts to standardize the procedure of saline instillation and collection, the BAL return in each bronchoscopy is variable. While this may result in variably concentrated samples, our results indicate that the variation in bacterial DNA burden among subjects is many-fold higher than that of variation in saline return (**Figure 1**), and any confounding effect of dilution is not enough to overwhelm the clear correlations apparent between bacterial DNA burden and important clinical parameters (**Figures 4E, 6C**). Variation in dilution between BAL samples should have no impact on relative abundance of bacteria, from which most of this study's findings are derived. The use of 40 cycles in our PCR protocol is a potential source of bias, but our touchdown protocol (described in Methods) is optimized for low biomass samples and produces a low fraction of spurious priming [49].

Our results suggest that future analyses of the lung transplant microbiome should distinguish between *P. aeruginosa* and other *Pseudomonas* species, as well as between symptomatic and asymptomatic subjects and those with evidence of acute respiratory infection.

Acknowledgments

The authors thank Zachary Britt, Sean Crudgington, Nicole Falkowski, Dayana Rojas and Chinmay Pandit for assistance in tissue processing. The authors wish to thank Rick Bushman and his lab at the University of Pennsylvania for providing the 16S qPCR protocol and Duane Newton for obtaining data on *P. fluorescens* isolates from the University of Michigan Clinical Microbiology Laboratory.

Author Contributions

Conceived and designed the experiments: RPD JRE BSS JMB JLC VNL GBH. Performed the experiments: RPD CMF NW JMB JLC VNL GBH. Analyzed the data: RPD JRE BSS GBH. Contributed reagents/materials/analysis tools: RPD JRE FJM JLC VNL GBH. Wrote the paper: RPD GBH.

References

1. Dickson RP, Erb-Downward JR, Huffnagle GB (2013) The role of the bacterial microbiome in lung disease. Expert Rev Respir Med 7: 245–257.
2. Erb-Downward JR, Thompson DL, Han MK, Freeman CM, McCloskey L, et al. (2011) Analysis of the lung microbiome in the "healthy" smoker and in COPD. PLoS One 6: e16384.
3. Hilty M, Burke C, Pedro H, Cardenas P, Bush A, et al. (2010) Disordered microbial communities in asthmatic airways. PLoS One 5: e8578.
4. Zhao J, Schloss PD, Kalikin LM, Carmody LA, Foster BK, et al. (2012) Decade-long bacterial community dynamics in cystic fibrosis airways. Proc Natl Acad Sci U S A109: 5809–5814.
5. Christie JD, Edwards LB, Kucheryavaya AY, Benden C, Dipchand AI, et al. (2012) The Registry of the International Society for Heart and Lung Transplantation: 29th adult lung and heart-lung transplant report-2012. J Heart Lung Transplant 31: 1073–1086.
6. Botha P, Archer L, Anderson RL, Lordan J, Dark JH, et al. (2008) Pseudomonas aeruginosa colonization of the allograft after lung transplantation and the risk of bronchiolitis obliterans syndrome. Transplantation 85: 771–774.
7. Husain S, Singh N (2002) Bronchiolitis obliterans and lung transplantation: evidence for an infectious etiology. Semin Respir Infect 17: 310–314.
8. Khalifah AP, Hachem RR, Chakinala MM, Schechtman KB, Patterson GA, et al. (2004) Respiratory viral infections are a distinct risk for bronchiolitis obliterans syndrome and death. Am J Respir Crit Care Med 170: 181–187.
9. Duncan MD, Wilkes DS (2005) Transplant-related immunosuppression: a review of immunosuppression and pulmonary infections. Proc Am Thorac Soc 2: 449–455.
10. Kotloff RM, Thabut G (2011) Lung transplantation. Am J Respir Crit Care Med 184: 159–171.
11. Willner DL, Hugenholtz P, Yerkovich ST, Tan ME, Daly JN, et al. (2013) Re-Establishment of Recipient-Associated Microbiota in the Lung Allograft is Linked to Reduced Risk of Bronchiolitis Obliterans Syndrome. Am J Respir Crit Care Med.
12. Vos R, Vanaudenaerde BM, Geudens N, Dupont LJ, Van Raemdonck DE, et al. (2008) Pseudomonal airway colonisation: risk factor for bronchiolitis obliterans syndrome after lung transplantation? Eur Respir J 31: 1037–1045.
13. Gottlieb J, Mattner F, Weissbrodt H, Dierich M, Fuehner T, et al. (2009) Impact of graft colonization with gram-negative bacteria after lung transplantation on the development of bronchiolitis obliterans syndrome in recipients with cystic fibrosis. Respir Med 103: 743–749.
14. Charlson ES, Diamond JM, Bittinger K, Fitzgerald AS, Yadav A, et al. (2012) Lung-enriched organisms and aberrant bacterial and fungal respiratory microbiota after lung transplant. Am J Respir Crit Care Med 186: 536–545.
15. Borewicz K, Pragman AA, Kim HB, Hertz M, Wendt C, et al. (2012) Longitudinal Analysis of the Lung Microbiome in Lung Transplantation. FEMS Microbiol Lett.
16. Lozupone C, Cota-Gomez A, Palmer BE, Linderman DJ, Charlson ES, et al. (2013) Widespread Colonization of the Lung by Tropheryma whipplei in HIV Infection. Am J Respir Crit Care Med.
17. Morris A, Beck JM, Schloss PD, Campbell TB, Crothers K, et al. (2013) Comparison of the respiratory microbiome in healthy nonsmokers and smokers. Am J Respir Crit Care Med 187: 1067–1075.
18. Estenne M, Maurer JR, Boehler A, Egan JJ, Frost A, et al. (2002) Bronchiolitis obliterans syndrome 2001: an update of the diagnostic criteria. J Heart Lung Transplant 21: 297–310.
19. Mason KL, Erb Downward JR, Mason KD, Falkowski NR, Eaton KA, et al. (2012) Candida albicans and bacterial microbiota interactions in the cecum during recolonization following broad-spectrum antibiotic therapy. Infect Immun 80: 3371–3380.
20. Charlson ES, Bittinger K, Haas AR, Fitzgerald AS, Frank I, et al. (2011) Topographical continuity of bacterial populations in the healthy human respiratory tract. Am J Respir Crit Care Med 184: 957–963.
21. Hill DA, Hoffmann C, Abt MC, Du Y, Kobuley D, et al. (2009) Metagenomic analyses reveal antibiotic-induced temporal and spatial changes in intestinal microbiota with associated alterations in immune cell homeostasis. Mucosal Immunol 3: 148–158.
22. Wilmotte A, Van der Auwera G, De Wachter R (1993) Structure of the 16 S ribosomal RNA of the thermophilic cyanobacterium Chlorogloeopsis HTF ('Mastigocladus laminosus HTF') strain PCC7518, and phylogenetic analysis. FEBS Lett 317: 96–100.
23. Jumpstart Consortium Human Microbiome Project Data Generation Working Group (2010) Human Microbiome Consortium 16S 454 Sequencing Protocol. 4.2.2 ed.

24. Daigle D, Simen BB, Pochart P (2011) High-throughput sequencing of PCR products tagged with universal primers using 454 life sciences systems. Curr Protoc Mol Biol Chapter 7: Unit7 5.

25. Schloss PD, Westcott SL, Ryabin T, Hall JR, Hartmann M, et al. (2009) Introducing mothur: open-source, platform-independent, community-supported software for describing and comparing microbial communities. Appl Environ Microbiol 75: 7537–7541.

26. Spilker T, Coenye T, Vandamme P, LiPuma JJ (2004) PCR-based assay for differentiation of Pseudomonas aeruginosa from other Pseudomonas species recovered from cystic fibrosis patients. J Clin Microbiol 42: 2074–2079.

27. Scarpellini M, Franzetti L, Galli A (2004) Development of PCR assay to identify Pseudomonas fluorescens and its biotype. FEMS Microbiol Lett 236: 257–260.

28. Katoh K, Misawa K, Kuma Ki, Miyata T (2002) MAFFT: a novel method for rapid multiple sequence alignment based on fast Fourier transform. Nucleic Acids Res 30: 3059–3066.

29. Ingenito EP, Solway J, McFadden ER Jr, Pichurko B, Bowman HF, et al. (1987) Indirect assessment of mucosal surface temperatures in the airways: theory and tests. J Appl Physiol 63: 2075–2083.

30. Bernstein DI, Lummus ZL, Santilli G, Siskosky J, Bernstein IL (1995) Machine operator's lung. A hypersensitivity pneumonitis disorder associated with exposure to metalworking fluid aerosols. Chest 108: 636–641.

31. Bahrani-Mougeot FK, Paster BJ, Coleman S, Barbuto S, Brennan MT, et al. (2007) Molecular analysis of oral and respiratory bacterial species associated with ventilator-associated pneumonia. J Clin Microbiol 45: 1588–1593.

32. Mulet M, Lalucat J, GarcíaValdés E (2010) DNA sequence-based analysis of the Pseudomonas species. Environ Microbiol 12: 1513–1530.

33. Loper JE, Hassan KA, Mavrodi DV, Davis II EW, Lim CK, et al. (2012) Comparative genomics of plant-associated Pseudomonas spp.: insights into diversity and inheritance of traits involved in multitrophic interactions. PLoS genetics 8: e1002784.

34. Silby MW, Winstanley C, Godfrey SA, Levy SB, Jackson RW (2011) Pseudomonas genomes: diverse and adaptable. FEMS Microbiol Rev 35: 652–680.

35. Diaz PI, Hong BY, Frias-Lopez J, Dupuy AK, Angeloni M, et al. (2013) Transplantation-Associated Long-Term Immunosuppression Promotes Oral Colonization by Potentially Opportunistic Pathogens without Impacting Other Members of the Salivary Bacteriome. Clin Vaccine Immunol 20: 920–930.

36. Patel SK, Pratap CB, Verma AK, Jain AK, Dixit VK, et al. (2013) Pseudomonas fluorescens-like bacteria from the stomach: A microbiological and molecular study. World J Gastroenterol 19: 1056–1067.

37. Paulsen IT, Press CM, Ravel J, Kobayashi DY, Myers GS, et al. (2005) Complete genome sequence of the plant commensal Pseudomonas fluorescens Pf-5. Nat Biotechnol 23: 873–878.

38. Gershman MD, Kennedy DJ, Noble-Wang J, Kim C, Gullion J, et al. (2008) Multistate outbreak of Pseudomonas fluorescens bloodstream infection after exposure to contaminated heparinized saline flush prepared by a compounding pharmacy. Clin Infect Dis 47: 1372–1379.

39. Mortensen JE, Fisher MC, LiPuma JJ (1995) Recovery of Pseudomonas cepacia and other Pseudomonas species from the environment. Infect Control Hosp Epidemiol: 30–32.

40. Leung RK, Zhou JW, Guan W, Li SK, Yang ZF, et al. (2012) Modulation of potential respiratory pathogens by pH1N1 viral infection. Clin Microbiol Infect.

41. Bossuyt X (2006) Serologic markers in inflammatory bowel disease. Clin Chem 52: 171–181.

42. Wei B, Huang T, Dalwadi H, Sutton CL, Bruckner D, et al. (2002) Pseudomonas fluorescens encodes the Crohn's disease-associated I2 sequence and T-cell superantigen. Infect Immun 70: 6567–6575.

43. Baader A, Garre C (1887) Über Antagonisten unter den Bacterien. Correspondenz-Blatt für Schweizer Ärzte 13: 385–392.

44. Sutherland R, Boon R, Griffin K, Masters P, Slocombe B, et al. (1985) Antibacterial activity of mupirocin (pseudomonic acid), a new antibiotic for topical use. Antimicrob Agents Chemother 27: 495–498.

45. Turnbaugh PJ, Hamady M, Yatsunenko T, Cantarel BL, Duncan A, et al. (2008) A core gut microbiome in obese and lean twins. Nature 457: 480–484.

46. Yatsunenko T, Rey FE, Manary MJ, Trehan I, Dominguez-Bello MG, et al. (2012) Human gut microbiome viewed across age and geography. Nature 486: 222–227.

47. Human Microbiome Project Consortium (2012) Structure, function and diversity of the healthy human microbiome. Nature 486: 207–214.

48. Twigg HL, Morris A, Ghedin E, Curtis JL, Huffnagle GB, et al. (2013) Use of bronchoalveolar lavage to assess the respiratory microbiome: signal in the noise. The Lancet Respiratory Medicine 1: 354–356.

49. Don R, Cox P, Wainwright B, Baker K, Mattick J (1991) 'Touchdown'PCR to circumvent spurious priming during gene amplification. Nucleic Acids Res 19: 4008.

Radiologic and Clinical Bronchiectasis Associated with Autosomal Dominant Polycystic Kidney Disease

Teng Moua[1]*, Ladan Zand[2], Robert P. Hartman[3], Thomas E. Hartman[3], Dingxin Qin[2], Tobias Peikert[1], Qi Qian[2]

1 Division of Pulmonary/Critical Care, Mayo Clinic Rochester, Rochester, Minnesota, United States of America, 2 Division of Nephrology, Mayo Clinic Rochester, Rochester, Minnesota, United States of America, 3 Department of Radiology, Mayo Clinic Rochester, Rochester, Minnesota, United States of America

Abstract

Background: Polycystin 1 and 2, the protein abnormalities associated with autosomal dominant polycystic kidney disease (ADPKD), are also found in airway cilia and smooth muscle cells. There is evidence of increased radiologic bronchiectasis associated with ADPKD, though the clinical and functional implications of this association are unknown. We hypothesized an increased prevalence of both radiologic and clinical bronchiectasis is associated with APDKD as compared to non-ADPKD chronic kidney disease (CKD) controls.

Materials and Methods: A retrospective case-control study was performed at our institution involving consecutive ADPKD and non-ADPKD chronic kidney disease (CKD) patients seen over a 13 year period with both chest CT and PFT. CTs were independently reviewed by two blinded thoracic radiologists. Manually collected clinical data included symptoms, smoker status, transplant history, and PFT findings.

Results: Ninety-two ADPKD and 95 non-ADPKD CKD control patients were compared. Increased prevalence of radiologic bronchiectasis, predominantly mild lower lobe disease, was found in ADPKD patients compared to CKD control (19 vs. 9%, P = 0.032, OR 2.49 (CI 1.1–5.8)). After adjustment for covariates, ADPKD was associated with increased risk of radiologic bronchiectasis (OR 2.78 (CI 1.16–7.12)). Symptomatic bronchiectasis occurred in approximately a third of ADPKD patients with radiologic disease. Smoking was associated with increased radiologic bronchiectasis in ADPKD patients (OR 3.59, CI 1.23–12.1).

Conclusions: Radiological bronchiectasis is increased in patients with ADPKD particularly those with smoking history as compared to non-ADPKD CKD controls. A third of such patients have symptomatic disease. Bronchiectasis should be considered in the differential in ADPKD patients with respiratory symptoms and smoking history.

Editor: Emmanuel A. Burdmann, University of Sao Paulo Medical School, Brazil

Funding: These authors have no support or funding to report.

Competing Interests: The authors have declared that no competing interests exist.

* E-mail: moua.teng@mayo.edu

Introduction

Autosomal dominant polycystic kidney disease (ADPKD) characteristically manifests with progressive fluid filled renal cysts leading to end-stage renal disease in approximately 50% of patients [1,2]. The contributing genetic defects are found in polycystin-1 and 2, two transmembrane regulatory proteins responsible for mechanoreception, cell polarization, and orientation [3,4].

Multiple non-pulmonary extra-renal manifestations of ADPKD have been described [5,6,7]. Interestingly, polycystins are expressed in the cilia of both human airway epithelial [8] and airway smooth muscle cells [9]. Consequently, functional abnormalities in polycystins may result in radiological bronchiectasis due to decreased mucociliary clearance or impaired airway injury repair [8]. The functional and clinical significance of this radiologic association remains mostly unexplored.

In the current study we investigated the possible association of radiologic bronchiectasis with abnormal PFT and increased clinical pulmonary disease in a retrospective review of consecutive ADPKD patients seen at our institution as case patients compared to non-ADPKD CKD controls.

Materials and Methods

IRB approval was obtained (Mayo Clinic IRB#: 09-002623) regarding study of patients giving written consent to have their stored medical records reviewed for the purposes of research. Clinical records of consecutive adult ADPKD patients seen at Mayo Clinic, Rochester, who underwent both high resolution chest computed tomography (HRCT) and pulmonary function testing (PFT) between 1998 and 2011, were reviewed. Patients were excluded if they had a known secondary etiology for clinical or radiologic bronchiectasis as reviewed in the available record, specifically cystic fibrosis (CF), prior mechanical airway obstruction, chest trauma or surgery resulting in focal lung injury, recurrent or severe pneumonia, or clinical immunodeficiencies

such as common variable immunodeficiency (CVID) resulting in proclivity towards recurrent infection. Patients who underwent transplantation of any organ other than lung (solid and hematological) were included in the study. Non-ADPKD chronic kidney disease (CKD) patients who also underwent chest CT and PFT during the same study period were selected as consecutive unmatched controls. The most recent chest CT in the record was used if multiple studies were completed.

Collected demographics were manually obtained from the primary medical record for both study groups including age, gender, smoker status (active, former, and non-smoker), pack years, and transplant history. Laboratory data included stable GFR and creatinine within one year of the selected study CT. Clinical pulmonary diagnoses or symptoms of individual study patients at the time of CT were categorized in the following manner: Group 0 = None or no longstanding clinical pulmonary disease, Group 1 = idiopathic clinical bronchiectasis defined as presenting symptoms of chronic productive cough, dyspnea, and/or other constitutional symptoms such as fever, weight loss, not explained by a secondary or underlying pulmonary diagnosis, Group 2 = All other airways disease (COPD, asthma, bronchial or small airways disease), and Group 3 = All other parenchymal, pleural, or pulmonary vascular disease (acute infection, interstitial lung disease or fibrosis, granulomatous disease, malignant and non-malignant nodules or masses, pulmonary emboli, vasculitis, and pleural disease). For patients with multiple pulmonary diagnoses, idiopathic clinical bronchiectasis (Group 1) was selected first as a primary categorization if present followed by all other airways disease (Group 2), then all other parenchymal/pleural/pulmonary vascular disease (Group 3). Our rationale was to categorize or capture existing clinical bronchiectasis or airways disease in the setting of radiologic findings.

CT criteria for radiologic bronchiectasis included one or more of the following: 1) an enlarged bronchial diameter greater than that of the accompanying blood vessel (Signet ring sign), 2) failure of airway tapering at least 2 cm beyond the last branch point, or 3) visible airway within one centimeter of the lung periphery [10,11,12]. All selected CT scans were independently reviewed by two experienced thoracic radiologists (RH & TH) who were blinded to the presence of ADPKD and CKD with agreement on presence and severity of radiologic bronchiectasis by consensus.

Pulmonary function testing done within one year of the selected chest CT was categorized based on standard criteria [13,14,15] into one of four diagnostic findings: 1) Normal, 2) Obstructive, 3) Restrictive, or 4) Other (mixed restrictive and obstructive, non-specific pattern, and isolated low diffusing capacity for carbon monoxide (DLCO)); interpreted previously in the record by an experienced non-study pulmonologist. No further revision or reinterpretation of PFT findings was done by study investigators. If PFT was not available within one year of the selected scan, the most recent PFT in the clinical record was reviewed. Selected PFT measurements, including pre-bronchodilator percent predicted forced expiratory volume in 1 second (FEV_1) and forced vital capacity (FVC), total lung capacity (TLC), forced expiratory flow at 25–75% of the FVC (FEF_{25-75}), FEV1/FVC ratio, and diffusing capacity for carbon monoxide (DLCO) were also collected and compared between the two cohorts.

Statistical analysis was performed using JMP Software Version 9.4 (Cary, NC) with Chi-square or Fisher's exact test applied to proportional or categorical data, and a Two Sample T-test with 2-sided P value used for comparison of continuous or mean data. Chi-square and ANOVA were used to compare proportion and means among multiple groups. For predictors of a dichotomous outcome, univariable and multivariable logistic regression was

applied adjusting for a priori selected covariates of age, gender, GFR, smoker status, and transplant history. Two-tailed P values<0.05 were considered statistically significant.

No external funding was involved in the hypothesis, study design, data collection, or analysis, of this work.

Results

Ninety-two consecutive ADPKD patients and 95 consecutive non-ADPKD CKD patients underwent both chest CT and PFT and were ultimately included in the study and control groups, respectively. Comparison baseline demographic and clinical characteristics are presented in Table 1. Of the initial screening cohort fitting radiologic criteria for bronchiectasis, two were excluded from the ADPKD group secondary to history of prior severe pneumonia as likely causes of radiologic findings, and one was excluded from the CKD group due to concomitant cystic fibrosis diagnosis.

Compared to ADPKD there were more men in the consecutively selected CKD control group (67% vs. 46%, P = 0.003). Mean FEV_1, FVC, and DLCO were statistically lower in the CKD group compared to ADPKD, though smoking status and summary PFT findings were not statistically different (P = 0.35 and P = 0.121, respectively). Frequency of organ transplantation of both solid and hematological origin was similar (P = 0.123). The majority of CT scans in both groups was obtained for assessment of clinical respiratory symptoms or previously established pulmonary disease, with none obtained for incidental findings found initially on lower lung cuts of abdominal CTs. In those whom underwent organ transplantation, 25% of reviewed CTs occurred prior to transplantation. The median time from date of transplant to CT was 35.4 (range −121 to 291) months, with no statistical difference between the two groups (P = 0.62).

Subgroup comparison data for baseline clinical features among APDKD patients with and without radiologic bronchiectasis is presented in Table 2. Smoking history was more prevalent in ADPKD patients with radiological bronchiectasis (74% vs. 44%, P = 0.04) without difference in other baseline characteristics.

Radiologic changes of bronchiectasis were more frequent in ADPKD patients (19 (21%) vs. 9 (9%); P = 0.032, OR 2.49 (CI 1.1–5.8)), with no difference in prevalence of clinically symptomatic disease (6 (7%) vs. 3 (3%), P = 0.32) (Table 1.) Univariate logistic regression for selected covariates is presented in Table 3 for the whole cohort and Table 4 for subgroup analysis of the ADPKD group. The presence of ADPKD was associated with radiologic bronchiectasis, even after adjusting for age, gender, GFR, transplant history, and smoking by multivariate regression (OR 2.78, CI 1.16–7.12). Smoking history among ADPKD patients after adjustment for age, gender, GFR, and transplant history, was associated with increased risk of radiologic bronchiectasis (OR 4.79, CI 1.43–19.58) despite similar rates of smoking between ADPKD and CKD patients. Smoking was not associated with increased clinical disease among the two groups (ADPKD 5/6 (83%) vs. 41/86 (47%), P = 0.09 vs. Control 1/3 (33%) vs. 53/92 (57%), P = 0.40).

Distribution of summary PFT patterns and frequency of clinical pulmonary diagnoses were similar among ADPKD patients and controls (Table 5). Statistically lower percent predicted mean FEV_1, FVC, and DLCO were noted in CKD controls (Table 1) despite increased prevalence of active smokers in ADPKD patients. Abnormal FEF 25–75 was primarily associated with concomitant obstructive physiology in those clinically diagnosed with COPD or emphysema followed by advanced restriction seen in interstitial lung disease. There were no isolated low FEF 25–75

Table 1. Demographics and baseline characteristics.

	ADPKD (N=92)	Control (N=95)	P value
Characteristic			
Age, mean (SD)	59.84 (12.6)	61.59 (12.9)	0.35
Gender, M/F (%)	42/50 (46/54)	64/31 (67/33)	**0.003**
BMI, mean (SD)	29.21 (6.9)	30.06 (6.1)	0.37
Smoker Status;			0.35
Non-smoker N (%)	46 (50)	41 (43)	
Former N (%)	38(41)	52 (55)	
Active N (%)	8(9)	2(2)	
Pack years, mean (SD)	31.41 (20.7)	37.32 (29.5)	0.26
Creatinine, mean (SD)	2.10 (1.9)	1.93 (1.2)	0.47
GFR, mean (SD)	50.1 (28.7)	46.92 (25.4)	0.43
Radiologic bronchiectasis, N (%)	19 (21)	9 (9.1)	**0.032**
Clinical bronchiectasis, N (%)	6 (7)	3 (3)	0.32
Summary PFT dx			0.121
Normal, N (%)	42 (46)	29 (31)	
Obstructive, N (%)	26 (28)	30 (31)	
Restrictive, N (%)	6 (6)	13 (14)	
Other, N (%)	18 (20)	23 (24)	
FEV1 % predicted, mean (SD), range	79.28 (21.5), (36–119)	71.96 (24), (22–121)	**0.032**
FVC % predicted, mean (SD), range	86.78 (18.7), (36–134)	77.15 (22.6), (24–119)	**0.003**
FEV1/FVC, mean (SD), range	72.2 (10.1), (35.2–88.5)	72.3 (10.2), (33.9–95.2)	0.98
FEF 25–75 % predicted, mean (SD), range	67.2 (33.1), (13–152)	61 (36.8), (6–174)	0.23
TLC % predicted, mean (SD), range	96.25 (22.4), (53–164) (N=52)	89.64 (20.1), (47–130) (N=56)	0.112
DLCO % predicted, mean (SD), range	76.11 (19.3), (34–134) (N=85)	68.24 (23.4), (17–125) (N=80)	**0.022**
Transplant of any kind, N (%)	37 (40)	28 (29)	0.123
Time from Transplant to Study CT, months, median (range)	35.4 (−121–291) (N=37)	31.4 (−30–163.5) (N=28)	0.63

values with normal FEV1/FVC and TLC to suggest early or small airways disease. Indications for PFT testing were no different between those with APDKD and CKD, primarily done for assessment of acute or chronic respiratory symptoms or those with known pulmonary disease (63%) followed by perioperative assessment for surgical clearance or related pulmonary complications of organ transplantation (37%). There was no difference in final clinical pulmonary diagnoses.

All ADPKD patients with clinical bronchiectasis (6 patients) had at least one or more years (range 14–60 months) of symptoms by the time of their CT assessment. Symptoms included productive cough, recurrent rhinosinusitis, and intermittent dyspnea. Chronic rhinosinusitis was seen in two APDKD patients with clinical bronchiectasis and none without radiologic disease, while occurring in only one patient from the CKD cohort who did not have radiologic disease. No other etiologies for bronchiectasis were evident at the time of clinical assessment. All were treated with various antibiotic and/or inhaler regimens previously or at the time of reviewed CT.

ADPKD-associated bronchiectasis most commonly represented mild bilateral lower lobe radiologic disease as opposed to more focal disease (Table 6) observed in control patients. Cylindrical bronchiectasis was the predominant radiological pattern in both groups (Figure 1).

Discussion

Our study confirms previously reported [8,16] increased prevalence of radiologic bronchiectasis associated with ADPKD (21% vs. 9%, P = 0.032). We observed similarly mild bilateral lower lobe disease using only chest CT studies. In the majority of cases, such radiologic findings were not identified during initial CT interpretation. Approximately one third of ADPKD patients with radiologic bronchiectasis (6 of 19, 32%) also had clinical idiopathic bronchiectasis however there was no difference in PFT pattern or prevalence of other pulmonary diagnoses. Finally, in ADPKD patients, smoking was associated with an increased risk of radiologic bronchiectasis (OR 4.79, CI 1.43–19.58) in our cohort even after adjustment for a priori covariates.

In the US, prevalence of clinically diagnosed bronchiectasis increases with age and ranges between 4.2 per 100,000 (age 18–34) and 271.8 cases per 100,000 individuals (age 75 and older) [17]. A recent trend analysis based on Medicare ICD-9 claims data between 2000 and 2007, found bronchiectasis prevalence to be 8.7% per year (period prevalence of 1,106 cases per 100,000 people) [18]. However, in the absence of universally accepted clinical and radiologic disease definitions, reliable prevalence studies are lacking [19,20]. Kwak and colleagues [21] investigated the prevalence of radiologic bronchiectasis in 1409 Korean adult patients who underwent CT scanning as part of general health assessment. They reported radiologic disease in 129 (9.1%) and

Table 2. Subgroup Analysis of ADPKD with and without radiologic bronchiectasis.

	ADPKD Bronchiectasis (N = 19)	ADPKD No Bronchiectasis (N = 73)	P value
Characteristic			
Age, mean (SD)	62.63 (12.2)	59.1 (12.7)	0.28
Gender, M/F (%)	11/8 (58/42)	31/42 (42/58)	0.23
BMI, mean (SD)	27.52 (5.4)	29.66 (7.3)	0.24
Smoker status;			**0.021**
Non-smoker N (%),	5 (26)	41 (56)	
Former N (%)	12 (63)	26 (36)	
Active N (%)	2 (11)	6 (8)	
Creatinine, mean (SD)	1.62 (1.1)	2.23 (2.1)	0.24
GFR, mean (SD)	52.26 (22.7)	49.53 (30.2)	0.71
PFT dx			0.52
Normal, N (%)	8 (42)	34 (47)	
Obstructive, N (%)	6 (32)	20 (27)	
Restrictive, N (%)	0 (0)	6 (8)	
Other, N (%)	5 (26)	13 (18)	
FEV1 % predicted, mean (SD), range	81.42 (19.9), (39–108)	78.73 (22.1), (36–119)	0.63
FVC % predicted, mean (SD), range	87.68 (14.6), (53–105)	86.55 (19.7), (36–134)	0.81
FEV1/FVC (SD), range	72.32 (9.9), (55.6–86.5)	72.22 (10.3), (35.2–88.5)	0.96
FEF 25–75 % predicted (SD), range	60.5 (33.2), (15–136)	68.9 (33.1), (13–152)	0.33
TLC % predicted, mean (SD), range	99.7 (13.6), (79–122) (N = 10)	95.43 (24.1), (53–164) (N = 42)	0.59
DLCO % predicted, mean (SD), range	71.83 (19), (45–107) (N = 18)	77.25 (19.4), (34–134) (N = 67)	0.29
Transplant of any kind (N, %)	10 (53)	27 (37)	0.22
Time from Transplant to study CT, months, median (range)	67. 4 (−37–268)	22.8 (−120–292)	0.27

more than half were clinically symptomatic (53.7%) [21]. Female gender, increased age, and history of prior tuberculosis were risk factors for the presence of radiologic disease in the study. Despite comprehensive medical evaluation the cause of bronchiectasis frequently remained unidentified and such cases were subsequently classified as idiopathic. While we used a non-ADPKD CKD control cohort in our study, currently available evidence does not suggest a higher risk of radiological or clinical bronchiectasis in such patients. We did find a similar rate of radiologic bronchiectasis (9%) in our control patients as compared to the general population studied by Kwak et al.

Table 3. Univariate logistic regression analysis for predictors of radiologic bronchiectasis for the entire cohort (N = 187).

	Odds Ratio	95% Confidence Intervals	P value
Age	0.98	0.94–1.01	0.202
Gender	1.21	0.54–2.83	0.64
Smoker status	1.69	0.75–4.0	0.21
Presence of ADPKD	2.49	1.1–6.1	**0.031**
Creatinine	0.98	0.73–1.24	0.88
GFR	1.0	0.98–1.01	0.92
FEV1	1.42	0.25–8.32	0.69
FVC	1.0	0.99–1.02	0.52
TLC	1.0	0.98–1.03	0.50
DLCO	0.99	0.97–1.01	0.161
Transplant Hx	1.25	0.54–2.85	0.59
Time from Transplant to Study CT	1.01	0.99–1.02	0.141

Table 4. Subgroup univariate logistic regression analysis for predictors of radiologic bronchiectasis in patients with ADPKD (N = 92).

	Odds Ratio	95% Confidence Intervals	P value
Age	1.02	0.98–1.07	0.27
Gender	1.86	0.68–5.33	0.23
Smoker status	3.59	1.23–12.1	**0.026**
Creatinine	0.80	0.51–1.10	0.185
GFR	1.0	0.99–1.02	0.71
FEV1	1.0	0.98–1.03	0.62
FVC	1.0	0.98–1.03	0.81
TLC	1.0	0.97–1.04	0.59
DLCO	0.98	0.95–1.01	0.28
Transplant Hx	1.89	0.68–5.34	0.22
Time from Transplant to Study CT	1.0	0.99–1.01	0.26

Jain et al. recently reviewed the clinical and radiologic features of ADPKD associated bronchiectasis in 163 transplanted and non-transplanted patients [16]. They found older age as predictive of radiologic disease using a modified scoring system with the majority of presenting radiologic features similarly mild in nature. Although demographic data was not available in all studied patients, only older age was again seen as a significant risk factor for bronchiectasis based on multivariable analysis. There was also noted increased frequency and severity of radiologic disease among those with renal transplantation compared to non-transplanted patients (52.4% vs 31.4%, P = 0.02). In contrast, our study noted significant correlation of radiologic bronchiectasis with active and prior smoking history, without difference in age distribution among our more highly selected cohort using chest CT and PFT findings. Including both solid (excluding lung transplant) and hematologic organ transplants in both case and control cohorts, we noted no difference in frequency of both radiologic and clinical bronchiectasis.

The spectrum of clinical disease among those with radiologic bronchiectasis was mild to moderate at most and not statistically different between the two groups in our study. Although symptoms were reported on average greater than a year prior to selected study CT, none had history of significant weight loss, recurrent fevers, or hemoptysis. Even among those with persistent clinical symptoms, severity of radiologic disease was not advanced, with

the majority of all patients with radiologic disease presenting as mild cylindrical bilateral lower lobe disease.

While the overall rate of smoking was similar between ADPKD and control patients, subgroup analysis revealed that radiologic bronchiectasis occurred more frequently in ADPKD smokers than non-smokers. This association is intriguing in the setting of known airway epithelial injury with exposure to cigarette smoke including impaired mucociliary clearance, stunned ciliary function, and decreased ciliary growth [22,23,24,25,26]. Smoking may further hasten these effects in patients with ADPKD whom perhaps have intrinsic ciliary dysfunction as compared to CKD controls whom did not see an association of radiologic bronchiectasis with smoking history in our study. Further work is needed to confirm this association while smoking cessation should be generally encouraged in all patients.

Interestingly we observed statistically lower mean FEV_1, FVC, and DLCO among CKD patients compared to ADPKD despite comparable smoking status. As CKD patients were consecutively allocated based on presence of HRCT and PFT without matching, such findings were unlikely explained by smoking having a protective effect on PFT findings in ADPKD patients or a much more severe effect in CKD. Smoking over the entire cohort was not associated with increased radiologic or clinical bronchiectasis, but again with subgroup analysis of ADPKD patients, significantly associated with radiologic disease even after correction for a priori covariates. Summary PFT findings (normal, obstructive,

Table 5. Frequency and distribution of summary respiratory diagnoses.

	No Clinical Respiratory Disease (Group 0)	Idiopathic clinical bronchiectasis (Group 1)	All Other Airways Diseases (Group 2)	Other Respiratory (Group 3)
ADPKD¶				
Radiologic Bronchiectasis (N = 19)	2	6	5	6
No bronchiectasis (N = 73)	15	0	22	36
Control¶				
Radiologic Bronchiectasis (N = 9)	2	3	0	4
No bronchiectasis (N = 86)	22	0	20	44

¶P values were not significant for distribution of clinical respiratory diagnoses between ADPKD cohort and control.

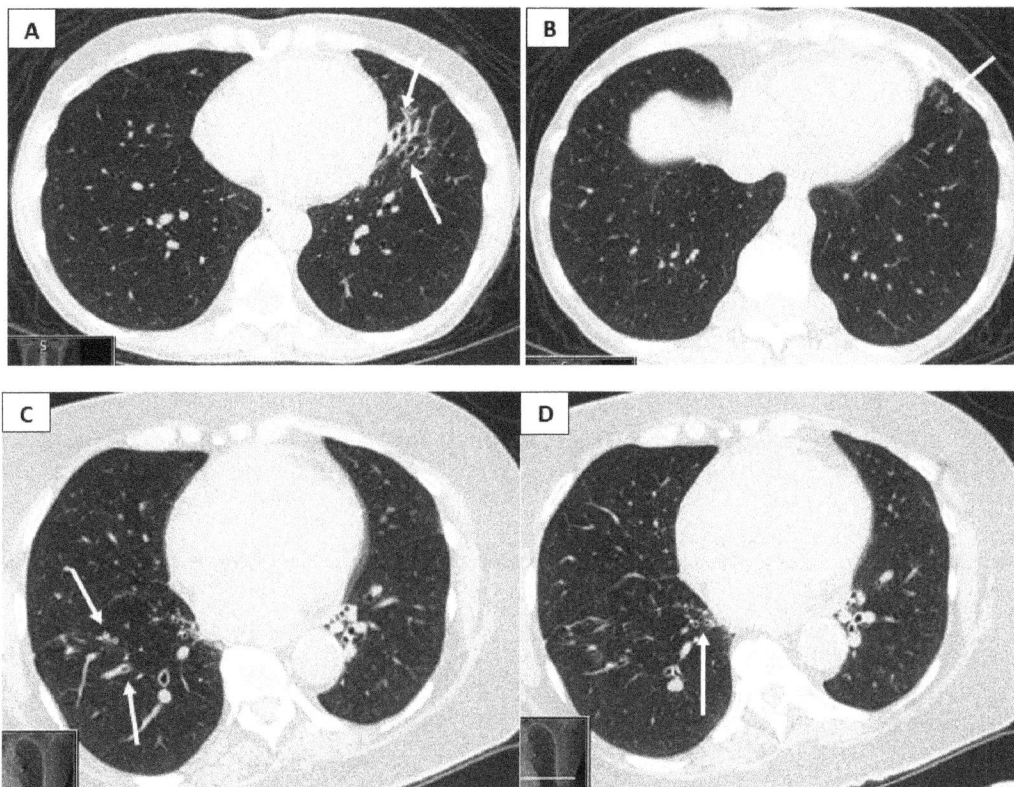

Figure 1. Radiologic and clinical bronchiectasis associated with ADPKD. Top panels (A and B) represent bronchiectasis in a 65 yo ADPKD female with productive cough and dyspnea on exertion, without a known secondary etiology. Panel B delineates enlarged airways visible within 1 cm of the lung periphery. Second panels (C and D) represent radiologic bronchiectasis manifesting predominantly in the right lower lobe of a 70 yo ADPKD female without clinical disease.

restrictive, and other) were not statistically different between ADPKD and CKD patients, or among ADPKD patients with or without radiologic or clinical bronchiectasis.

A proposed mechanism for the development of bronchiectasis in patients with ADPKD may be linked to abnormalities in polycystin-1 and 2, the gene products of PKD1 and PKD 2 located on chromosomes 16 and 4 respectively. Although alterations of these genes are responsible along with other genetic abnormalities for renal cyst formation [1,27,28], expression of both of these genes have been reported in various cell types involved in the extra-renal manifestations of ADPKD, including valvular heart disease, vascular aneurysm, gut diverticula, and hepatic cysts [1,28]. The presence of functional polycystin-1 in the motile cilia of human airway epithelial cells [8] and primary cilia of human airway smooth muscle cells [9] has also been demonstrated. These particular cells have been implicated in

airway ciliary function and injury repair with decreased function due to polycystin abnormality, perhaps an underlying mechanism by which ADPKD patients develop radiologic and clinical bronchiectasis. The negative impact of cigarette smoke may possibly hasten these effects. Although suggestive, more directed studies are needed to confirm this mechanism at a cellular level.

Strengths of our study include the review of ADPKD patients with both high resolution chest CT (as opposed to abdominal CT with lower lung cuts) and comprehensive PFT, allowing assessment and comparison of both radiologic and functional characteristics. While our cohort provided a more specific assessment of ADPKD-associated clinical and radiologic bronchiectasis, exclusion of ADPKD and control patients whom did not undergo CT and PFT may have underestimated the true prevalence of radiologic disease, explaining our lower prevalence of radiologic findings as compared to Driscoll and colleagues [8]. As well, such

Table 6. Location and distribution of ADPKD-associated radiologic bronchiectasis.

Lobe	Focal	Unilateral Multilobe	Diffuse (bilateral multilobe)	RUL*	RML	RLL	LUL	LML (lingula)	LLL
Group									
ADPKD (N)	7	2	10	1	6	13	0	2	13
Control (N)	6	1	2	2	3	3	1	1	4

*RUL = right upper lobe; RML = right middle lobe; RLL = right lower lobe; LUL = left upper lobe; LML = left middle lobe; LLL = left lower lobe.

selection may bias towards patients with other respiratory symptoms or pulmonary disease whose presentation may be difficult to differentiate from clinical bronchiectasis, and may not represent again a true estimate of less symptomatic bronchiectatic disease where chest CT and PFT would not have been obtained. However, our methodology was less likely to have missed ADPKD patients with more advanced or clinically relevant bronchiectasis, one of our study objectives. Another possible confounder is the inclusion of transplanted patients, whose immunosuppression may have led to increased risk of both radiologic and clinical bronchiectasis. While immunosuppression may be contributory, clinical bronchiectasis was infrequent and similar between the two groups with both groups having similar transplantation rates. As well, median time from date of transplantation to study CT was statistically similar making duration of transplantation over time less likely contributory to increased risk of infection or immuno-suppression related radiologic or clinical bronchiectasis. Finally, our study has all the limitations associated with retrospective data collection and reflects the patient population of a tertiary referral center. It did allow though for maximal accrual of selected patients for a meaningful analysis using more strict radiologic and functional inclusion criteria.

In conclusion, we observed an increased prevalence of radiologic bronchiectasis among ADPKD patients who underwent high resolution chest CT. These changes most frequently involved mild-to-moderate cylindrical bronchiectasis with bilateral lower lung predominance. There were no differences in summary PFT abnormalities or frequency of clinical disease. A history of smoking in patients with APDKD may predispose to the development of radiologic and clinical bronchiectasis and smoking cessation should be generally encouraged. Radiologic bronchiectasis may be regarded as an extra-renal manifestation of ADPKD with further studies needed to explore this association.

Author Contributions

Conceived and designed the experiments: TM LZ DQ RH TH TP QQ. Performed the experiments: TM LZ RH TH. Analyzed the data: TM LZ QQ TP TH RH DQ. Wrote the paper: TM TP QQ.

References

1. Torres VE, Harris PC (2006) Mechanisms of Disease: autosomal dominant and recessive polycystic kidney diseases. Nature clinical practice Nephrology 2: 40–55; quiz 55.
2. Barua M, Pei Y (2010) Diagnosis of autosomal-dominant polycystic kidney disease: an integrated approach. Seminars in nephrology 30: 356–365.
3. Hopp K, Ward CJ, Hommerding CJ, Nasr SH, Tuan HF, et al. (2012) Functional polycystin-1 dosage governs autosomal dominant polycystic kidney disease severity. The Journal of clinical investigation 122: 4257–4273.
4. Gallagher AR, Germino GG, Somlo S (2010) Molecular advances in autosomal dominant polycystic kidney disease. Advances in chronic kidney disease 17: 118–130.
5. Qian Q, Hartman RP, King BF, Torres VE (2007) Increased occurrence of pericardial effusion in patients with autosomal dominant polycystic kidney disease. Clinical journal of the American Society of Nephrology: CJASN 2: 1223–1227.
6. Qian Q, Younge BR, Torres VE (2007) Retinal arterial and venous occlusions in patients with ADPKD. Nephrology, dialysis, transplantation : official publication of the European Dialysis and Transplant Association - European Renal Association 22: 1769–1771.
7. Kumar S, Adeva M, King BF, Kamath PS, Torres VE (2006) Duodenal diverticulosis in autosomal dominant polycystic kidney disease. Nephrology, dialysis, transplantation : official publication of the European Dialysis and Transplant Association - European Renal Association 21: 3576–3578.
8. Driscoll JA, Bhalla S, Liapis H, Ibricevic A, Brody SL (2008) Autosomal dominant polycystic kidney disease is associated with an increased prevalence of radiographic bronchiectasis. Chest 133: 1181–1188.
9. Wu J, Du H, Wang X, Mei C, Sieck GC, et al. (2009) Characterization of primary cilia in human airway smooth muscle cells. Chest 136: 561–570.
10. Naidich DP, McCauley DI, Khouri NF, Stitik FP, Siegelman SS (1982) Computed tomography of bronchiectasis. Journal of computer assisted tomography 6: 437–444.
11. Muller NL, Bergin CJ, Ostrow DN, Nichols DM (1984) Role of computed tomography in the recognition of bronchiectasis. AJR American journal of roentgenology 143: 971–976.
12. Kim JS, Muller NL, Park CS, Grenier P, Herold CJ (1997) Cylindrical bronchiectasis: diagnostic findings on thin-section CT. AJR American journal of roentgenology 168: 751–754.
13. Miller MR, Hankinson J, Brusasco V, Burgos F, Casaburi R, et al. (2005) Standardisation of spirometry. The European respiratory journal 26: 319–338.
14. Wanger J, Clausen JL, Coates A, Pedersen OF, Brusasco V, et al. (2005) Standardisation of the measurement of lung volumes. The European respiratory journal 26: 511–522.
15. Pellegrino R, Viegi G, Brusasco V, Crapo RO, Burgos F, et al. (2005) Interpretative strategies for lung function tests. The European respiratory journal 26: 948–968.
16. Jain R, Javidan-Nejad C, Alexander-Brett J, Horani A, Cabellon MC, et al. (2012) Sensory functions of motile cilia and implication for bronchiectasis. Frontiers in bioscience 4: 1088–1098.
17. Weycker D, Edelsberg J., Oster G., and Tino G. (2005) Prevalence and economic burden of bronchiectasis. Clinical Pulmonary Medicine 12: 205–209.
18. Seitz AE, Olivier KN, Adjemian J, Holland SM, Prevots R (2012) Trends in bronchiectasis among medicare beneficiaries in the United States, 2000 to 2007. Chest 142: 432–439.
19. Barker AF (2002) Bronchiectasis. The New England journal of medicine 346: 1383–1393.
20. O'Donnell AE (2008) Bronchiectasis. Chest 134: 815–823.
21. Kwak HJ, Moon JY, Choi YW, Kim TH, Sohn JW, et al. (2010) High prevalence of bronchiectasis in adults: analysis of CT findings in a health screening program. The Tohoku journal of experimental medicine 222: 237–242.
22. Tamashiro E, Xiong G, Anselmo-Lima WT, Kreindler JL, Palmer JN, et al. (2009) Cigarette smoke exposure impairs respiratory epithelial ciliogenesis. American journal of rhinology & allergy 23: 117–122.
23. Leopold PL, O'Mahony MJ, Lian XJ, Tilley AE, Harvey BG, et al. (2009) Smoking is associated with shortened airway cilia. PloS one 4: e8157.
24. Maestrelli P, Saetta M, Mapp CE, Fabbri LM (2001) Remodeling in response to infection and injury. Airway inflammation and hypersecretion of mucus in smoking subjects with chronic obstructive pulmonary disease. American journal of respiratory and critical care medicine 164: S76–80.
25. Simet SM, Sisson JH, Pavlik JA, Devasure JM, Boyer C, et al. (2010) Long-term cigarette smoke exposure in a mouse model of ciliated epithelial cell function. American journal of respiratory cell and molecular biology 43: 635–640.
26. Bhatta N, Dhakal SS, Rizal S, Kralingen KW, Niessen L (2008) Clinical spectrum of patients presenting with bronchiectasis in Nepal: evidence of linkage between tuberculosis, tobacco smoking and toxic exposure to biomass smoke. Kathmandu University medical journal 6: 195–203.
27. Chapin HC, Caplan MJ (2010) The cell biology of polycystic kidney disease. The Journal of cell biology 191: 701–710.
28. Al-Bhalal L, Akhtar M (2005) Molecular basis of autosomal dominant polycystic kidney disease. Advances in anatomic pathology 12: 126–133.

3

Cross-Reactive Anti-Viral T Cells Increase Prior to an Episode of Viral Reactivation Post Human Lung Transplantation

Thi H. O. Nguyen[1,2], Glen P. Westall[1,2], Tara E. Bull[1,2], Aislin C. Meehan[1,2], Nicole A. Mifsud[1,2*9], Tom C. Kotsimbos[1,29]

1 Department of Medicine, Monash University, Central Clinical School, The Alfred Centre, Melbourne, Victoria, Australia, 2 Department of Allergy, Immunology and Respiratory Medicine, The Alfred Hospital, Melbourne, Victoria, Australia

Abstract

Human Cytomegalovirus (CMV) reactivation continues to influence lung transplant outcomes. Cross-reactivity of anti-viral memory T cells against donor human leukocyte antigens (HLA) may be a contributing factor. We identified cross-reactive HLA-A*02:01-restricted CMV-specific cytotoxic T lymphocytes (CTL) co-recognizing the NLVPMVATV (NLV) epitope and HLA-B27. NLV-specific CD8+ T cells were expanded for 13 days from 14 HLA-A*02:01/CMV seropositive healthy donors and 11 lung transplant recipients (LTR) then assessed for the production of IFN-γ and CD107a expression in response to 19 cell lines expressing either single HLA-A or -B class I molecules. In one healthy individual, we observed functional and proliferative cross-reactivity in response to B*27:05 alloantigen, representing approximately 5% of the NLV-specific CTL population. Similar patterns were also observed in one LTR receiving a B27 allograft, revealing that the cross-reactive NLV-specific CTL gradually increased (days 13–193 post-transplant) before a CMV reactivation event (day 270) and reduced to basal levels following viral clearance (day 909). Lung function remained stable with no acute rejection episodes being reported up to 3 years post-transplant. Individualized immunological monitoring of cross-reactive anti-viral T cells will provide further insights into their effects on the allograft and an opportunity to predict sub-clinical CMV reactivation events and immunopathological complications.

Editor: Hidde L. Ploegh, Whitehead Institute, United States of America

Funding: This study was funded by the National Health and Medical Research Council of Australia (NHMRC) and The Margaret Pratt Foundation. N.A.M was supported by a Peter Doherty NHMRC postdoctoral fellowship. The funders had no role in study design, data collection and analysis, decision to publish, or preparation of the manuscript.

Competing Interests: The authors have declared that no competing interests exist.

* E-mail: nicole.mifsud@monash.edu

9 These authors contributed equally to this work.

Introduction

Viral infections, in particular human CMV infection, continue to influence clinical outcomes following lung transplantation. Whilst intensive anti-viral prophylactic and pre-emptive strategies following transplantation have reduced the incidence of symptomatic CMV disease in "at-risk" patients, subclinical CMV reactivation in the lung allograft remains associated with poor long term allograft survival [1].

Following a HLA-mismatched lung transplant, alloreactive T cells can infiltrate the lung allograft, resulting in episodes of acute cellular rejection, despite the administration of aggressive immunosuppression. Persistent activities of the same T cells are believed to be the major risk factor for chronic rejection or Bronchiolitis Obliterans Syndrome (BOS) in LTR [2,3]. There is now clear evidence demonstrating that the total alloreactive T cell repertoire consists of both allo-specific T cells and varying amounts of virus-specific memory T cells [4] that are capable of cross-reactivity towards unrelated HLA alloantigens [5]. In this setting, specific viral infections can potentially heighten immune mechanisms

leading to adverse clinical outcomes above and beyond any indirect viral effects.

The capacity of virus-specific memory T cells to cross-react with HLA alloantigens is facilitated by the T cell receptor (TCR), which has been shown to mediate immunological responses in individuals otherwise considered to have been "naïve" to allogeneic stimulation, thereby accounting for the presence of alloreactive memory T cells in individuals with no prior sensitization [6–9]. Importantly, cross-reactive anti-viral memory T cells are likely to be less susceptible to immunosuppression regimens and may exponentially expand in the setting of specific viral reactivation. It has been previously proposed that the presence of cross-reactive anti-viral T cells may contribute to a less controllable and easily magnified immunological response that can influence allograft function and survival.

In patients undergoing lung transplantation, we recently described an EBV model of T cell cross-reactivity [10] and explored whether HLA-B*08:01-restricted FLRGRAYGL (FLR)-specific CD8+ T cells cross-recognizing the alloantigen HLA-B*44:02 [11,12] contributed to allograft dysfunction. Although we demonstrated that cross-reactive FLR-specific CD8+ T cells were detectable and functional in HLA-B8/EBV seropositive LTR that received a HLA-B*44:02 allograft, they did not contribute to allograft dysfunction in the absence of an active EBV infection [10]. Based on this and our previous study showing that low levels of CMV reactivation were sufficient to prime and recruit CMV-specific CD8+ T cells to the lung allograft [13], we suggest that there may be a threshold level of viral reactivation(s) (i.e. magnitude and/or frequency) that is required for cross-reactive virus-specific T cells to become activated and exert deleterious effects on the allograft. Therefore, we now shift our focus towards identifying alloreactive anti-viral T cells in the CMV setting due to its tendency to reactivate much more frequently in our patients compared to EBV.

CMV was a major cause of morbidity and mortality in the early days of lung transplantation when anti-viral prophylaxis was not available. Despite anti-viral prophylaxis however, CMV continues to have a propensity to reactivate post-transplantation in the immunosuppressed host [14,15], thereby providing a source of ongoing antigenic stimulation. The relatively high frequency of circulating CMV-specific memory T cells [13,16] and the previously reported cross-reactive nature of T cells towards unrelated HLA alloantigens [4,17–20], produces an immunological environment where increasing viral reactivation may drive recognition of the HLA mismatched allograft. We believe that such a scenario provides further insights to previously reported links between allograft rejection and DNA virus reactivation following transplantation [21–23].

The cross-reactive potential of CD8+ T cells specific for the HLA-A*02:01-restricted immunodominant CMV pp65$_{495-503}$ epitope NLVPMVATV (NLV) has been previously reported by independent investigators in healthy individuals, although the specificity of some HLA alloantigens were not completely defined [4,18,20]. However, this study showcases a fully characterized novel model of CMV cross-reactivity of NLV-specific CD8+ T cells towards the HLA-B27 molecule (HLA-A-restricted T cells recognizing HLA-B molecules) in both a healthy immunocompetent individual as well as an immunosuppressed LTR. We report for the first time in a clinical setting following lung transplantation that cross-reactive NLV-specific CD8+ T cells remain stable in the setting of persistent alloantigen but significantly increase prior to detectable CMV reactivation. However, in a specific example of CMV reactivation driven increase in cross-reactive anti-viral T cells we did not demonstrate an association between cross-reactive T cells and adverse long term lung allograft outcomes.

Methods

Cohort demographics and ethics approval

Eleven HLA-A2 LTR receiving either a HLA-A30, -A31, -A32 or -B27 donor lung allograft between March 2008 and December 2010 (Table 1) and fourteen HLA-A2 healthy individuals (Table 2) were recruited to the study. All LTR received standard triple-therapy immunosuppression and underwent routine surveillance bronchoscopy at approximately 14, 30, 60, 90, 180, 270 and 365 days post-transplant or if clinically indicated [13]. Transbronchial biopsies were assessed for acute cellular rejection and/or CMV pneumonitis according to standard histopathological criteria [24,25]. Both LTR and healthy controls (HC) provided written consent, with ethics approval granted by The Alfred Hospital (Victoria, Australia) and the Australian Bone Marrow Donor Registry (New South Wales, Australia).

CMV prophylaxis and monitoring

LTR at risk of CMV reactivation (recipient and/or donor CMV+; R+ and/or D+) received 2 weeks of intravenous ganciclovir treatment (5 mg/kg body density) followed by 5 months of oral valganciclovir anti-viral prophylaxis. In addition, primary D+/R− CMV-mismatch patients received a course of CMV hyperimmune globulin daily in the first month post-transplant. CMV load was measured in bronchoalveolar lavage (BAL) fluid (copies/ml) with the semi-automated COBAS Amplicor CMV monitor test (Roche Diagnostic Systems, NSW, Australia) as described elsewhere [26].

Lung function

All LTR had routine monitoring of lung function [Spirometry - forced expiratory volume in one second (FEV$_1$)] with chronic rejection/BOS defined as a sustained and irreversible loss of FEV$_1$ below 80% of Personal Best achieved post-transplant [24,27].

Blood samples

Peripheral blood samples from healthy individuals and LTR (taken pre-transplant and at the time of routine bronchoscopy) were collected in heparinized vacutainer tubes. PBMC were isolated by Ficoll-Paque (GE Healthcare, Uppsala, Sweden) density gradient centrifugation and cryopreserved at −180°C until required.

Cell lines and culture

B-lymphoblastoid cell lines (B-LCL) and HLA class I-transfected cell lines derived from class 1 reduced (C1R) and 721.221 Parental cells (Table 3) were maintained in RPMI (GIBCO, Grand Island, NY), 10% FBS (SAFC Biosciences, Victoria, Australia) and supplements as previously described [28].

Generation of HLA class I transfectants

Retroviral transduction of C1R.B*27:03, C1R.B*27:05 and C1R.B*27:09 cell lines were carried out as described [29]. Firstly, HLA-B*27:05 cDNA was extracted from the RSV5neoB*27:05 plasmid (kind gift from Dr L. Kjer-Nielsen, The University of Melbourne, Victoria, Australia) using forward and reverse primers: 5′-CCGGAATTCGCCACCATGCGGGTCACGGCGCCCCG-AACCCTCC-3′ and 3′-CCGCTCGAGTCAAGCTGTGAGA-GACACATCAGAGCCCTGGGCACTGTCG-5′, respectively. HLA-B*27:05 cDNA was cloned into the pGEM-T Easy Vector following manufacturer's instructions (Promega, Madison, WI, USA) before co-transferring into the pMIG vector, (kind gift from Professor D. Vignali, St Jude Children's Research Hospital, Memphis, USA) using EcoR1 and XhoI digestion and ligation techniques to generate pMIG.B*27:05. Site-directed mutagenesis was performed on pMIG.B*27:05 using *PfuTurbo*® DNA polymerase according to manufacturer's instructions (Stratagene, La Jolla, CA, USA) to generate pMIG.B*27:03 (5′ primer: GAGGGGCCG-GAGCATTGGGACCGG; 3′ primer: CCGGTCCCAATGCTC-CGGCCCCTC) and pMIG.B*27:09 (5′ primer: CGGGTAC-CACCAGCACGCCTACGACGGC; 3′ primer: GCCGTCGT-AGGCGTGCTGGTGGTACCCG) alleles. Retrovirus production was performed via 293T cells for subsequent transduction of C1R Parental cells [29].

HLA-A2/NLV class I tetramer

R-PE-conjugate tetramer comprising of the HLA-A*02:01/ NLVPMVATV (A2/NLV-tetramer) complex was generated as previously described [30]. NLV peptide was synthesized by Genscript (Piscataway, NJ, USA).

Table 1. Patient demographics.

Patient	Age	Gender (D/R)	Primary Disease	CMV status (D/R)	HLA-A, -B (R)	HLA-A, -B (D)
LTR1	62	F/F	COPD	−/−	A2, 24; B27, 44	A3, 30; B18, 65
LTR2	41	M/M	CF	−/−	A2, 3; B7, 62	A1, 32; B8, 27
LTR3	64	F/F	COPD	+/+	A2; B27, 44	A2, 32; B13, 27
LTR4	51	F/M	IPF	−/−	A2, 3; B7, 37	A24, 30; B44, 60
LTR5	35	M/F	IPF	+/+	A2, 3; B7, 18	A11, 33; B27, 58
LTR6	29	F/F	IPF	−/+	A2, 11; B13, 35	A3; B18, 27
LTR7	45	M/M	OB	+/+	A2, 31; B35	A24, 31; B55, 62
LTR8	60	M/M	COPD	+/+	A1, 2; B8, 44	A2, 30; B7, 62
LTR9	64	M/M	COPD	−/+	A2, 24; B13, 40	A2, 31; B40, 57
LTR10	39	M/M	CF	+/−	A1, 2; B7, 27	A11, 31; B51, 55
LTR11	29	F/F	CF-Bronchiectasis	+/−	A2; B39, 44	A2402, 31; B55, 61

Abbreviations: donor (D), recipient (R), female (F), male (M), cystic fibrosis (CF), chronic obstructive pulmonary disease (COPD), idiopathic pulmonary fibrosis (IPF), idiopathic bronchiolitis obliterans (OB).

T cell cultures and functional assays

T cell cultures were generated by stimulating PBMC from healthy individuals or LTR with either NLV-pulsed autologous PBMC (irradiated at 3000 Rad) or B-LCL (irradiated at 10,000 Rad) for 13 days ($37°C$, 5% CO_2) at a 2:1 ratio [31]. The functionality of T cell cultures were assessed by (i) proliferation (CFSE assay), (ii) cytokine production (intracellular cytokine staining [ICS] assay) or cytotoxic potential (cell surface expression of degranulation marker CD107a). For proliferation, responder PBMC were stained with CFSE (1 µM, Sigma, St Louis, MO, USA) for exactly 5 minutes at $37°C$ then washed in the presence of FBS prior to culturing with stimulator cells. Both cytokine production and cytotoxic potential were assessed using a combined CD107a staining and ICS assay [10]. Briefly, PBMC or day 13 T cell cultures (2×10^5 cells) were stimulated with each cell line (10^5 cells) for a total of 6 hours in which Brefeldin A (10 µg/ml, Sigma) was added at 2 hours. In CD107a/ICS assays, anti-CD107a FITC (1:20, clone H4A3, Becton Dickinson [BD], CA, USA) and monensin (3.5 µg/ml, Sigma) were also added at 0 and 1 hour

Table 2. Healthy controls (HC) demographics and NLV expansion profiles.

HC	HLA-A or -A*	HLA-B or -B*	CMV serology	NLV-specific CD8+ T cells	
				% *Ex vivo*	% *In vitro*
HC1	2	51, 61	−	NT	0.2
HC2	2, 3	14, 27	−	NT	0.1
HC3	2, 24	07:02, 56:01	+	0.1	23.4
HC4	02:01	15, 44:02	+	1.2	90.5
HC5	02:01, 11	51, 61	+	0.1	69.9
HC6	1, 02:01	07:02, 44:02	+	NT	9.1
HC7	1, 2	08:01, 44:03	+	NT	14
HC8	02:01, 29:02	07:02, 44:03	+	NT	37.6
HC9	2	8, 62	+	NT	97.2
HC10	2	8, 57	+	NT	93.2
HC11	2, 32	35, 44	+	NT	65.95
HC12	2, 3	8, 18	+	2.1	16.3
HC13	2, 3	7, 8	+	1	0.4
HC14	02:01, 03:01	07:02, 45:01	+	1.4	0.2
Average				1.0	43.2
±SD				0.8	35.6
Range				0.1–2.1	0.2–97.2

HLA class I typing, CMV serology status and NLV-specific T cell expansion profiles of healthy individuals. Molecular resolution of HLA class I antigens was available as indicated (4-digit). *In vitro* T cell cultures were derived by autologous stimulation of PBMC with NLV peptide (1 µM) for 13 days in the presence of IL-2 (20 U/ml). Percentages of A2/NLV-tetramer+ T cells were based on the total CD8+ T cell population. HC1 and 2 were excluded from the average, SD and range calculations. Abbreviation: not tested (NT).

Table 3. HLA class I typing of cell lines.

Cell Line	HLA-A or -A*	HLA-B or –B*	HLA-C or -C*
9009	01:01	37:01	06:02
9026	26:01	38:01	12:03
9063	32:01	44:02	05:01
9072	31:01	15:01	01:02
T102	2, 29	57, 65	
75083	1, 30	13, 35	6
C1R Parental[a]	**02:01**	**35:03**	**04:01**
C1R.A*01:01	01:01		
C1R.A*02:01	02:01		
C1R.A*03:01	03:01		
C1R.B*08:01		08:01	
C1R.B*18:01		18:01	
C1R.B*27:03		27:03	
C1R.B*27:05		27:05	
C1R.B*27:09		27:09	
C1R.B*35:01		35:01	
C1R.B*35:02		35:02	
C1R.B*35:03		35:03	
C1R.B*44:02		44:02	
C1R.B*44:03		44:03	
C1R.B*57:01		57:01	
721.221 Parental			
721.221.A*29:02	29:02		
721.221.A68	68		
721.221.B53		53	

Molecular resolution of HLA class I antigens was available as indicated (4-digit).
[a]C1R Parental cell line has no detectable surface expression of HLA-A, low levels of HLA-B35 and normal levels of HLA-Cw4 [51].

time points, respectively. Stimulation with NLV-pulsed C1R.A*02:01 or NLV peptide (1 μM) were included as positive controls. Negative controls included the background C1R Parental cell line, non-pulsed C1R.A*02:01 or autologous T cells alone. Cells were then labelled with anti-CD8 PE-Cy5 (1:20, clone HIT8a, BD) and A2/NLV-tetramer (1:100–200), fixed in 1% paraformaldehyde (ProSciTech, Queensland, Australia) and then permeabilized with 0.3% saponin (Sigma) containing either anti-IFN-γ FITC (1:50, clone 25723.11, BD) or anti-IFN-γ APC (1:1000, clone B27, BD) before acquisition using a FACSCalibur (BD). All flow cytometry data was analysed using FlowJo software (Tree Star, Inc., Ashland, OR, USA).

Results

Panning for cross-reactive NLV-specific CD8+ T cells towards common HLA molecules

Currently there is a very limited number of human studies characterizing NLV-specific CD8+ T cell cross-reactivity towards unrelated HLA alloantigens [4,18], which have been shown to demonstrate specificity towards the class I antigens A30, A31, A32 [20]. Considering that following exposure to primary CMV infection there is an establishment of a pool of potentially cross-reactive CMV-specific memory T cells, we sought to define new T

cell cross-reactivities towards high frequency HLA alloantigens expressed within the Australian population (Table 3).

An expanded pool of day 13 NLV-specific CD8+ T cells from HC3-5 (Table 2) were re-stimulated in a 6 hour ICS assay with a panel of either transfected cell lines or EBV-B-LCL encompassing six HLA-A (A*01:01, A*02:01, A*03:01, A*26:01, A*29:02 and A68) and thirteen HLA-B (B*08:01, B*18:01, B*27:05, B*35:01, B*35:02, B*35:03, B*37:01, B*38:01, B*44:02, B*44:03, B53, B*57:01 and B65). Cross-reactivity was determined by the percentage of NLV-tetramer+ CD8+ T cells producing IFN-γ in response to the cell lines. High levels of IFN-γ production were generated towards the positive controls: NLV-pulsed C1R.A*02:01 (HC3-5; 65.8%, 38.4% and 32.3%, respectively) and NLV peptide alone (HC3-5; 68.8%, 40.7% and 46.1%, respectively). Negative controls were all below 0.1%, except for HC5 with C1R Parental (0.4%) (Figure 1). Background levels of IFN-γ production was only observed in the tetramer-negative CD8+ T cell population in response to B27 alloantigen. High background levels in HC5 are a common occurrence as observed over many independent investigations (data not shown). Of the 19 alloantigens screened, cross-reactivity was only detected towards B*27:05 in HC5, with 3.7% of NLV-specific CD8+ T cells producing IFN-γ upon stimulation with the C1R.B*2705 cell line (Figure 1). As anticipated based on the CMV oligoclonal TCR usage [32,33], analysis of NLV-specific CD8+ T cells expanded from HC6-11 did not reveal cross-reactivity towards B*27:05 (data not shown).

In addition to panning for new cross-reactive alloantigens recognised by NLV-specific CD8+ T cells, we explored whether HLA-A30, A31 or A32 molecules identified by Morice et al. [20] were also present in our cohort of healthy individuals (HC3-11). Day 13 in vitro expanded NLV-specific CD8+ T cells were restimulated with three different B-LCL 75083, 9072, 9063 that expressed A30, A31 and A32, respectively (Table 3). However, no evidence of T cell cross-reactivity was observed (data not shown).

Due to the relatively low numbers of ex vivo tetramer+ CD8+ T cells in most of our healthy donors (Table 2) and transplant patients, NLV-specific CD8+ T cells were expanded from PBMC in order to increase cell numbers sufficient for the cross-reactivity assays. We have previously compared ex vivo versus in vitro-expanded cross-reactivity profiles using the public HLA-B*08:01/FLR model and showed that cross-reactivity towards B*44:02 was detected in both conditions, but was more amplified using in vitro cultures enabling further functional characterisation [10]. In vitro culturing methods have also been used by others to assess cross-reactivity due to the low numbers of tetramer+ CD8+ T cells [4,20]. Unfortunately for HC5, we were unable to detect any ex vivo cross-reactivity (data not shown) due to very low numbers of NLV-tetramer+ CD8+ T cells (≤0.1%).

Characterising HLA-A*02:01-restricted NLV-specific CD8+ T cell cross-reactivity towards HLA-B*27:05

Phenotypic identification. To confirm our previous findings, four independent experiments of HC5 were conducted at different intervals within a one year time period. PBMC were in vitro expanded with NLV-pulsed autologous PBMC for 13 days. NLV-specific CD8+ T cells significantly increased in magnitude from very low (below threshold of detection) baseline ex vivo frequencies of 0.09±0.06% (range: 0.0–0.1%) to 65.4±16.4% (range: 46.2–80.5%) of the total CD8+ T cell population on day 13. Of these NLV-specific CD8+ T cells cross-reactivity towards B*27:05, measured by IFN-γ production following stimulation with C1R.B*27:05 transfected cell line, was observed with frequencies of 4.9±1.0% (range: 3.7–6.1%) including the initial screening experiment (data not shown).

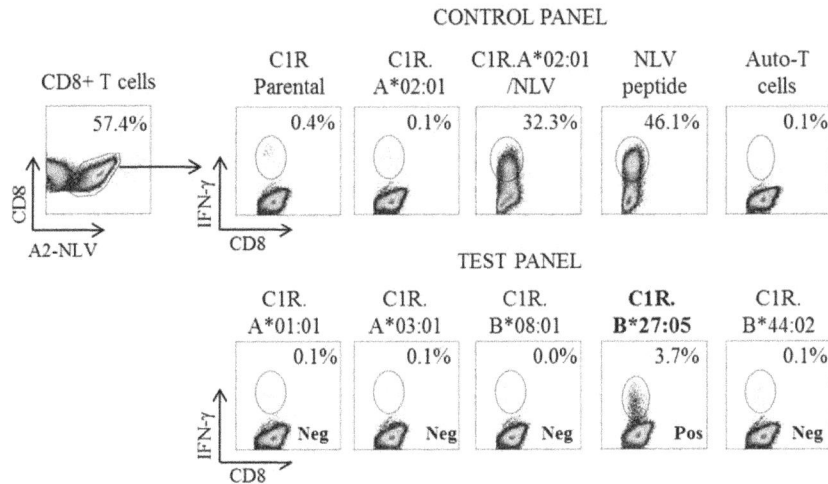

Figure 1. Cross-reactive NLV-specific CD8+ T cells via IFN-γ production. NLV-specific CD8+ T cells from HC5 were expanded for 13 days before performing a 6 hour ICS assay against a panel of transfected cell lines and EBV-LCLs encompassing 6 HLA-A and 13 HLA-B antigens. Cross-reactivity was measured by the production of IFN-γ in response to HLA antigenic stimulation after gating on tetramer+CD8+ T cells. Both the positive controls (C1R.A*02:01/NLV, NLV peptide) and negative controls (C1R Parental, C1R.A*02:01, T cells alone) responded as expected. No cross-reactivity was observed with the test panel, albeit C1R.B*27:05 which had a positive IFN-γ response well above background levels. IFN-γ responses towards 9009, 9026, T102, C1R.B*18:01, C1R.B*35:01, C1R.B*35:02, C1R.B*35:03, C1R.B*44:03, C1R.B*57:01, 721.221 Parental, 721.221.A*29:02, 721.221.A68 and 721.221.B53 were also negative (data not shown).

Functional assessment. The day 13 cross-reactive pool of NLV-specific CD8+ T cells were examined for their capacity to (i) induce cytotoxicity, via cell surface expression of degranulation marker CD107a [34], (ii) proliferate, via dilution of CFSE staining [35] and (iii) secrete Th1 cytokine, via production of IFN-γ following stimulation with B*27:05 alloantigen. T cell subsets differentiated by functionality were described as being either single-positive (IFN-γ+ or CD107a+) or double-positive (IFN-γ+CD107a+) in terms of their cytokine production and/or cytotoxic response, respectively. Of the total NLV-specific CD8+ T cell population, responses to C1R.B*27:05 elicited 4.2% IFN-γ+, 0.8% IFN-γ+CD107a+ and 0.1% CD107a+ subset populations, thus suggesting that these cells were dominated by a cytokine producing profile. Both the positive (C1R.A*02:01/NLV; 55.0% IFN-γ+, 18.0% IFN-γ+CD107a+ and 0.9% CD107a+) and negative (C1R.A*02:01; ≤0.2% all subsets) controls generated immune responses as expected (Figure 2A). The entire NLV-specific CD8+ T cell population had proliferated after 13 days as shown by the decreased CFSE expression including the 4.8% cross-reactive CD8+ T cell population following C1R.B*27:05 restimulation (Figure 2B). Collectively, this data demonstrated both confirmation and functionality of our model of HLA-A*02:01-restricted NLV-specific CD8+ T cell cross-reactivity in response to HLA-B*27:05.

HLA-B27 allelic variation influences the magnitude of CD8+ T cell cross-reactivity

In a well-characterized model of EBV TCR cross-reactivity, HLA-B*08:01-restricted FLR-specific CD8+ T cells were able to recognise the B*44:02 alloantigen, but not B*44:03 [11,12]. These two B44 allelic subtypes differ by a single amino acid substitution, aspartate (D) for B*44:02 or leucine (L) for B*44:03, at position 156 of the alpha 2 domain, which contributes to disparate alloreactive profiles [28] as well as impacting on clinical transplant outcomes [36,37]. To determine whether the A*02:01/NLV cross-reactivity model was influenced by B27 allelic variation, day 13 *in vitro* expanded NLV-specific CD8+ T cells generated from HC5 were restimulated with C1R transfectants expressing either B*27:03, B*27:05 or B*27:09 in a 6 hour ICS assay (Table 3). Using B*27:05 as the consensus sequence, B*27:03 and B*27:09 alleles differ by a single amino acid substitution at position 59 (tyrosine (Y) to histidine (H)) and position 116 (D to H), respectively (Figure 3). Site-directed mutagenesis of B*27:05 cDNA was used to generate the C1R transfectants for B*27:03 and B*27:09 subtypes. Comparison of immune reactivity of NLV-specific CD8+ T cells directed against each of the B27 alleles demonstrated that the B*27:09 allele (4.1%) generated the strongest frequency of IFN-γ production, followed by B*27:05 (0.9%) and then B*27:03 (0.5%) (Figure 3). The same cross-reactive T cell immune hierarchy of B*27:09>B*27:05>B*27:03 was observed in three independent experiments (data not shown).

Measuring the cross-reactive T cell potential in HLA mismatched lung allografts

To determine the potential impact of NLV-specific CD8+ T cell cross-reactivity on the specific clinical allograft outcomes of lung function and acute rejection, as well as CMV primary infection or reactivation and survival following transplantation, 11 HLA-A*02:01 LTR who received either an HLA-A30 (LTR1, 4, 8), A31 (LTR7, 9–11), A32 (LTR2, 3) or B27 (LTR2, 3, 5, 6) bilateral lung allograft (Table 1) were investigated for (i) the presence and expansion of NLV-specific CD8+ T cells and (ii) their ability to recognise HLA alloantigens based on our newly identified model of A*02:01/NLV T cell cross-reactivity (B27) and the previously published models (A30, A31, A32) [20].

Firstly, levels of circulating NLV-specific CD8+ T cells were measured from pre-transplant up to 12 months post-transplant, where available. *Ex vivo* analysis of A*02:01/NLV-tetramer+ cells revealed undetectable levels (<0.1%) in one CMV seropositive (+) LTR (LTR7) and as expected in four CMV seronegative (−) LTR (LTR1, 4, 10, 11). However, a range of 0.1–17.6% was detected in four CMV+ LTR (LTR3, 5, 8, 9) (Figure 4A). LTR2 (CMV−) and LTR6 (CMV+) were not evaluated. Following antigen-specific expansion of the memory T cell pool, the presence of NLV-specific CD8+ T cells was detected in all six CMV+ LTR (range 0.1–

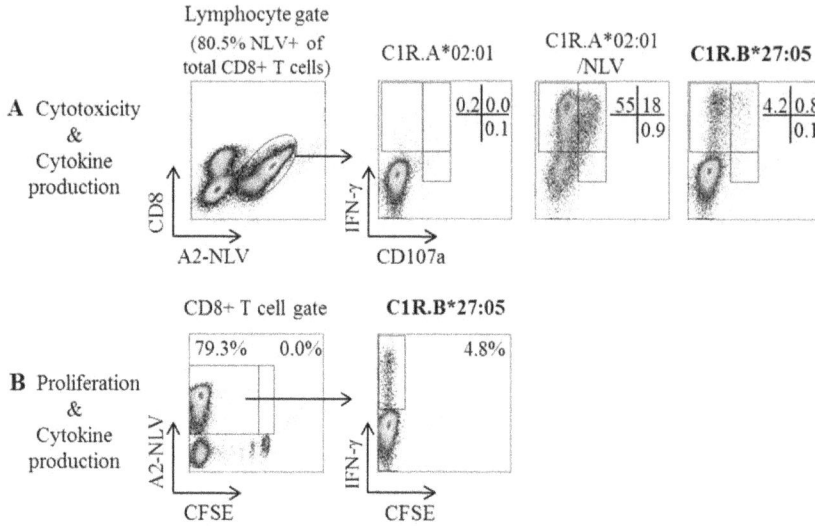

Figure 2. Functional analyses of new cross-reactivity towards B^x27:05. Flow cytometric analyses of IFN-γ and CD107a expression were performed after 13 days of NLV-specific T cell expansion from HC5. T cell cultures were stimulated with C1R.A*02:01 (negative control), NLV-pulsed C1R.A*02:01 (positive control) or C1R.B*27:05 (cross-reactive target) for 6 hours in a combined CD107a staining and ICS assay revealing that cross-reactivity was mainly via cytokine production (IFN-γ+) and to a lesser extent dual cytokine/cytotoxic ability (IFN-γ+/CD107a+) (A). Both proliferation and cytokine production were measured in a parallel experiment after CFSE-labelled PBMCs from HC5 were cultured with autologous irradiated NLV-pulsed PBMCs for 13 days before performing a 6 hour ICS assay (B). The lymphocyte gate was based on side scatter versus forward scatter. CD8+ T cells were then gated from lymphocytes using side scatter versus anti-CD8 PE-Cy5.

88.1%; LTR3, 5–9) (Figure 4B). Although LTR10 and LTR11 received CMV+ allografts, we did not detect any NLV-specific CD8+ T cells within the first 3.5 months post-transplant.

Secondly, quantitation of NLV-specific CD8+ T cell cross-reactivity toward the HLA alloantigens A30, A31, A32 or B27 was measured (IFN-γ production) following *in vitro* stimulation of the expanded pool of NLV-specific CD8+ T cells with B-LCL expressing the respective mismatched HLA molecules. Of the 11

LTR, T cell cross-reactivity was only detected in LTR5 and LTR8, who had received a B27 and an A30 lung allograft, respectively (Figure 5).

In LTR5, *ex vivo* levels of NLV-specific CD8+ T cells ranged between 0.0–0.1% from pre-transplant to 193 days post-transplant (Figure 4A). However, peptide-induced *in vitro* expansion of NLV-specific CD8+ T cells yielded frequencies of 2.5% pre-transplant to 62.3% at 193 days post-transplant (Figure 5A, total NLV-

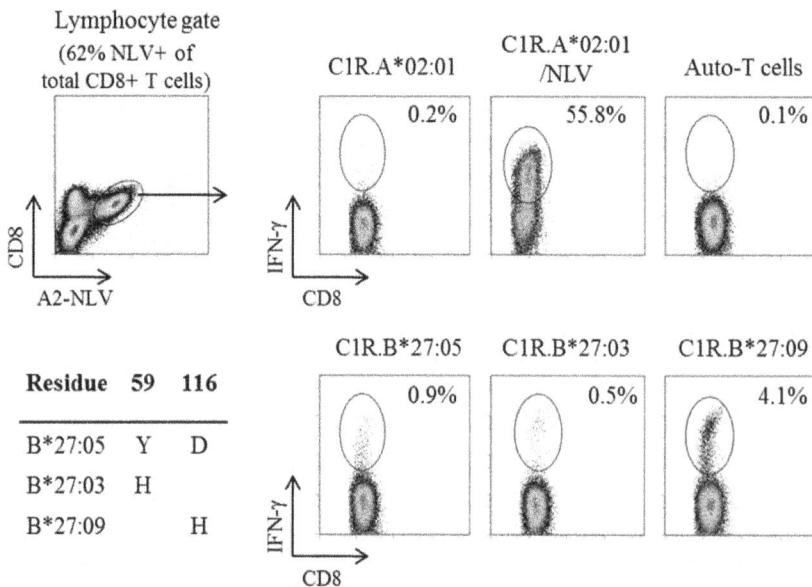

Figure 3. Influence of cross-reactivity by B27 allelic subtypes. Site-directed mutagenesis of the pMIG.B*27:05 vector was performed to generate B*27:03- and B*27:09-specific retroviruses for transducing C1R Parental cells. Comparison of cross-reactive NLV-specific IFN-γ responses between B*27:05, B*27:03 and B*27:09 was then carried out following a 6 hour stimulation and ICS assay of day 13 NLV-specific CD8+ T cells (HC5) with the B27-specific cell lines as well as positive (C1R.A*02:01/NLV) and negative controls (C1R.A*02:01, Auto-T cells).

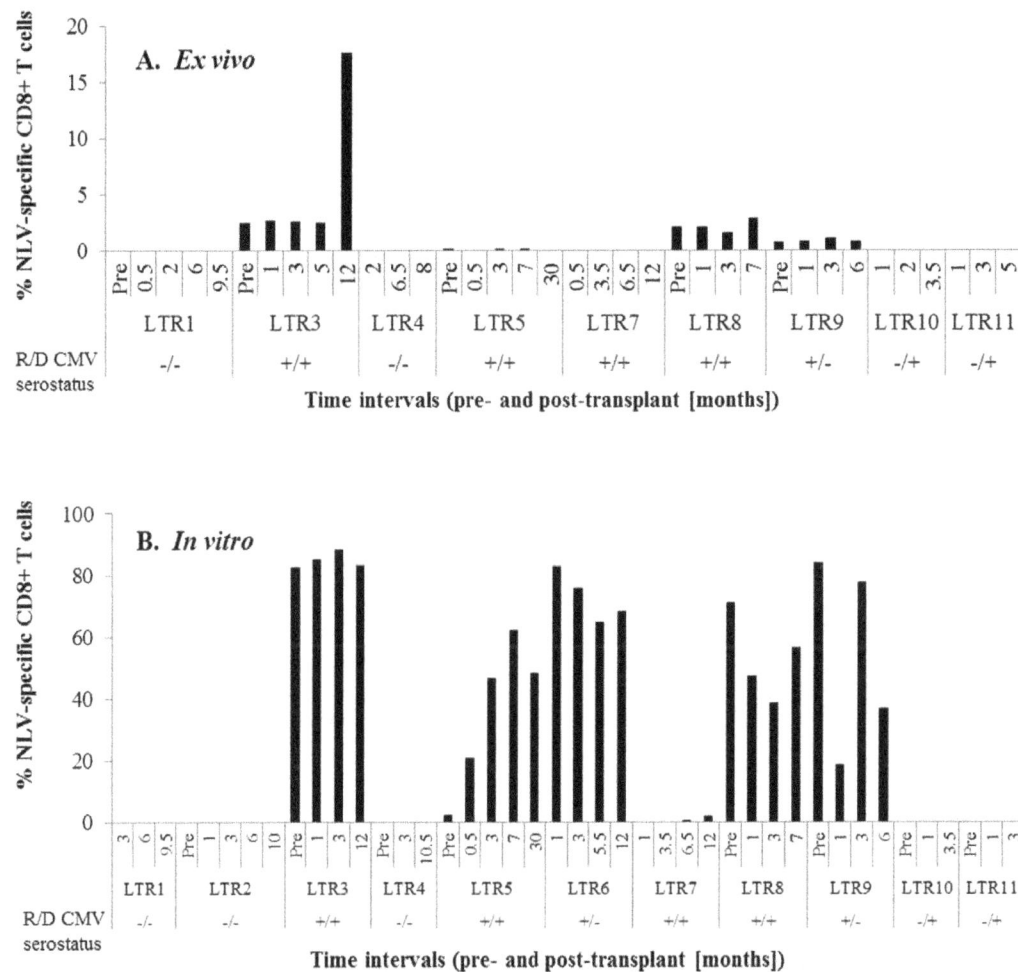

Figure 4. Expansion profiles of NLV-specific CD8+ T cells in LTR. NLV-specific CD8+ T cell frequencies were measured on day 0 (A) and after 13 days of NLV peptide stimulation (B) based on the total CD8+ T cell population, where available. CMV serostatus of the recipients and donors are indicated in the graphs.

specific CD8+ T cells). More importantly, cross-reactivity of NLV-specific CD8+ T cells towards two of the three B27 alleles tested was observed, with B*27:09 cross-reactivity gradually increasing from 2.3% to 34.9% of NLV-specific CD8+ T cells producing IFN-γ from pre-transplant to 193 days post-transplant. Although, cross-reactivity towards B*27:05 was evident the level remained relatively stable over time (Figure 5A). This data suggested that the B*27:09 allele was the most favourable cross-reactive alloantigen.

For LTR8, *ex vivo* levels of 1.6–2.9% of NLV-specific CD8+ T cells (data not shown) expanded upon antigenic stimulation to 38.8–71.3% from pre-transplant to 219 days post-transplant (Figure 5B, total NLV-specific CD8+ T cells). Based on a report of NLV-specific CD8+ T cell cross-reactivity towards A30 alloantigen [20] we showed a minimal IFN-γ response of 0.4–1.0% that remained stable throughout the pre-transplant to 219 days post-transplant time period (Figure 5B). No NLV-specific CD8+ T cell cross-reactivity was observed towards A31 or A32 alloantigens in this group of LTR.

Increase in cross-reactive T cells is dependent on availability of an antigen source

Of the 11 LTR, 2 (18%) were at risk of experiencing primary CMV disease despite anti-viral prophylaxis (R−/D+: LTR10, 11),

6 (55%) were at risk of CMV reactivation (R+/D− or R+/D+; LTR3, 5–9), whilst 3 (27%) were of no risk (R−/D−; LTR1, 2, 4) and hence did not receive CMV prophylaxis (Table 1). In all LTR, except LTR5, there was no primary CMV infection or reactivation event within the first 12 months post-transplant based on CMV viral load monitoring, although LTR10 and LTR11 were only assessed to 3 months post-transplant due to sample availability. For LTR5, CMV reactivation was detected on day 270 post-transplant by a positive PCR for CMV DNA and a viral titre of 18,600 copies/ml. Interestingly, CMV pneumonitis was also evident on day 270 in the transbronchial biopsy sample. However, negative PCR results and undetectable viral loads were recorded both prior to (days 13–193) and following (day 375) the CMV reactivation episode (Figure 6A). Although routine CMV prophylaxis had ceased on day 159 (5 months post-transplant), LTR5 received an additional 2 weeks of intravenous ganciclovir treatment from day 270 of CMV reactivation (9 months), followed by oral valganciclovir treatment (450 mg: morning and evening) up until 24 months post-transplant.

Although CMV viremia in LTR5 was undetectable in BAL samples on days 13, 35, 60, 88 and 193 post-transplantation, we quantitatively observed an increase in both conventional and cross-reactive, towards HLA-B*27:09, NLV-specific CD8+ T cells

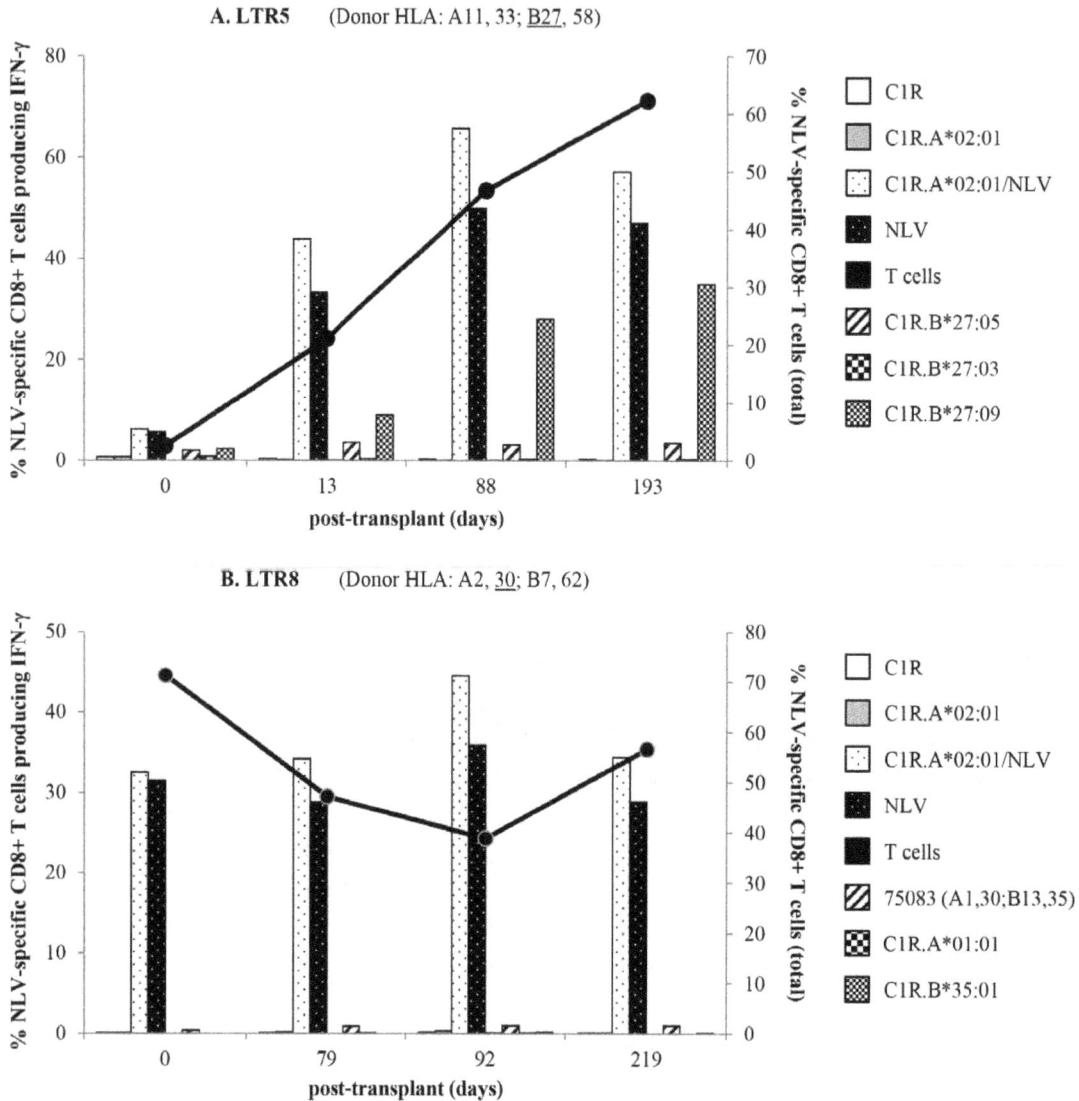

A. LTR5 (Donor HLA: A11, 33; B27, 58)

B. LTR8 (Donor HLA: A2, 30; B7, 62)

Figure 5. Longitudinal analysis of LTR cross-reactivity. NLV-specific cross-reactivity responses against B27 and A30 were measured against time after lung transplant in LTR5 ([A] top) and LTR8 ([B] bottom), respectively. Following a 6 hour ICS assay of day 13 T cell cultures, B*27:09 cross-reactivity significantly increased over time in LTR5, whereas A30 cross-reactivity remained stable post-transplant in LTR8. Percentages were based on IFN-γ production of NLV-specific +CD8+ T cells. The secondary axis represents the percentage of NLV-specific CD8+ T cells gated on total CD8+ T cells (circles).

(Figure 6A). A clinically relevant active CMV reactivation was measured on day 270 post-transplantation and following CMV treatment intervention strategies and clearance of the virus, only the cross-reactive NLV-specific CD8+ T cell pool returned to baseline frequencies (day 909) (Figure 6A). Conversely, in the absence of CMV viremia there was no increase in cross-reactive NLV-specific CD8+ T cells as demonstrated by LTR8 (Figure 6B).

Clinical dynamics of lung function, acute cellular rejection and pulmonary associated survival were not influenced by presence of cross-reactive T cells

Of the 11 LTR, NLV-specific CD8+ T cell cross-reactivity was detected only in LTR5 (B*27:09 and B*27:05) and LTR8 (A30). Our *in vitro* studies demonstrated that the presence of either exogenous peptide (LTR5, 8) or CMV viremia (LTR5) significantly magnified the frequency of these cross-reactive T cells,

which raises the possibility that these cells can contribute to adverse clinical events against the lung allograft expressing the target HLA alloantigen. To determine the impact of NLV-specific CD8+ T cell cross-reactivity on allograft function we monitored longitudinal measurements of lung function, acute cellular rejection and survival on the background of potent immunosuppression.

There was no association between the potential cross-reactive T cell dynamics and physiological lung function (as measured by % Personal Best) in either LTR5 and LTR8, who both exhibited excellent lung function (>90%) up to 24 months post-transplant (data not shown). Transbronchial biopsy samples were evaluated for the presence of acute cellular rejection within the first 12 months post-transplant. There was no evidence of cellular infiltrate or change in tissue architecture reported for either LTR5 or LTR8. Indeed, all LTR were alive at 24 months following transplantation.

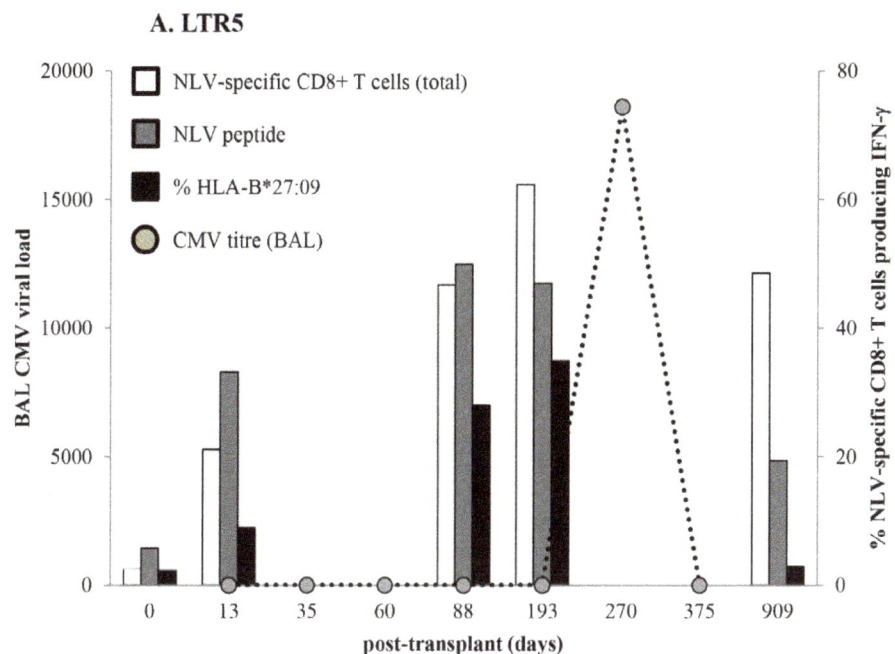

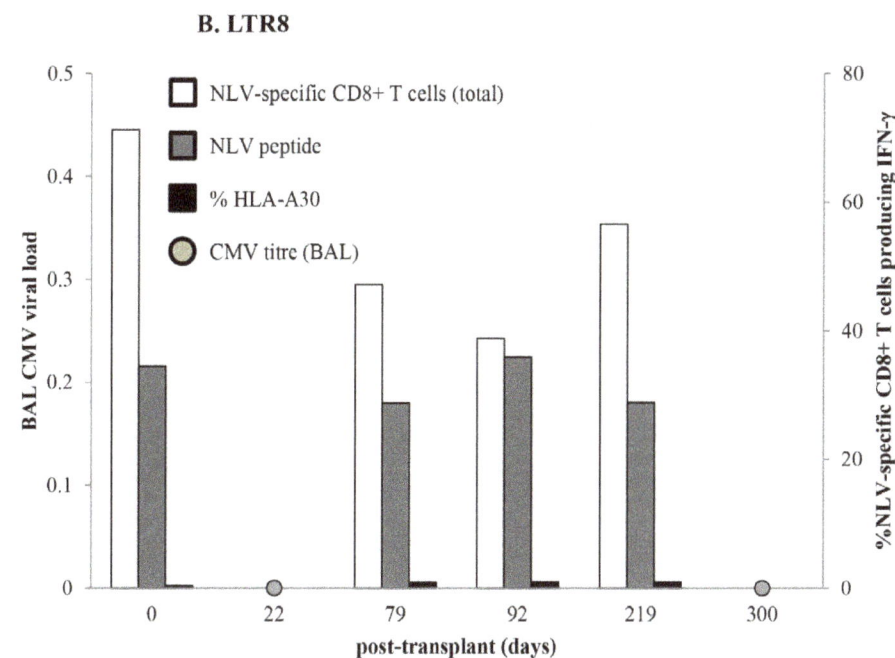

Figure 6. Presence of CMV reactivation increases magnitude of cross-reactivity against the allograft. Comparison of CMV viral load in the BAL (grey circles, left y-axis) and NLV-specific cross-reactivity responses towards B27 and A30 (6 hour ICS assay using day 13 T cells) were measured against time after lung transplant in LTR5 (top) and LTR8 (bottom), respectively. A CMV reactivation episode was classified for viral titres above 10,000. LTR5 experienced CMV reactivation at day 270 post-transplant but had ceased after day 375. A steady increase in B*27:09-cross-reactivity response based on %IFN-γ production of tetramer+CD8+ gated cells (black bars, right y-axis) and %tetramer+CD8+ cells of total CD8+ T cells (white bars, right y-axis) were observed prior to CMV reactivation event at day 193 but had dropped to pre-transplant levels after CMV reactivation had ceased. For LTR8, BAL CMV viral titre was not detected post-transplant. In alignment, A30 cross-reactivity and %tetramer+CD8+ cells of total CD8+ T cells remained consistent post-transplant.

Collectively these data show that cross-reactive NLV-specific CD8+ T cells did not necessarily contribute to any clinical manifestations of allograft dysfunction in the single CMV reactivation scenario that could be examined. Whilst we observed a significant increase in cross-reactive T cells frequency following CMV reactivation, we suspect that a single viral reactivation event (particularly if it is low level and relatively short lived) may not be sufficient to drive cross-reactivity associated destructive lung immunopathology in adequately immunosuppressed LTR.

Discussion

Since the first human report of a cross-reactive EBV-specific CD8+ T cell recognizing the unrelated HLA alloantigen B*4402 [11] was described, there have been an array of publications identifying human cross-reactive virus-specific T cells directed towards both class I and class II HLA alloantigens in CMV [4,17–20], EBV [4,11,12,38], HSV-2 [39], Influenza [4] and Varicella zoster virus (VZV) [4] models. However, these reports examined T cell cross-reactivity in healthy individuals and could only speculate about the implications of this mechanism in contributing to destructive immunopathology associated with either allograft rejection or graft versus host disease (GvHD) in a transplant setting.

Only recently have there been two human reports in a real clinical setting examining the contribution of cross-reactive virus-specific T cells towards either allograft dysfunction in LTR (from our group) [10] or GvHD in hematopoietic stem cell transplant recipients [40]. Whilst both studies demonstrated the presence of cross-reactive virus-specific T cells and their contribution to the alloreactive T cell pool in patient cohorts, we and Melenhorst et al. were unable to associate cross-reactive virus-specific T cells with either episodes of allograft dysfunction and rejection or incidences of GvHD, respectively. In our study [10], we specifically measured EBV reactivation in order to better frame our T cells cross-reactivity results. However, as there was no active EBV infection in our patient cohort we concluded that the presence of cross-reactive T cells was not enough to mediating allograft rejection alone and that the frequency and extent of active viral infection was likely to be important. Hence, we have since focussed on a CMV study in the setting of either primary infection (CMV mismatch) or reactivation, which occurs much more frequently (7.2% or 17.5%, respectively from 2006–2008; n = 97) and constitutes severe morbidity and mortality associated complications following lung transplantation. In this setting, we proposed that viral antigenic stimulation in vivo has the potential to magnify cross-reactive CMV-specific T cell responses towards specifically targeted HLA alloantigen(s), thereby contributing to a destructive immunopathology and promoting allograft rejection or loss. In support, we have previously reported that CMV-specific memory T cells can account for up to 20% of the total circulating T cells early post-transplantation and uniformly increases following episodes of significant CMV reactivation [13,41].

For the first time, we describe the cross-reactivity of HLA-A*02:01-restricted CMV-specific CD8+ T cell towards the common HLA-B27 antigen. Functional characterisation of NLV-specific CD8+ T cell cross-reactivity was determined by both IFN-γ production and cell surface expression of CD107a. Our model utilizes the predominance of HLA-A*02:01 in our general population (over 40%) and our lung transplant cohort (37%) as well as the immunodominant nature of the NLV epitope [42,43]. Cross-reactivity between HLA-A and -B groups is a new paradigm for CTL recognition with only one other example reported recently whereby HLA-A*02:01-restricted VZV-specific

CTLs cross-reacted with HLA-B*55:01 cell lines in one VZV-seropositive healthy individual [4] and one VZV-seronegative kidney transplant patient following VZV vaccination [44]. The fact that we observed similar HLA-A to -B cross-reactivity in both a healthy donor and a LTR suggests that this mechanism of T cell recognition may be more common than previously considered.

We assessed the clinical interrelationships between the presence and dynamics of cross-reactive CD8+ T cells against clinical outcomes including lung function, acute cellular rejection and pulmonary associated survival following lung transplantation. As only LTR5 had increasing cross-reactive NLV-specific CD8+ T cells in the setting of a CMV reactivation profile, but stable lung allograft function at 24 months we were limited in making any sweeping conclusions regarding increased anti-viral cross reactivity and poorer lung allograft outcomes. Importantly, the proportion of cross-reactive CD8+ T cells in relation to the total NLV-specific CD8+ T cell population in LTR5 declined back to pre-transplant levels once the virus was cleared. This poses an important question; should these cross-reactive T cells continue to dominate in the setting of multiple hits of CMV reactivation, then would this accelerate allograft loss? To address this critical question, future studies measuring cross-reactive T cells in cohorts experiencing multiple CMV-related events would be useful, as well as the expansion of known cross-reactivities between CMV and HLA molecules.

The presence of stable circulating cross-reactive CD8+ T cells seen in LTR8 with no CMV reactivation may suggest that there may be compartmental issues in terms of using peripheral blood for our assays rather than BAL mononuclear cells that reside within the lung allograft, however there are technical difficulties associated with obtaining sufficient cell numbers for these investigations. In support, we have previously reported that CMV-specific CD8+ T cell dynamics in both the blood and the lung allograft reflect viral reactivation following lung transplantation [13]. Another consideration is that our experiments involved primarily in vitro cultures to enhance the signal from very low starting numbers of ex vivo virus-specific (tetramer+) T cells. Our previous study in the EBV model compared ex vivo and in vitro FLR-specific cross-reactive responses towards B*44:02 and although they were functionally different (cytotoxic versus cytolytic, respectively), the strength and hierarchy of the response was highly comparable [10].

Moving from the classic T cell cross-reactivity model of the EBV gamma herpesvirus to a more evolved CMV beta herpesvirus raises a very different immunological scenario for consideration. The EBV-specific TCR repertoire that recognises the HLA-B*08:01-restricted FLR peptide is widely public and predominantly consists of either the cross-reactive LC13 clone, expressed by almost all individuals who do not co-express HLA-B*44:02/05, or the non-cross-reactive CF34 clone [11,12,45]. Whereas, the CMV-specific TCR repertoire for the HLA-A2-restricted NLV epitope is much more diverse [43,46,47] and may be an important mechanism to counteract CMV's highly evolved immune evasion strategies. Although public NLV-specific TCRs have been described [47,48], the oligoclonal nature helps explain why we and others have identified the relatively private specificity of NLV-specific T cell cross-reactivity between individuals of either undefined HLA alloantigens [4,18] or A30, A31, A32 [20] and B27 (this study). Yet, the allopeptide(s) presented by these HLA molecules remain unknown. By chance, we were still able to detect comparative B27 T cell cross-reactivity in a healthy donor and a lung transplant patient as well as confirm A30 directed T cell cross-reactivity as reported by Morice et al. [20] in one patient using a limited sample size, suggesting that these cross-reactive T cells may not be so "private". This now leads to question whether we would find more commonality between NLV-specific T cell cross-reactivity profiles as we increasing our cohort numbers or whether these cross-reactive TCR's are truly private and only unique to a few individuals. Further studies are currently being investigated to determine whether HC5 and LTR5 share a common TCR profile.

The cross-reactivity hierarchy between the B27 subtypes may be explained by the location of the variant residues. For example, B*27:05 and B*27:09 differ by a single substitution at residue 116 (D to H, respectively) which is located on the floor of the peptide binding groove. Structural studies by Fiorillo and colleagues show CD8+ T cell functional disparities between B*27:05 and B*27:09 in their engagement of self and viral peptides [49]. However, a full understanding of the mechanistic basis of our B27-cross-reactivity model with structural studies will require the discovery of the allopeptide.

We observed one LTR example of a single episodic increase of cross-reactive NLV-specific CD8+ T cells was not associated with adverse clinical lung immunopathology and allograft deterioration. Interestingly, these cross-reactive T cells significantly increased in frequency prior to the onset of a clinically significant CMV reactivation and were then shown to decrease back to baseline levels following CMV viremia clearance. In contrast, significant increases of the cross-reactive T cell pool were not seen in the setting of persistent alloantigen exposure under current immunosuppression strategies. The findings of this study suggest that at the very least a threshold level of anti-viral cross-reactivity may be required to mediate allograft rejection. Whilst the findings of this study does not directly support recent experimental evidence in a murine model examining T cell cross-reactivity, where Lymphocytic Choriomeningitis Virus-specific T cells were shown to mediate skin allograft rejection [50], it should be remembered that these murine studies were performed in a highly artificial and controlled environment, without the administration of immunosuppression.

Our previous studies showed the ability of cross-reactive EBV-specific T cells to induce immune reactivity towards HLA molecules expressed on both PBMC and BAL mononuclear cells [10,28,31]. However, we were unable to demonstrate the clinical impact of these T cells in mediating allograft dysfunction [10]. In addition to the requirement for active viral infection, cross-reactive T cells may exert tissue-specific recognition of HLA alloantigens.

A seminal study by D'Orsogna et al. [44] confirmed that recognition of allogeneic HLA molecules by virus-specific memory T cells is dependent on self-peptide presentation by the allogeneic target cell. The more readily testable EBV model yielded key observations with EBNA3A-specific T cells showing weak recognition of HLA-B*44:02 target cells due to lack of EEYLQAFTY peptide presentation in specific tissues. Further studies examining the ability of differential lung allograft tissue (epithelial versus endothelial) to (i) naturally process and present HLA/self-peptide complexes and (ii) decipher their ability to be specifically targeted by cross-reactive anti-viral T cells are currently being explored.

In conclusion, we have demonstrated that cross-reactive NLV-specific CD8+ T cells remain stable in the setting of persistent alloantigen but significantly increase prior to a clinically relevant CMV reactivation event. We speculate that a series of immunological events may be required to align in order for cross-reactive virus-specific T cells to exert physiological damage on transplanted allograft, especially in the setting of potent immunosuppressive regimens. These events include (i) an active viral infection as a sustainable antigen source, (ii) the magnitude (high titres) and frequency (more than one episode) of viremia requiring clinical intervention, (iii) the significant increase in frequency of cross-reactive T cells and (iv) the tissue-specific expression of the targeted HLA/peptide complex. Finally, we speculate that discordance between persistently increased cross-reactive anti-viral T cells and CMV viremia that has subsided may be the first sign that these anti-viral T cells are influencing allograft immunopathology.

Acknowledgments

We gratefully acknowledge the generous support of Prof. Greg Snell and all the clinicians, nurses and allied health professionals associated with the Lung Transplant Service at The Alfred Hospital, especially the patients recruited for this study. Thank you to Prof. Dario Vignali (St Jude Children's Research Hospital) and Dr. Lars Kjer-Nielsen (The University of Melbourne) for generous gift of reagents and guidance for the retroviral transduction experiments.

Author Contributions

Conceived and designed the experiments: THON NAM. Performed the experiments: THON TEB ACM NAM. Analyzed the data: THON GPW NAM TCK. Contributed reagents/materials/analysis tools: GPW TCK. Wrote the paper: THON GW NAM TCK.

References

1. Paraskeva M, Bailey M, Levvey BJ, Griffiths AP, Kotsimbos TC, et al. (2011) Cytomegalovirus Replication Within the Lung Allograft Is Associated With Bronchiolitis Obliterans Syndrome. Am J Transplant 10: 2190–2196.
2. Brugiere O, Thabut G, Suberbielle C, Reynaud-Gaubert M, Thomas P, et al. (2008) Relative impact of human leukocyte antigen mismatching and graft ischemic time after lung transplantation. J Heart Lung Transplant 27: 628–634.
3. Chalermskulrat W, Neuringer IP, Schmitz JL, Catellier DJ, Gurka MJ, et al. (2003) Human leukocyte antigen mismatches predispose to the severity of bronchiolitis obliterans syndrome after lung transplantation. Chest 123: 1825–1831.
4. Amir AL, D'Orsogna LJ, Roelen DL, van Loenen MM, Hagedoorn RS, et al. (2010) Allo-HLA reactivity of virus-specific memory T cells is common. Blood 115: 3146–3157.
5. Macdonald WA, Chen Z, Gras S, Archbold JK, Tynan FE, et al. (2009) T cell allorecognition via molecular mimicry. Immunity 31: 897–908.
6. Bendjelloul F, Desin TS, Shoker AS (2004) Donor non-specific IFN-gamma production by primed alloreactive cells as a potential screening test to predict the alloimmune response. Transpl Immunol 12: 167–176.
7. Heeger PS, Greenspan NS, Kuhlenschmidt S, Dejelo C, Hricik DE, et al. (1999) Pretransplant frequency of donor-specific, IFN-gamma-producing lymphocytes is a manifestation of immunologic memory and correlates with the risk of posttransplant rejection episodes. J Immunol 163: 2267–2275.
8. Lombardi G, Sidhu S, Daly M, Batchelor JR, Makgoba W, et al. (1990) Are primary alloresponses truly primary? Int Immunol 2: 9–13.
9. Merkenschlager M, Terry L, Edwards R, Beverley PC (1988) Limiting dilution analysis of proliferative responses in human lymphocyte populations defined by the monoclonal antibody UCHL1: implications for differential CD45 expression in T cell memory formation. Eur J Immunol 18: 1653–1661.
10. Mifsud NA, Nguyen TH, Tait BD, Kotsimbos TC (2010) Quantitative and functional diversity of cross-reactive EBV-specific CD8+ T cells in a longitudinal study cohort of lung transplant recipients. Transplantation 90: 1439–1449.
11. Burrows SR, Khanna R, Burrows JM, Moss DJ (1994) An alloresponse in humans is dominated by cytotoxic T lymphocytes (CTL) cross-reactive with a single Epstein-Barr virus CTL epitope: implications for graft-versus-host disease. J Exp Med 179: 1155–1161.
12. Burrows SR, Silins SL, Cross SM, Peh CA, Rischmueller M, et al. (1997) Human leukocyte antigen phenotype imposes complex constraints on the antigen-specific cytotoxic T lymphocyte repertoire. Eur J Immunol 27: 178–182.
13. Westall G, Kotsimbos T, Brooks A (2006) CMV-specific CD8 T-cell dynamics in the blood and the lung allograft reflect viral reactivation following lung transplantation. Am J Transplant 6: 577–584.
14. Wong JY, Tait B, Levvey B, Griffiths A, Esmore DS, et al. (2004) Epstein-Barr virus primary mismatching and HLA matching: key risk factors for post lung transplant lymphoproliferative disease. Transplantation 78: 205–210.
15. Wreghitt T (1989) Cytomegalovirus infections in heart and heart-lung transplant recipients. J Antimicrob Chemother 23 Suppl E: 49–60.
16. Maecker HT, Maino VC (2004) Analyzing T-cell responses to cytomegalovirus by cytokine flow cytometry. Hum Immunol 65: 493–499.

17. Elkington R, Khanna R (2005) Cross-recognition of human alloantigen by cytomegalovirus glycoprotein-specific CD4+ cytotoxic T lymphocytes: implications for graft-versus-host disease. Blood 105: 1362–1364.
18. Gamadia LE, Remmerswaal EB, Surachno S, Lardy NM, Wertheim-van Dillen PM, et al. (2004) Cross-reactivity of cytomegalovirus-specific CD8+ T cells to allo-major histocompatibility complex class I molecules. Transplantation 77: 1879–1885.
19. Rist M, Smith C, Bell MJ, Burrows SR, Khanna R (2009) Cross-recognition of HLA DR4 alloantigen by virus-specific CD8+ T cells: a new paradigm for self-/nonself-recognition. Blood 114: 2244–2253.
20. Morice A, Charreau B, Neveu B, Brouard S, Soulillou JP, et al. (2010) Cross-reactivity of herpesvirus-specific CD8 T cell lines toward allogeneic class I MHC molecules. PLoS One 5: e12120.
21. Westall GP, Michaelides A, Williams TJ, Snell GI, Kotsimbos TC (2003) Bronchiolitis obliterans syndrome and early human cytomegalovirus DNAaemia dynamics after lung transplantation. Transplantation 75: 2064–2068.
22. Westall GP, Brooks AG, Kotsimbos T (2007) CD8+ T-cell maturation following lung transplantation: the differential impact of CMV and acute rejection. Transpl Immunol 18: 186–192.
23. Cainelli F, Vento S (2002) Infections and solid organ transplant rejection: a cause-and-effect relationship? Lancet Infect Dis 2: 539–549.
24. Estenne M, Maurer JR, Boehler A, Egan JJ, Frost A, et al. (2002) Bronchiolitis obliterans syndrome 2001: an update of the diagnostic criteria. J Heart Lung Transplant 21: 297–310.
25. Yousem SA, Berry GJ, Cagle PT, Chamberlain D, Husain AN, et al. (1996) Revision of the 1990 working formulation for the classification of pulmonary allograft rejection: Lung Rejection Study Group. J Heart Lung Transplant 15: 1–15.
26. Michaelides A, Facey D, Spelman D, Wesselingh S, Kotsimbos T (2003) HCMV DNA detection and quantitation in the plasma and PBL of lung transplant recipients: COBAS Amplicor HCMV monitor test versus in-house quantitative HCMV PCR. J Clin Virol 28: 111–120.
27. Estenne M, Hertz MI (2002) Bronchiolitis obliterans after human lung transplantation. Am J Respir Crit Care Med 166: 440–444.
28. Macdonald WA, Purcell AW, Mifsud NA, Ely LK, Williams DS, et al. (2003) A naturally selected dimorphism within the HLA-B44 supertype alters class I structure, peptide repertoire, and T cell recognition. J Exp Med 198: 679–691.
29. Holst J, Szymczak-Workman AL, Vignali KM, Burton AR, Workman CJ, et al. (2006) Generation of T-cell receptor retrogenic mice. Nat Protoc 1: 406–417.
30. Nguyen TH, Sullivan LC, Kotsimbos TC, Schwarer AP, Mifsud NA (2010) Cross-presentation of HCMV chimeric protein enables generation and measurement of polyclonal T cells. Immunol Cell Biol 88: 676–684.
31. Mifsud NA, Purcell AW, Chen W, Holdsworth R, Tait BD, et al. (2008) Immunodominance hierarchies and gender bias in direct T(CD8)-cell alloreactivity. Am J Transplant 8: 121–132.
32. Turner SJ, Doherty PC, McCluskey J, Rossjohn J (2006) Structural determinants of T-cell receptor bias in immunity. Nat Rev Immunol 6: 883–894.
33. Wynn KK, Fulton Z, Cooper L, Silins SL, Gras S, et al. (2008) Impact of clonal competition for peptide-MHC complexes on the CD8+ T-cell repertoire selection in a persistent viral infection. Blood 111: 4283–4292.
34. Betts MR, Brenchley JM, Price DA, De Rosa SC, Douek DC, et al. (2003) Sensitive and viable identification of antigen-specific CD8+ T cells by a flow cytometric assay for degranulation. J Immunol Methods 281: 65–78.
35. Mannering SI, Morris JS, Jensen KP, Purcell AW, Honeyman MC, et al. (2003) A sensitive method for detecting proliferation of rare autoantigen-specific human T cells. J Immunol Methods 283: 173–183.
36. Fleischhauer K, Kernan NA, O'Reilly RJ, Dupont B, Yang SY (1990) Bone marrow-allograft rejection by T lymphocytes recognizing a single amino acid difference in HLA-B44. N Engl J Med 323: 1818–1822.
37. Keever CA, Leong N, Cunningham I, Copelan EA, Avalos BR, et al. (1994) HLA-B44-directed cytotoxic T cells associated with acute graft-versus-host disease following unrelated bone marrow transplantation. Bone Marrow Transplant 14: 137–145.
38. D'Orsogna IJ, Amir AL, Zoet YM, van der Meer-Prins PM, van der Slik AR, et al. (2009) New tools to monitor the impact of viral infection on the alloreactive T-cell repertoire. Tissue Antigens 74: 290–297.
39. Koelle DM, Chen HB, McClurkan CM, Petersdorf EW (2002) Herpes simplex virus type 2-specific CD8 cytotoxic T lymphocyte cross-reactivity against prevalent HLA class I alleles. Blood 99: 3844–3847.
40. Melenhorst JJ, Leen AM, Bollard CM, Quigley MF, Price DA, et al. (2010) Allogeneic virus-specific T cells with HLA alloreactivity do not produce GVHD in human subjects. Blood 116: 4700–4702.
41. Westall GP, Mifsud NA, Kotsimbos T (2008) Linking CMV serostatus to episodes of CMV reactivation following lung transplantation by measuring CMV-specific CD8+ T-cell immunity. Am J Transplant 8: 1749–1754.
42. Wills MR, Carmichael AJ, Mynard K, Jin X, Weekes MP, et al. (1996) The human cytotoxic T-lymphocyte (CTL) response to cytomegalovirus is dominated by structural protein pp65: frequency, specificity, and T-cell receptor usage of pp65-specific CTL. J Virol 70: 7569–7579.
43. Khan N, Cobbold M, Keenan R, Moss PA (2002) Comparative analysis of CD8+ T cell responses against human cytomegalovirus proteins pp65 and immediate early 1 shows similarities in precursor frequency, oligoclonality, and phenotype. J Infect Dis 185: 1025–1034.
44. D'Orsogna IJ, van Besouw NM, van der Meer-Prins EM, van der Pol P, Franke-van Dijk M, et al. (2011) Vaccine-induced allo-HLA-reactive memory T cells in a kidney transplantation candidate. Transplantation 91: 645–651.
45. Gras S, Burrows SR, Kjer-Nielsen L, Clements CS, Liu YC, et al. (2009) The shaping of T cell receptor recognition by self-tolerance. Immunity 30: 193–203.
46. Venturi V, Chin HY, Asher TE, Ladell K, Scheinberg P, et al. (2008) TCR beta-chain sharing in human CD8+ T cell responses to cytomegalovirus and EBV. J Immunol 181: 7853–7862.
47. Price DA, Brenchley JM, Ruff LE, Betts MR, Hill BJ, et al. (2005) Avidity for antigen shapes clonal dominance in CD8+ T cell populations specific for persistent DNA viruses. J Exp Med 202: 1349–1361.
48. Trautmann L, Rimbert M, Echasserieau K, Saulquin X, Neveu B, et al. (2005) Selection of T cell clones expressing high-affinity public TCRs within Human cytomegalovirus-specific CD8 T cell responses. J Immunol 175: 6123–6132.
49. Fiorillo MT, Ruckert C, Hulsmeyer M, Sorrentino R, Saenger W, et al. (2005) Allele-dependent similarity between viral and self-peptide presentation by HLA-B27 subtypes. J Biol Chem 280: 2962–2971.
50. Brehm MA, Daniels KA, Priyadharshini B, Thornley TB, Greiner DL, et al. (2010) Allografts stimulate cross-reactive virus-specific memory CD8 T cells with private specificity. Am J Transplant 10: 1738–1748.
51. Zemmour J, Little AM, Schendel DJ, Parham P (1992) The HLA-A,B "negative" mutant cell line C1R expresses a novel HLA-B35 allele, which also has a point mutation in the translation initiation codon. J Immunol 148: 1941–1948.

4

"Glowing Head" Mice: A Genetic Tool Enabling Reliable Preclinical Image-Based Evaluation of Cancers in Immunocompetent Allografts

Chi-Ping Day[1], John Carter[2], Zoe Weaver Ohler[4], Carrie Bonomi[2], Rajaa El Meskini[4], Philip Martin[4], Cari Graff-Cherry[5], Lionel Feigenbaum[5], Thomas Tüting[6], Terry Van Dyke[3], Melinda Hollingshead[7], Glenn Merlino[1]*

1 Laboratory of Cancer Biology and Genetics, National Cancer Institute, Bethesda, Maryland, United States of America, 2 In Vivo Evaluation, Leidos Biomedical Research Inc., Frederick National Laboratory for Cancer Research, Frederick, Maryland, United States of America, 3 Center for Advanced Preclinical Research of The Center for Cancer Research, National Cancer Institute, Frederick, Maryland, United States of America, 4 Center for Advanced Preclinical Research of Leidos Biomedical Research Inc., Frederick National Laboratory for Cancer Research, Frederick, Maryland, United States of America, 5 Laboratory Animal Science Program, Leidos Biomedical Research Inc., Frederick National Laboratory for Cancer Research, Frederick, Maryland, United States of America, 6 Department of Dermatology and Allergy, University Hospital Bonn, Bonn, Germany, 7 Biological Testing Branch, Developmental Therapeutics Program, National Cancer Institute, Frederick, Maryland, United States of America

Abstract

Preclinical therapeutic assessment currently relies on the growth response of established human cell lines xenografted into immunocompromised mice, a strategy that is generally not predictive of clinical outcomes. Immunocompetent genetically engineered mouse (GEM)-derived tumor allograft models offer highly tractable preclinical alternatives and facilitate analysis of clinically promising immunomodulatory agents. Imageable reporters are essential for accurately tracking tumor growth and response, particularly for metastases. Unfortunately, reporters such as luciferase and GFP are foreign antigens in immunocompetent mice, potentially hindering tumor growth and confounding therapeutic responses. Here we assessed the value of reporter-tolerized GEMs as allograft recipients by targeting minimal expression of a luciferase-GFP fusion reporter to the anterior pituitary gland (dubbed the "Glowing Head" or GH mouse). The luciferase-GFP reporter expressed in tumor cells induced adverse immune responses in wildtype mouse, but not in GH mouse, as transplantation hosts. The antigenicity of optical reporters resulted in a decrease in both the growth and metastatic potential of the labeled tumor in wildtype mice as compared to the GH mice. Moreover, reporter expression can also alter the tumor response to chemotherapy or targeted therapy in a context-dependent manner. Thus the GH mice and experimental approaches vetted herein provide concept validation and a strategy for effective, reproducible preclinical evaluation of growth and response kinetics for traceable tumors.

Editor: Devanand Sarkar, Virginia Commonwealth University, United States of America

Funding: This project has been funded in whole or in part with federal funds from the National Cancer Institute, National Institutes of Health, under Contract No. HHSN261200800001E. This work was supported in part by the Developmental Therapeutics Program in the Division of Cancer Treatment and Diagnosis and Intramural Research Program of the Center for Cancer Research, NCI, NIH. Leidos Biomedical Research Inc. provided support in the form of salaries for authors John Carter, Zoe Weaver-Ohler, Carrie Bonomi, Rajaa El Meskini, Philip Martin, Cari Graff-Cherry, and Lionel Feigenbaum, but did not have any additional role in the study design, data collection and analysis, decision to publish, or preparation of the manuscript. The specific roles of these authors are articulated in the 'author contributions' section.

Competing Interests: Co-authors John Carter, Zoe Weaver-Ohler, Carrie Bonomi, Rajaa El Meskini, Philip Martin, Cari Graff-Cherry and Lionel Feigenbaum are employed by Leidos Biomedical Research Inc. Leidos Biomedical Research Inc., is dedicated to a single contract to operate the Frederick National Laboratory for Cancer Research (FNLCR), a Federally Funded Research and Development Center. It is not involved in any employment, consultancy, patents, products in development or marketed products etc. related to this study.

* Email: gmerlino@helix.nih.gov

Introduction

The average drug developed by major pharmaceutical companies has been estimated to cost between 4 and 11 billion dollars [1], costing the average cancer patient approximately $100,000 per year. These staggering costs are driven in part by an inability early in the developmental pipeline to reliably identify drugs that will be efficacious, and the overall approval rate for an oncological compound is currently about 5% [2]. Much of this failure can be attributed to the inadequacy of preclinical models used in therapeutic evaluation. Historically, preclinical animal studies have utilized decades-old established human cell lines, transplanted as xenografts subcutaneously into immunocompromised mice [3]. Unfortunately, these models have had limited efficacy-predictive value for drug development, yet have been deemed critical for improving pharmaceutical productivity and patient care [4].

The proficiency of preclinical cancer studies is linked to the appropriateness of the animal model itself. Paramount is the presence of a fully functional immune system, which is involved in virtually every step of disease development, and critically determines treatment responses [5]. Tumor cells interact reciprocally and dynamically with immune and other microenvironmental cells throughout the course of metastatic progression and also following therapeutic intervention [6]. This interaction is appropriately modeled both in autochthonous genetically engineered mouse (GEM) cancer models and by orthotopic transplantation of GEM-derived allografts (GDAs) into fully immunocompetent host mice [7], but not effectively in current human cancer xenograft models. Finally, therapeutic and biomarker evaluation should ideally rely on preclinical cancer models recapitulating *naturally occurring* metastasis, the most deadly cancer phase.

Tractable preclinical models require the ability to accurately monitor disease progression and therapeutic response, facilitating the adoption of relevant clinical endpoints [8]. Disease monitoring is essential for metastases and otherwise undetectable tumors. Optical imaging of cells expressing light-generating proteins currently dominates monitoring technologies due to their ability to measure real-time events, cost-effectiveness and time-efficiency [9]. However, most traceable marker proteins, including the popular firefly luciferase (ffLuc) and jellyfish enhanced green fluorescent protein (eGFP), are xenobiotic to mammals. Their expression naturally induces various immune responses in immunocompetent animals, resulting in inconsistent activity [10,11], rejection of grafts [12] and suppression of metastatic activity [13], confounding the validity of preclinical conclusions. Thus, the effective use of xenobiotic reporters is restricted to either short-term studies, or fully immunocompromised animal models, limiting preclinical options [9,13].

To overcome these problems, we have developed a GEM model that is immune-tolerant to both ffLuc and eGFP to serve as a host for transplantation of labeled syngeneic tumors. Using the rat growth hormone (rGH) promoter, expression of a ffLuc-eGFP fusion protein was targeted to the anterior pituitary, a non-immune privileged site distant from commonly monitored organs in preclinical studies, thereby creating the "Glowing Head" (GH) mouse [14]. We demonstrate that in wildtype mice immune responses induced by xenobiotic reporters substantially affect the progression and therapeutic responses of imageable transplanted tumors. Importantly, the use of pre-tolerized GH mice minimizes or eliminates these aberrations, resulting in more reliable, tractable preclinical models.

Materials and Methods

Lentiviral Vectors

The lentiviral vector that expresses the firefly luciferase-enhanced green fluorescent protein fusion protein (FerH-ffLuc-eGFP) was described previously [10]. It was here modified to remove eGFP and insert an internal ribosome binding site (IRES) and histone H2B-tagged eGFP (H2B-eGFP) to generate FerH-ffLuc-IRES-H2B-eGFP, which targets the expression of ffLuc and eGFP to the cytoplasm and nucleus, respectively. Detailed information on the vector sequence will be provided upon request to Dr. Dominic Esposito (e-mail: espositod@mail.nih.gov), Leidos Biomedical Research, Frederick, MD, USA.

Animals

To reduce bioluminescence absorption and experimental variation, albino 6- to 8-week-old inbred female mice on a C57BL/6 (C57BL/6$^{c-brd/c-brd}$/Cr) or FVB/N background were used as hosts for transplantation studies. F1 mice from the breeding of C57BL/6 with 129 (B6;129) mice were used as isogenic hosts in the study of NRas^{Q61K}/p19^{ARF}-null melanoma,

which was derived from a mixed genetic background [15,16]. All animals used in this research project were cared for and used humanely according to the following policies: The U.S. Public Health Service Policy on Humane Care and Use of Animals (1996); the Guide for the Care and Use of Laboratory Animals (1996); and the U.S. Government Principles for Utilization and Care of Vertebrate Animals Used in Testing, Research, and Training (1985). All mouse experiments were performed in strict accordance with Animal Study Protocols approved by the Animal Care and Use Committee (ACUC), NCI, at the Frederick National Laboratory for Cancer Research, which is accredited by AAALACi and follows the Public Health Service Policy on the Care and Use of Laboratory Animals. The following protocols were approved by the ACUC for performing this study: ASP# 08–084, 11–044, and 11–058.

The mice in this study were euthanized by CO2 asphyxiation following NCI-approved ACUC guidelines: (1) Transfer the mice to a CO2 chamber right before euthanasia. (2) Turn on the CO2 at 2 liters per minute for a standard sized of chamber. (3) Within approximately two to three minutes, adult mice should be immobile and unresponsive; when this is evident, increase the flow rate to high or approximately 10 liters/min. (4) When breathing ceases for all animals seen through the cage, set the timer for 2 minutes. At the end of two minutes, the mice may be removed from the CO2-filled cage. Ensure death by making sure there are no movements of any kind for an additional 60 seconds outside the CO2-filled cage, using the timer.

Generation of the "Glowing Head" mouse

The rGH-hGH construct [17] (a gift of Dr. Rhonda Kineman, University of Illinois-Chicago, Chicago, IL) was modified by insertion of an ffLuc-eGFP fusion gene to generate the anterior pituitary gland-targeting vector, which was used to generate transgenic mice in both the C57BL/6 and FVB/N genetic backgrounds by blastocyst microinjection. Small colonies of homozygous transgenic mice were maintained for breeding purposes, and their heterozygous progeny used for all preclinical studies. All the transgenic and breeding work was performed through the Laboratory Animal Science Program, Frederick National Laboratory.

Murine tumors, cancer cell lines, and their labeling

The Lewis Lung Carcinoma (LLC) tissue was maintained only *in vivo* since its derivation from the original lung tumor of C57BL/6 mice [8]. The spontaneously metastasizing serial Hgf-tg/CDK4^{R24C} melanoma skin transplant was generated from a primary melanoma induced in Hgf-tg/CDK4^{R24C} C57BL/6 mice by epicutaneous application of the carcinogen DMBA [18]. HGF-tg/CDKN2A$^{-/-}$ melanoma was derived from tumors induced in HGF-tg/CDKN2A$^{-/-}$ FVB mice by UV irradiation [19]. These tumors were maintained only in syngeneic mice. For transplantation, the harvested tumor tissues were divided into 3 mm ×3 mm pieces and each one was inserted into a 5-mm cut on skin of a mouse. Mvt-1 murine breast cancer cells were derived from mammary tumors of the MMTV-c-Myc/MMTV-Vegf bi-transgenic mouse on an FVB/N inbred background [20]. They were established as a cell line and maintained through in vitro culture. For transplantation, 1.0×10^6 cells were prepared from culture and injected subcutaneously into each mouse. Mutant NRas^{Q61K}/p19^{ARF}-null melanoma cells were generated as described [15,16]. In the first passage, 1.0×106 cells from in vitro culture were inoculated into C57BL/6x129 F1 mice to form tumors. In the following passages, the fragments divided from harvested tumor were used for transplantation, as described above.

To label the *in vivo* maintained tumors, cell suspensions prepared from *in vivo*-expanded tumors were infected *ex vivo* with lentivirus by *ex vivo* spinoculation [10,21]. LLC tissue was infected with lentivirus encoding ffLuc-eGFP or ffLuc-IRES-H2B-eGFP and then subjected to *in vivo* cycling to obtain uniformly-labeled tumors, as described previously [8]. Cell lines were labeled with ffLuc-eGFP lentivirus *in vitro*, and the eGFP+ populations were isolated using the fluorescence-activated cell sorter (FACS).

Preclinical studies and pathological analysis

For preclinical studies, a cryogenically preserved labeled tumor was revived and expanded by subcutaneous transplantation into mice. These tumors were resected upon reaching 500 mm^3 and expanded through passage into the requisite number of mice for the actual studies described in the text. Tumor size was measured manually and calculated by V (mm^3) $= 0.5 \times L \times W^2$, where L is length and W is width in mm. For the preclinical modeling of primary tumors, mice were randomized into groups according to study design when their tumors reached 125 mm^3. The control group received vehicle solution, and the experimental group received treatments of chemotherapeutic agents. The dose and schedule in each experiment have been specified in the Results. When tumors grew to 2000 mm^3, mice had reached their endpoints and were euthanized for further study.

For preclinical models of spontaneous metastasis, primary tumors were surgically removed upon reaching 500 mm^3, and the mice were randomized into groups according to the study design. Metastasis and recurrence were monitored periodically by imaging using the Xenogen IVIS system [8] to measure BL flux (photon/sec/radial degree). The control group received vehicle solution, and the experimental group received treatments of chemotherapeutic agents. The dose and schedule in each experiment have been specified in the Results. When mice showed signs of morbidity, defined by the animal study protocol (e.g. short of breathiness, difficulty in moving), they reached their endpoint and were euthanized for further study.

The drugs used in this study were obtained from the Drug Synthesis & Chemistry Branch, DTP, NCI (Bethesda, MD). Paclitaxel was dissolved at 10x the desired concentration in 100% ethanol, diluted with an equal volume of Cremaphor EL and then diluted to the 1x concentration with saline before intravenous injection into mice. Gemcitabine was dissolved in water and injected intraperitoneally into mice. Crizotinib was resuspended in 0.5% methylcellulose in 0.9% saline, and given once daily by oral gavage (PO) over a 3-week period at 10 ml/Kg. Mice carrying subcutaneous tumors were randomized into 3 groups based on tumor measurement (200–500 mm^3), and treated with vehicle alone, crizotinib at 50 mg/kg, or Crizotinib at 100 mg/kg.

Harvested tissues were fixed in 10% formaldehyde and paraffin-embedded. Adjacent serial sections were stained with hematoxylin and eosin (H&E) for histological analysis, or used for GFP immunohistochemistry (ab6556, Abcam, Cambridge, MA, USA). Histopathology was performed by Dr. Miriam Anver (Pathology and Histotechnology Laboratory, Leidos Biomedical Research, Frederick, MD). For quantitative analysis, slides were scanned using the ScanScope XT system and images were analyzed by Spectrum Plus pathology analysis software (Aperio Technologies, Vista, CA).

Hormone and immunological marker analysis

Sera were prepared from the collected whole blood following conventional protocols and stored at −80°C. To analyze anti-GFP antibody in serum, ELISA plates (Nunc MaxiSorp, cat# 439454, Thermo Scientific, Waltham, MA, USA) were coated with 31.25 ng of recombinant GFP (MB-0752, Vector Laboratory, Burlingame, CA, USA) in each well overnight at 4°C. The next day, sera and control monoclonal anti-GFP antibody (11814460001, Roche Applied Science, Indianapolis, IN, USA) were subjected to serial dilution with blocking solution (3% milk in phosphate-buffered saline [PBS]) to reach the range 1:25–1:2000 for the former and 6.25–200 ng/ml for the latter. 50 μl of diluted sera or control antibody were added to the coated wells, followed by incubation for an hour at room temperature. After washing with PBS containing 0.05% Tween 20 (PBST). Horse reddish peroxidase (HRP)-conjugated goat anti-mouse antibody (115-035-062, Jackson ImmunoResearch Laboratories) at 1:1000 dilution in blocking solution was then added into each well, followed by the addition of peroxidase substrate (TMB 2-Component Microwell Peroxidase Substrate Kit, 50-76-00, KPL, Gaithersburg, MD, USA) for color development according to the manufacturer's instruction. The A450 absorption of the plates was measured using a microplate reader (VMax Kinetic ELISA Absorbance Microplate Reader, 97059-546, VWR Corp., Radnor, PA, USA). Mouse growth hormone levels in sera were analyzed using the Growth Hormone (GH) ELISA kit (M0934, Biotang Inc., CA, USA) according to the manufacturer's instruction as following. Sera were diluted 2-fold with RPMI1640 medium, and standard solutions were prepared for the concentration range 0.3125–100 ng/ml. The standards and samples were added into the provided ELISA plate, which was incubated at 37°C for 40 min and washed with washing buffer. Each well was then added with 50 μl of water and 50 μl of biotinylated anti-GH antibody, and incubated at 37°C for 20 min. After washing, 100 μl of streptavidin-conjugated HRP was added into each well and incubated at 37°C for 10 min. After another washing, 100 μl of HRP substrate solution was added to each well, incubated at 37°C for 15 min, followed by adding 100 μl of stop solution. The A450 absorption of the plates was measured using the VMax microplate reader.

To analyze cell surface markers, single-cell suspensions were prepared from harvested mouse spleens and incubated with 5 μl/ml of Fcγ Receptor antibody (14-0161-85, eBiosciences, San Diego, CA, USA) for blocking for 20 min. Following a wash with staining solution (PBS containing 1% bovine serum albumin [BSA]), they were incubated with 0.3 μl/ml of rat anti-mouse CD4 (550728, BD-Pharmingen, San Jose, CA, USA) or CD8α (550281, BD-Pharmingen antibody, or isotype control antibody (559073, BD-Pharmingen) at 4°C for 1 hr, followed by washing with staining solution for three times. The cells were then incubated with 4 μl/ml of Alexa 488-conjugated goat anti-rat secondary antibody (A11006, Invitrogen, Grand Island, NY, USA) at 4°C for 20 min. After washing with staining solution for three times, the cells were subjected to FACS analysis (FACSCalibur, BD Biosciences, San Jose, CA, USA) or Cell Analyzer equipped with a filter optics module for FITC detection to quantitate the expression of cell markers (Cellometer Vision, Nexcelom Bioscience, Lawrence, MA, USA). The data generated from FACS and Cellometer Vision were analyzed and quantitated with software FlowJo (TreeStar, Inc. Ashland, OR, USA) and FCS Express (De Novo Software, Los Angeles, CA, USA), respectively.

Statistical analysis

Differences in quantity distribution (e.g. tumor size, bioluminescence intensity, CD8/CD4 ratio) between study groups were analyzed using the parametric unpaired t test. For preclinical studies, the end point was overall survival, defined as the time until mouse morbidity according to the animal study protocol. Mice alive at the end of the study were censored at that date. The

Kaplan-Meier method and Mantel-Cox logrank-test were performed to compare survival rates of the mouse groups. Statistical significance was established at the P-value <0.05. The median survival time was calculated as the smallest survival time for which the survivor function reached 50%. The computations were done with GraphPad Prism 6 (La Jolla, CA).

Results

Reporter activity of ffLuc-eGFP-labeled murine tumors is inconsistent in immunocompetent syngeneic mice

The subcutaneously transplanted Lewis Lung Carcinoma (LLC) is a well-characterized metastatic model that has recently been exploited in several high profile preclinical studies [22–24]. We recently retrieved archived LLC tissue never adapted to cell culture, and showed that following transplantation and resection metastasis occurred with very short latency in >90% of syngeneic WT C57BL/6 host mice [8]. Here we labeled LLC with an ffLuc-eGFP-encoded lentivirus ex vivo [10]. Since viral transduction results in heterogeneous cell population [25], we subject this labeled tumor to in vivo cycling to render them uniformly labeled [8,26]. Briefly, mice bearing transplanted tumors are monitored for metastasis, and metastatic nodules will be harvested for subcutaneous transplantation to initiate next cycle. Since each nodule was derived from a single cell, the tumor derived from it is presumably clonal. Therefore, homogeneity will be enhanced through each cycle. As shown in Fig. 1A, following subcutaneously transplantation and resection of the labeled LLC in five mice, arising metastases were readily detected by in vivo bioluminescence (BL) imaging. In this passage, although tumors grew in all hosts, metastases were detected in only one (#160 in Fig. 1A, lower panel). We harvested lungs from that mouse and examined it with ex vivo imaging (Fig. 1B, upper panel). The unevenly distributed BL intensity reflected the heterogeneity of transduced cells in primary tumor (Fig. 1B, upper panel). We collected from host mice three individual well-labeled lung metastases, presumed to be clonal, dividing them into five fragments for transplantation into five C57BL/6 mice. Labeled pulmonary nodules from that mouse were collected and transplanted into another five C57BL/6 mice; however, these tumors then grew very slowly and/or exhibited no detectable reporter activity (Fig. 1B). These results demonstrate that reporter activity in labeled cells could not be consistently maintained over passages in syngeneic immunocompetent mice, even after clonal selection.

To determine if reporter consistency was dependent on tumor type, we extended our analysis to mouse melanoma. An NRas^{Q61K}-transformed, p19^{ARF}-deficient melanocytic cell line [15,16] was labeled using the ffLuc-eGFP lentivirus and transplanted subcutaneously into syngeneic immunocompetent mice. Following resection one high-BL pulmonary nodule was selected for subcutaneous transplantation into two mice (Fig. S1A, left panels). Both tumors exhibited a significant reduction in normalized BL activity during subcutaneous growth (Fig. S1A, right panels). We corroborated these results in two other models. Melanoma cells harvested directly from an HGF-transgenic/CDKN2A-knockout FVB/N mouse were transduced with the ffLuc-eGFP gene ex vivo, and transplanted subcutaneously into syngeneic FVB/N mice. While all tumors grew, BL intensity was either reduced or increased more slowly (Fig. S1B), and BL intensity/size ratio, serving as the labeling retention indicator, was reduced in three of five tumors. In another model, ffLuc-eGFP-expressing mouse Mvt-1 breast cancer cells transplanted orthotopically into mammary fat pads of syngeneic FVB/N mice also demonstrated poor retention of BL signaling (see below). We

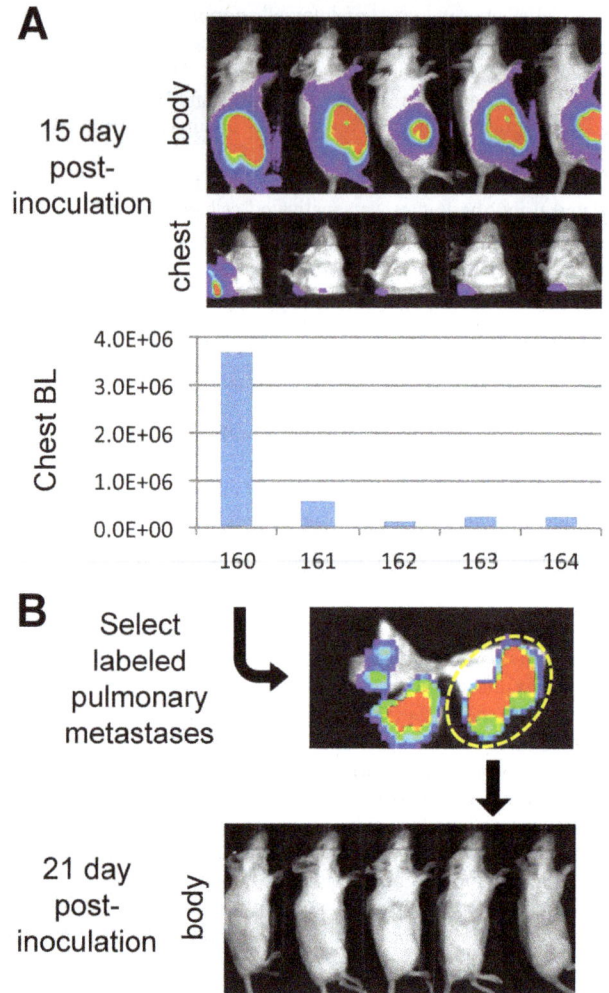

Figure 1. Inconsistency of ffLuc-eGFP reporter activity in labeled tumors during passages in syngeneic immunocompetent mice. **A**, Murine Lewis Lung Carcinoma (LLC) cells were infected with ffLuc-eGFP-expressing lentivirus ex vivo, and subcutaneously transplanted into five syngeneic albino C57BL/6 (c-Brd) mice (#160-164). Reporter activity was monitored by BL imaging of subcutaneous tumor growth (body) and pulmonary metastasis (chest). At day 15 after inoculation, a metastatic BL signal was found in one of the mice (#160 in the lower panel). **B**, The lung was harvested from #160, and a single glowing metastatic nodule selected using ex vivo imaging (upper panel) was transplanted into five c-Brd mice in the second passage. Imaging results showed that the reporter activity could not be consistently maintained in the resulting palpable tumors (lower panel).

conclude that ffLuc-eGFP expression in allografts in immunocompetent wildtype (WT) mice is inconsistently maintained between mice and/or passages, irrespective of tumor type, genetic background or transplantation site.

Generation of a GEM model immunologically tolerant to GFP and luciferase reporters

Our results suggested that immunogenicity of xenobiotic reporter gene products is largely responsible for their inconsistency in the context of a fully functional immune system. To circumvent this issue, we generated C57BL/6- and FVB/N-based GEM models recognizing ffLuc and eGFP proteins as self. For its high specificity, rGH gene sequences [17] (Fig. 2A) were employed to

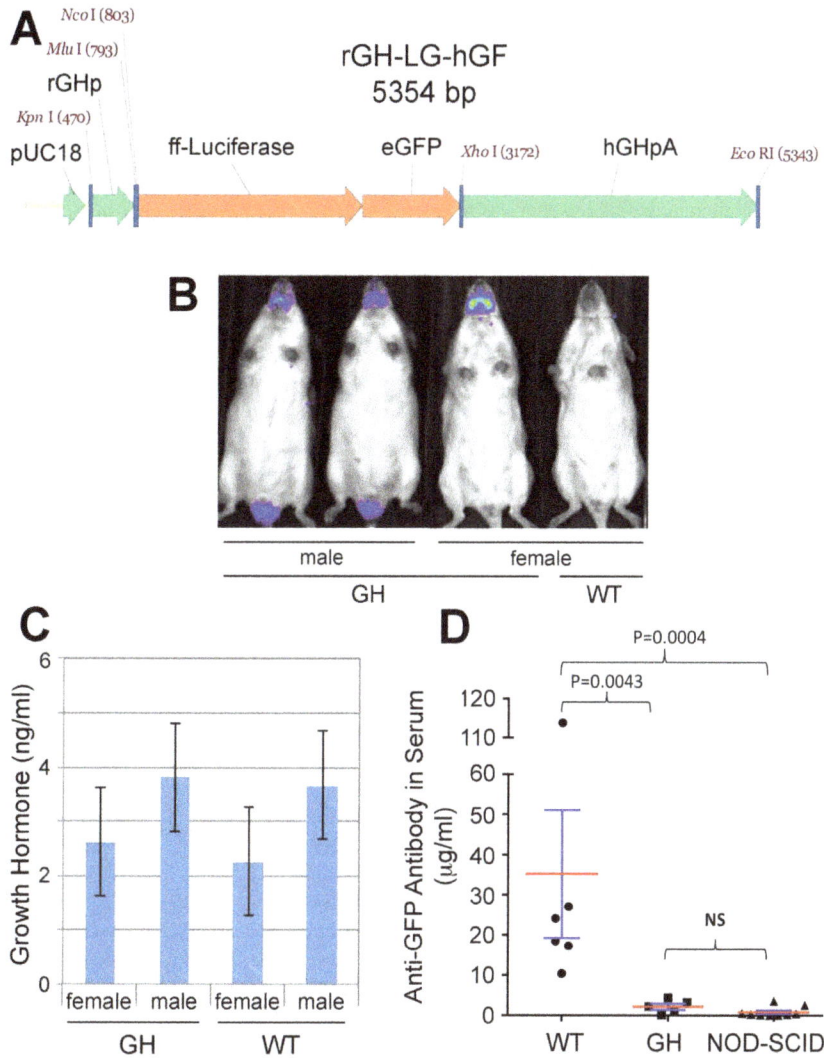

Figure 2. Generation of the rGH-ffLuc-eGFP ("Glowing Head") genetically engineered mouse. A, Structure of the expression vector for generation of Glowing Head (GH) transgenic mice. Expression of a firefly luciferase-eGFP fusion gene (ffLuc-eGFP) was targeted to the mouse anterior pituitary gland by using the rat growth hormone promoter (rGH) and human growth hormone gene sequences, which include a polyadenylylation site (hGHpA)[20]. **B**, Optical expression pattern of transgene in GH mice as visualized by BL imaging. Reporter activity was detected in the anterior pituitary gland of both genders and the testes of male mice. **C**, Serum levels of growth hormone from age-matched GH mice and wildtype (WT) c-Brd mice was assessed by ELISA (mean ± SE). Blood was withdrawn at the same time of day. No significant differences in circulating growth hormone levels between the GH and WT mice were found. **D**, ffLuc-eGFP-labeled LLC tumors were subcutaneously transplanted into WT, GH, and NOD-SCID mice. Blood was withdrawn to prepare sera when tumors reached 500 mm³, and the serum levels of anti-GFP antibody were analyzed by ELISA. The levels of anti-GFP antibody in WT mice are significantly higher than those in GH and NOD-SCID mice (p<0.005), but no difference was found between those in GH and NOD-SCID mice (p = 0.19). The sera from healthy mice without tumor transplantation served as controls to define zero point.

target expression of an ffLuc-eGFP fusion gene to the anterior pituitary gland of the mouse, thereby avoiding interfering signaling from the most common metastatic sites.

The anterior pituitary gland is not an immune-privileged site and is thus part of systemic circulation [27]. The transgene-encoded ffLuc and eGFP proteins expressed in the anterior pituitary gland during embryonic development therefore participate in the selection of T and B cells and are recognized as self-antigens, resulting in their tolerization. To reduce light adsorption by pigment the ffLuc-eGFP transgene was bred into the albino C57BL/6F (c-Brd) background. Founder lines were chosen from each strain that demonstrated Mendelian transgene inheritance and normal fecundity. In our previous study, we identified the

detection limit of BL signal from in vivo mouse imaging was 1.5×10^5 photon/sec/rad [8]. To avoid possible confounding effects associated with high transgene expression, those founder lines exhibiting low but consistent BL signal above background reading (about 2–6×10^5 photon/sec/rad) were selected (Fig. S2A). Consistent with targeting reported for the rGH promoter [17], BL signal was evident in the head and testes of transgenic lines (Fig. 2B); modest signal could also be detected in the thyroid glands, but only by using *ex vivo* imaging (not shown). The BL levels in the body of GH mice are close to those in WT mice, indicating the high specificity of the transgene (Fig. S2B). Based on the site of reporter activity and rGH promoter used for targeting these GEMs were dubbed "Glowing Head" (GH) mice.

The possible impact of transgene expression on pituitary function was evaluated by comparing circulating growth hormone levels in GH and WT C57BL/6 mice. We found that serum growth hormone levels were not significantly different between transgenic and WT (Fig. 2C), irrespective of gender, indicating that expression of the ffLuc-eGFP transgene does not overtly affect anterior pituitary function in GH mice.

To assess the immunological consequences of reporter expression, cells from ffLuc-eGFP-labeled LLC tumors were transplanted subcutaneously into GH and WT C57BL/6 mice, as well as MHC-unmatched, immunocompromised non-obese diabetic/severe combined immunodeficiency (NOD/SCID) mice (BALB/c background). When tumors reached 500 mm^3 blood was withdrawn and sera tested for the presence of anti-GFP antibody. While tumor-bearing WT mice possessed significant levels of circulating anti-GFP antibody (Fig. 2D and Fig. S2C), no significant difference was found between tumor-bearing GH and NOD-SCID mice, which is known incompetent to produce antibody (Fig. S2C). These data show that while immunogenic in WT mice, ffLuc-eGFP is tolerated and recognized as self in GH mice.

Growth and metastasis of tumor cells expressing imageable xenobiotic reporters are altered in WT and NOD/SCID mice compared to GH mice

To test the function of GH mice, we implanted ffLuc-EGFP-labeled tumors subcutaneously into syngeneic WT and GH mice. Although tumor size increased similarly in both types of host mice, BL increases in tumors were significantly delayed in WT mice as compared to GH mice (Fig. S3A). This result suggested that using GH mice as allograft recipients could help correct the inconsistencies observed in BL signals from labeled tumors transplanted into immunocompetent mice. To validate this point, we tested GH mouse in a larger scale study involving both primary tumor and metastasis. Metastatic Mvt-1 breast cancer cells [20,28] were transduced with ffLuc-eGFP lentivirus and transplanted orthotopically into mammary fat pads of GH or WT syngeneic FVB/N recipient mice. Labeled Mvt-1 cells exhibited a significant enhancement in BL signaling over time when transplanted into GH mice vs. WT, which failed to retain signaling (Fig. 3A and higher panels of Fig. S4A). Since imageable reporters are essential for monitoring metastasis, responsible for the vast majority of cancer patient deaths, primary Mvt-1 tumors were resected and host mice followed over time. BL imaging showed that metastases were present after a few days and grew efficiently in GH mice (Fig. 3B and lower right panels of Fig. S4A). In contrast, metastases were first detected in a small percentage of WT mice at day 20, while most mice remained BL-free for over 2 months (Fig. 3C and lower left panel of Fig. S4A). Notably, at the experimental endpoint ex vivo imaging revealed that metastases were found at multiple sites in GH mice, but only in the lungs of WT mice (Fig. S4B). The survival of WT mice was also significantly prolonged compared to GH mice (Fig. 3D; p = 0.0025). These results indicate that immunity against xenobiotic reporters can suppress the metastatic potential of transplanted labeled cancer cells, and highlight the advantages provided by the GH mouse for monitoring cancer progression and cell tracking.

We corroborated and expanded our assessment of the GH mouse using ffLuc-eGFP-expressing LLC cells. Well-labeled LLC cells were transplanted subcutaneously into GH, WT and also NOD/SCID mice, which have residual innate immune activity, and arising tumors resected at the same size. In the first imaging after resection (day 3 in Fig. 3E to 3G and Fig. S5), metastases arose with higher BL levels in GH mice relative to those in WT

and NOD/SCID mice. Subsequent monitoring revealed that metastases progressed efficiently and caused the death of all GH mice from day 9 to 15. As compared to GH mice, the overall disease progression was delayed in NOD/SCID and even more in WT mice. Accordingly, all the NOD/SCID mice died from day 13 to 18, while two of five WT mice were still alive at day 18 (Fig. S5). Importantly, the median survival time of GH mice was significantly shorter than that of either WT or NOD/SCID mice (Fig. 3H; P = 0.0037). These results demonstrate that immune responses against xenobiotic reporters can restrict the growth and metastatic potential of labeled tumors in immunocompetent and even partly immunocompromised mice, a problem that could be overcome through the use of GH host mice.

Immunogenicity associated with imageable reporter expression influences the therapeutic outcome of preclinical mouse studies

The advantages illustrated above suggest that GH mice would constitute a superior preclinical model for drug assessment. We have shown that chemotherapeutic paclitaxel has no significant effect on growth of subcutaneous LLC tumors in syngeneic C57BL/6 hosts, irrespective of doses ranging between 6.7–22 mg/kg, QDx5 (Fig. S6). In this study syngeneic GH and WT mice carrying subcutaneous ffLuc-eGFP-labeled LLC tumors were randomized to receive vehicle or paclitaxel at 7.5 mg/kg, QDx5, considered to be a dose mimicking human treatment [8,29]. As with unlabeled LLC growing in WT mice, paclitaxel had no effect on tumors growing in GH mice (Fig. 4A); in contrast, growth of the ffLuc-eGFP-labeled tumor was significantly delayed in treated WT mice (Fig. 4B). Interestingly, the spleens of paclitaxel-treated WT mice were significantly larger relative to the other three groups (Fig. 4C), and exhibited enlarged, disrupted lymphatic follicles (Fig. S7). Accordingly, the CD8/CD4 ratio of splenocytes increased in paclitaxel-treated WT mice (Fig. 4D), correlating with spleen size in all groups (Fig. 4E). There was no difference in the growth or response to paclitaxel of unlabeled LLC cells growing in WT vs. GH mice (not shown). These data suggest that paclitaxel treatment could produce a false-positive preclinical outcome by inducing a cytotoxic T cell response against a xenobiotic tumor antigen, but only in WT mice that had not been pre-tolerized to that antigen. Taken more broadly, our results show that tumor antigens can significantly influence preclinical tumor response to chemotherapy.

To assess the effects of antigenic reporters on response to molecularly-targeted therapeutic agents, we employed the melanoma GDA model HCmel12 (derived from an HGF/CDK4^{R24C}-transgenic mouse [18]), labeled ex vivo with ffLuc-eGFP, and transplanted subcutaneously into syngeneic GH or WT c-Brd mice. Upon reaching 125 mm^3, mice were randomized to receive either vehicle or crizotinib, a drug targeting the HGF receptor (MET). Crizotinib effected insignificant or modest changes on tumor growth in GH and WT recipients, respectively (Fig. 5A). Pathological analysis revealed that in GH, but not WT, host mice crizotinib significantly reduced inflammation and tumor invasiveness at the primary site (Fig. 5B and Fig. S8). Moreover, crizotinib significantly reduced the number of pulmonary metastases in a dose-dependent manner only in GH mice (Fig. 5C). In this case, our data indicate that immunity against xenobiotic reporters can produce a false-negative response in WT mice, which can be avoided by using GH mice as hosts.

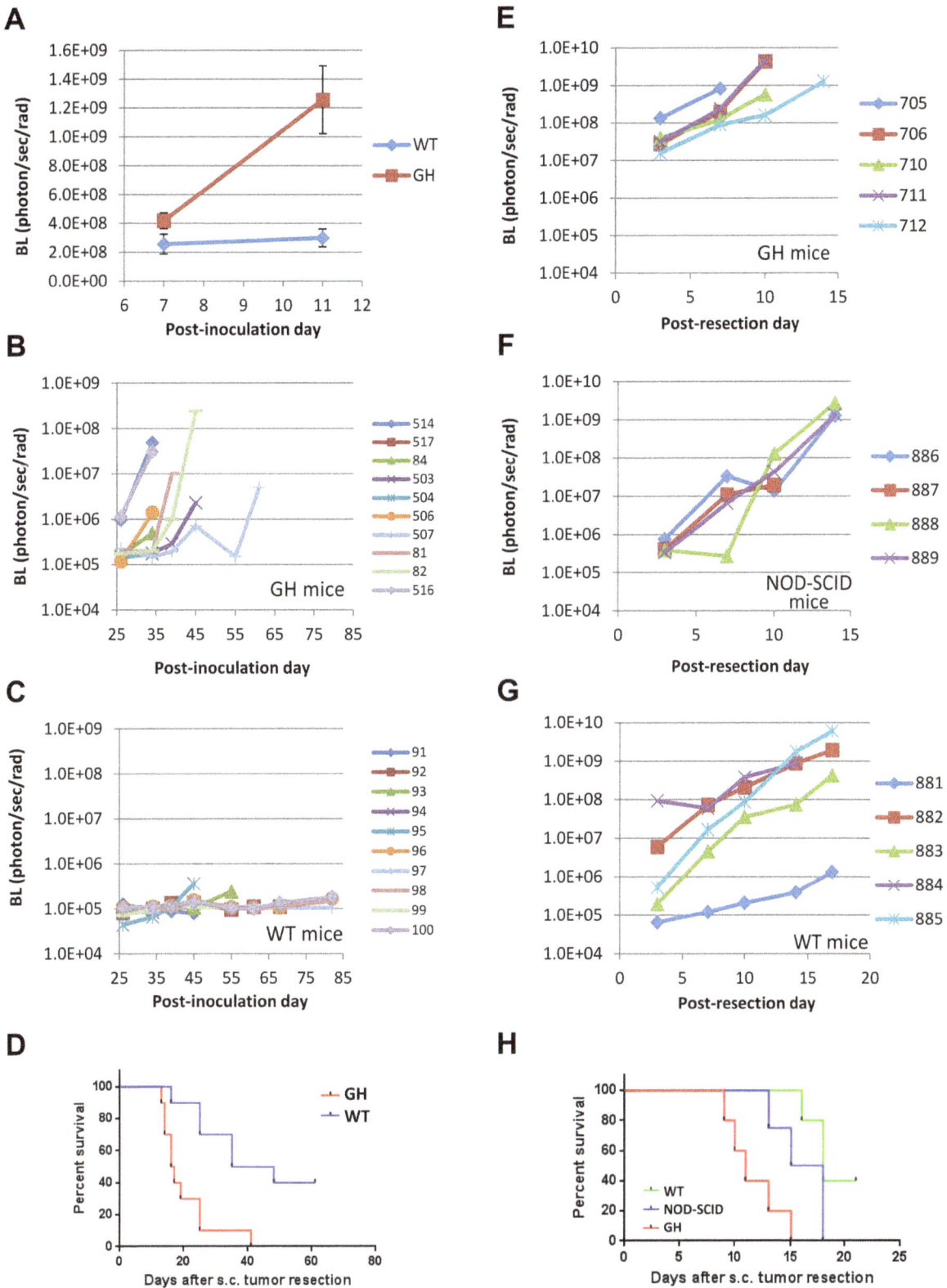

Figure 3. Reporter activity and metastasis of ffLuc-eGFP-labeled cancer cells are consistent in GH mice but suppressed in immunocompetent wildtype mice. A–D, Functional comparison of GH and WT mice as transplantation hosts using a breast cancer model. The GFP$^+$ population from ffLuc-eGFP-transduced Mvt1 mouse breast cancer cells was isolated and expanded in culture. 1×10^5 cells were injected into the mammary fat pads (m.f.p.) of WT and GH syngeneic FVB/N mice, followed by BL imaging to monitor tumor growth. Though tumors grew in the fat pads of both groups, the BL intensity (mean $\pm$ SE) of those in WT mice was highly suppressed relative to GH mice (**A**). *, $P = 0.083$; **, $P < 0.001$. (**B–C**) Upon reaching 500 mm^3 m.f.p. tumors were resected, and BL imaging was used to monitor metastatic progression, which is visualized by body BL signal in each mouse. Metastatic disease progressed consistently in GH mice (**B**), while being suppressed in WT mice (**C**); the sign and number at side

refer to individual mice in each figure. Kaplan-Meier survival analysis showed that GH mice exhibited significantly shorter survival times than WT mice ($P = 0.0025$). Median survival times in GH and WT groups were 16.5 and 41.5 days, respectively (**D**). **E–H**, Behavioral inconsistency of labeled tumors in WT and immunocompromised mice as compared to GH mice. ffLuc-eGFP-labeled LLC tumors were transplanted subcutaneously into syngeneic GH mice, strain-unmatched immunocompromised NOD/SCID (BALB/c) mice, and syngeneic c-Brd (WT) mice. Upon reaching 500 mm³ subcutaneous tumors were resected, and mice were subjected to periodic BL imaging to monitor metastasis. The growth curves representing metastatic growth in GH (**E**), NOD/SCID (**F**), and c-Brd WT mice (**G**) are shown; the sign and number at side refer to individual mice in each figure. Compared to those in GH mice, the metastatic growth in the other two groups exhibited heterogeneous and delayed patterns. In accordance with their more efficient metastatic progression, Kaplan-Meyer survival analysis showed that GH mice exhibited significantly shorter survival time than the other two strains of mice ($P = 0.0037$). Median survival times in WT, NOD/SCID, and GH groups were 18 days, 16.5 days and 11 days, respectively (**H**).

GH mice enable the ability to reliably track metastatic disease progression and therapeutic response in fully immunocompetent preclinical models

Previously, we demonstrated the feasibility of tracking cancer recurrence and progression with BL imaging in metastatic models [8]. Our initial studies using ffLuc-eGFP LLC tumors transplanted into GH mice showed that in vivo BL increases within the range of 1.5×10^5 to 5×10^7 photon/sec/rad reliably represent metastatic

growth following resection of subcutaneous tumors (Fig. S9A). Encouraged by the demonstrated ability of GH mice to detect therapeutic differences in metastatic disease, we tested a first-line chemotherapeutic drug in a post-resection adjuvant setting. Tumors from ffLuc-eGFP-labeled LLC were transplanted subcutaneously into syngeneic GH mice and resected at 500 mm³, after which mice were randomized to receive vehicle or gemcitabine. BL imaging showed that metastasis progressed efficiently in mice

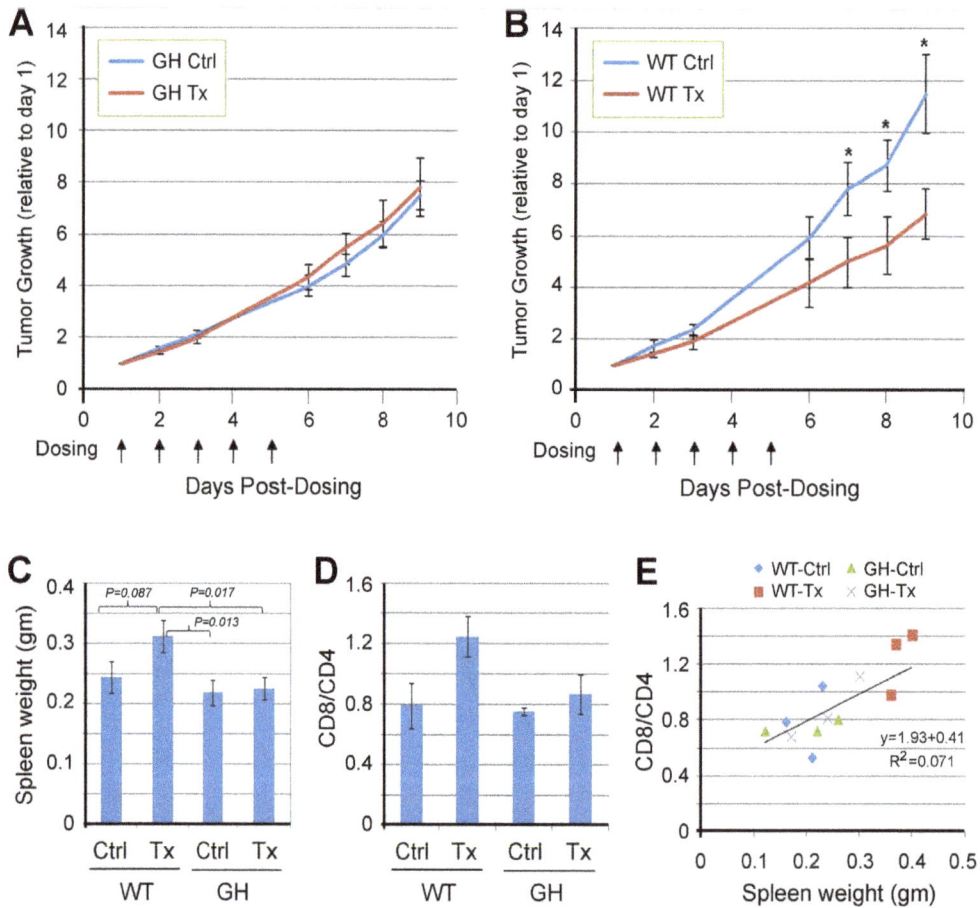

Figure 4. Immunogenicity of ffLuc-eGFP alters the response of tumors to chemotherapeutic agents in wildtype mice compared to GH mice. Labeled LLC tumors were inoculated subcutaneously into WT and GH c-Brd mice. When the average tumor size reached 125 mm³, each strain of mice was randomized into two groups to receive either control vehicle (Cremophor EL + saline) or paclitaxel. Tumor size was measured periodically. **A and B**, Tumor growth (fold-increase relative to day 1) in WT and GH c-Brd mice (mean ± SE). Paclitaxel treatment was inefficacious in GH mice (**A**), but delayed tumor growth in WT mice (*, $P<0.05$ in a two-tailed T-test) (**B**). Ctrl, control vehicle; Tx, paclitaxel treatment. **C**, Spleen size in each group (mean ± SE). Spleens in paclitaxel-treated WT c-Brd mice were marginally bigger than those in vehicle-treated c-Brd mice but significantly bigger than those in both groups of GH mice. No significant difference was found between the two GH mouse groups. **D and E**, Enlarged spleens in paclitaxel-treated WT mice correspond to higher CD8/CD4 ratios. Splenocytes were prepared from spleens harvested from mice from each treatment group. These were stained with anti-mouse CD4 or CD8 antibodies, and analyzed by flow cytometry and Cellometer to obtain the ratio of the CD8+ to CD4+ subpopulation (CD8/CD4) in WT and GH c-Brd host mice (mean ± SE) (**D**). **E**, Regressional analysis demonstrated a significant correlation between CD8/CD4 ratio and spleen size ($P<0.01$).

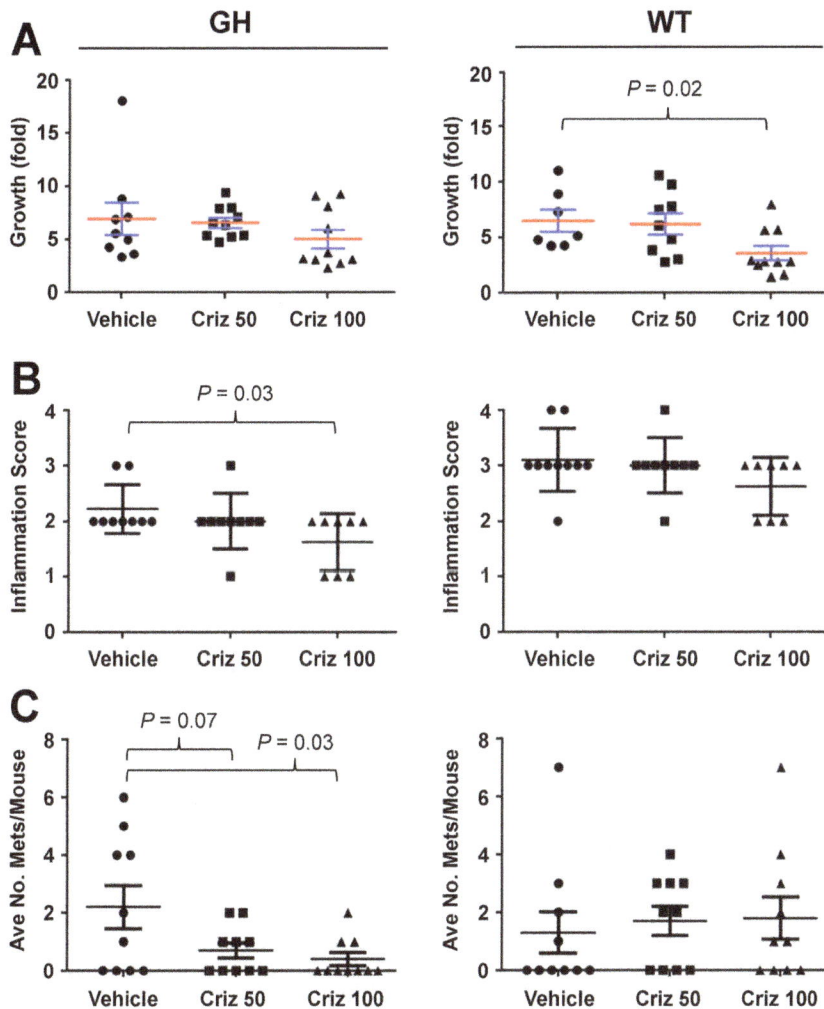

Figure 5. Immunogenicity of ffLuc-eGFP alters the response of tumors, including metastases, to targeted therapy in wildtype mice compared to GH mice. Labeled melanoma tissues from the HGF/CDK4^{R24C}-transgenic mouse [18] were subcutaneously inoculated into WT and GH c-Brd mice. When the average tumor size reached 125 mm^3, mice from each strain were randomized into two groups to receive either control vehicle (saline) or the MET inhibitor crizotinib (Criz). Tumor size was measured periodically. **A**, Fold-tumor growth in WT and GH c-Brd mice (mean ± SE). 100 mg/kg Criz treatment delayed tumor growth in WT mice (right panel, $P<0.02$ in two-tailed T-test), but no efficacy was found in GH mice (left panel). **B**, When primary tumors reached 2000 mm^3, the mice were euthanized to harvest tumors and lungs. Tumors were subjected to pathological analysis of inflammatory infiltrates according to the scoring system: minimal = 1, mild = 2, moderate = 3, severe = 4. Criz at 100 mg/kg significantly reduced inflammatory infiltration of the primary tumors in GH mice (left panel), but not in WT mice (right panel). **C**, The fixed lungs were subjected to the quantitation of metastatic foci. Criz reduced the number of pulmonary metastases in GH mice in a dose-dependent manner (left panel), but had no effect in WT mice (right panel).

from the control treatment group (Fig. 6A), but was greatly suppressed by gemcitabine (Fig. 6B). Accordingly, gemcitabine significantly prolonged mouse disease-free survival ($P<0.0001$, time median undecided vs. 11 days in control; Fig. 6C). BL signals from *in vivo* imaging well corresponded to the metastatic nodules identified in harvested lungs by visual observation and *ex vivo* imaging (Fig. 6D). At the endpoint, the metastatic burden detected by in vivo BL imaging was also validated by ex vivo imaging of the harvested lungs (Fig. S10A). To determine if fluorescence could be exploited to isolate tumor cells for molecular analyses, whole lung single cell suspensions from untreated GH mice were subjected to FACS. The eGFP$^+$ LLC cells were readily separated from all stromal cells by FACS (Fig. 6E), and formed well-labeled tumors upon re-transplantation (Fig. S10B).

Discussion

Based on recent clinical breakthroughs in immunotherapy [30], and the ever-expanding evidence that the immune system plays numerous key roles in tumorigenesis, the need for immunocompetent preclinical mouse models has become acute. Immunocompetent GDA transplantation models offer significant advantages, allowing: incorporation of human-relevant genomic alterations and environmental insults into GEM-derived allografts; appropriate microenvironmental interactions between the transplanted tumor and host; preclinical and molecular analyses of metastatic lesions and perfectly matched sets of pre- and post-treatment samples; and industry-friendly experimental turnaround time. Immunocompromised patient-derived xenograft (PDX) models have shown promise as preclinical tools for testing chemotherapy

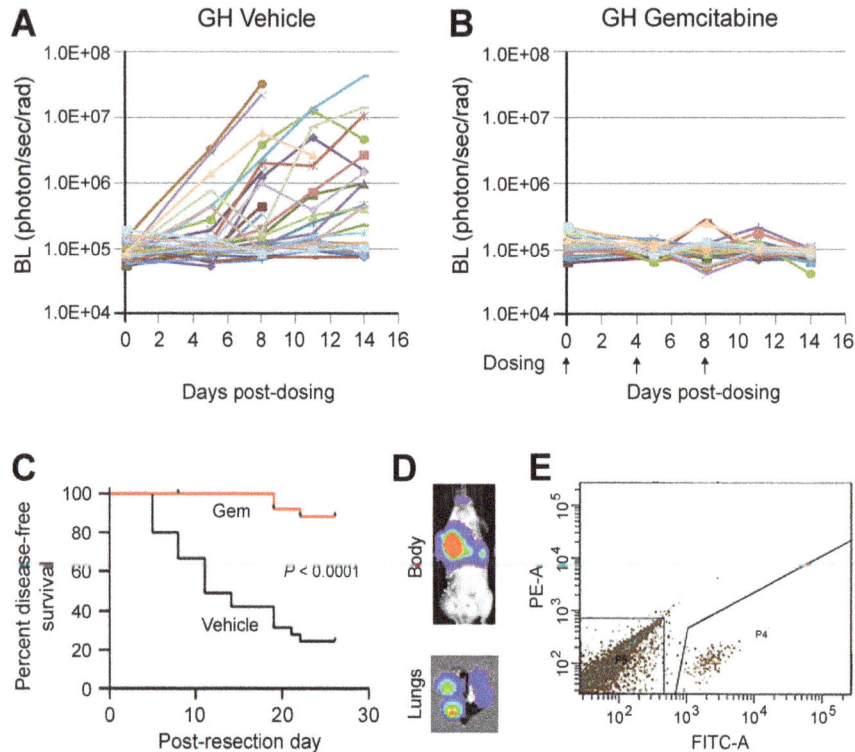

Figure 6. The GH mouse allows for consistent tracking of the progression of labeled metastases, their therapeutic responses and isolation in a preclinical adjuvant study. ffLuc-eGFP-labeled LLC tumors were transplanted subcutaneously into GH mice. Upon reaching 500 mm³, the primary tumors were resected. **A and B**, GH mice were randomized into control and treated groups to receive vehicle and gemcitabine at 25 mg/kg, respectively. Metastatic progression in mice was periodically monitored by BL imaging. Metastatic growth was efficient in untreated GH mice (**A**) but suppressed by gemcitabine (**B**). **C**, Kaplan-Meyer analysis showed that survival was significantly shorter in control compared to treated GH mice. **D and E**, GFP+ cancer cells can be readily isolated from whole lungs of GH mice. The lungs were harvested from control GH mice, made into a single-cell suspension, and subjected to sorting by FACS to isolate GFP$^+$ cells. The representative result from mouse #806 is shown. The *in vivo* image of mice and *ex vivo* image of lung (**D**) showed BL signal from pulmonary metastases and individual lung nodules, respectively. The GFP$^+$ cancer cells were successfully isolated from whole lung by FACS sorting (P4 subpopulation in **E**).

[31], but the approach to modify host mice to bear a "humanized" immune system is prohibitively expensive and mostly untested.

The full value of any preclinical model can only be realized if cancerous lesions can be accurately monitored longitudinally. On balance optical reporters offer superior qualities and are widely used; unfortunately, their xenobiotic nature confounds their use in the context of a fully competent murine immune system. In fact, any xenobiotic gene introduced into immunocompetent animals poses a potential problem [32,33], including other reporters [34], recombinases [35], transactivating factors [36] and viral oncogenes [37]. In this report we demonstrate that xenobiotic reporters induce problematic immune responses in immunocompetent mice, causing inconsistent activity and altered tumor behavior. We also describe a new GEM model immunologically tolerant to ffLuc and eGFP, which can serve as a transplantation host for any so-labeled syngeneic tumors. Immune responses induced by optical markers substantially affected growth, progression, and therapeutic responses of tumors transplanted into WT hosts, problems that were minimized or eliminated by using pre-tolerized GH mice. This difference was most notable with metastatic disease. GH mice enable consistent ffLuc-eGFP reporter activity, accurate monitoring throughout longitudinal studies, and tumor cell isolation for molecular analyses, all in the context of a normal immune system. Moreover, GEMs pre-tolerized to virtually any imageable marker can now be developed and exploited.

Most notably, immunity against reporter genes expressed in labeled tumors could significantly alter the outcome of preclinical therapeutic studies. Our first study showed that, relative to GH mice, paclitaxel delayed the growth of ffLuc-eGFP-expressing LLC tumors in WT hosts, where it induced a cytotoxic T cell response. Consistent with our observations, the immunogenicity of cell death induced by cytotoxic agents has been reported to be a critical determinant of chemotherapeutic efficacy [5]. However, we were surprised to observe that labeled tumors transplanted into WT mice could also be less responsive to drugs relative to those transplanted into GH hosts, indicating that the precise consequence of xenobiotic reporter expression is context-dependent (e.g. tumor type, tumor location, drug). The impact of such preclinical uncertainty on cancer patients is the possible inclusion of an ineffective drug *or* the exclusion of an efficacious drug in clinical trials. Therefore, results obtained from preclinical studies using labeled tumors transplanted into immunocompetent WT mice must be interpreted with great caution.

Interestingly, we found that reporter activity and growth of labeled transplanted tumors were altered not only in syngeneic WT, but also in partially immunocompromised NOD/SCID mice. Similarly, while progressing efficiently in GH mice, spontaneous metastasis was delayed or suppressed in NOD/SCID as well as WT mice. NOD/SCID mice are defective in adaptive immunity, but retain some innate immune function, including NK cell activity [38]. These findings suggest that xenobiotic reporters activate innate immunity, and indicate that immunocompromised mice with residual immunity cannot fully overcome the labeling inconsistency observed in WT mice.

The results above have demonstrated the complicated interaction between tumor antigens and immune system. The antibody reaction in WT vs. GH mice observed in Fig. 2D indicated that ffLuc-eGFP is an antigen capable of activating B cells. The results that tumor progression was delayed in NOD-SCID mice as compared to GH mice suggested that NK cells are involved, since the former still exhibits residual NK cell activity [38]. We further demonstrated that cytotoxic T cell response induced by ffLuc-eGFP induced was significantly enhanced by paclitaxel treatment (Fig. 6). Importantly, chemotherapy and targeted drug may modify the response against tumor antigen, as proposed by many studies [5]. The results above have suggested that immune system may respond to xenobiotic antigens in multiple, inter-dependent mechanisms, including adaptive (B and T cells) and innate (NK cells) immunity. In fact, a routine practice for the analysis of immune response is to compare antigenic responses between a specific mouse strain and a pre-tolerized control strain. In this regard, GH mice serve as "control" strain to study the immune response. Therefore, GH mice can also be a useful tool for immunological studies. Our complex immune system is involved to varying degrees in virtually all aspects of health and disease. Inclusion of an immune system in any preclinical model is clearly highly desirable, and of course essential when assessing highly promising immunotherapies. Preclinical cancer models become more valuable and versatile when tumor progression and drug response can be accurately and longitudinally monitored, an ability that represents an imposing challenge with the most relevant models where tumors are evaluated at orthotopic and/or metastatic sites. The Glowing Head mouse enables the consistent and reliable tracking of the progression and therapeutic response of tumors in the context of a normal immune system. We anticipate that the use of this GEM model will facilitate the assessment of metastatic and recurrent disease, permit the evaluation of immunomodulatory drugs both alone and in combination with small molecule inhibitors, and enhance the ability of preclinical models to predict clinical efficacy.

Acknowledgments

We thank Drs. Rhonda Kineman (University of Illinois-Chicago, USA) for providing the rGH-Cre vector and Richard Palmiter (University of Washington, Seattle, WA) for his permission. We also thank Drs. Dominic Esposito (Leidos Biomedical Research, Inc., Frederick, MD, USA) for lentiviral vector production and Miriam Anver (Leidos Biomedical Research, Inc., Frederick, MD, USA) for histopathology. We are also grateful to Drs. Jude Alsarraj and Kent Hunter (National Cancer Institute, Bethesda, MD, USA) for providing the ffLuc-eGFP-labeled Mvt-1 breast cancer cells for the metastatic model. The content of this publication does not necessarily reflect the views or policies of the Department of Health and Human Services, nor does mention of trade names, commercial products, or organizations imply endorsement by the U.S. Government.

Supporting Information

Figure S1 Expression of the ffLuc-eGFP reporter cannot be consistently maintained in labeled melanoma cells transplanted into strain-matched WT immunocompetent mice. **A**, Melanoma cells derived from mutant NRas-expressing p19ARF-null transformed mouse melanocytes were transplanted subcutaneously into isogenic F1 mice from C57BL/6 X 129 crosses, followed by periodic BL imaging and tumor measurement. The primary tumors were resected at day 25, and metastases were found in #38 and 39 the day after by imaging. The lungs were harvested from #38, and a single glowing metastatic nodule selected via the guidance of ex vivo imaging was transplanted into two isogenic mice in the second passage (P2). Imaging results showed that the reporter activity could not be consistently maintained in P2 mice, indicating that the inconsistency of reporter activity in immunocompetent mice could not be rescued by selection of a high-expressing tumor clone. **B**, Melanoma cells harvested from a HGF-transgenic/CDKN2A-knockout mouse were dissociated and transduced with the ffLuc-eGFP gene ex vivo, followed by subcutaneous transplantation of 10,000 cells into syngeneic FVB/N mice. The mice were periodically subjected to tumor measurement and bioluminescence (BL) imaging for reporter activity (upper panel). All tumors grew from day 14 to day 18 (lower left panel). However, BL intensity was reduced in #62 (red line) and extinguished in #63 (green line), while slowly increasing in the other three tumors (lower middle panel). The labeling retention of the tumors, measured as BL intensity/size ratio, was actually reduced in three of five tumors (lower right panel). These results indicate that ffLuc-eGFP activity in the labeled tumor could not be consistently maintained in syngeneic immunocompetent mice.

Figure S2 Generation of rGH-ffLuc-eGFP transgenic (GH) mouse. **A**, Selection of germline GH mice. Founders G6 and D8 were bred with wildtype (WT) mice to generate germline GH mice. In the examples of bioluminescence (BL) imaging shown here, pups #1–5 and #6–10 were generated from founder G6 and D8, respectively. Mouse #3 had head BL 2.3×10^6 photon/sec/rad, which is more than 20-fold higher than the WT background (1.0×10^5) shown in B. In contrast, #7 and #8 exhibited head BL 2–6 fold over WT background. Therefore, pups derived from Line D8 were selected for further breeding. This line shows stable transgene expression through generations. **B**, rGH targeted reporter gene expression to pituitary gland is highly specific. Sixteen GH and seven WT FVB/N mice from the same colonies used in this study were subjected to BL imaging for 1 min under anesthesia in ventral position. These results show the high specificity of BL signal in the head of GH mice.

Figure S3 Comparison of tumor labeling consistency in wildtype and GH mice. The ffLuc-eGFP-labeled LLC tumor selected from in vivo cycling in GH mice was transplanted into syngeneic wildtype (c-Brd) and GH mice. The tumor size (left panel; mm3 ± SE) and BL signal (right panel; photon/sec/rad ± SE) were measured periodically following transplantation. At day 10, no significant difference in tumor size was found between c-Brd and GH mice (p = 0.86). However, BL intensities from tumors in GH were significantly higher than that in c-Brd (p = 0.036).

Figure S4 BL images of mice from the study in Fig. 3A to 3D. **A**, Comparison of progression of ffLuc-eGFP-labeled mammary tumors in GH and WT mice. Mvt1 mouse breast cancer cells were transduced with ffLuc-eGFP-encoded lentivirus and the GFP+ tumor cells FACS isolated and expanded in culture. These cells were injected into mammary fat pads in syngeneic WT and GH FVB/N mice. Time as days after inoculation were indicated here. Images of primary tumors at day 7 and 11 and post-resection images from day 26 to 45 are shown here. D-number indicates the day that mouse morbidity was first diagnosed or noted (e.g. D26 is day 26). **B**, Metastatic pattern in WT and GH mice. At the endpoint, mice were injected with the luciferase substrate luciferin and euthanized. The internal organs were exposed and subjected to ex vivo imaging. In WT mice, metastases were detected almost exclusively in lungs (left panels). In GH mice, metastases were often detected in the thyroid, pleural, spleen, and/or peritoneum, as well as the lung (right panels).

Figure S5 BL images of mice from the study in Fig. 3E to 3G. Time as days after primary tumor resection are indicated. Post-resection images from day 3 to 14 are shown here. D-number indicates the day that mouse morbidity was first diagnosed or noted (e.g. D9 is day 9).

Figure S6 Responses of subcutaneous LLC tumors to paclitaxel within the dose range of 6.7–22.5 mg/kg. LLC cells from in vitro culture were inoculated subcutaneously. Upon reaching 125 mm^3 at day 5, treatments with the indicated doses were initiated. A single dose was given each day for five days. Tumor sizes were measured by caliper. No significant efficacy was observed.

Figure S7 Representative hematoxylin and eosin staining of spleen sections from each treatment group. Note that spleens from the paclitaxel-treated WT c-Brd mice exhibited more lymphoid follicles (deep purple region) with disrupted structures, corresponding hematopoiesis and splenomegaly.

Figure S8 Pathological analyses of inflammation and invasion in melanoma allografts transplanted into GH and WT mice. **A–C**, representative images of tumors in GH mice receiving vehicle control, 50 mg/kg, or 100 mg/kg crizotonib (Criz). A, In vehicle control group, tumor invades into the deep subcutaneous tissue (arrows), but does not reach the level of the deep cutaneous skeletal muscle. Note that there are scattered mild inflammatory infiltrates throughout the deep subcutaneous tissue. B, Treatment of crizotinib at 50 mg/kg slightly reduced invasion into the deep subcutaneous adipose tissue (arrows) as compared to A. Mild to moderate inflammation surrounds this invasive front. C, In the treated group of 100 mg/kg crizotinib there are no distinct invasive foci, and mild inflammatory infiltrates are present along the tumor/subcutaneous tissue interface. **D–F**, representative images of tumors in WT mice receiving vehicle control, 50 mg/kg, or 100 mg/kg crizotonib. D, In vehicle control group, deep invasion into the underlying cutaneous skeletal muscle (arrows) can be observed in WT mice. However, this degree of invasion is very

rare in GH mice. E, In the treated group of 50 mg/kg crizotinib deep invasive tumor foci are still observed (arrows), as well as large regions of dense inflamed granulation tissue (*), which was commonly observed at the deep invasive front in tumors in WT mice. F, In tumors from mice receiving 100 mg/kg crizotinib, dense granulation tissue (*) to the primary subcutaneous tumor, as well as a deeper invading melanoma (M) that contains abundant hemorrhage, are occasionally observed.

Figure S9 Correlation between disease burden and in vivo BL in the metastatic model. ffLuc-eGFP-labeled LLC tumors were subcutaneously transplanted into GH mice. Upon reaching 500 mm^3, primary tumors were resected from mice, which were subjected to BL imaging periodically. Mice were selected at different in vivo BL intensities to be euthanized. The harvested lungs were fixed and sectioned for pathological analysis. **A**, H&E staining of lung sections from mice transplanted with fLuc-eGFP-labeled LLC tumors (the same used in Fig. 2-1). Under each panel is the chest BL intensity of each mouse from in vivo imaging. **B**, The disease burden in A was quantified with an Aperio slide image analysis system (Leica Biosystems). The correlation between in vivo BL signal and area of metastases in lung section follows a logarithmic function in regression analysis, a result similar to our previous study (Int. J. Cancer 2012, 130: 190–9).

Figure S10 Validation of the function of the metastatic model based on transplantation of labeled tumors into GH mice. **A**, At the endpoint of the study in Fig. 6, following in vivo BL imaging, the mice were euthanized, and the freshly harvested lungs were subjected to ex vivo BL and bright field imaging to identify metastatic nodules. The higher in vivo BL intensity was associated with either more or bigger sized nodules. The results validated quantitation by in vivo BL imaging. **B**, The GFP$^+$ cells isolated in Fig. 6D and E were subcutaneously inoculated into three GH mice. After 7 days, the mice were subjected to tumor size measurement and BL imaging. The results showed that FACS-isolated cells were able to grow tumors.

Author Contributions

Conceived and designed the experiments: CPD TVD ZWO MH GM. Performed the experiments: CPD JPC CB ZWO REM CGC LF. Analyzed the data: CPD TVD MH GM PM TT. Wrote the manuscript: CPD GM.

References

1. Herper M (2012) The Truly Staggering Cost Of Inventing New Drugs. Forbes. Available: http://www.forbes.com/sites/matthewherper/2012/02/10/the-truly-staggering-cost-of-inventing-new-drugs/.
2. Sharpless NE, Depinho RA (2006) The mighty mouse: genetically engineered mouse models in cancer drug development. Nat Rev Drug Discov 5: 741–754.
3. Suggitt M, Bibby MC (2005) 50 years of preclinical anticancer drug screening: empirical to target-driven approaches. Clin Cancer Res 11: 971–981.
4. Administration USFaD (2004) Innovation or Stagnation: Challenge and Opportunity on the Critical Path to New Medical Products.
5. Zitvogel L, Apetoh L, Ghiringhelli F, Kroemer G (2008) Immunological aspects of cancer chemotherapy. Nat Rev Immunol 8: 59–73.
6. Holzel M, Bovier A, Tuting T (2013) Plasticity of tumour and immune cells: a source of heterogeneity and a cause for therapy resistance? Nat Rev Cancer 13: 365–376.
7. Merlino G, Flaherty K, Acquavella N, Day CP, Aplin A, et al. (2013) Meeting report: The future of preclinical mouse models in melanoma treatment is now. Pigment Cell Melanoma Res.
8. Day CP, Carter J, Bonomi C, Hollingshead M, Merlino G (2012) Preclinical therapeutic response of residual metastatic disease is distinct from its primary tumor of origin. Int J Cancer 130: 190–199.
9. Baker M (2010) Whole-animal imaging: The whole picture. Nature 463: 977–980.
10. Day CP, Carter J, Bonomi C, Esposito D, Crise B, et al. (2009) Lentivirus-mediated bifunctional cell labeling for in vivo melanoma study. Pigment Cell Melanoma Res 22: 283–295.
11. Stripecke R, Carmen Villacres M, Skelton D, Satake N, Halene S, et al. (1999) Immune response to green fluorescent protein: implications for gene therapy. Gene Ther 6: 1305–1312.
12. Andersson G, Denaro M, Johnson K, Morgan P, Sullivan A, et al. (2003) Engraftment of retroviral EGFP-transduced bone marrow in mice prevents rejection of EGFP-transgenic skin grafts. Mol Ther 8: 385–391.
13. Steinbauer M, Guba M, Cernaianu G, Kohl G, Cetto M, et al. (2003) GFP-transfected tumor cells are useful in examining early metastasis in vivo, but immune reaction precludes long-term tumor development studies in immunocompetent mice. Clin Exp Metastasis 20: 135–141.
14. Day CP, Merlino G (2011) Immunocompetent Mouse Model for Tracking Cancer Progression (HHS Reference No. E-173-2010/0). Federal Register 76: 40382.

15. Ha L, Ichikawa T, Anver M, Dickins R, Lowe S, et al. (2007) ARF functions as a melanoma tumor suppressor by inducing p53-independent senescence. Proc Natl Acad Sci U S A 104: 10968–10973.

16. Mishra PJ, Ha L, Rieker J, Sviderskaya EV, Bennett DC, et al. (2010) Dissection of RAS downstream pathways in melanomagenesis: a role for Ral in transformation. Oncogene 29: 2449–2456.

17. Luque RM, Amargo G, Ishii S, Lobe C, Franks R, et al. (2007) Reporter expression, induced by a growth hormone promoter-driven Cre recombinase (rGHp-Cre) transgene, questions the developmental relationship between somatotropes and lactotropes in the adult mouse pituitary gland. Endocrinology 148: 1946–1953.

18. Bald T, Quast T, Landsberg J, Rogava M, Glodde N, et al. (2014) Ultraviolet-radiation-induced inflammation promotes angiotropism and metastasis in melanoma. Nature 507: 109–113.

19. Recio JA, Noonan FP, Takayama H, Anver MR, Duray P, et al. (2002) Ink4a/arf deficiency promotes ultraviolet radiation-induced melanomagenesis. Cancer Res 62: 6724–6730.

20. Pei XF, Noble MS, Davoli MA, Rosfjord E, Tilli MT, et al. (2004) Explant-cell culture of primary mammary tumors from MMTV-c-Myc transgenic mice. In Vitro Cell Dev Biol Anim 40: 14–21.

21. O'Doherty U, Swiggard WJ, Malim MH (2000) Human immunodeficiency virus type 1 spinoculation enhances infection through virus binding. J Virol 74: 10074–10080.

22. Gao D, Nolan DJ, Mellick AS, Bambino K, McDonnell K, et al. (2008) Endothelial progenitor cells control the angiogenic switch in mouse lung metastasis. Science 319: 195–198.

23. Hiratsuka S, Watanabe A, Aburatani H, Maru Y (2006) Tumour-mediated upregulation of chemoattractants and recruitment of myeloid cells predetermines lung metastasis. Nat Cell Biol 8: 1369–1375.

24. Kaplan RN, Riba RD, Zacharoulis S, Bramley AH, Vincent L, et al. (2005) VEGFR1-positive haematopoietic bone marrow progenitors initiate the pre-metastatic niche. Nature 438: 820–827.

25. Biffi A, Bartolomae CC, Cesana D, Cartier N, Aubourg P, et al. (2011) Lentiviral vector common integration sites in preclinical models and a clinical trial reflect a benign integration bias and not oncogenic selection. Blood 117: 5332–5339.

26. Fidler IJ (2003) The pathogenesis of cancer metastasis: the 'seed and soil' hypothesis revisited. Nat Rev Cancer 3: 453–458.

27. de Jersey J, Carmignac D, Barthlott T, Robinson I, Stockinger B (2002) Activation of CD8 T cells by antigen expressed in the pituitary gland. J Immunol 169: 6753–6759.

28. Crawford NP, Alsarraj J, Lukes L, Walker RC, Officewala JS, et al. (2008) Bromodomain 4 activation predicts breast cancer survival. Proc Natl Acad Sci U S A 105: 6380–6385.

29. Sparreboom A, van Tellingen O, Nooijen WJ, Beijnen JH (1996) Nonlinear pharmacokinetics of paclitaxel in mice results from the pharmaceutical vehicle Cremophor EL. Cancer Res 56: 2112–2115.

30. Couzin-Frankel J (2013) Breakthrough of the year 2013. Cancer immunotherapy. Science 342: 1432–1433.

31. Tentler JJ, Tan AC, Weekes CD, Jimeno A, Leong S, et al. (2012) Patient-derived tumour xenografts as models for oncology drug development. Nat Rev Clin Oncol 9: 338–350.

32. Bessis N, GarciaCozar FJ, Boissier MC (2004) Immune responses to gene therapy vectors: influence on vector function and effector mechanisms. Gene Ther 11 Suppl 1: S10–17.

33. Michou AI, Santoro L, Christ M, Julliard V, Pavirani A, et al. (1997) Adenovirus-mediated gene transfer: influence of transgene, mouse strain and type of immune response on persistence of transgene expression. Gene Ther 4: 473–482.

34. Yang Y, Jooss KU, Su Q, Ertl HC, Wilson JM (1996) Immune responses to viral antigens versus transgene product in the elimination of recombinant adenovirus-infected hepatocytes in vivo. Gene Ther 3: 137–144.

35. Agah R, Frenkel PA, French BA, Michael LH, Overbeek PA, et al. (1997) Gene recombination in postmitotic cells. Targeted expression of Cre recombinase provokes cardiac-restricted, site-specific rearrangement in adult ventricular muscle in vivo. J Clin Invest 100: 169–179.

36. Latta-Mahieu M, Rolland M, Caillet C, Wang M, Kennel P, et al. (2002) Gene transfer of a chimeric trans-activator is immunogenic and results in short-lived transgene expression. Hum Gene Ther 13: 1611–1620.

37. Melief CJ, Kast WM (1993) Potential immunogenicity of oncogene and tumor suppressor gene products. Curr Opin Immunol 5: 709–713.

38. Shultz LD, Schweitzer PA, Christianson SW, Gott B, Schweitzer IB, et al. (1995) Multiple defects in innate and adaptive immunologic function in NOD/LtSz-scid mice. J Immunol 154: 180–191.

5

Elevated Peptides in Lung Lavage Fluid Associated with Bronchiolitis Obliterans Syndrome

Matthew D. Stone[1,2,◗], Stephen B. Harvey[2,◗], Gary L. Nelsestuen[2], Cavan Reilly[3], Marshall I. Hertz[4], Chris H. Wendt[4,5]*

1 Waters Corporation, Milford, Massachusetts, United States of America, 2 Department of Biochemistry, Molecular Biology and Biophysics, University of Minnesota, Minneapolis, Minnesota, United States of America, 3 Department of Biostatistics, University of Minnesota, Minneapolis, Minnesota, United States of America, 4 Department of Medicine, University of Minnesota, Minneapolis, Minnesota, United States of America, 5 Department of Medicine, Veterans Administration Medical Center, University of Minnesota, Minneapolis, Minnesota, United States

Abstract

Objective: The objective of this discovery-level investigation was to use mass spectrometry to identify low mass compounds in bronchoalveolar lavage fluid from lung transplant recipients that associate with bronchiolitis obliterans syndrome.

Experimental Design: Bronchoalveolar lavage fluid samples from lung transplant recipients were evaluated for small molecules using ESI-TOF mass spectrometry and correlated to the development of bronchiolitis obliterans syndrome. Peptides associated with samples from persons with bronchiolitis obliterans syndrome and controls were identified separately by MS/MS analysis.

Results: The average bronchoalveolar lavage fluid MS spectrum profile of individuals that developed bronchiolitis obliterans syndrome differed greatly compared to controls. Controls demonstrated close inter-sample correlation (R = 0.97+/−0.02, average+/−SD) while bronchiolitis obliterans syndrome showed greater heterogeneity (R = 0.86+/−0.09, average+/−SD). We identified 89 features that were predictive of developing BOS grade 1 and 66 features predictive of developing BOS grade 2 or higher. Fractions from MS analysis were pooled and evaluated for peptide content. Nearly 10-fold more peptides were found in bronchiolitis obliterans syndrome relative to controls. C-terminal residues suggested trypsin-like specificity among controls compared to elastase-type enzymes among those with bronchiolitis obliterans syndrome.

Conclusions: Bronchoalveolar lavage fluid from individuals with bronchiolitis obliterans syndrome has an increase in low mass components detected by mass spectrometry. Many of these features were peptides that likely result from elevated neutrophil elastase activity.

Editor: Aric Gregson, University of California Los Angeles, United States of America

Funding: This work was supported in part by grant HL080041 from the National Institutes of Health. Instruments used for metabolome and peptide analysis were in the Center for Mass Spectrometry and Proteomics (CMSP), University of Minnesota and were purchased with partial support from the NIH, NSF and from Hatch funds and the CMSP receives operational support from the College of Biological Sciences, Academic Health Center, Medical School, College of Food, Agriculture and Natural Resource Sciences and from the Office of the Vice President for Research, University of Minnesota. The funders had no role in study design, data collection and analysis, decision to publish, or preparation of the manuscript.

Competing Interests: Dr. Stone was a post-doctoral fellow at the University of Minnesota at the time the experiments were performed, the data was analyzed and interpreted. Subsequently, Dr. Stone has taken employment with Waters, Inc. Since employment with Waters, Inc., Dr. Stone has been involved in manuscript editing as usual for a contributing author.

* E-mail: wendt005@umn.edu

◗ These authors contributed equally to this work.

Introduction

Lung transplantation has become a widely accepted therapeutic modality for many end-stage lung diseases. Unfortunately, chronic rejection remains a major barrier to long-term survival with 50–60% of lung transplant recipients affected at 5 years [1,2]. The clinical surrogate of chronic allograft rejection is bronchiolitis obliterans syndrome (BOS), which manifests as a decline, often progressive, of lung function [3]. In addition to a peribronchial infiltration of lymphocytes, neutrophilia also is a predominant finding in BOS [4–9]. These neutrophils release factors of the innate immune system, along with proteases [4,10–12]. Despite the high incidence of BOS, the underlying pathogenesis remains unknown and no clinical biomarker has been found to predict its onset.

Bronchoalveolar lavage fluid (BALF) is a rich source of potential biomarkers. Although invasive, BALF is collected on a routine basis for surveillance after lung transplant. In addition to cells and proteins, small molecules or metabolites are sampled in BALF. These small molecules can represent the end product of metabolism, lipids, drugs and peptide byproducts of protease digestion. Identification of metabolites unique to BOS has the potential to provide novel biomarkers and to provide insight into

Table 1. Subject underlying diseaseunderlying Disease.

Underlying Disease	Controls (n = 50)	BOS (n = 95)
COPD/Emphysema	19 (38.0%)	38 (40%)
Alpha -1- Antitrypsin Deficiency	13 (26.0%)	37 (38.9%)
Pulmonary Hypertension	3 (6.0%)	12 (12.2%)
Cystic Fibrosis/Bronchiectasis	9 (18.0%)	0 (0%)
Pulmonary Fibrosis	4 (8.0%)	8 (8.4%)
Other	2 (4.0%)	0 (0%)

mechanism of disease. This report describes a discovery-level study of BALF samples from individuals at various times before and after the diagnosis of BOS. While specific metabolites were targeted, it became clear that many were peptides generated by protease activity.

Materials and Methods

Study Population

The samples studied were excess cell-free BALF collected between 1993–1996 and 2003–2007 at the time of clinically obtained bronchoscopies as previously described [10]. Written informed consent was obtained from all subjects. Briefly, bronchoalveolar lavage consisted of 100–140 ml normal saline instilled in either the right middle lobe or left upper lobe (lingula), then aspirated. Samples were collected and immediately placed on ice, cells were removed by centrifugation and supernatants were stored at –80°C [10]. For this case-control study we chose 145 BALF samples (summarized in Table 1) from 64 individuals ages 27–63 (median 49, 48% female, average 2.25 BALF samples/individual, range 1–8). Of these samples, 76 were from the 1993–1996 source described previously [10] and 69 were from the 2003–2007 source. The sample size was determined by the number that could be accommodated in a single MS run. Cases (n = 95) consisted of individuals that developed BOS within 18 months of BALF sample acquisition. Controls (n = 50) were defined as those who did not progress to any grade of BOS within 6 years or more from BALF collection. Due to differences in column properties and elution times, LC-MS data from the two experiments could not be combined, whereas peptide and protein identifications were combined.

Ethics Statement

This study was approved by the University of Minnesota Institutional Review Board Human Subjects Committee (# 0107M04822).

Sample Preparation and Initial LC-MS Analysis

BALF samples (0.80 mL) were prepared for LCT-MS analysis by application to a disposable C18 spin column (MacroSpin, C18, The Nest Group Inc.). Columns were conditioned with 500 μL acetonitrile (ACN) followed by 500 μL water with centrifugation (4 minutes, 2000×g) each time. Samples were acidified to pH 2 with formic acid and applied to the conditioned column. The columns were rinsed twice with 400 μL of water/ACN/formic acid (95/5/0.1). The sample was eluted first with 200 μL of water/ACN/formic acid (50/50/0.1) followed by 200 μL of water/ACN/formic acid (10/90/0.1). The combined 400 μL was concentrated by vacuum centrifugation to approximately 50 μL. Samples were

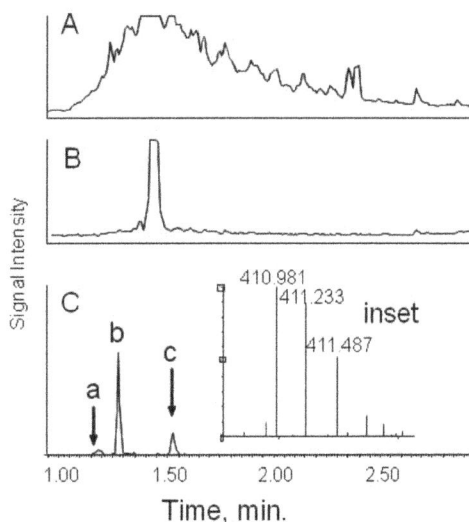

Figure 1. UPLC separation of BALF fluid. Panel A. Total ion current for a typical sample from an individual with BOS. Panel B. Total ion current for a control subject who did not develop BOS within at least 100 months. The intensity has been adjusted to the same maximum as Panel A. The large peak at 1.48 minutes corresponded to lidocaine. Panel C. Extracted ion current for the +4 charge state of a component at m/z = 410.98. Only peak b represented a monoisotopic ion. Peaks a and c were isotopes of other compounds.

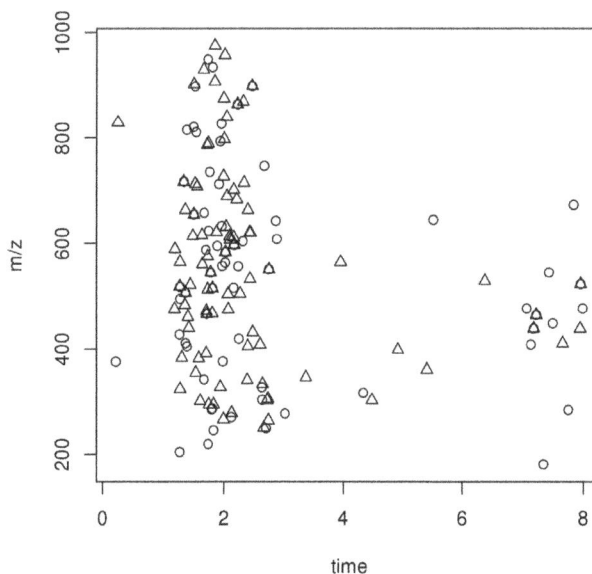

Figure 2. Features predictive of BOS. The median intensity of each feature is represented by the mass/charge (m/z) and retention time (time). Using a false discovery rate of 10%, the circles indicate features that are predictive of time to BOS 1 (triangles, n = 89) and those that are predictive of time to BOS 2 or 3 (circles, n = 66).

brought up to 100 μL with water/ACN/formic acid (95/5/0/1). Analysis was performed with the Waters, Inc. Acquity UPLC system and an Acquity UPLC BEH C18 1.7 μm 2.1×100 mm column. The flow rate was 0.5 mL/minute with a column temperature of 40°C. Injected sample (7 μL) was eluted using an increasing gradient of ACN/water in 0.1% formic acid: 0.5

minutes of initial buffer (water:can,98:2), a gradient to 20% ACN (over 0.5 minutes) and a linear gradient to 100% ACN (over 7 minutes). The column was washed with 100% ACN (two minutes) and then re-equilibrated with the starting buffer. This protocol provided acceptable peak separation with minimal carry-over. Mass spectrometry utilized the Waters LCT Premier XE TOF operated in positive, double reflectron mode with dynamic range enhancement. The scan rate was 0.1/s with continual calibration by a lock spray. Leucine enkaphalin was the lock spray reagent (557.2802 lock mass and 556.2771 attenuated lock mass) sampled every ten scans. Capillary and cone voltages were 2500 and 30 V, respectively. Features (accurate mass and retention time pair) of the profile were compiled using MarkerLynx software and were expressed as either raw intensity or normalized to 10,000 total counts per profile. Features of the background (>0.1-times the sample average) were disregarded. A feature is defined by a specific mass/charge (m/z) and retention time. Due to multiple charge states and possible adducts, a metabolite may be represented by more than one feature.

Peptide Identification by LC-MS/MS

Peptide identification required pooling of samples from the LCT-MS run to reach adequate concentrations for MS/MS analysis. In two separate experiments we pooled aliquots (20 µL each) from: 1) 6 BOS samples and from 16 control samples (1993–96 samples) and 2) 15 controls and 5 BOS samples (2003–2007 samples). UPLC (elution as above) fractions were collected at 0.5

minute intervals (0.25 mL) between 1.0 and 3.5 minutes. Each fraction was submitted for MS/MS analysis in the Orbitaltrap mass spectrometer for peptide identification. Sample loading, HPLC, and mass spectrometry were performed as previously described [13] with the following exceptions: Electrospray mass spectrometry was performed using a LTQ-Orbitrap XL (Thermo-Scientific) with spray voltage set to 1.95 kV. Charge state screening was enabled so that undetermined charge states were excluded for data dependent fragmentation. Each sample was run in duplicate to enhance coverage.

Database Searching and Data Processing

Raw mass spectrometric data obtained from Xcalibur software (ThermoScientific) were extracted using ReAdw (Institute of Systems Biology) to generate mzXML files. Data were searched with SEQUEST V27 against a composite database consisting of the NCBI human database V200806 and its reversed complement and common contaminating protein sequences totaling 70711 entities. A total of 42242 spectra were searched from the control dataset and 65124 spectra were searched from the BOS dataset. Search parameters included no enzyme specification, 100 ppm precursor molecular mass tolerance, 0.8 amu fragment ion mass tolerance, a precursor ion mass range from 700–3600 Da and Met oxidation. SEQUEST output was organized and peptide probabilities were calculated through Peptide Prophet [14] using Scaffold (Proteome Software, Inc., Portland, OR). Peptide identifications were filtered using the following parameters: 95%

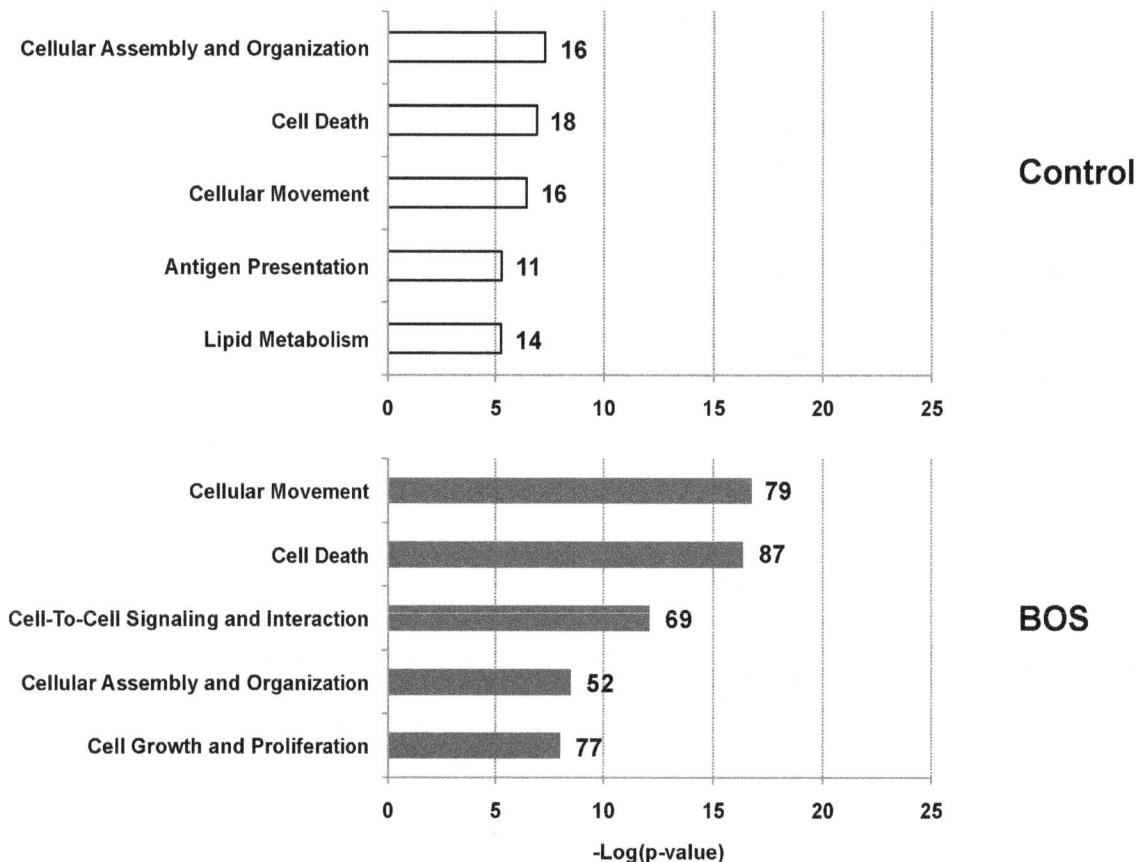

Figure 3. Top molecular and cellular biofunctions identified from protein substrates. Proteins identified from the sequenced peptides were used in Ingenuity Pathway Analysis to determine the molecular and cellular function of the substrate proteins. The number of proteins associated with each function is listed next to the bar.

Table 2. C-Terminal amino acid comparison of unique endogenous peptides identified in BALF of transplant patients, control compared to BOS.

c-terminal residue	frequency	% frequency	% of frequency normalized to naturally occuring AA frequency	frequency	% frequency	% of frequency normalized to naturally occuring AA frequency
	Controls			BOS		
A	22	6.1	4.5	321	**9.4**	**7.1**
C	1	0.3	0.7	6	0.2	0.4
D	11	3.0	3.5	118	3.5	4.1
E	12	3.3	2.6	132	3.9	3.1
F	21	5.8	7.7	209	6.1	8.3
G	13	3.6	2.8	128	3.8	3.0
H	4	1.1	2.2	14	0.4	0.8
I	6	1.7	1.8	385	**11.3**	**12.5**
K	38	10.5	10.1	187	5.5	5.4
L	66	18.3	9.0	420	12.3	6.2
M	12	3.3	6.9	111	3.3	6.9
N	9	2.5	3.5	36	1.1	1.5
P	2	0.6	0.5	19	0.6	0.5
Q	19	5.3	6.0	74	2.2	2.5
R	43	11.9	11.6	86	2.5	2.5
S	33	9.1	5.7	141	4.1	2.6
T	8	2.2	2.0	232	**6.8**	**6.2**
V	14	3.9	3.4	617	**18.1**	**16.0**
W	5	1.4	4.9	21	0.6	2.2
Y	22	6.1	10.8	154	4.5	8.1
total	361			3411		

peptide probability and 7 ppm for precursor mass tolerance. Estimated false positive rates were calculated from identified spectra using the equation: (2 × reverse database identifications/ (forward+reverse database identifications)*100). Protein false discovery rates were determined using the following calculation: (reverse database identifications/(forward+reverse database identifications)*100). All identified MS/MS spectra (Table S1) can be downloaded from Tranche (https://proteomecommons.org/tranche/) with the following hash: haakgsT9g6Fl4waTlcLGNCD7NJepCE2t0YG6oZCvq6dvkBc7uwf25BFEtTZ9hff0szXET8NK-sODQcM3SeC0gkdaLGoUAAAAAAAACbA = =. These annotated spectra can be viewed using the freely available Scaffold Viewer software from www.proteomesoftware.com.

Statistical Analysis

Regression analysis was used to obtain correlation coefficients for comparison of total LCT-MS profiles. To test if a metabolomic feature was predictive of time to development of BOS, the median intensity of each feature was used to dichotomize the feature values. The log rank test was used to test for a difference in the time to development of BOS between the dichotomized feature values. The p-values produced by the log rank test were then adjusted for multiple comparisons using the q-value approach of Storey [15]. Features were declared of interest by setting the threshold for the false discovery rate at 10%. This analysis was conducted separately for BOS grade 1 and BOS grade 2 or 3.

Results

LCT-MS Analysis

The total ion current from LCT-MS analysis of organic solvent-soluble materials revealed a very intense peak at 1.48 minutes with $m/z = 235.34$. This was consistent with lidocaine, the local anesthetic used in the bronchoscopy. Excluding that feature, profiles were widely divergent between controls and those with BOS. An individual with BOS (Figure 1A) showed very high total ion current between 1.2 to 3.5 minutes while many control samples showed low intensity for most of the profile (example in Figure 1B).

From visual observation it was apparent that the average profile for BOS differed greatly from the average profile for controls. To determine reproducibility, replicate experimental runs were performed at a 24-hour interval on 6 BOS samples and 6 controls. Reproducibility was excellent as illustrated by high correlation coefficients of 0.996–0.999 between experimental runs. Inter-sample comparisons gave high correlation coefficients as well, especially for controls (R = 0.97+/−0.02). All combinations among six BOS samples showed somewhat lower correlation (R = 0.86+/−0.09). Most surprising was that BOS samples had similar correlation to control samples (R = 0.86+/−0.07). Overall, correlation coefficients indicated that the novel features of BOS samples differed widely, whereas control samples contained similar features.

To test if a feature was predictive of developing BOS we used the log rank test to look for a difference in the time to develop BOS. Since we had multiple samples from individuals (average 2.25 BALF samples/individual) we used the first BALF sample obtained from an individual for analysis. We identified 89 features that were predictive of developing BOS grade 1 and 66 features predictive of developing BOS grade 2 or higher (Figure 2). Most of these features had elution times, mass ranges (m/z) and charge states that were suggestive of peptides.

One limitation of the LCT-MS is that it provided m/z and retention times but not structural identities. Circumstantial factors such as elution times and the presence of multiply charged features suggested that many of the features predictive of BOS were peptides. An example was a feature at +4 charge that eluted at 1.33 minutes (peak b, Figure 1C). A peptide of the same m/z and charge state was found in separate MS/MS analysis of pooled samples and was assigned IRNDEELNKLLGKV of Histone cluster 1, H2ah (Table S2). The extracted ion profile showed two minor peaks with the same m/z (Figure 1C, lower case a and c). However, these were easily distinguished as isotopes of other compounds. We sought to identify endogenous peptides in our samples since the retention times and charge pattern of many of the features that predicted BOS suggested that they were peptides.

Identification of Endogenous Peptides of BALF

To have adequate sample volume we used pooled samples from the BOS and control sample UPLC chromatograms to identify endogenous peptides. Fractions were collected from two column runs from each sample source and were analyzed in the LTQ-Orbitrap mass spectrometer. Peptide identifications were stringently filtered to give an estimated false positive rate of 0.16%, corresponding to a protein false discovery rate of 1.2%. A comprehensive list of all unique peptide identifications is given in Table S2. Controls provided 196 unique peptides from 349 assigned spectra. From these peptides we identified 45 proteins. The BOS samples had 1739 unique peptides from 3424 identified spectra and a total of 228 unique proteins identified from the peptides (Table S3). The majority (84%) of the 45 proteins identified in controls were also found in BOS. There was less commonality among peptides; only 34% of the peptides found in the control samples were identified in BOS. Therefore, although there appears to be some common substrates (i.e. proteins) that generate the various peptides, the peptides themselves are heterogeneous.

To categorize the protein substrates that generated the peptides, Ingenuity Pathways Analysis™ (IPA) was performed using unique accession numbers of each identified peptide. The top biofunctions that the proteins identified in the BOS samples were: cellular movement, cell death, cell-to-cell signaling and interaction, cellular assembly and organization and cell growth and proliferation (Figure 3). There was overlap in biofunctions between BOS and control samples, however, there were significantly less proteins in the control samples.

Analysis of the C-terminal residues of the identified peptide sequences showed further differences between controls and BOS. C-terminals were tabulated and normalized to the natural amino acid distribution of the human genome (Table 2). Peptides from the control samples had the highest occurrence of basic C-terminal residues: 10.1 and 11.6% for K and R, respectively. BOS samples had comparatively high C-terminal frequencies of V (16.0%), I (12.5%), A (7.1%), and T (6.2%). The latter cleavage site specificity implicated an increase of elastase 2-like activity [16]. Furthermore, a peptide from elastase- 2 or human neutrophil elastase was identified in the BOS sample.

Discussion

One initial goal of this study was to further characterize BALF of lung transplant recipients and to identify potential biomarkers for BOS. Metabolite biomarkers offer several advantages over proteins that are subject to degradation, modification and aggregation, which may confound antibody-based assays. In contrast, many small molecules are stable and easily measured. As this study progressed, it became apparent that many features of the metabolite profile were peptides. These offered the advantages of easy identification by MS/MS. The combination of peptide identity and substrate identification provides important information regarding the basis and mechanism of these peptides in BOS.

Global MS analysis revealed many components that were more abundant in patients with BOS. There was high inter-sample correlation among controls suggesting relatively uniform components of the BALF. However, profiles from BOS showed lower correlation whether compared with controls or with other BOS samples. This suggested that, while considerable similarity existed among all BALF samples, BOS samples were substantially diverse.

MS/MS analysis of pooled samples identified many peptides and their protein substrates. Ingenuity pathway analysis revealed that, while protein substrates were similar for BOS and controls, BOS samples provided 10-fold more peptides. Cellular movement, cell death and cell growth and proliferation were among the top five biofunctions of the substrates seen in BOS. This was consistent with BOS being a disease marked by loss of normal cellular function with subsequent proliferation, specifically fibroproliferation. The protein substrates present in BALF were consistent with those proteins likely to be involved in the pathogenesis of BOS.

Although we, and others, have identified the presence of certain proteases, such as matrix metalloprotease 9 and proteinase 3 as biomarkers for the diagnosis and prediction of BOS [17–19], specific protease activity has not been documented. Interestingly, examination of C-terminal residues indicated an elastase-2 type activity in BOS. In fact, a peptide from human neutrophil elastase was found in pooled BOS samples. Neutrophilia has been associated with BOS [4–6,11,12] and generalized protease activity has been noted to increase in BOS along with a decrease in anti-protease activity [4,12]. Our findings suggest that although other proteases are present, the neutrophil elastase is the predominant active protease.

Overall, there were an enormous number of features in the BALF, especially in the BOS samples. Many of these features were identified as peptide metabolites generated by cleavage from neutrophil elastase. No peptide pattern specific to BOS was identified. It is possible that many other classes of small molecules are also altered in BOS and were not identified in this study. Further studies of low mass compounds may expand the number of metabolites that can be linked to the development of BOS.

Supporting Information

Table S1   All identified MS/MS features identified by retention time and m/z.

Table S2   Summary of Unique Identified Peptides from Control Samples (2–199) and BOS2 Samples (202–1940).

Table S3   Peptides matched to LCT mass spectrometry experiment.

Acknowledgments

The authors are indebted to Allison Tisdale and Matthew Wroblewski for excellent technical assistance and to the Minnesota Supercomputing Institute for software support and data storage.

References

1. Estenne M, Hertz MI (2002) Bronchiolitis obliterans after human lung transplantation. Am J Respir Crit Care Med 166: 440–444.
2. Boehler A, Kesten S, Weder W, Speich R (1998) Bronchiolitis obliterans after lung transplantation: a review. Chest 114: 1411–1426.
3. Estenne M, Maurer JR, Boehler A, Egan JJ, Frost A, et al. (2002) Bronchiolitis obliterans syndrome 2001: an update of the diagnostic criteria. J Heart Lung Transplant 21: 297–310.
4. Meyer KC, Nunley DR, Dauber JH, Iacono AT, Keenan RJ, et al. (2001) Neutrophils, Unopposed Neutrophil Elastase, and Alpha(1)-Antiprotease Defenses Following Human Lung Transplantation. Am J Respir Crit Care Med 164: 97–102.
5. DiGiovine B, Lynch JP, Martinez FJ, Flint A, Whyte RI, et al. (1996) Bronchoalveolar lavage neutrophilia is associated with obliterative bronchiolitis after lung transplantation: role of IL-8. J Immunol 157(9): 4194–4202.
6. Henke JA, Golden JA, Yelin EH, Keith FA, Blanc PD (1999) Persistent increases of BAL neutrophils as a predictor of mortality following lung transplant. Chest 115: 403 409.
7. Riise GC, Andersson BA, Kjellstrom C, Martensson G, Nilsson FN, et al. (1999) Persistent high BAL fluid granulocyte activation marker levels as early indicators of bronchiolitis obliterans after lung transplant. Eur Respir J 14: 1123–1130.
8. Riise GC, Williams A, Kjellstrom C, Schersten H, Andersson BA, et al. (1998) Bronchiolitis obliterans syndrome in lung transplant recipients is associated with increased neutrophil and decreased antioxidant status in the lung. Eur Respir J 12: 82–88.
9. Zheng L, Walters EH, Ward C, Wang N, Orsida B, et al. (2000) Airway neutrophilia in stable and bronchiolitis obliterans syndrome patients following lung transplantation. Thorax 55: 53–59.
10. Nelsestuen GL, Martinez MB, Hertz MI, Savik K, Wendt CH (2005) Proteomic identification of human neutrophil alpha-defensins in chronic lung allograft rejection. Proteomics 5: 1705–1713.
11. Elssner A, Vogelmeier C (2001) The role of neutrophils in the pathogenesis of obliterative bronchiolitis after lung transplantation. Transpl Infect Dis 3: 168–176.
12. Nunley D, Dauber J, Iacono A, Keenan R, Zeevi A, et al. (1999) Unopposed neutrophil elastase in bronchoalveolar lavage from transplant recipients with cystic fibrosis. American Journal of Respiratory & Critical Care Medicine 159: 258–261.
13. Bandhakavi S, Stone MD, Onsongo G, Van Riper SK, Griffin TJ (2009) A dynamic range compression and three-dimensional peptide fractionation analysis platform expands proteome coverage and the diagnostic potential of whole saliva. J Proteome Res 8: 5590–5600.
14. Keller A, Nesvizhskii AI, Kolker E, Aebersold R (2002) Empirical statistical model to estimate the accuracy of peptide identifications made by MS/MS and database search. Anal Chem 74: 5383–5392.
15. Storey JD (2002) A direct approach to false discovery rates. Journal of the Royal Society Statistical Society B: 479–498.
16. Rawlings ND, Barrett AJ, Bateman A (2010) MEROPS: the peptidase database. Nucleic Acids Re 38: D227–D233.
17. Zhang Y, Wroblewski M, Hertz MI, Wendt CH, Cervenka TM, et al. (2005) Analysis of chronic lung transplant rejection by MALDI-TOF profiles of bronchoalveolar lavage fluid. Proteomis in press.
18. Hubner RH, Meffert S, Mundt U, Bottcher H, Freitag S, et al. (2005) Matrix metalloproteinase-9 in bronchiolitis obliterans syndrome after lung transplantation. Eur Respir J 25: 494–501.
19. Smith GN, Jr., Mickler EA, Payne KK, Lee J, Duncan M, et al. (2007) Lung transplant metalloproteinase levels are elevated prior to bronchiolitis obliterans syndrome. Am J Transplant 7: 1856–1861.

Author Contributions

Conceived and designed the experiments: GLN CHW. Performed the experiments: MDS SBH. Analyzed the data: MDS GLN CR CHW. Contributed reagents/materials/analysis tools: GLN MIH CR CHW. Wrote the paper: MDS GLN CHW. Edited the manuscript: MH.

6

A Critical Role for the mTORC2 Pathway in Lung Fibrosis

Wenteh Chang[1], Ke Wei[1], Lawrence Ho[2], Gerald J. Berry[3], Susan S. Jacobs[1], Cheryl H. Chang[1], Glenn D. Rosen[1]*

1 Division of Pulmonary and Critical Care Medicine, Stanford University School of Medicine, Stanford, California, United States of America, 2 Division of Pulmonary and Critical Care Medicine, University of Washington School of Medicine, Seattle, Washington, United States of America, 3 Department of Pathology, Stanford University School of Medicine, Stanford, California, United States of America

Abstract

A characteristic of dysregulated wound healing in IPF is fibroblastic-mediated damage to lung epithelial cells within fibroblastic foci. In these foci, TGF-β and other growth factors activate fibroblasts that secrete growth factors and matrix regulatory proteins, which activate a fibrotic cascade. Our studies and those of others have revealed that Akt is activated in IPF fibroblasts and it mediates the activation by TGF-β of pro-fibrotic pathways. Recent studies show that mTORC2, a component of the mTOR pathway, mediates the activation of Akt. In this study we set out to determine if blocking mTORC2 with MLN0128, an active site dual mTOR inhibitor, which blocks both mTORC1 and mTORC2, inhibits lung fibrosis. We examined the effect of MLN0128 on TGF-β-mediated induction of stromal proteins in IPF lung fibroblasts; also, we looked at its effect on TGF-β-mediated epithelial injury using a Transwell co-culture system. Additionally, we assessed MLN0128 in the murine bleomycin lung model. We found that TGF-β induces the Rictor component of mTORC2 in IPF lung fibroblasts, which led to Akt activation, and that MLN0128 exhibited potent anti-fibrotic activity in vitro and in vivo. Also, we observed that Rictor induction is Akt-mediated. MLN0128 displays multiple anti-fibrotic and lung epithelial-protective activities; it (1) inhibited the expression of pro-fibrotic matrix-regulatory proteins in TGF-β-stimulated IPF fibroblasts; (2) inhibited fibrosis in a murine bleomycin lung model; and (3) protected lung epithelial cells from injury caused by TGF-β-stimulated IPF fibroblasts. Our findings support a role for mTORC2 in the pathogenesis of lung fibrosis and for the potential of active site mTOR inhibitors in the treatment of IPF and other fibrotic lung diseases.

Editor: Ana Mora, University of Pittsburgh, United States of America

Funding: This work was supported by a grant from the Takeda Corporation. The funders had no role in data collection, and analysis or decision to publish. They did provide MLN-0128, made suggestions about its formulation for animal studies, and proofread the manuscript.

Competing Interests: This work was supported by a grant from the Takeda Corporation.

* Email: grosen@stanford.edu

Introduction

Idiopathic Pulmonary Fibrosis (IPF) is a devastating disease, which afflicts over 200,000 patients in the United States and Europe [1]. The pathogenesis is unknown but a dysregulated wound healing response to lung epithelial injury, which leads to progressive interstitial fibrosis, is a hallmark of the disease. Activated fibroblasts in fibroblastic foci secrete a variety of pro-fibrotic proteins in response to TGF-β, such as type I and type III collagen, fibronectin (FN), and the matricellular family members, secreted protein acidic and rich in cysteine (SPARC) and connected tissue growth factor (CTGF) [2].

The evolutionary conserved serine/threonine protein kinase mTOR is a member of the phosphatidylinositol 3-kinase (PI3K)-related kinase (PIKK) family [3]. mTOR integrates both extracellular and intracellular signals and acts as a central regulator of cell metabolism, growth, proliferation and survival [4]. In mammalian cells, mTOR resides in two physically and functionally distinct signaling complexes: mTOR complex 1 (mTORC1), a rapamycin-sensitive complex, and mTOR complex 2 (mTORC2) [5,6]. The mTORC1 complex consists of at least five components: (i) mTOR, the catalytic subunit of the complex; (ii) Raptor; (iii) mLS8; (iv) PRAS40; and (v) Deptor; mTORC1 phosphorylates the ribosomal S6K1 (protein S6 kinase 1) and 4E-

BP1 (eukaryotic translation initiation factor eIF4E binding protein 1) proteins, which regulate growth and protein synthesis, respectively [7]. Rapamycin and related rapalogs are known allosteric inhibitors of mTORC1 but do not generally directly inhibit mTORC2, although prolonged treatment with rapamycin suppresses mTORC2 in some cell types [8]. Also, the inhibition of mTORC1 by rapamycin can activate mTORC2 and thereby activate Akt [9]. A recent study showed that rapamycin failed in an IPF clinical trial [10].

The mTORC2 complex consists of six different known proteins: (i) mTOR; (ii) Rictor; (iii) mSIN1; (iv) Protor-1; (v) mLST8; and (vi) Deptor. Rictor and mSIN1 mutually stabilize each other, thus establishing the structural foundation of the complex [7]. The mTORC2 complex mediates the phosphorylation of Akt on Ser473 and thereby activates the downstream Akt pathway, which regulates multiple cellular responses, including increased cell growth and proliferation, a shift to glycolytic metabolism, and increased cell migration [11]. In response to growth factors, PI3K stimulates phosphorylation of Akt at Thr308 through activation of phosphoinositide-dependent protein kinase 1 (PDK1) [11]. We showed previously that SPARC produced by IPF fibroblasts activates Akt by phosphorylation of serine 473 (Ser473) leading to inhibition of glycogen synthase kinase 3β (GSK-3β), which resulted in activation of the β-catenin pathway and inhibition of apoptosis [12]. Other studies have shown that loss of phosphate and tensin homolog (PTEN) in IPF fibroblasts also causes activation of Akt, through phosphorylation at Ser473 [13,14]. We hypothesized, therefore, that Akt activation in IPF lung fibroblasts is mediated by the mTORC2 component of the mTOR pathway.

The discovery of active site ATP-competitive mTORC1/2 inhibitors was recently reported by several research groups, although a selective mTORC2 inhibitor has yet to be developed. Several active site mTOR inhibitors, that block both mTORC1 and mTORC2, such as MLN0128 (previously known as INK128), have progressed to clinical trials for cancer [5,15–17]. In this study, we show that the Rictor component of mTORC2 is induced by TGF-β in lPF lung fibroblasts, which was coincident with Akt activation. Also, we show that the active site mTOR inhibitor MLN0128 exhibits several properties, which suggest it may have antifibrotic activity in a clinical setting: (i) it inhibits expression of stromal proteins by IPF fibroblasts; (ii) it inhibits lung injury and fibrosis in a murine bleomycin model, and (iii) it protects lung epithelial cells from TGF-β-induced toxicity originating from IPF fibroblasts. These data suggest a role for mTORC2 as a mediator of lung fibrosis and suggest that active site mTOR inhibitors may hold promise for the treatment of fibrotic disease.

Materials and Methods

Ethics Statement

Informed consent was obtained with a Stanford IRB-approved protocol to obtain explant lung tissue from patients undergoing surgical lung biopsy for the diagnosis of an idiopathic interstitial pneumonia or lung transplant for IPF. Fibroblasts were isolated from the surgical lung explants.

All mice used in this research project are maintained in two animal rooms in the Division of Laboratory Animal Medicine. All mice are maintained under filter-top, barrier isolation and all cages are changed in a laminar flow hood. Critically important strains are maintained in rooms in which the cages, filter tops, bedding and food are autoclaved. At the present time, the mice are free of all known murine viruses and free of ecto- and endoparasites. Experimental mice are monitored on a daily basis for morbidity and are sacrificed if there is evidence of suffering. The colony as a whole are monitored every 2–3 months for the presence of antibodies to a standard panel of murine viruses, cultured for the presence of pathogenic bacteria and examined for parasites regularly. Every effort is made to ensure that the animals do not suffer any discomfort, distress, pain or injury beyond what is unavoidable in the conduct of this research. Animals that are part of a treatment group are evaluated on a daily basis for evidence of morbidity and are sacrificed if there is any appearance of suffering. Mice that are to be sacrificed for specific studies are euthanized by CO_2 inhalation. Following any surgical procedures, the animals are warmed on a heating pad until they are awake and ambulating. All of the methods of euthanasia and anesthesia are consistent with the recommendations of the Panel of Euthanasia of the American Veterinary Medical Association.

Cells and reagents. Reagents were from Sigma-Aldrich (St. Louis, MO) or otherwise indicated. Lung fibroblasts were isolated from IPF patients obtained from surgical lung biopsy or lung transplant and cultured in DMEM/10% fetal bovine serum (Invitrogen, Grand Island, NY) as previously described [12]. All protocols were approved by Stanford Institutional Review Board and Administrative Panel on Biosafety. Cells were starved in 0.1% serum medium for 24 hours, before TGF-β (5 ng/ml) stimulation. A549 and RLE-6TN cells were from the American Type Culture

Collection (Manassas, VA) and maintained following supplier's instructions. PP242 and MLN0128 were from Chemdea (Ridgewood, NJ), and Takeda Pharmaceuticals (Deerfield, IL), respectively.

Western blot analysis. Western blot analysis was described previously [18] with following antibodies; type I collagen (Millipore, Billerica, MA), EDA-fibronectin (MP Biochemicals, Aurora, OH), α-SMA (American Research Products, Belmont, MA), SPARC (Biodesign International, Saco, ME), p-Akt (Ser473 or Thr308), Akt, p-S6, p-Smad2, p-Smad3, Raptor (Cell Signaling Technology, Danvers, MA), Smad2/3 (BD Biosciences, Franklin Lakes, NJ), Smad3 (Zymed, Life Technologies, Grand Island, NY), Smad4, Rictor (Santa Cruz Biotechnology, Dallas, Texas), Smad7 (Imgenex/Novus, Littleton, CO) and α-tubulin (Calbiochem/Millipore, Billerica, MA).

RNA interference. Constructs of raptor and rictor shRNA were from Addgene (plasmids 1857 and 1853, respectively) [11]. The SPARC shRNA, scramble, cell transduction, and selection procedures were described previously [12].

Bleomycin lung model. The murine bleomycin lung toxicity model was used as described previously [19]. Mice received intratracheal bleomycin (MP Biomedicals, Santa Ana, CA) at 1.0 U/kg body weight. Mice were treated by intraperitoneal delivery of vehicle (40% PEG400) or MLN0128 (0.75 mg/kg body weight) daily (6/7 days) starting at Day 0 (prevention model) or Day 7 (therapeutic model) after bleomycin. For the prevention model, three mice were used in saline, or MLN0128 groups, and six mice were used in bleomycin, or bleomycin+MLN0128 groups. Body weight was measured at day −1 (receiving treatment), day 0 (receiving bleomycin), day 4, 7, 11, and 14 when all surviving animals were collected from four independent experiments. For the therapeutic model, three mice were used in saline, or MLN0128 groups, six mice were used in each bleomycin group, and five mice were used in each bleomycin+MLN0128 group. Body weight for the therapeutic model was collected at day 0 (receiving bleomycin), day 3, 7 (the first day receiving treatment), 10, 14, 17, and day 21 when all surviving animals were collected from five independent experiments. One mouse from the bleomycin group was harvested at day 7 from each experiment to access lung histology prior to MLN0128 treatment. For the Sircoll collagen assay and Ashcroft analysis, data from surviving mice is combined from experiments, which are described above.

Histological analysis. The mouse left lung was assessed for fibrosis by the Ashcroft scale [20] as previously described [19].

Sircoll collagen assay. Collagen content of the right lung was determined per the manufacturer's instructions (Biocolor Ltd., UK). In the prevention model, 2/3 of mice were used for the Sircoll collagen assay and 1/3 for gene expression analysis.

Transwell culture. Fibroblasts (before passage 8) were seeded in a 24-well plate at 5×10^4 cells/well. After starvation, cells were pre-treated with inhibitors for 30 minutes before TGF-β treatment for 16 hours. A549 or RLE-6TN cells were plated at 1×10^4 cells per transwell (BD Biosciences, Franklin Lakes, NJ), and starved for 24 hours. Treated-fibroblasts were washed twice with PBS and placed in starvation media before the insertion of epithelia-containing transwells. After a 48 hour incubation, the epithelia-containing transwells were transferred into new vessels and the viability of epithelia was determined by Alamar blue assay [21].

Measurement of H_2O_2 release. H_2O_2 release was measured through the conversion of Amplex Red reagent by peroxidase to produce the red-fluorescent oxidation product, resorufin [22]. Following treatment, IPF fibroblasts were washed twice, and incubated with a reaction mixture (100 μM Amplex red

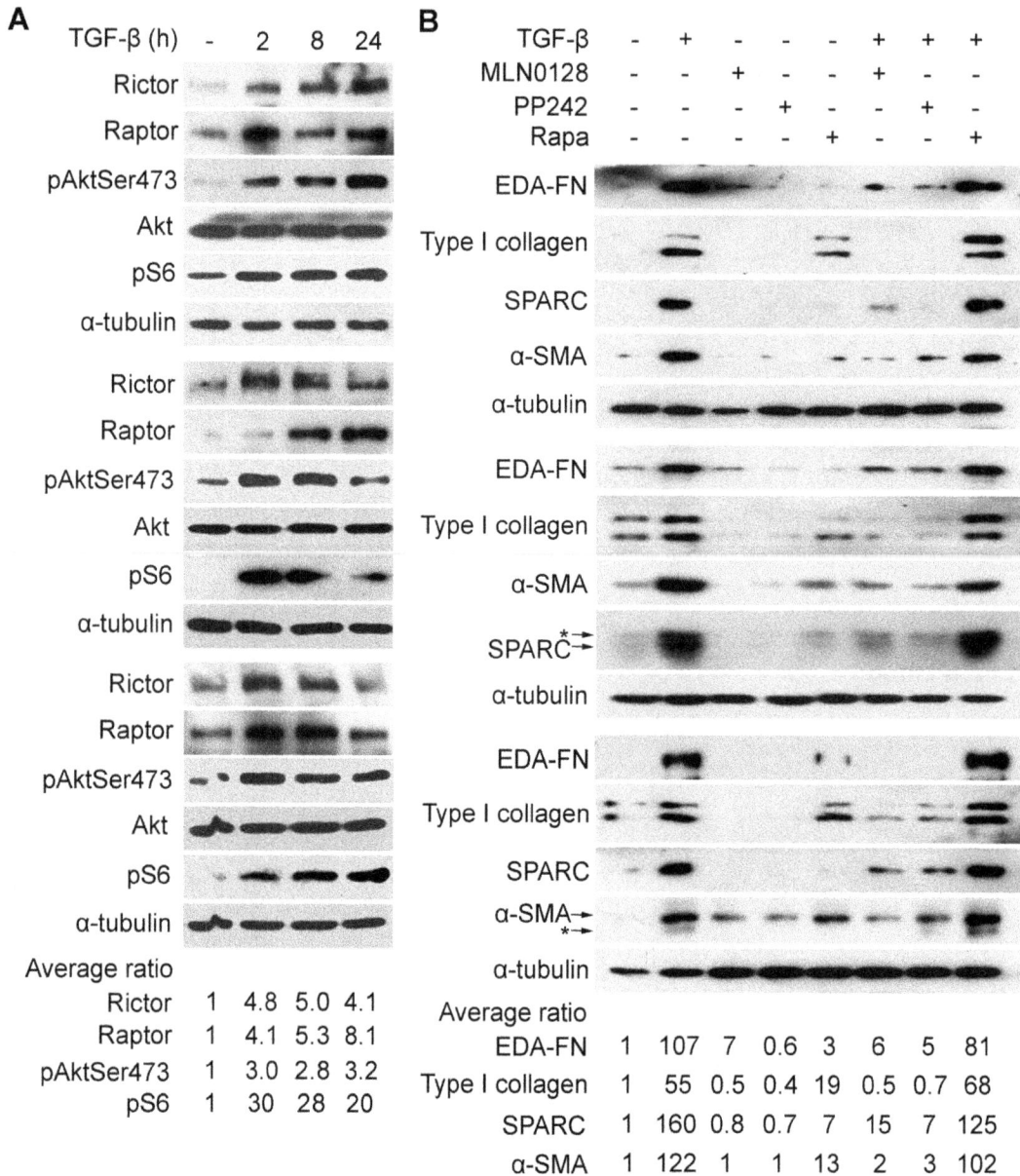

Figure 1. Rictor is a target of TGF-β and the effect of mTOR inhibitors on TGF-β signaling in IPF lung fibroblasts. IPF fibroblasts (< passage 8) isolated from surgical lung biopsy (top panel) or lung transplant patients (middle and lower panels) were serum-starved for 24 hours prior to treatment. In (A) cells were treated with TGF-β (5 ng/ml) for time as shown; (B) cells were treated with TGF-β (5 ng/ml) overnight or left untreated in the presence or absence of indicated inhibitors MLN0128 (0.2 μM), PP242 (2 μM), or rapamycin (Rapa, 0.05 μM), which were added 30 minutes prior to TGF-β. Total cell lysates were prepared and equal amounts of protein were analyzed by Western blot analysis with specific antibodies as indicated. α-tubulin was used as a loading control. Asterisk indicates the carry-over signals between the western blots of α-SMA and SPARC. Band intensity was determined by using Image J software from the NIH. Data was presented as band intensity relative to untreated samples. EDA-FN, extra domain A fibronectin; SPARC, secreted protein acidic and rich in cysteine; α-SMA, α-smooth muscle actin.

[Cayman Chemical, Ann Arbor, MI], 5 U/ml horseradish peroxidase, 1 mM HEPES in Hank's Balanced Salt Solution without phenol red). After a 90 minute incubation, signals were measured with excitation and emission wavelengths at 544 and 590 nm, respectively. H_2O_2 concentrations were calculated by plotting against a standard curve.

Statistical Analysis. Results are expressed as mean ± standard deviation (SD). One-way analysis of variance and the Student's t Test were used for inter-group comparison. A probability level of $p < 0.05$ was considered significant.

Results

Akt is activated by TGF-β and has recently been shown to be a target of mTORC2, so we first examined if TGF-β activates mTORC2 in IPF lung fibroblasts. Rictor is unique to the mTORC2 complex and Raptor to the mTORC1 complex, we looked at the effect of TGF-β on expression of Rictor and/or Raptor- a recent study showed that Rictor is a TGF-β target [23]. We saw that TGF-β induces Rictor in IPF fibroblasts, obtained from patients undergoing surgical lung biopsy (Fig. 1A, upper panel) or lung transplant (Fig. 1A, middle and lower panels). The

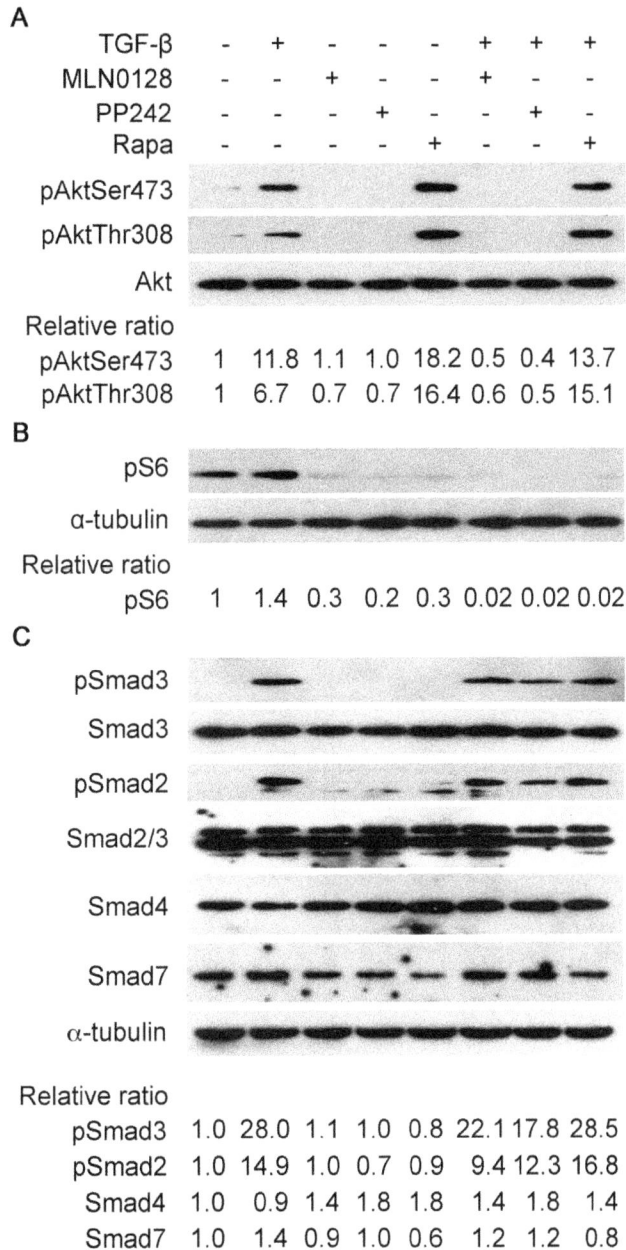

Figure 2. Effect of mTOR inhibitors on TGF-β activation of mTOR and Smad pathways. Serum-deprived IPF fibroblasts were treated with TGF-β for 60 minutes or left untreated in (A), followed by Western blot analysis with anti-phospho Akt (Ser473 or Thr 308) and anti-total Akt antibodies, or in (B) for 6 hours in the presence or absence of indicated inhibitors MLN0128 (0.2 μM), PP242 (2 μM), or rapamycin (0.02 μM), followed by Western blot analysis with anti-phospho-S6 and anti-α-tubulin antibodies. (C) Serum-deprived IPF fibroblasts were treated with or without TGF-β for 15 minutes in the presence or absence of indicated inhibitors followed by Western blot analysis with an anti-phospho-Smad2 or Smad3 antibody. Expression of total Smad-2, 3, 4 and 7 was analyzed by Western blot. Experiment was done on three lines, which are shown in Figure 1; results were similar between the three lines and results from the IPF fibroblasts isolated from surgical lung biopsy are shown here.

induction of Rictor coincided temporally with the activation of Akt (phosphorylation at Ser473); levels of Rictor and Akt activation were maximal at 2–8 h in the transplant lines and at 24 h in the biopsy line (Fig. 1A). Raptor was also induced by TGF-β but the induction did not mirror the activation of S6 kinase, a target of mTORC1. Since Rictor is induced by TGF-β in IPF lung fibroblasts and Akt (Ser473) phosphorylation is an mTORC2 target, we surmised that mTORC2 is a downstream target of TGF-β in IPF fibroblasts; therefore, we turned to examine if blocking mTORC2 inhibits TGF-β-mediated induction of an

activated fibroblast or myofibrolast phenotype, which is characterized by the induction of alpha smooth muscle actin (α-SMA) and matricellular proteins such as fibronectin, type I collagen, and secreted protein acidic and rich in cysteine (SPARC), also known as osteonectin. However, only inhibitors that target the shared active site of mTORC1 and mTORC2 have been developed; we began our initial studies with the mTORC1 and mTORC2 inhibitor, PP242, an active site mTOR inhibitor, and subsequently advanced to MLN0128, which is structurally similar to PP242 but is approximately 10-fold more potent [24]. In the three IPF

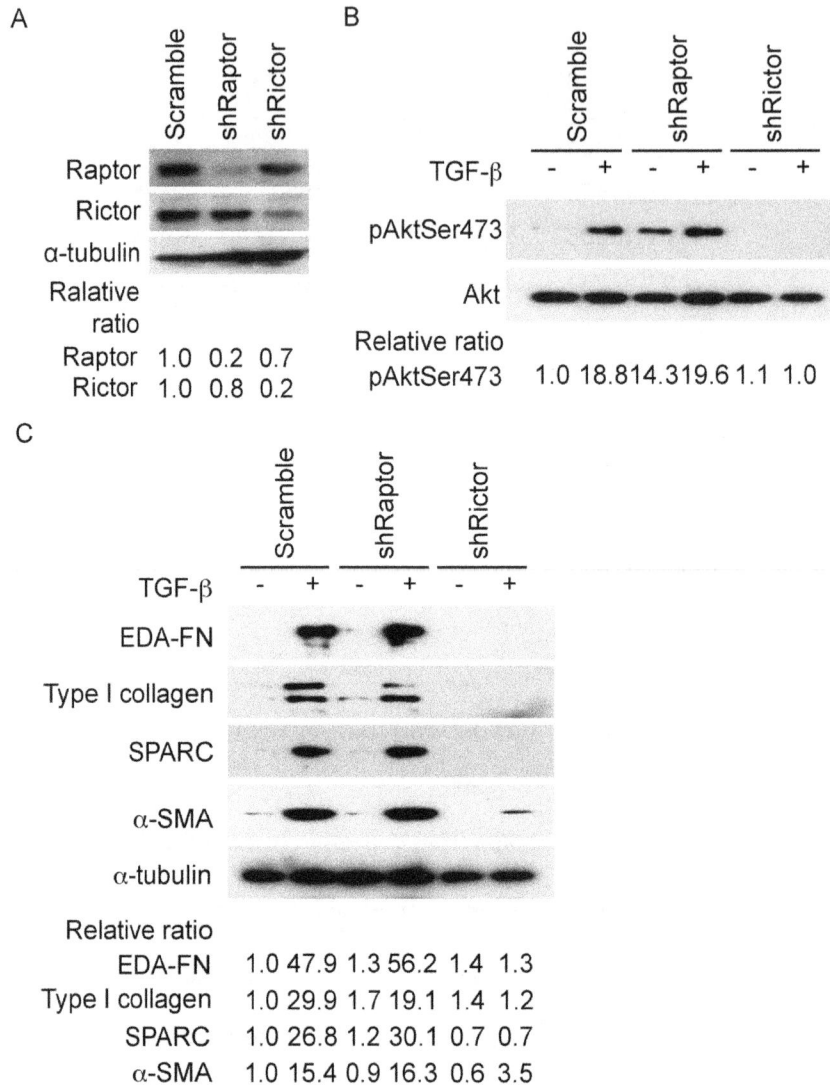

Figure 3. Rictor but not Raptor regulates Akt phosphorylation (Ser473) and the expression of matrix regulatory proteins. In (A) IPF fibroblasts isolated from surgical lung biopsy were infected with lentivirus-derived shRNA against raptor or rictor, or control (scramble) as described in Materials and Methods. Western blot analysis was performed with the indicated antibodies. α-tubulin was used as a loading control. (B) Serum-starved IPF fibroblasts were treated with TGF-β for 60 minutes followed by an analysis of Akt phosphorylation by Western blot analysis. Total Akt was used as a loading control. (C). Serum-deprived IPF fibroblasts were treated overnight with TGF-β followed by analysis of matrix-regulatory proteins by Western blot analysis. α-tubulin was used as a loading control. Experiments with the three IPF lines showed similar results and representative results from the surgical lung biopsy fibroblasts are shown.

fibroblast primary cell lines, we found that PP242 (2.5 μM) and MLN0128 (0.2 μM), but not rapamycin (0.05 μM), suppressed by 50%–80% the basal and TGF-β-inducible expression of type I collagen, the alternatively spliced extra type III domain A fibronectin variant (EDA-FN), α-SMA, and SPARC (Fig. 1B). The selected dose of each inhibitor, i.e., rapamycin, PP242, or MLN0128, mirrors the effective concentration observed in cellular and mouse studies and is in the range of doses being tested in clinical trials [15,16,25,26]. The IC50 of MLN0128 for suppression of stromal proteins by TGF-β is 0.03 μM–0.1 μM (data not shown). Since Akt (Thr308) is a target of PI3K-mediated, PDK1-dependent activation of Akt, we determined if TGF-β also induces phosphorylation of Akt at Thr308 in these cells. We observed that PP242 and MLN0128 blocked TGF-β-induced phosphorylation of Akt at both Ser473 and Thr308, whereas rapamycin caused hyperphosphorylation of Akt (Fig. 2A). All inhibitors blocked the

activation of S6 kinase, i.e., phosphorylation, an mTORC1-dependent target (Fig. 2B). Since the canonical TGF-β pathway involves activation of Smad proteins, we examined if any of the mTOR inhibitors block TGF-β-dependent phosphorylation of Smads. Activation of Smad2 or Smad3 by TGF-β was not affected by PP242, MLN0128, or rapamycin (Fig. 2C). Also, TGF-β did not affect expression of Smad4 or Smad7 in these cells (Fig. 2C).

In order to confirm mTORC2 as a target of TGF-β, we investigated the effect of depleting Rictor or Raptor by RNA interference. Depletion of Rictor, but not Raptor suppressed TGF-β activation of Akt; interestingly, shRaptor increased the basal activation of Akt, (Fig. 3A), similar to what we had observed with rapamycin (Fig. 2A). Moreover, the downregulation of Rictor, but not Raptor, inhibited the expression of markers of activated fibroblasts (Fig. 3B), similar to our observed inhibitory effect of

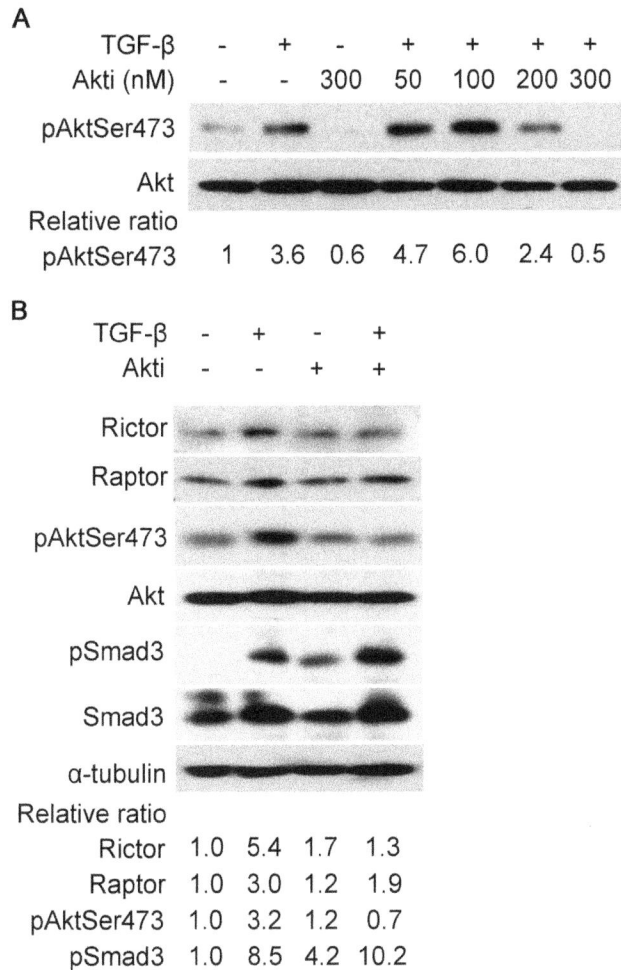

Figure 4. Akt inhibition suppresses induction of Rictor by TGF-β. Serum-starved IPF fibroblasts were pre-treated with Akti (Akt inhibitor VIII/124018) for 30 minutes or left untreated prior to TGF-β (5 ng/ml) treatment for two hours. In (A) cells were pre-treated with Akti at indicated concentration as shown, then followed by TGF-β treatment; (B) cells were pre-treated with Akti at 300 nM prior to TGF-β treatment or left untreated. Total cell lysates were prepared and equal amounts of protein were analyzed by Western blot analysis with specific antibodies as indicated. α-tubulin was used as a loading control.

MLN0128 (Fig. 1B). MLN0128 alone caused a 15%–20% reduction in the viability of IPF lung fibroblasts (Fig. S1).

To ascertain if Rictor induction by TGF-β is mediated by Akt, we applied the specific Akt inhibitor, Akti (Akt inhibitor VIII/124018, Millipore, Billerica, MA). Akti caused a dose-dependent inhibition of Akt activation (Fig. 4A). Also, Akti (300 nM) suppressed Rictor induction by TGF-β; inhibition of Akt, however, did not suppress the induction of Raptor (Fig. 4B).

To explore the anti-fibrotic activity of MLN0128 *in vivo* we examined its effect in the murine lung bleomycin model. MLN0128 was administered as part of a prevention strategy, i.e., treatment initiation on Day −1, one day prior to bleomycin insult, or a delayed therapeutic strategy, i.e., treatment starting at Day 7 after bleomycin (Fig. 5A). We chose intraperitoneal injection for MLN0128, even though it is orally administered in clinical trials with cancer patients, because mice ailing from bleomycin treatment did not tolerate oral gavage with the vehicle routinely used to dissolve MLN0128 (15% polyvinylpyrrolidone K30). An MLN0128 dose of 0.75 mg/kg/d was selected based on its efficacy and lack of toxicity in animal murine cancer models [15,26]. Mice were treated daily (6/7 days) with MLN0128, and sacrificed at Day 14 in the prevention model or at Day 21 in the

therapeutic model, respectively. There was no significant difference in mortality in the bleomcyin control versus MLN0128 treatment group (Fig. 5B). However, body weight significantly improved in MLN0128 treatment groups in both the prevention (Day 14) and therapeutic models (Day 21) (Fig. 5C). In both the prevention and therapeutic models, MLN0128 significantly inhibited bleomycin-induced lung fibrosis (Fig. 6) and collagen content (Fig. 7A); also, MLN0128-treated mice had a significantly lower Ashcroft score (Fig. 7B). Moreover, MLN0128 reduced picosirius red staining, another measure of collagen content (Fig. S2 and Text S1). There was no observable lung toxicity with MLN0128 (Fig. S4).

We then examined the effect of MLN0128 in the prevention model on mRNA expression of known TGF-β responsive genes (Fig. S3 and Text S1). There was no significant increase in Type I collagen, Type III collagen, SPARC, or α-SMA at Day 14 after bleomycin administration (Fig. S3). However, bleomycin caused a significant increase in matrix-regulatory genes, plasminogen activator inhibitor 1 (PAI-1), S100A4, also known as fibroblast specific protein-1 (FSP-1) or metastasin1 (MTS1), and FN gene expression, which were all significantly inhibited by MLN0128 (Fig. S3) [27].

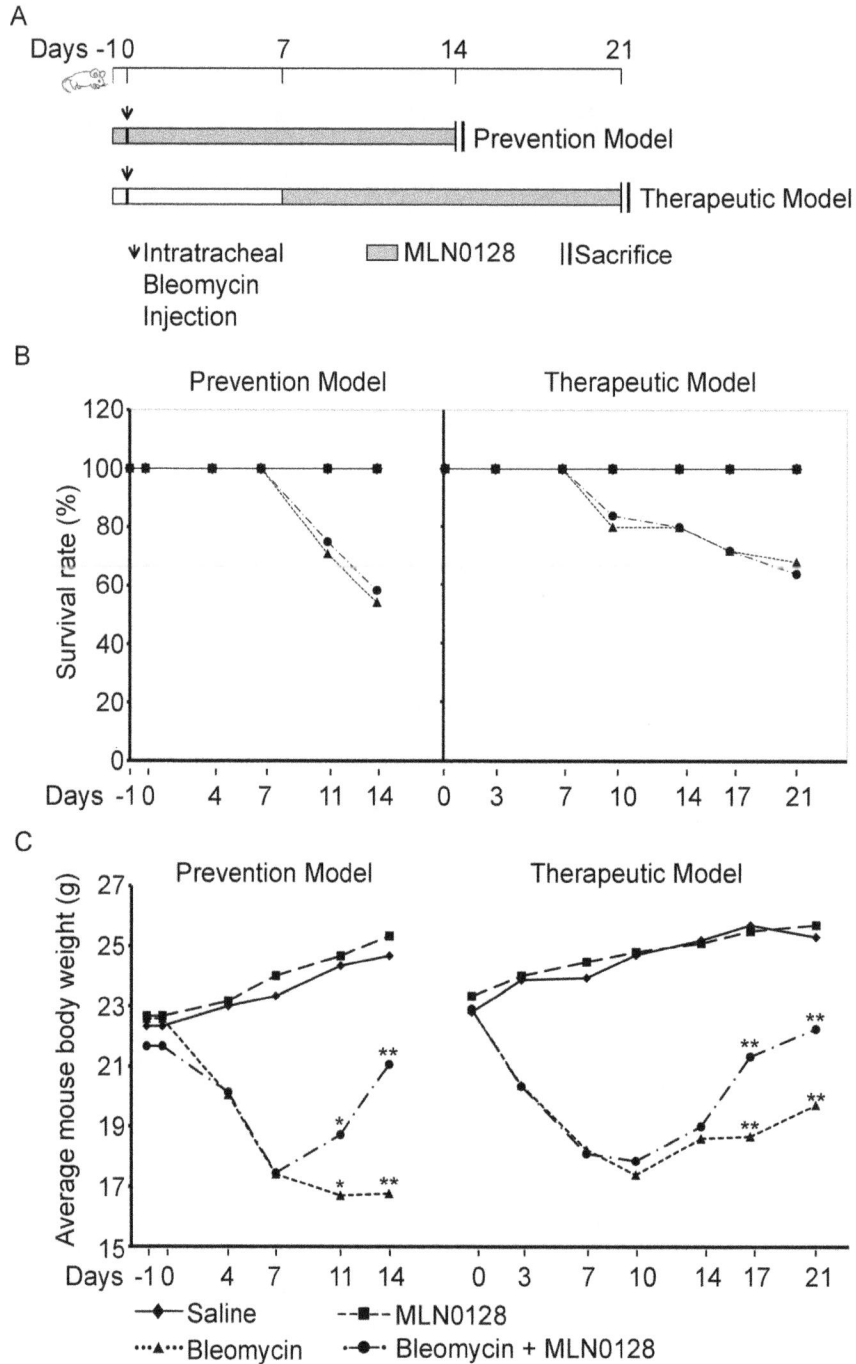

Figure 5. (A) Schematic of bleomycin prevention and therapeutic protocols. (B) Mouse survival rates are from four independent experiments for the prevention model (n = 3 for Saline or MLN groups and n = 6 for Bleo or Bleo + MLN groups) and from five independent experiments for the therapeutic model (n = 3 for Saline or MLN groups, n = 6 for Bleo, and n = 5 for Bleo + MLN groups). (C) Mouse body weights are from bleomycin prevention and therapeutic model experiments (*P<0.05. and **P<0.005) as in (B). Each point represents the mean body weight of mice in the respective treatment group from each experiment.

In IPF fibroblastic foci, it is generally believed that type II alveolar epithelial cells are damaged by activated fibroblasts. It has previously been shown in a Transwell co-culture system that TGF-β-stimulated fibroblasts impair the viability of lung epithelial cells [28]. We utilized this assay to determine if MLN0128 attenuates the TGF-β-mediated reduction in lung epithelial viability. We saw a 25%–30% reduction in lung epithelial viability of A549 or

RLE-6TN cells, which were co-cultured with TGF-β-stimulated IPF lung fibroblasts (Fig. 8A, B). Also, treatment of unstimulated IPF fibroblasts with rapamycin reduced lung epithelial viability in both cell lines and rapamycin did not protect against the reduction in viability by TGF-β (Fig. 8A, B). In contrast, treatment of TGF-β-stimulated IPF fibroblasts with MLN0128 blocked the TGF-β-mediated reduction in epithelial viability (Fig. 8A, B). Using the

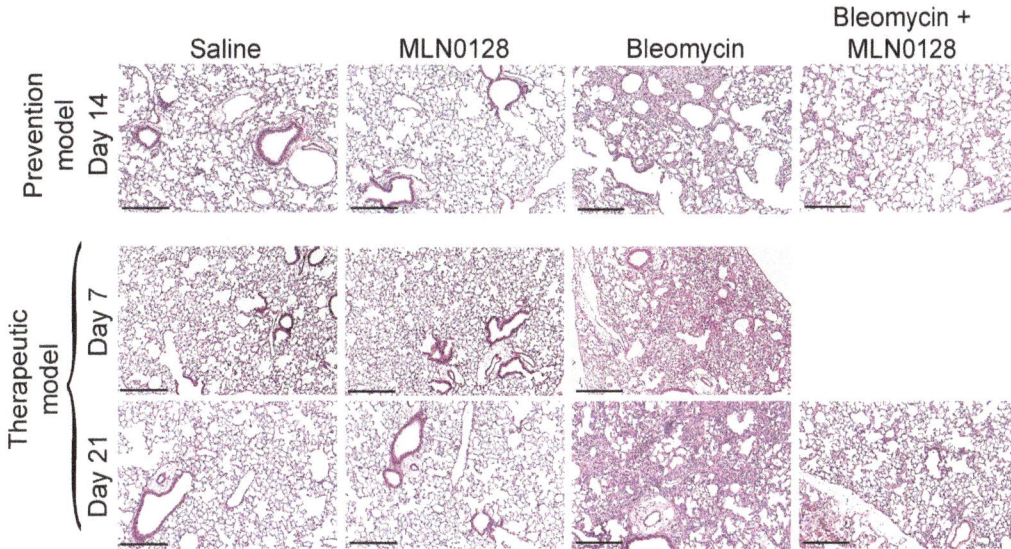

Figure 6. MLN0128 inhibits bleomycin-induced lung fibrosis. Mice were treated according to the schematic shown in Fig. 5A. Mice lungs were harvested at Day 14 (prevention model) or Day 21 (therapeutic model) followed by H&E staining. Scale bar = 100 micron.

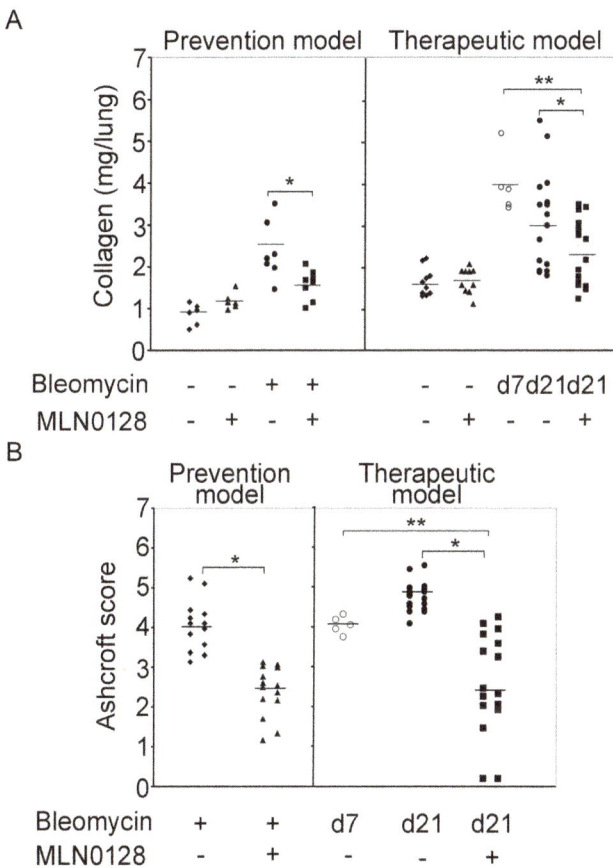

Figure 7. MLN0128 inhibits bleomycin-induced fibrosis. In (A) mice were treated as described in Fig. 5A followed by harvest of the right lung for a Sircoll collagen assay. The horizontal bar represents the mean value of collagen content (mg/lung) for each sample group. *$P<$ 0.05. (B) Analysis of Ashcroft score in left lung of mice from (A); *$P<$ 0.001. Data shown is combined from four independent prevention model and five independent therapeutic model experiments.

Transwell co-culture assay, a recent paper by Shibata, et al, showed that the SPARC secreted by TGF-β-treated normal lung fibroblasts impairs lung epithelial viability [29]. We extended this analysis to IPF fibroblasts, where we depleted SPARC by RNA interference [12]. Downregulation of SPARC almost completely restored A549 or RLE-6TN viability following the TGF-β treatment of IPF fibroblasts (Fig. 8C, D). Since the mTORC2 pathway likely regulates SPARC expression in IPF fibroblasts (Fig. 1B and 3), we examined the effect of downregulation of Rictor in TGF-β-treated IPF lung fibroblasts on lung epithelial viability. Similar to turning down SPARC, the downregulation of Rictor almost completely restored A549 or RLE-6TN viability (Fig. 8C, D).

In the study by Shibata, et al, the authors contend that a SPARC-mediated induction of hydrogen peroxide (H_2O_2) production by lung fibroblasts impaired lung epithelial viability [29]. Since SPARC is a target of the mTORC2 pathway, we examined a role for mTORC2 by adding MLN0128 or by Rictor downregulation in this co-culture system. We found that MLN0128 or Rictor downregulation causes a 90% and 80% reduction in H_2O_2 release respectively ($P<0.05$) (Fig. 9A). Also, the downregulation of SPARC suppressed H_2O_2 production by 95% ($P<0.05$); rapamycin decreased H_2O_2 production by 40% ($P>0.05$) (Fig. 9B).

Discussion

The mTOR pathway has a broad regulatory role in metabolism, cell growth, tumorigenesis, and development. However, until recently, the majority of research and published studies have focused on the rapamycin-sensitive mTORC1 component of the pathway. Once it was revealed that Akt is activated by mTORC2, there have been several recent studies defining functions of mTORC2, which are distinct from mTORC1 [6]. For example, mTORC2 regulates growth factor dependent signaling, glycolysis, and epithelial-mesenchymal transition (EMT) [6]; most recently, a study by Goncharov, et al, showed that mTORC2 regulates the glycolytic pathway and mediates increased proliferation and survival of pulmonary artery vascular smooth muscle cells in Idiopathic Pulmonary Arterial Hypertension (IPAH) [30]. Also,

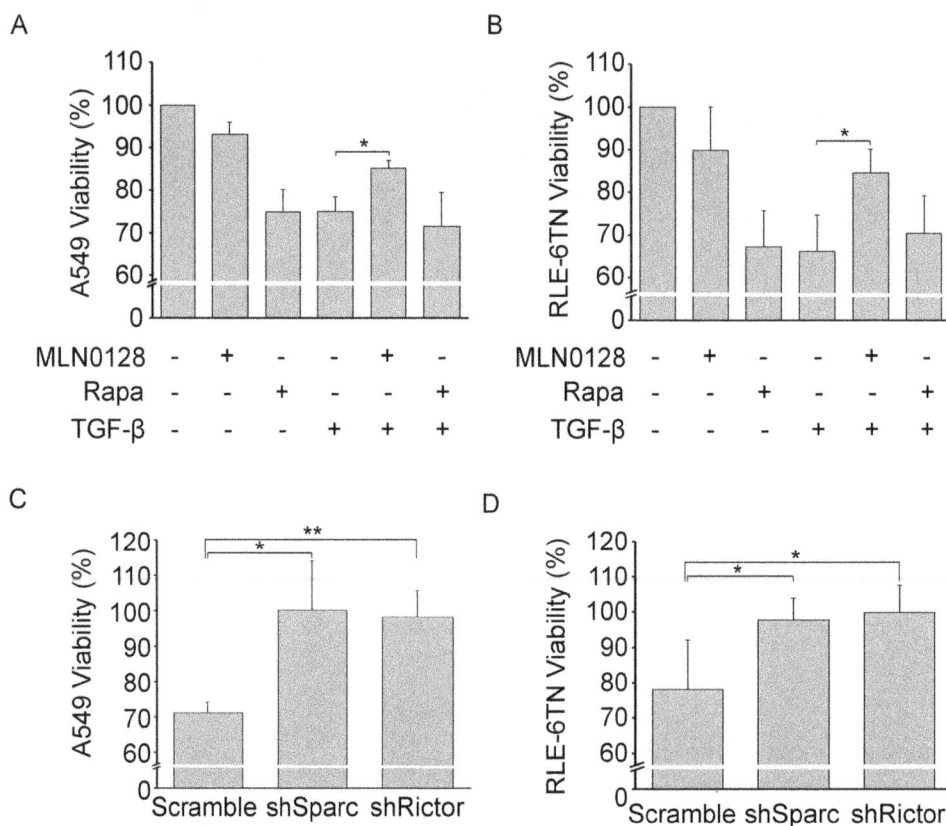

Figure 8. MLN0128 blocks TGF-β-mediated attenuation of lung epithelial cell viability. (A) A transwell culture protocol, as described in detail in Materials and Methods, using IPF fibroblasts co-cultured with A549 cells (*P<0.005) or **(B)** RLE-6TN cells (*P<0.001), which was followed by analysis of A549 or RLE-6TN viability by an Alamar Blue assay. **(C)** Downregulation of SPARC or Rictor in A549 (*P<0.05; **P<0.005) or **(D)** RLE-6TN cells (*P<0.05) by RNA interference in TGF-β-treated IPF fibroblasts was followed by an Alamar Blue assay of A549 or RLE-6TN cells. Data is expressed as mean +/− standard deviation from two IPF fibroblast lines (isolated from surgical lung biopsy and lung transplant) in three independent experiments.

evidence is emerging for both transcriptional and translational regulation of Rictor expression. For example, a study showed that Forkhead box (FoxO) transcription factors induce Rictor expres-sion during oxidative or nutrient stress [31,32]. Also, recent study showed that Rictor is upregulated during S phase of the cell cycle, leading to mTORC2 activation, which is necessary for accurate

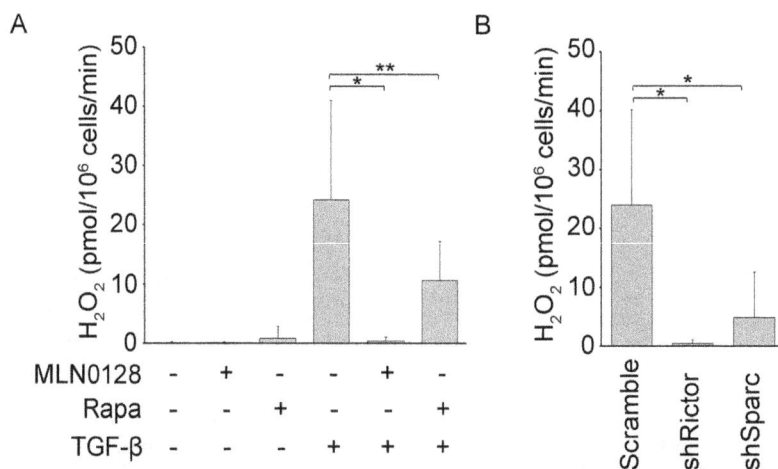

Figure 9. H₂O₂ release from IPF fibroblasts is mediated by SPARC and mTORC2. (A) IPF fibroblasts were treated for 16 h with TGF-β alone or in combination with MLN0128 (0.2 μM) or rapamycin (0.05 μM) followed by measurement of H₂O₂ (*P<0.05, **P>0.05), as described in detail in Materials and Methods. **(B)** SPARC or Rictor was downregulated by RNA interference in TGF-β-treated IPF fibroblasts followed by measurement of H₂O₂; *P<0.05. Data is expressed as mean +/− standard deviation from same two fibroblast lines as in Figure 8, in three independent experiments.

cell cycle progression [33]. A study by Serrrano, I., et al, showed that TGF-β induces Rictor in cancer cells, that was accompanied by formation of an ILK/Rictor complex, which promoted migration and EMT in mammary cancer cells [23]. Interestingly, the late, but not early (up to 2 h), phase of Akt activation (>24 h) was required for EMT. Moreover, downregulation of the MicroRNAs MiR-424 and MiR503 was shown to upregulate Rictor, which promotes colon cancer progression [34]. In the study here, we found that TGF-β induces Rictor in IPF fibroblasts, and its induction coincides with Akt activation. Our results suggest that Rictor upregulation leads to an mTORC2-dependent sustained activation of Akt in IPF fibroblasts. It is possible that this sustained activation is required for regulation of the activated fibroblast, ie, myofibroblast, phenotype.

We targeted mTORC2-dependent activation of Akt with MLN0128, an active site mTOR inhibitor. Other downstream targets of mTORC2 include AGC kinases, such as PKC-δ, which is downstream of lysophosphatidic acid receptor (LPA)-mediated activation of the G protein, $G\alpha_{12}$ [35]. LPA appears to play a significant role in lung fibrosis, in part through its induction of fibroblast migration [36]. However, we did not see activation of PKC-δ by TGF-β in IPF lung fibroblasts, suggesting a more prominent role possibly for inhibition of Akt by active site mTOR inhibitors, not PKC-δ, in the inhibition of fibroblast activation and lung fibrosis.

Interestingly, we observed hyperactivation of Akt with rapamycin- other studies have also found that blocking mTORC1 alone with agents like rapamycin or everolimus can lead to undesirable activation of mTORC2 [37]. This may be an underlying cause why everolimus failed in a clinical trial of IPF patients; also, it may be that activation of mTORC2 by rapamycin or everolimus is involved in the pathogenesis of interstitial pneumonitis, which has been observed in 10%–15% of patients treated with these agents [38]. Finally, active site mTOR inhibitors, through targeting the ATP binding motif in mTOR, are also more active in blocking mTORC1 than rapamycin, which is an allosteric partial inhibitor of mTORC1 [39].

Our data from cultured IPF fibroblasts demonstrate the superiority of active site mTOR inhibitors over rapamycin in suppression of expression of pro-fibrotic matrix regulatory proteins, such as type I collagen, EDA-FN, and SPARC, all of which are targets of TGF-β. We show here that the dual inhibitor MLN0128 significantly inhibits fibrosis in a prevention and therapeutic murine model of bleomycin-induced lung fibrosis. It is arguable whether administration of an inhibitor, such as MLN0128, remotely from bleomycin injury is in fact a "therapeutic" model, but it is administered after the peak of the inflammatory and injury phase and therefore targets the fibrotic phase of repair. A study by Peng, R. et al also suggests that the bleomycin therapeutic model may be a more clinically relevant model of IPF than the prevention model [40]. We did not observe any evidence of lung or systemic toxicity of MLN0128 at the dose of 0.75 mg/kg/d IP, a dose that yields serum levels analogous to those seen in the higher dose ranges currently being tested in Phase I and Phase II cancer clinical trials. This dose was also well tolerated in a murine tuberous sclerosis model, but there was significant weight loss at a higher dose of MLN0128 (1 mg/kg/d) [26]. Identifying potential biomarkers of targeted inhibition by MLN0128 will be important for designing clinical trials in pulmonary fibrosis patients- PAI-1, FN, and S100A4 are potential biomarkers since they are inhibited by MLN0128 in the bleomycin model (Figure S3). Investigating the inhibition of Akt activation in peripheral blood and bronchoalveolar lavage cells (BAL) could be a logical readout of mTORC2 inhibition. In fact, a new Phase I study of a specific PI3K inhibitor in IPF by GlaxoSmithKline proposes to look at Akt activation in platelet-rich plasma and BAL cells as a biomarker of drug activity (ClinicalTrials.gov-NCT1725139).

There is no well-described *in vitro* mimic of the epithelial-fibroblastic crosstalk, which occurs in fibroblastic foci in IPF lung and other fibrotic lung diseases. Injury and depletion of the type II AEC likely contributes to the unrelenting process of dysregulated repair and progressive fibrosis in IPF; however, the precise role of the fibroblast in mediating epithelial injury and its loss is incompletely understood. Since secreted matricellular proteins like PAI-1 and SPARC are expressed by fibroblasts in fibroblastic foci, they are in the perfect biological context in IPF lung to influence lung epithelial cell behavior; therefore, we set out to recapitulate epithelial-fibroblast crosstalk using a compartmentalized Transwell system. Surprisingly, rapamycin alone led to a reduction in epithelial viability suggesting that rapamycin causes the fibroblast to secrete a factor(s) that is harmful to lung epithelium (Fig. 8). Since SPARC is downstream of TGF-β-mediated activation of mTORC2 signal transduction, we speculated that mTORC2 and SPARC plays a role in mediating the protective effect of MLN0128; this was especially likely in that Shibata, S., and Ishiyama, J., recently published that fibroblast-derived SPARC causes a loss of lung epithelial cell viability [29]. In accordance with this, we observed that mTORC2 and SPARC regulate A549 or RLE-6TN lung epithelial viability and their production of H_2O_2- a similar amount of H_2O_2 was shown to damage small airway lung epithelia using the same Transwell model system [29]. These data suggest a possible *in vivo* correlation in IPF: TGF-β induces SPARC production through mTORC2 and Akt activation in IPF fibroblasts, which then activates H_2O_2 production by the fibroblasts, leading to a loss of viability of neighboring type II alveolar epithelial cells.

The failure of multiple clinical trials in IPF of several therapeutic agents has been disheartening; however, two recent trails showed that pirfenidone and nintedanib appeared to slow disease progression in IPF [41,42]. We present an argument for further investigation of the active site mTOR inhibitors, like MLN0128 in IPF based on its pleiotropic effects, which include the inhibition of production of pro-fibrotic proteins by IPF fibroblasts, efficacy in the murine bleomcyin model, and protection of lung epithelium. However, the safety profile of an antiproliferative agent like MLN0128 needs to be carefully examined in the IPF population. An obvious question and concern is whether active site mTOR inhibitors will cause interstitial pneumonitis in humans which has been observed with mTORC1 inhibitors such as rapamycin or everolimus. Even though rapamycin-mediated activation of Akt and mTORC2 may be the culprit, lung toxicity may be due to mTORC1 inhibition, which is a target of both rapamycin and active site mTOR inhibitors. Ideally, an active site mTOR inhibitor or another agent in clinical trials for IPF will not only delay physiologic evidence of disease progression but will also be disease modifying.

Supporting Information

Figure S1 Effect of MLN0128 on viability of IPF fibroblasts. Serum-starved IPF fibroblasts were treated with TGF-β (5 ng/ml) for overnight or left untreated in the presence or absence of MLN0128 (0.2 μM), followed by an Alamar Blue assay. The results from untreated or TGF-β treated samples are set as the maximal growth (100%), and the effects of MLN0128 are presented as relative percentage change. Results are presented as mean +/− standard deviation from three IPF fibroblast lines (*P< 0.001).

Figure S2   MLN0128 inhibits collagen expression in the bleomycin lung therapeutic model. H&E and Picrosirus Red staining of formalin fixed paraffin-embedded lung section harvested at Day 21 after the treatments is shown. The quantification of bleomycin vs. bleomycin + MLN0128 yielded the color difference of 9.05% vs. 3.37%, respectively from an analysis by Image J software from the NIH. Scale bar = 100 micron.

Figure S3   Effect of MLN0128 on gene expression in the bleomycin model. Expression of several matrix-regulatory genes was examined by harvesting RNA from right lung at Day 14 of bleomycin prevention model followed by analysis of genes indicated by reverse transcriptase reaction and quantitative PCR (n = 4–6 mice per group; *P<0.05, **P<0.005). Results are

presented as mean +/− standard deviation, and are combined from four independent experiments. α-SMA, α-smooth muscle actin; COL1a, collagen Ia; COL3a, collagen IIIa.

Figure S4   Effect of MLNO128 on mouse lung. H&E staining of formalin fixed paraffin embedded lung section harvested at Day 7 and 14 after the treatments in the prevention model was shown. Scale bar = 100 micron.

Author Contributions

Conceived and designed the experiments: WC GDR. Performed the experiments: WC KW GJB CHC. Analyzed the data: WC KW LH GJB GDR. Contributed reagents/materials/analysis tools: SSJ GJB. Wrote the paper: WC GDR. IRB Approval and Informed Consent: SSJ.

References

1. Zisman DA, Keane MP, Belperio JA, Strieter RM, Lynch JP 3rd (2005) Pulmonary fibrosis. Methods Mol Med 117: 3–44.
2. Ask K, Martin GE, Kolb M, Gauldie J (2006) Targeting genes for treatment in idiopathic pulmonary fibrosis: challenges and opportunities, promises and pitfalls. Proceedings of the American Thoracic Society 3: 389–393.
3. Moritz A, Li Y, Guo A, Villen J, Wang Y, et al. (2010) Akt-RSK-S6 kinase signaling networks activated by oncogenic receptor tyrosine kinases. Sci Signal 3: ra64.
4. Gibbons JJ, Abraham RT, Yu K (2009) Mammalian target of rapamycin: discovery of rapamycin reveals a signaling pathway important for normal and cancer cell growth. Semin Oncol 36 Suppl 3: S3–S17.
5. Bhagwat SV, Crew AP (2010) Novel inhibitors of mTORC1 and mTORC2. Curr Opin Investig Drugs 11: 638–645.
6. Oh WJ, Jacinto E (2011) mTOR complex 2 signaling and functions. Cell Cycle 10: 2305–2316.
7. Proud CG (2009) mTORC1 signalling and mRNA translation. Biochem Soc Trans 37: 227–231.
8. Sarbassov DD, Ali SM, Sengupta S, Sheen JH, Hsu PP, et al. (2006) Prolonged rapamycin treatment inhibits mTORC2 assembly and Akt/PKB. Mol Cell 22: 159–168.
9. Li Y, Wang X, Yue P, Tao H, Ramalingam SS, et al. (2013) Protein phosphatase 2A and DNA-dependent protein kinase are involved in mediating rapamycin-induced Akt phosphorylation. The Journal of biological chemistry.
10. Malouf MA, Hopkins P, Snell G, Glanville AR (2011) An investigator-driven study of everolimus in surgical lung biopsy confirmed idiopathic pulmonary fibrosis. Respirology 16: 776–783.
11. Sarbassov DD, Guertin DA, Ali SM, Sabatini DM (2005) Phosphorylation and regulation of Akt/PKB by the rictor-mTOR complex. Science 307: 1098–1101.
12. Chang W, Wei K, Jacobs SS, Upadhyay D, Weill D, et al. (2010) SPARC suppresses apoptosis of idiopathic pulmonary fibrosis fibroblasts through constitutive activation of beta-catenin. The Journal of biological chemistry 285: 8196–8206.
13. Xia H, Khalil W, Kahm J, Jessurun J, Kleidon J, et al. (2010) Pathologic caveolin-1 regulation of PTEN in idiopathic pulmonary fibrosis. Am J Pathol 176: 2626–2637.
14. Huang SK, White ES, Wettlaufer SH, Grifka H, Hogaboam CM, et al. (2009) Prostaglandin E2 induces fibroblast apoptosis by modulating multiple survival pathways. FASEB J.
15. Janes MR, Vu C, Mallya S, Shieh MP, Limon JJ, et al. (2013) Efficacy of the investigational mTOR kinase inhibitor MLN0128/INK128 in models of B-cell acute lymphoblastic leukemia. Leukemia 27: 586–594.
16. Gokmen-Polar Y, Liu Y, Toroni RA, Sanders KL, Mehta R, et al. (2012) Investigational drug MLN0128, a novel TORC1/2 inhibitor, demonstrates potent oral antitumor activity in human breast cancer xenograft models. Breast Cancer Res Treat 136: 673–682.
17. Wilson-Edell KA, Yevtushenko MA, Rothschild DE, Rogers AN, Benz CC (2014) mTORC1/C2 and pan-HDAC inhibitors synergistically impair breast cancer growth by convergent AKT and polysome inhibiting mechanisms. Breast Cancer Res Treat 144: 287–298.
18. Chang WT, Kang JJ, Lee KY, Wei K, Anderson E, et al. (2001) Triptolide and chemotherapy cooperate in tumor cell apoptosis. A role for the p53 pathway. J Biol Chem 276: 2221–2227.
19. Krishna G, Liu K, Shigemitsu H, Gao M, Raffin TA, et al. (2001) PG490-88, a derivative of triptolide, blocks bleomycin-induced lung fibrosis. Am J Pathol 158: 997–1004.
20. Ashcroft T, Simpson JM, Timbrell V (1988) Simple method of estimating severity of pulmonary fibrosis on a numerical scale. J Clin Pathol 41: 467–470.
21. Ahmed SA, Gogal RM, Jr., Walsh JE (1994) A new rapid and simple non-radioactive assay to monitor and determine the proliferation of lymphocytes: an alternative to [3H]thymidine incorporation assay. Journal of immunological methods 170: 211–224.
22. Zhou M, Diwu Z, Panchuk-Voloshina N, Haugland RP (1997) A stable nonfluorescent derivative of resorufin for the fluorometric determination of trace hydrogen peroxide: applications in detecting the activity of phagocyte NADPH oxidase and other oxidases. Analytical biochemistry 253: 162–168.
23. Serrano I, McDonald PC, Lock FE, Dedhar S (2013) Role of the integrin-linked kinase (ILK)/Rictor complex in TGFbeta-1-induced epithelial-mesenchymal transition (EMT). Oncogene 32: 50–60.
24. Richard DJ, Verheijen JC, Zask A (2010) Recent advances in the development of selective, ATP-competitive inhibitors of mTOR. Curr Opin Drug Discov Devel 13: 428–440.
25. Janes MR, Limon JJ, So L, Chen J, Lim RJ, et al. Effective and selective targeting of leukemia cells using a TORC1/2 kinase inhibitor. Nat Med 16: 205–213.
26. Guo Y, Kwiatkowski DJ (2013) Equivalent benefit of rapamycin and a potent mTOR ATP-competitive inhibitor, MLN0128 (INK128), in a mouse model of tuberous sclerosis. Molecular cancer research: MCR.
27. Pandit KV, Corcoran D, Yousef H, Yarlagadda M, Tzouvelekis A, et al. (2010) Inhibition and role of let-7d in idiopathic pulmonary fibrosis. American journal of respiratory and critical care medicine 182: 220–229.
28. Waghray M, Cui Z, Horowitz JC, Subramanian IM, Martinez FJ, et al. (2005) Hydrogen peroxide is a diffusible paracrine signal for the induction of epithelial cell death by activated myofibroblasts. FASEB J 19: 854–856.
29. Shibata S, Ishiyama J (2013) Secreted protein acidic and rich in cysteine (SPARC) is upregulated by transforming growth factor (TGF)-beta and is required for TGF-beta-induced hydrogen peroxide production in fibroblasts. Fibrogenesis & tissue repair 6: 6.
30. Goncharov DA, Kudryashova TV, Ziai H, Ihida-Stansbury K, Delisser H, et al. (2013) mTORC2 Coordinates Pulmonary Artery Smooth Muscle Cell Metabolism, Proliferation and Survival in Pulmonary Arterial Hypertension. Circulation.
31. Guertin DA, Stevens DM, Thoreen CC, Burds AA, Kalaany NY, et al. (2006) Ablation in mice of the mTORC components raptor, rictor, or mLST8 reveals that mTORC2 is required for signaling to Akt-FOXO and PKCalpha, but not S6K1. Dev Cell 11: 859–871.
32. Chen CC, Jeon SM, Bhaskar PT, Nogueira V, Sundararajan D, et al. (2010) FoxOs inhibit mTORC1 and activate Akt by inducing the expression of Sestrin3 and Rictor. Dev Cell 18: 592–604.
33. Stumpf CR, Moreno MV, Olshen AB, Taylor BS, Ruggero D (2013) The translational landscape of the Mammalian cell cycle. Mol Cell 52: 574–582.
34. Oneyama C, Kito Y, Asai R, Ikeda J, Yoshida T, et al. (2013) MiR-424/503-Mediated Rictor Upregulation Promotes Tumor Progression. PLoS One 8: e80300.
35. Gan X, Wang J, Wang C, Sommer E, Kozasa T, et al. (2012) PRR5L degradation promotes mTORC2-mediated PKC-delta phosphorylation and cell migration downstream of Galpha12. Nature cell biology 14: 686–696.
36. Tager AM, LaCamera P, Shea BS, Campanella GS, Selman M, et al. (2008) The lysophosphatidic acid receptor LPA1 links pulmonary fibrosis to lung injury by mediating fibroblast recruitment and vascular leak. Nature medicine 14: 45–54.

37. Rodriguez-Pascual J, Cheng E, Maroto P, Duran I (2010) Emergent toxicities associated with the use of mTOR inhibitors in patients with advanced renal carcinoma. Anticancer Drugs 21: 478–486.

38. Lee HS, Huh KH, Kim YS, Kim MS, Kim HJ, et al. (2012) Sirolimus-induced pneumonitis after renal transplantation: a single-center experience. Transplantation proceedings 44: 161–163.

39. Syed F, Sherris D, Paus R, Varmeh S, Pandolfi PP, et al. (2012) Keloid disease can be inhibited by antagonizing excessive mTOR signaling with a novel dual TORC1/2 inhibitor. The American journal of pathology 181: 1642–1658.

40. Peng R, Sridhar S, Tyagi G, Phillips JE, Garrido R, et al. (2013) Bleomycin induces molecular changes directly relevant to idiopathic pulmonary fibrosis: a model for "active" disease. PLoS ONE 8: e59348.

41. King TE, Jr., Bradford WZ, Castro-Bernardini S, Fagan EA, Glaspole I, et al. (2014) A phase 3 trial of pirfenidone in patients with idiopathic pulmonary fibrosis. N Engl J Med 370: 2083–2092.

42. Richeldi L, du Bois RM, Raghu G, Azuma A, Brown KK, et al. (2014) Efficacy and safety of nintedanib in idiopathic pulmonary fibrosis. N Engl J Med 370: 2071–2082.

7

Conventional vs. Tablet Computer-Based Patient Education following Lung Transplantation – A Randomized Controlled Trial

Hendrik Suhling[1]*, Jessica Rademacher[1], Imke Zinowsky[1], Jan Fuge[1], Mark Greer[1], Gregor Warnecke[2], Jacqueline M. Smits[3], Anna Bertram[4], Axel Haverich[2], Tobias Welte[1], Jens Gottlieb[1]

1 Dept. of Respiratory Medicine, Hannover Medical School, Hannover, Germany, 2 Dept. of Cardiothoracic, Transplantation and Vascular Surgery, Hannover Medical School, Hannover, Germany, 3 Eurotransplant International Foundation, Leiden, The Netherlands, 4 Dept. of Nephrology and Hypertension, Hannover Medical School, Hannover, Germany

Abstract

Background: Accurate immunosuppression is of critical importance in preventing rejection, while avoiding toxicity following lung transplantation. The mainstay immunosuppressants are calcineurin inhibitors, which require regular monitoring due to interactions with other medications and diet. Adherence to immunosuppression and patient knowledge is vital and can be improved through patient education. Education using tablet-computers was investigated.

Objective: To compare tablet-PC education and conventional education in improving immunosuppression trough levels in target range 6 months after a single education. Secondary parameters were ratio of immunosuppression level measurements divided by per protocol recommended measurements, time and patient satisfaction regarding education.

Design: Single-centre, open labelled randomised controlled trial.

Participants: Patients >6 months after lung-transplantation with <50% of calcineurin inhibitor trough levels in target range.

Intervention: Tablet-pc education versus personal, nurse-led education.

Measurements: Calcineurin inhibitor levels in target range 6 months after education, level variability, interval adherence, knowledge and adherence was studied. As outcome parameter, renal function was measured and adverse events registered.

Results: Sixty-four patients were 1:1 randomised for either intervention. Levels of immunosuppression 6 months after education were equal (tablet-PC 58% vs. conventional 48%, p = 0.27), both groups improved in achieving a CNI trough level within target range by either education method (delta tablet-PC 29% vs. conventional 20%). In all patients, level variability decreased (−20.4%), whereas interval adherence remained unchanged. Knowledge about immunosuppression improved by 7% and compliance tests demonstrated universal improvements with no significant difference between groups.

Conclusion: Education is a simple, effective tool in improving adherence to immunosuppression. Tablet-PC education was non-inferior to conventional education.

Trial Registration: ClinicalTrials.gov NCT01398488 http://clinicaltrials.gov/ct2/show/NCT01398488?term = gottlieb+tablet+pc+education&rank = 1.

Editor: Aric Gregson, University of California Los Angeles, United States of America

Funding: The authors have no support or funding to report.

Competing Interests: The authors have declared that no competing interests exist.

* E-mail: suhling.hendrik@mh-hannover.de

Introduction

It has been previously demonstrated in a variety of chronic diseases that non-adherence to medication and other forms of treatment is a major problem [1], which may impact on long-term outcomes [2,3]. Numerous reasons for non-adherence have been reported, including insufficient information, anxiety of side-effects, treatment cost, forgetfulness and lack of perceived benefit [4]. Patient education and awareness is considered pivotal in improving adherence, with various concepts having already been developed to address this [5,6]. Patient educational needs vary greatly depending on their underlying condition, with diseases demanding precise medication dosing (diabetes mellitus) or modifications in health-related behaviour (COPD) appearing to profit most from educational programs [7–10].

Following organ transplantation, patients require highly complex treatment regimes based on various immunosuppressant drugs that have small therapeutic ranges and profound side-effect profiles [11]. Sub-therapeutic immunosuppression remains a leading cause of allograft rejection, graft loss, and death [12]. Indirectly it is associated with decreased quality of life and inevitably increased health care costs. Previous studies have demonstrated non-adherence rates in calcineurin inhibitors (CNI) ranging between 13 and 22% [13]. Non-adherence increases over time after transplantation [13,14].

Conventional patient-education requires a trained specialist, a suitable location and is time-intensive [15]. Computer-based patient education has been attempted, with reports suggesting that it can provide a more cost-effective method of educating patients [16]. Tablet-PCs, with their user-friendly interfaces and large screens improve simplicity and can be handled even by chronically ill or elderly patients. This study investigated whether tablet-PC education could improve immunosuppression adherence amongst lung transplant recipients compared to conventional education strategies.

Materials and Methods

Study design and patient collective

A prospective randomized open labelled control trial was undertaken at a single university centre (Hannover Medical School, Germany), comparing tablet–PC to conventional patient education. Patient recruitment occurred between August 2011 and July 2012. After inclusion, patients first answered a questionnaire assessing their understanding of the various important aspects related to CNI treatment (further described below), before being randomized 1:1 into either of the 2 education groups. At the same visit, patients then participated either in self-directed tablet-PC education or were counselled by a trained nurse (I.Z.). Both education content was identical. Six months later they completed the initial questionnaire for a second time.

Follow-up was 6 months after start of the education (Figure 1).

All patients provided written informed consent. The study was approved by the Internal Review Board of the Hannover Medical School (No. 1019–2011) and registered under clinicaltrials.gov, No. NCT01398488.

Inclusion and exclusion criteria

All patients aged ≥18 years, who had undergone a single, double or heart-lung-transplantation ≥6 months and who regularly participated in our post-transplantation surveillance program were screened for eligibility. Our program provides exclusive centralized monitoring of calcineurin inhibitors (CNI) for all patients at our central lab. Local physicians mail patient blood samples at specified intervals for analysis. To qualify for study participation, patients required a minimum of 10 CNI trough levels in the preceding 6 months, of which less than 50% were in the target range. Patients who were hospitalized during the previous 3 months, who had advanced chronic lung allograft dysfunction (stage 3), chronic kidney disease K/DOQI stage V (eGFR <15 ml/min/1.73 m^2), oxygen requirement at rest or pulsed steroids in the previous 4 weeks (>500 mg methylprednisolone per day) were excluded. Illiteracy, limited German language skills, need for isolation (multi- or pan-resistant organisms) or other factors limiting patient communication or computer handling were considered additional exclusion criteria.

Immunosuppression

Standard maintenance immunosuppression consisted of a triple drug regimen including CNI, prednisolone and mycophenolate mofetil [17]. Ciclosporine A (CSA) was the 1st line CNI, with exception of combined-organ recipients who received tacrolimus. Patients with recurrent or steroid-resistant rejection episodes or CSA intolerance were switched to tacrolimus. Target CSA trough levels, as measured by liquid chromatography were 180 ng/ml (0–6 months), 140 ng/ml (6–12 months), 100 ng/ml (12–24 months) and 60 ng/ml (>24 months). A target range of ±20 ng/ml was defined. Target trough levels for tacrolimus were 12 ng/ml (0–6 months), 10 ng/ml (6–12 months), 8 ng/ml (12–24 months) and 6 ng/ml (>24 months). A target range of ±2 ng/ml was defined for tacrolimus. Patients demonstrating variable trough levels were required to send control samples every 1–2 weeks. Levels out of target range were re-checked after 1 week following dose adjustment. In stable patients, control intervals were gradually lengthened to a maximum of every 4 weeks.

Intervention: Education materials and education content

Educational material was devised by lung-transplant specialists (J.G., H.S), and paper- and computer-based presentations of identical content were designed (J.F.). Content differed slightly depending on whether patients were receiving cyclosporine or tacrolimus, necessitating two sets of educational aids. An iPad (Apple Inc., second generation) was used in the tablet-pc group for education. A Keynote presentation (Apple Inc.) consisting of 30 slides and 4 video clips totalling 12:45 min were included. Patients unfamiliar with using an iPad received short instruction before commencing their tutorial. In the conventional group, a trained nurse-specialist (I.Z.) using the designated written material provided patient instruction.

Educational content comprised of highlighting the importance of regular medication and side-effects (e.g. rejection or infection) and subsequently provided practical tips on how to achieve stable drug levels (Table S1). Incorporated video clips emphasized evidence for immunosuppression and the importance of ongoing adherence. This included a patient explaining regular CNI intake, another illustrating correct storage of immunosuppressive drugs and one explaining common causes of variation in drug levels (Figure S1).

All patients received a single page summary sheet to take home and were encouraged to ask further questions during follow-up.

The iPads were cleaned between patients according to standard recommendations obtained from the deBac-App (available via iTunes, PLRI MedAppLab, Hannover). All software used was regularly updated to latest versions.

Outcome measurement

Primary objective was percentage of immunosuppression levels in target range 6 months after education and the comparison between the table-pc and the conventional education group. Secondary objectives were interval adherence, which is defined as the number of measurements in which the target level is reached out of the total number of measurements and time required completing the questionnaire and documentation. The glomerular filtration rate before inclusion and at 6 months was compared and adverse events, hospitalisation, rejection or infection were monitored (Table 1).

Questionnaires for medication intake adherence

To assess patient medication intake adherence, all participants completed the Basel assessment of adherence with immunosup-

A

B

C

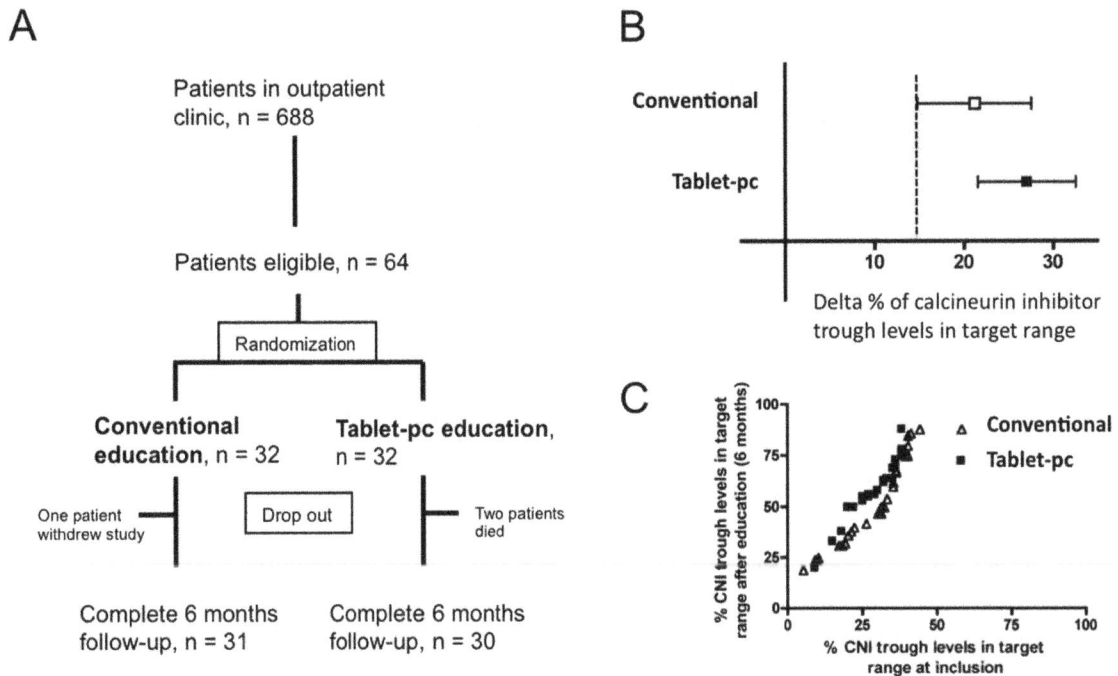

Figure 1. Flow chart of inclusion and improvement of immunosuppression. Flow chart of inclusion (**A**). Delta % of calcineurin inhibitor trough levels in target range 6 months after patient education compared to 6 months before patient education (**B**). Dashed line marks cut-off of non-inferiority (lower 95% CI of conventional group, p = 0.17). Visualization of calcineurin inhibitor levels at inclusion (x-axis) and after 6 months (y-axis) (**C**).

pressive medication scales (BAASIS) [18–20], the immunosuppressant therapy adherence barrier instrument (ITBS) [21] and the Morisky Score [22]. The BAASIS questionnaire included 4 questions (0–4 points) evaluating missed CNI consumption in the last 4 weeks, consecutive occasions were CNI medication was missed, delays of ≥2 hours in CNI consumption and autonomous CNI dose alteration. The Morisky score has been described previously (0–4 points) [22]. Higher scores in all tests correlated with better adherence. The ITBS examines 13 items using a

Likert-type scale (1 = 'strongly disagree' to 5 = 'strongly agree') as previously described [21].

Physicians' valuation of adherence

Physicians independently ranked patient adherence in five categories, including drug levels, physical fitness, communication with the transplantation centre, completion of daily home-spirometry and general health awareness. Good, moderate and bad adherence was differentiated.

Table 1. End points.

Primary endpoint:
Percentage of calcineurin inhibitor trough levels in target range 6 months after patient education
Secondary endpoints:
Improvement of percentage of calcineurin inhibitor trough levels in target range (Delta %) of the next 10 measurements after patient education compared to the last 10 measurements before patient education
Trough level variability 6 months after patient education compared to 6 months before patient education
Number of immunosuppression level measurements vs. recommended measurements
Total time of education
Total time of answering questionnaire
Improvement of patient knowledge on immunosuppressive after patient education
Patient satisfaction
Self rated adherence to immunosuppressive medication (BAASIS scale)
Therapy adherence 6 months after patient education compared to 6 months before patient education
Glomerular filtration rate 6 months after patient education compared to baseline

Questions evaluating satisfaction and knowledge

Questions relating to patient satisfaction regarding educational training and questionnaire satisfaction were also incorporated. Knowledge pertaining to immunosuppressant medication was assessed using 20 yes/no questions derived directly from the educational material. Knowledge was rated to be 0–100%.

The questionnaire was completed either electronically via tablet-PC or in written form and was provided before education and 6 months subsequently.

Tablet-PC usage and link to local database

Patients in the tablet-PC group could use an AluPen (Just mobile, Germany) for data entry. Questionnaires were completed using FileMaker Go (v. 11, FileMaker Inc., USA) installed on the iPads, with data being transferred via WiFi in real time to a study database in FileMaker Pro 10 Server hosted on the local intranet.

Methods against bias

All patients attending our outpatient clinic were screened for eligibility. Blinding was not undertaken. Randomisation involved an allocation sequence using numbered containers (created by J.F. using www.random.org), with patients being assigned to groups based on their inclusion number. Stratification was performed for cystic fibrosis (CF) patients due to comparatively younger age (median 27 years vs. 55 years for other diagnoses) to minimize bias due to better computer literacy among younger patients as well as their increased susceptibility to variable drug absorption that can profoundly influence drug pharmacokinetics, leading to greater fluctuation in trough levels [23].

Statistical analysis

Our calculations indicated that a cohort of 62 patients was required to achieve statistical power of 95% in detecting a 20% difference therapeutic trough-levels between both groups. This estimation of improvement was derived from previous studies. All continuous variables are presented as median with inter-quartile ranges (25% and 75%). Likert-scales with less than 5 points (satisfaction and Morisky Score) were expressed as mean ± standard deviation. Variables were compared between the groups using student's t-test (Table 2 and 3 for numeric data) or non-parametric testing (Mann-Whitney U) (Table 4) in cases of non-normal distribution. Categorical variables were compared between the groups using the chi-square test. All reported P values are two-sided and the level of significance was set at $p<0.05$.

Results

Sixty-four patients were enrolled between 5.8.2011 and 15.5.2012, with 32 patients being randomly assigned to each group. Three patients did not complete the study: two died and one withdrew from study. In total, 30 patients completed the study in the tablet-PC and 31 in the conventional group. Patient characteristics were similar between the groups (Table 2).

Endpoint outcomes

Primary endpoint: there was no difference between the groups in regard to levels of immunosuppression in target range after 6 months ($p = 0.27$), see Table 3.

Following any educational intervention, significant improvements of immunosuppression levels in target range (31% to 55%; $p<0.001$) were observed. Absolute improvement in percentage of calcineurin inhibitor trough levels ($\Delta\%$) in target range in the 6 months before and after patient education showed no significant difference in a two-sided t-test between the groups. Overall, a 26% absolute improvement of CNI levels in target range was observed, with an interesting trend towards better performance in the tablet-PC group (20% vs. 29%, $p = 0.17$). Secondary end-points are displayed in Table 3.

Knowledge and renal function

There was no difference between groups and between time-points for renal function or knowledge (Table 3 and 4).

Self-reported and measured adherence

Results from questionnaires relating to adherence revealed no differences between inclusion and at 6 months in either group.

Three patients reported drug holidays in the preceding 4 weeks but no autonomous changes in dosage (BAASIS questionnaire). On 15 occasions prior to education, CNI intake fell outside the recommended 2-hour window, with no differences observed between groups. Following training only six patients admitted this. In ITBS, 3 patients reported that they could hardly remember taking their CNI although all knew when they should take them. Two patients reported problems correctly timed CNI dosing resulting from changes in daily schedule.

Physicians' judgment of adherence

Physicians rated most patients as adherent at inclusion (Table 1). There was no significant improvement after 6 months ($p = 0.5$) and no intergroup differences were observed.

Evaluation of tablet-PC usage

All patients participating in tablet-PC training successfully completed both the tutorial and the questionnaire. All patients rated training with the tablet-PC as good.

Sub-group analysis

All study participants considered themselves treatment-adherent at the time of inclusion despite poor performance in achieving therapeutic trough-levels. We, therefore, examined the influence of knowledge levels at inclusion on drug level improvement (cut-off <80% knowledge corresponding to median). Low knowledge levels with regard to immunosuppression were identified in 24 patients. Analysis however revealed no significant differences in improvement in these patients compared to the remainder of the cohort (29% vs. 23% respectively; $p = 0.39$).

Patients rated as moderately or poorly adherent exhibited significantly lower knowledge levels ($p = 0.01$). Fifteen patients judged as non-adherent at inclusion displayed smaller improvements in therapeutic CNI levels compared to patients with good adherence (23% vs. 29% respectively; $p = 0.38$). Patients demonstrating poor existing knowledge and non-adherence ($n = 10$) displayed no difference in drug-level improvements based on education received ($p = 0.3$).

Existing level of knowledge influenced the time needed to complete the questionnaire (low knowledge: median 20 min (IQR 16–28), good knowledge: 17 min (IQR 14–20); $p = 0.005$), but not the duration of education (low knowledge: median 26 min (IQR 23–31), good knowledge: median 25 min (IQR 21–28); $p = 0.3$).

Hospitalization, rejection and infection during follow-up

Two patients died during follow-up, with both being in the tablet-PC group. Causes of death were lymphoma and myocardial infarction. Eight patients were hospitalized during follow-up (1 tablet-PC and 7 conventional education; $p = 0.05$), due to progression in chronic rejection ($n = 2$), infection ($n = 3$), oesophageal biopsy ($n = 1$) and vascular prosthesis ($n = 1$). Seventeen

Table 2. Demographics.

Variable	Subgroup	All patients, n = 64	Tablet-pc group, n = 32	Conventional group, n = 32	Significance
FEV1% baseline (%)		93 (84; 97)	93 (82; 97)	93.5 (88.3; 96.8)	0.4
Grade of chronic rejection (BOS grade)	0	52 (82.5)	24 (78)	28 (88)	0.34
	1	11 (17.5)	7 (22)	4 (12)	
Underlying disease, n (%)	Cystic fibrosis	22 (34)	9 (28)	13 (41)	0.8
	Pulmonary fibrosis	12 (19)	7 (22)	5 (16)	
	Emphysema	5 (8)	2 (6)	3 (9)	
	Pulm. Hypertension	7 (11)	4 (12)	3 (9)	
	other	18 (28)	10 (32)	8 (25)	
Transplantation, n (%)	Single lung-transplantation	2 (3)	1 (3)	1 (3)	0.75
	double lung transplantation	62 (97)	31 (97)	31 (97)	
Age, years		47 (34; 57)	52 (35.9; 57.6)	45 (33.3; 53.9)	0.18
Immunosuppression n (%)	Cyclosporine	36 (56)	19 (59)	17 (53)	0.8
	Tacrolimus	28 (44)	13 (41)	15 (47)	
Baseline adherence judged by physician at inclusion, n (%)	Good	49 (76)	27 (84)	22 (69)	0.3
	Moderate	12 (19)	4 (13)	8 (25)	
	Bad	3 (5)	1 (3)	2 (6)	
Adherence after 6 month) n (%)	Good	47 (77)	21 (70)	26 (84)	0.4
	Moderate	13 (21)	8 (27)	5 (16)	
	Bad	1 (2)	1 (3)	0	
Levels of immunosuppression in target range at inclusion, % (IQR)		31 (20; 36)	31 (20.5; 36)	31 (20; 38.3)	0.77
Absolute number of immunosuppression level within 6 months, n	before education	15 (13;22)	15 (13; 22)	16 (14; 21)	0.9
	after education	15 (13; 19)	15 (13; 20)	14 (13; 17)	0.1
Absolute number of immunosuppression levels in target range, n	before education	5 (3; 7)	5 (3; 7)	5 (2; 7)	0.9
	after education	8.5 (5; 12)	10 (5.8; 14)	7 (4.8; 9.5)	0.048

Patient demographics and characteristics. Categorical variables were compared using a chi-square test and numeric values were shown as median with IQR, using student's t-test.

patients suffered an infection, 9 of which were in the tablet-PC group (p = 1.0). Ten patients received pulsed steroids: 6 in the tablet-PC and 4 in the conventional group (median 123 days after inclusion, p = 0.5).

Cost-calculation

The creative time required for tablet-PC education and questionnaire compared to that for conventional education was assumed to be equal. The initial equipment outlay for tablet-PC education included an iPad (499 €), an Apple AirPort Express (79 €), the required software (Keynote for iPad, Filemaker Pro for iPad, Filemaker Server and Client, totalling 852 €). Short instruction in using the tablet-PC was usually required (5 min, performed by study nurse). Conventional education was provided by a study nurse (approx. 50 €/h employer costs) and lasted around 30 min per patient. Taken together, the cost of each educational session in tablet-PC group was 45 €, with conventional training costing 25 €. Seventy-two educational sessions were therefore required to render tablet-PC training cost-effective.

Discussion

In this randomized, controlled trial, tablet-PC education proved to be non-inferior in terms of improved immunosuppression-compliance compared to conventional education. Along with reduced variability in immunosuppression, significant improvements in patient knowledge were observed following further training. To our knowledge, this is the first study that studied tablet-PC education among lung-transplant recipients. Based on the described system, other educational themes after transplantation have been implemented.

Education part

Ongoing patient education has become an established medical instrument, aiming to improve patients' knowledge about their disease and its treatment [24,25]. Currently, structured programmes have been developed in a variety of chronic diseases (asthma, diabetes), augmenting medical therapy [26–29]. New concepts examining the role of e-learning have emerged in recent years and promises cost effectiveness [30–32]. In common with

Table 3. End point results.

Variable	Time point	All patients, n = 64	Tablet-pc group, n = 32	Conventional group, n = 32	Significance
Levels of immunosuppression in target range, % (IQR)	6 months	55 (38; 68)	58 (50; 69.3)	48.5 (36; 67.3)	0.27
Improvement of percentage of calcineurin inhibitor trough levels in target range (Delta %) of the next 10 measurements after patient education compared to the last 10 measurements before patient education		20 (10; 40)	30 (10; 40)	20 (7.5; 30)	0.27
Ratio of level measurements divided by recommended measurements *	inclusion	1.11 (0.96; 1.27)	1.09 (0.90; 1.21)	1.17 (97; 1.30)	0.21
	6 months	1.14 (1.00; 1.43)	1.24 (1.07; 1.51)	1.11 (0.96; 1.28)	0.48
Improvement of percentage of calcineurin inhibitor trough levels (Delta %) in target range 6 months after patient education compared to 6 months before patient education		26 (12.5; 36)	29 (17.3; 36.3)	20 (4.8; 36)	0.17
Total time of education (first visit) (min)	inclusion	25 (21.3; 29.5)	25 (22; 28)	25 (21; 30)	0.75
Total time of answering questionnaire (first visit) (min)	inclusion	18 (14.3; 21.6)	16.5 (14; 22)	19 (16; 22)	0.38
Estimated glomerular filtration rate (% improvement 6 months to baseline)		4 (−1.2; 15.1)	4 (−1.2; 18.5)	5 (−2.5; 13.3.)	0.37

*<1: less measurements than required, >1 more measurements than required.
Results from pre-defined end-points. All values are shown as median with IQR (student's t-test).

existing studies [30,33–35], we could demonstrate non-inferiority of tablet-PC education in patients with demonstrating poor therapeutic adherence of their immunosuppression following lung-transplantation. Effectiveness of self-directed, computer-based education may be explained by increased attention that patients require whilst interacting with the device [30]. This

Table 4. Adherence Scores.

Variable	Time point	All patients, n = 64	Tablet-pc group, n = 32	Conventional group, n = 32	Significance
BAASIS questions [a]	inclusion	4 (3; 4)	4 (3; 4)	3 (3; 4)	0.12
	after 6 months	4 (4; 4)	4 (3; 4)	4 (3; 4)	0.8
VAS [b]	inclusion	100 (96; 100)	100 (96.3; 100)	100 (96.3; 100)	
	after 6 months	100 (100; 100)	100 (93.8; 100)	100 (100;100)	
ITBS Score	inclusion	14 (12; 16)	14 (12; 15)	14 (12; 16)	0.56
	after 6 months	12 (12; 15)	13 (12; 15)	12 (12; 14)	0.8
Morisky Score [c]	inclusion	4 (0.29)	4 (0.25)	4 (0.34)	0.4
	after 6 months	4 (0.22)	4 (0.18)	4 (0.25)	0.5
Satisfaction education [d]	inclusion	1 (0.54)	1 (0.55)	1 (0.53)	0.6
	after 6 months	2 (0.78)	1 (0.9)	2 (0.64)	0.27
Satisfaction questionnaire	inclusion	2 (0.77)	2 (0.55)	2 (0.91)	0.09
	after 6 month	2 (0.98)	2 (0.94)	2 (0.99)	0.11
Baseline knowledge; n (%)	80–100%	40 (63)	19 (59)	21 (66)	0.8
	<80%	24 (37)	13 (41)	11 (34)	0.8
Knowledge %	inclusion	80 (71, 90)	80 (71; 90)	85 (71; 90)	0.6
	after 6 months	90 (81; 95)	90 (83; 95)	90 (78; 95)	0.6
Improvement of knowledge (%)		7 (0; 18)	7 (0; 19)	7 (−1; 18)	0.87

Results from subjective and objective adherence (BAASIS, VAS, ITBS and Morinsky scale). [a] Self reported adherence: 1–4 points; 1 poor adherence, 4 very good adherence. [b] VAS (visual analogue scale of BAASIS questionnaire) 0 to 100; 100 very good self rated adherence.
[c]Mann-Whitney-U-Test, Mean (SD); [d] Satisfaction, 1–5 points (1 very good to 5 very bad); Mean (SD), Mann-Whitney-U-Test.

repetition aids patients in retaining the information provided [30,31]. Although e-education is a more standardized method than face-to-face education [31], face-to-face education offers a more individual teaching that can focus on individual problems of a given patient.

To maximize the cohort of patients capable of participating in interactive education, we chose an iPad®, due to its simpler handling when compared to standard laptop computers [36]. Additionally, the physical design of the iPad® afforded straightforward decontamination (deBac-app), which was considered advantageous in a potentially infectious and simultaneously infect-susceptible patient cohort.

Cost

Computer-based, self-directed education helps reduce involvement of professional staff, which may result in economic benefits [31]. A cost-calculation revealed that e-education was however more expensive than conventional education with 45 vs. 25 € per session in this study. Beyond 72 patients however, e-education achieves cost-effectiveness and given that our center currently follows up almost 800 patients after lung-transplantation, the tablet-PC approach offers substantial savings, particularly given the continual expansion in educational themes being added to our repertoire. Positive effects of education (better immunosuppression drug levels) lead to lengthening intervals between drug measurements and reduced laboratory costs (24 € per measurement) as well as postal and the cost of calls to inform patients. If the number of required trough levels could be reduced by 50%, an annual saving of 300 € per patient would ensue.

Immunosuppression

After multiple studies evaluating adherence, potential risk factors and the consequences of non-adherence [37–40], this is the first study investigating two strategies to improve immunosuppression after lung-transplantation.

Aspects of patients medication adherence

Non-adherence can extend to other important aspects of patient cooperation e.g. communicating changes in health status between appointments and physical activity, which were not considered here. Stable therapeutic CNI drug levels result from patients' knowledge and discipline regarding medication consumption, correct intervals, drug metabolism and handling demanded by their inherent pharmacokinetics and –dynamics. All patients demonstrated good fundamental knowledge at inclusion in this trial (16/20 correct answers) and appeared to follow prescribed dosing of CNI. Adherence rating by physicians correlated with knowledge test results. Whereas patients with good adherence had better knowledge, there was no correlation of knowledge and improvement of therapeutic drug levels. Consequently, good knowledge about medication alone cannot prevent from non-

therapeutic drug levels. We conclude that practical advice for daily handling of immunosuppressants were highly important in achieving good compliance. Patient evaluation of the education they received illustrated this aspect clearly. Evaluation of long-term improvements on patient survival following this intervention should be evaluated in future studies.

Limitations

Larger trials testing for superiority are required to provide evidence of clinical benefit. Future studies are required to evaluate, whether education can help prevent acute and consecutively chronic lung allograft dysfunction [41].

Conclusion

This randomised study proves positive effects of patient education on achieving improvements in therapeutic immunosuppression levels. Tablet-PC based education proved non-inferior to personal conventional education and may help physicians to improve effectiveness of education. Due to limitations in computer literacy and handling of electronic devices, specialist input was still required. Tablet-PC education now represents an integral component in our routine management of outpatients demonstrating poor immunosuppressive treatment control. Once established, the same equipment may be used for different aspects of patient education (e.g., therapy with azithromycine or bronchial stenting), adding greatly to their cost effectiveness.

Supporting Information

Figure S1 **A** Patient with tablet-PC receiving education. **B – C** Screenshots from included video clips. **B** explanation of immunosuppression levels after intake and the consequences of missing or excessive intake. **C** patient with excellent drug levels and adherence describes tips. **D** demonstration of storage of immunosuppressive drugs in a car (influence of sunlight or cold). All individuals have given written informed consent, as outlined in the PLOS consent form, to publication of their photograph.

Author Contributions

Conceived and designed the experiments: HS JF TW JG. Performed the experiments: HS JR IZ JF TW JG. Analyzed the data: HS JF JS JG. Contributed reagents/materials/analysis tools: HS MG GW AB AH JG. Wrote the paper: HS JR MG AH TW JG. Designed the software for education: HS JG JF.

References

1. Osterberg L, Blaschke T (2005) Adherence to medication. N Engl J Med 353: 487–497.
2. Trueman JF (2000) Non-adherence to medication in asthma. Prof Nurse 15: 583–586.
3. Ho PM, Magid DJ, Masoudi FA, McClure DL, Rumsfeld JS (2006) Adherence to cardioprotective medications and mortality among patients with diabetes and ischemic heart disease. BMC Cardiovasc Disord 6: 48.
4. The Boston Consulting Group Website (2003) The hidden epidemic: finding a cure for unfilled prescriptions and missed doses. Available: http://www.bcg.com/impact_expertise/publications/files/Hidden_Epi- demic_Finding_Cure_Unfulfilled_Rx _Missed_Doses_Dec2003.pdf. in Accessed 2013 Apr 2.
5. Delgado PL (2000) Approaches to the enhancement of patient adherence to antidepressant medication treatment. J Clin Psychiatry 61 Suppl 2: 6–9.
6. De Bleser L, Matteson M, Dobbels F, Russell C, De Geest S (2009) Interventions to improve medication-adherence after transplantation: a systematic review. Transpl Int 22: 780–797.
7. Khunti K, Gray LJ, Skinner T, Carey ME, Realf K, et al. (2012) Effectiveness of a diabetes education and self management programme (DESMOND) for people with newly diagnosed type 2 diabetes mellitus: three year follow-up of a cluster randomised controlled trial in primary care. BMJ 344: e2333.
8. Dhein Y, Munks-Lederer C, Worth H (2003) [Evaluation of a structured education programme for patients with COPD under outpatient conditions – a pilot study]. Pneumologie 57: 591–597.
9. Gadoury MA, Schwartzman K, Rouleau M, Maltais F, Julien M, et al. (2005) Self-management reduces both short- and long-term hospitalisation in COPD. Eur Respir J 26: 853–857.

10. Clark NM, Feldman CH, Evans D, Millman EJ, Wailewski Y, et al. (1981) The effectiveness of education for family management of asthma in children: a preliminary report. Health Educ Q 8: 166–174.
11. Best NG, Trull AK, Tan KK, Spiegelhalter DJ, Cary N, et al. (1996) Pharmacodynamics of cyclosporine in heart and heart-lung transplant recipients. I: Blood cyclosporine concentrations and other risk factors for cardiac allograft rejection. Transplantation 62: 1429–1435.
12. Pollock-Barziv SM, Finkelstein Y, Manlhiot C, Dipchand AI, Hebert D, et al. (2010) Variability in tacrolimus blood levels increases the risk of late rejection and graft loss after solid organ transplantation in older children. Pediatr Transplant 14: 968–975.
13. Dew MA, Dimartini AF, De Vito Dabbs A, Zomak R, De Geest S, et al. (2008) Adherence to the medical regimen during the first two years after lung transplantation. Transplantation 85: 193–202.
14. Dharancy S, Giral M, Tetaz R, Fatras M, Dubel L, et al. (2012) Adherence with immunosuppressive treatment after transplantation: results from the French trial PREDICT. Clin Transplant 26: E293–299.
15. Donaghy D (1995) The asthma specialist and patient education. Prof Nurse 11: 160–162.
16. Miners A, Harris J, Felix L, Murray E, Michie S, et al. (2012) An economic evaluation of adaptive e-learning devices to promote weight loss via dietary change for people with obesity. BMC Health Serv Res 12: 190.
17. Gottlieb J, Mattner F, Weissbrodt H, Dierich M, Fuehner T, et al. (2009) Impact of graft colonization with gram-negative bacteria after lung transplantation on the development of bronchiolitis obliterans syndrome in recipients with cystic fibrosis. Respir Med 103: 743–749.
18. Walsh JC, Mandalia S, Gazzard BG (2002) Responses to a 1 month self-report on adherence to antiretroviral therapy are consistent with electronic data and virological treatment outcome. AIDS 16: 269–277.
19. Terebelo S, Markell M (2010) Preferential adherence to immunosuppressive over nonimmunosuppressive medications in kidney transplant recipients. Transplant Proc 42: 3578–3585.
20. Lennerling A, Forsberg A (2012) Self-reported non-adherence and beliefs about medication in a Swedish kidney transplant population. Open Nurs J 6: 41–46.
21. Chisholm MA, Lance CE, Williamson GM, Mulloy LL (2005) Development and validation of an immunosuppressant therapy adherence barrier instrument. Nephrol Dial Transplant 20: 181–188.
22. Morisky DE, Green LW, Levine DM (1986) Concurrent and predictive validity of a self-reported measure of medication adherence. Med Care 24: 67–74.
23. Del Tacca M (2004) Prospects for personalized immunosuppression: pharmacologic tools – a review. Transplant Proc 36: 687–689.
24. Arsham GM, Bartlett EE, Cohen EJ, Squyres WD, DuVal MK (1979) Symposium: Patient/health education: training for what? Annu Conf Res Med Educ 18: 407–416.
25. Squyres WD (1983) Challenges in health education practice. J Biocommun 10: 4–9.
26. Viswanathan M, Golin CE, Jones CD, Ashok M, Blalock SJ, et al. (2012) Interventions to improve adherence to self-administered medications for chronic diseases in the United States: a systematic review. Ann Intern Med 157: 785–795.
27. Deakin T, McShane CE, Cade JE, Williams RD (2005) Group based training for self-management strategies in people with type 2 diabetes mellitus. Cochrane Database Syst Rev: CD003417.
28. Duke SA, Colagiuri S, Colagiuri R (2009) Individual patient education for people with type 2 diabetes mellitus. Cochrane Database Syst Rev: CD005268.
29. Lee TI, Yeh YT, Liu CT, Chen PL (2007) Development and evaluation of a patient-oriented education system for diabetes management. Int J Med Inform 76: 655–663.
30. Keulers BJ, Welters CF, Spauwen PH, Houpt P (2007) Can face-to-face patient education be replaced by computer-based patient education? A randomised trial. Patient Educ Couns 67: 176–182.
31. Fox MP (2009) A systematic review of the literature reporting on studies that examined the impact of interactive, computer-based patient education programs. Patient Educ Couns 77: 6–13.
32. Sechrest RC, Henry DJ (1996) Computer-based patient education: observations on effective communication in the clinical setting. J Biocommun 23: 8–12.
33. Evans AE, Edmundson-Drane EW, Harris KK (2000) Computer-assisted instruction: an effective instructional method for HIV prevention education? J Adolesc Health 26: 244–251.
34. Wydra EW (2001) The effectiveness of a self-care management interactive multimedia module. Oncol Nurs Forum 28: 1399–1407.
35. Miller DP Jr, Kimberly JR Jr, Case LD, Wofford JL (2005) Using a computer to teach patients about fecal occult blood screening. A randomized trial. J Gen Intern Med 20: 984–988.
36. Kho A, Henderson LE, Dressler DD, Kripalani S (2006) Use of handheld computers in medical education. A systematic review. J Gen Intern Med 21: 531–537.
37. Bosma OH, Vermeulen KM, Verschuuren EA, Erasmus ME, van der Bij W (2011) Adherence to immunosuppression in adult lung transplant recipients: prevalence and risk factors. J Heart Lung Transplant 30: 1275–1280.
38. DeVito Dabbs A, Dew MA, Myers B, Begey A, Hawkins R, et al. (2009) Evaluation of a hand-held, computer-based intervention to promote early self-care behaviors after lung transplant. Clin Transplant 23: 537–545.
39. Ivarsson B, Ekmehag B, Sjoberg T (2012) Patients experiences of information and support during the first six months after heart or lung transplantation. Eur J Cardiovasc Nurs.
40. Korb-Savoldelli V, Sabatier B, Gillaizeau F, Guillemain R, Prognon P, et al. (2010) Non-adherence with drug treatment after heart or lung transplantation in adults: a systematic review. Patient Educ Couns 81: 148–154.
41. Husain AN, Siddiqui MT, Holmes EW, Chandrasekhar AJ, McCabe M, et al. (1999) Analysis of risk factors for the development of bronchiolitis obliterans syndrome. Am J Respir Crit Care Med 159: 829–833.

8

Association of Soluble HLA-G with Acute Rejection Episodes and Early Development of Bronchiolitis Obliterans in Lung Transplantation

Steven R. White[1]*, Timothy Floreth[1], Chuanhong Liao[1], Sangeeta M. Bhorade[2]

1 Departments of Medicine and Health Studies, University of Chicago, Chicago, Illinois, United States of America, **2** Department of Medicine, Northwestern University, Chicago, Illinois, United States of America

Abstract

Lung transplantation has evolved into a life-saving therapy for select patients with end-stage lung diseases. However, long-term survival remains limited because of bronchiolitis obliterans syndrome (BOS). Soluble HLA-G, a mediator of adaptive immunity that modulates regulatory T cells and certain classes of effector T cells, may be a useful marker of survival free of BOS. We conducted a retrospective, single-center, pilot review of 38 lung transplant recipients who underwent collection of serum and bronchoalveolar lavage fluid 3, 6 and 12 months after transplantation, and compared soluble HLA-G concentrations in each to the presence of type A rejection and lymphocytic bronchiolitis in the first 12 months and to the presence of BOS at 24 months after transplantation. Lung soluble HLA-G concentrations were directly related to the presence of type A rejection but not to lymphocytic bronchiolitis. Our data demonstrate that soluble HLA-G concentrations in bronchoalveolar lavage but not in serum correlates with the number of acute rejection episodes in the first 12 months after lung transplantation, and thus may be a reactive marker of rejection.

Editor: Peter Chen, Cedars-Sinai Medical Center, United States of America

Funding: Supported by HL-083527 by NHLBI (National Heart, Lung and Blood Institute) and AI-095230 by NIAID (National Institute of Allergy and Infectious Diseases). The funders had no role in study design, data collection and analysis, decision to publish, or preparation of the manuscript.

Competing Interests: The authors have declared that no competing interests exist.

* Email: swhite@medicine.bsd.uchicago.edu

Introduction

Lung transplantation (LT) remains the best hope for selected patients with end-stage lung diseases. Chronic allograft rejection, clinically manifested as bronchiolitis obliterans syndrome (BOS), remains a major limitation to long-term survival: BOS occurs in 40–60% of lung transplant recipients within 4 years and is the leading cause of death after the first year, despite advances in the use of immunosuppressive therapy [1]. Although several alloimmune-dependent and independent events have been considered as risk factors for BOS, the most common and consistently identified factor associated with the development of BOS is acute lung allograft rejection episodes and alloimmune T-cell reactivity [2,3].

HLA-G is a major histocompatibility complex class I antigen encoded by a gene on chromosome 6p21 [4]. Two HLA-G isoforms exist outside the placenta: membrane-bound G1 and soluble G5 (sHLA-G) that due to alternative splicing lacks the transmembrane and intracellular domains of G1 [5]. HLA-G binds the inhibitory receptor Ig-like transcript (ILT)2/LILRB1/CD85j, expressed by human NK cells, monocytes, T cells, B cells and dendritic cells [6], and the myeloid-specific ILT4/LILRB2/CD85d receptor [7]. HLA-G has effects on both CD4+FoxP3+ regulatory T (Treg) cells and on alloreactive recipient alloreactive CD4+ and CD8+ effector T (Teff) cells that may be beneficial in transplantation: it induces expansion of Treg cells [8], inhibits both NK cell- and CD8+ T cell-mediated cytolysis [9], suppresses CD4+ T cell alloproliferative responses [10], and induces

apoptosis of CD8+ T cells [11]. Perhaps more important for long-term tolerance, HLA-G-bearing antigen-presenting cells also induce the differentiation of CD4+ T cells into suppressor cells [12,13].

HLA-G has been demonstrated in heart transplant allografts: patients with higher HLA-G expression had fewer acute rejection episodes (AREs) and less evidence for chronic rejection [14,15]. Circulating sHLA-G was seen only in patients with HLA-G expression in the heart allograft, suggesting the allograft as the source [14]. Similar results were seen in patients following liver [16] and renal [17] transplantation. Suppressor T cells were present in increased number in liver and liver-kidney transplant patients who express HLA-G at high levels [18]. In one recent single-center, retrospective study of 64 LT recipients within the first year of transplant, HLA-G expression was seen in both bronchial and alveolar epithelial cells most frequently in stable patients but less so in patients with frequent AREs or in patients with BOS [19]. This study did not evaluate the presence of either circulating or local (lung) sHLA-G, however.

We have previously demonstrated that low numbers of FoxP3+ Treg cells are associated with accelerated rejection and the development of BOS in LT [20]. Other investigators have demonstrated that increasing the number/function of Treg cells is associated with less alloreactivity in GVHD [21]. Given the association between the presence of HLA-G and other solid-organ transplantation and the potential modulatory role of HLA-G on Treg and Teff function, we asked whether there was an association between HLA-G locally in the recipient lung in the first year after LT and subsequent BOS. To answer this question, we examined a respective cohort of LT recipients to compare the presence of sHLA-G in plasma and in bronchoalveolar lavage (BAL) fluid collected in the first year to the number of acute rejection episodes in the first year and the appearance of BOS after transplantation.

Methods

Ethics statement

Approval was obtained from the University of Chicago Institutional Review Board (IRB) for this study, and was continuously updated as required during the study. Informed written consent done on forms approved by the IRB was obtained from all patients included in this analysis prior to their participation.

Patient population

Adult subjects receiving a single or bilateral sequential lung transplant from June, 2006 to September, 2011 at the University of Chicago Hospitals were evaluated. Clinical data, blood samples, and BAL fluid collected by bronchoscopy in the first 12 months after transplantation, and clinical status and pathology samples to determine the presence or absence of acute rejection episodes and BOS in the first 48 months after transplantation, were evaluated. As the point of the study was to evaluate a potential marker for the development of BOS, patients had to survive for 12 months or longer after transplantation to be included in this study.

Immunosuppression

Baseline immunosuppression for all patients included tacrolimus (target trough level: 10 ng/mL), azathioprine (2 mg/kg/day), and prednisone (tapered to 5 mg/day by 3 months post-transplantation). Daclizumab induction therapy was administered to all patients per the manufacturer's instructions. Immunosuppression was changed because of declining pulmonary function per the discretion of the attending transplant physician.

Bronchoscopy samples

We have previously described these methods [20]. Specimens were collected during surveillance bronchoscopies in the first 12 months post-transplantation. For BAL, one 60 mL and one 30 mL aliquot were instilled into the distal airways and aspirated. In general, 40 to 50 mL of BAL fluid was recovered. An aliquot of this recovered fluid was processed by clinical laboratories to assess clinical infection. Fluid to be used for mediator analysis was centrifuged at $300\times g$ and $4°C$ for 10 min, after which the supernatant was removed, passed through a 1.2-μm filter, and frozen at $-80°C$ until used. Cell pellets were also frozen at $-80°C$ until analyzed. For transbronchial biopsies, samples were collected by standard technique from the recipient lung and processed for evaluation of rejection.

Plasma samples

Blood was collected on the same day as bronchoscopy in heparin-containing tubes and immediately placed on ice. Plasma was separated by centrifugation and stored in aliquots at $-80°C$ until use.

Acute rejection and BOS

Acute rejection was determined by histological analysis of transbronchial biopsies obtained during each surveillance bronchoscopy and clinical bronchoscopies. Acute rejection was graded

in accordance with International Society of Heart and Lung Transplantation (ISHLT) guidelines [22,23]. All analyses included episodes of both grade A rejection (RA) and lymphocytic bronchiolitis (LB). All rejection episodes that met criteria were included in the data analysis. Determination of BOS was done periodically at clinical encounters for each subject using standard spirometry definitions.

Measurement of sHLA-G

sHLA-G was measured in plasma and in BAL fluid using ELISA (Exbio, Inc., Czech Republic). The capture antibody, MEM-G/9, recognizes both shed G1 and soluble G5. The limit of sensitivity is ~1 U/ml. Concentrations in BAL fluid were not normalized for BAL fluid protein content or other markers.

Data analysis

Clinical data are expressed as the mean ± standard deviation or as the median with interquartile ranges. When HLA-G concentrations were below the limit of detection the value was recorded as '0'. Results were compared using the non-parametric Kruskal-Wallis test. The Spearman correlation was used to determine associations between HLA-G concentrations and grade A or B rejection. The associations between HLA-G, RA or LB and mortality or BOS-free survival were analyzed using Kaplan–Meier analysis and Cox regression model. The log-rank test was used to compare differences of groups. The survival time was measured from the beginning of lung transplant to the date of death or to the end of the study (Jan. 25, 2013) and BOS-free survival was calculated from lung transplant date to the first of observation of BOS or death or the end of study, whichever was earlier. A p value less than 0.05 was considered significant. The data was analyzed using the statistic software Stata/SE 13.0 and IBM SPSS Statistics 20.

Results

Demographics and survival

We performed 53 lung transplants in the time period of this study in which patients survived for 1 year or longer; of these 38 subjects were eligible for inclusion (Figure 1). Subjects characteristics are shown in Table 1. Of the 38 subjects, 28 survived the length of time recorded in the study (mean survival 4.12±1.73 years), whereas 10 subjects died after lung transplant (mean survival 2.77±1.81 years). These subjects were included in our data analysis. BOS-free survival was 3.22±1.49 years in the 15 subjects recorded as not having a clinical diagnosis of BOS during the study, and 1.07±1.62 years in the 23 subjects who did develop clinically-diagnosed BOS. There were no differences in overall survival based on gender, but median BOS-free survival was greater in male subjects: 3.84 years (1.94 to 5.75 years by 95% confidence interval) versus 1.73 years (1.03 to 2.43 years by 95% confidence interval) for female subjects. There were no significant differences in survival or BOS-free survival based on race, type of transplant (single versus bilateral sequential) or diagnosis at the time of transplantation.

Rejection

Both RA and LB were noted in a majority of subjects prior to the onset of BOS (Table 2). There was no difference in overall survival time based on either maximum grade RA or LB score in the first year after transplant. As the numbers of subjects with a RA grade of 2 or 3 were small, these were grouped in subsequent analysis. Three patients had a score of ≥2 for both RA and LB; two patients had a score of 1 for both RA and LB. The association

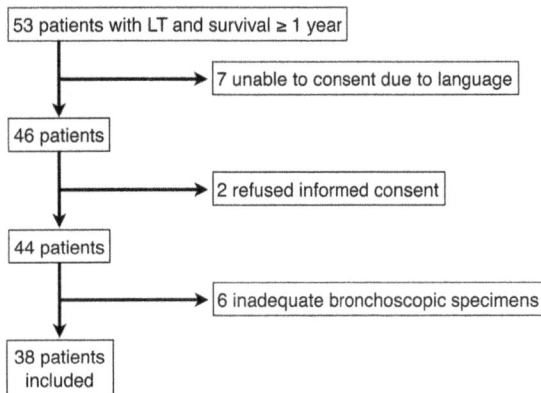

Figure 1. Study enrollment.

between RA and LB was not significant as measured using Kendall's Tau test. There was a significant correlation between BOS-free survival time and maximum RA grade after transplantation (Figure 2) (P = 0.030 for RA by Mantel-Cox log rank test).

sHLA-G concentrations and rejection

A total of 71 plasma and 85 BAL samples were collected in the first year after transplantation in 38 subjects. Plasma sHLA-G concentrations could be measured in every subject at every encounter, whereas 10 BAL samples had an sHLA-G concentration below the limit of sensitivity. Substantial variance was noted in both plasma and BAL maximum concentrations in the first year (Table 2).

There was no relation between either maximum plasma HLA-G concentration recorded in the first year, or in mean plasma HLA-G concentration of all first year samples, and overall survival or BOS-free survival. Likewise, there was no relation between

Table 1. Demographic characteristics of 38 subjects in study.

Age at time of transplantation, years (SD)	
	58.2 (12.3)
Gender, N (%)	
Female	10 (26.3)
Male	28 (73.7)
Type of transplant*, N (%)	
Single lung	24 (64.9)
Bilateral sequential lung	13 (35.1)
Race, N (%)	
European ancestry	24 (63.2)
African ancestry	4 (10.5)
Hispanic ancestry	4 (10.5)
Other	6 (15.7)
Diagnosis at time of transplantation, N (%)	
IPF	20 (52.6)
COPD	12 (31.6)
CF	3 (7.9)
Other	3 (7.9)

*1 missing.

either maximum BAL HLA-G concentration recorded in the first year, or in mean BAL HLA-G concentration of all first year samples, and overall survival. Contrary to our expectations, an increased maximum BAL HLA-G concentration was associated with a higher grade of RA prior to a clinical diagnosis of BOS (P = 0.006 by Kruskal-Wallis test) (Figure 3). In contrast, an increased maximum plasma HLA-G concentration was associated with a lower grade of LB prior to a clinical diagnosis of BOS (P = 0.044 by Kruskal-Wallis test), but not with any grade of RA (Figure 3).

sHLA-G concentrations and infection

Both blood and lung infection, as demonstrated by positive cultures in blood or BAL fluid respectively, were noted in a majority of subjects prior to the onset of BOS (Table 2). There was no significant correlation between the number of infections and either plasma or BAL HLA-G concentrations.

Discussion

Bronchiolitis obliterans syndrome remains the major limitation to long-term survival after lung transplantation despite advances in immunosuppressive therapy, infection control, and management of other complications. The poor prognosis associated with BOS reflects in part an inadequate understanding to date of disease processes which in turn leads either to under-treatment with immunosuppressive medications, and thus BOS progression, or to over-treatment or inappropriate treatment, and thus the increased number of infections and complications seen in this patient population. Our study demonstrates that the local (BAL) presence of HLA-G in the first year after transplantation in the lung correlates with the number of grade A rejection, and that circulating plasma HLA-G in the first year after transplantation correlates inversely with LB. Our study suggests that HLA-G may be a biological marker of rejection in a lung allograft. Such a marker, if confirmed in larger studies, would be useful to segregate those patients with a higher risk of rejection and BOS who require more intense immunosuppressive therapy from those in whom such therapy would entail increased risk without commensurate benefit.

Concentrations of sHLA-G were usually, but not always, detected in BAL fluid collected from LT recipients, and some variance was seen in BAL concentrations. We hypothesized that increased HLA-G levels in the lung would be associated with a lower rejection score as has been seen in patients following other solid-organ transplant [14–17]. Contrary to our hypothesis, however, the highest concentrations in BAL fluid were seen in patients with a RA score ≥2. The reasons for this are not clear: it may suggest that local production of HLA-G (by macrophages or by epithelial cells) is reactive and represent an attempt to induce the presence and generation of regulatory T cells [8]. Alternatively, it may reflect differences in the state of activation of airway macrophages and/or epithelial cells. Further evaluation of this will require studies in which local airway cell production can be ascertained over time.

There was variance also in circulating serum HLA-G concentrations in the first year after transplantation, and these were inversely associated with LB, but not RA, status. Serum HLA-G concentrations in subjects with a score of 1 in LB status was not different than that seen in recipients with a score of 0, while subjects with a score ≥2 had lower HLA-G concentrations. This suggests that mild lymphocytic bronchiolitis demonstrated on transbronchial biopsies may not be associated with changes in immune status sufficient to in turn decrease serum levels. The

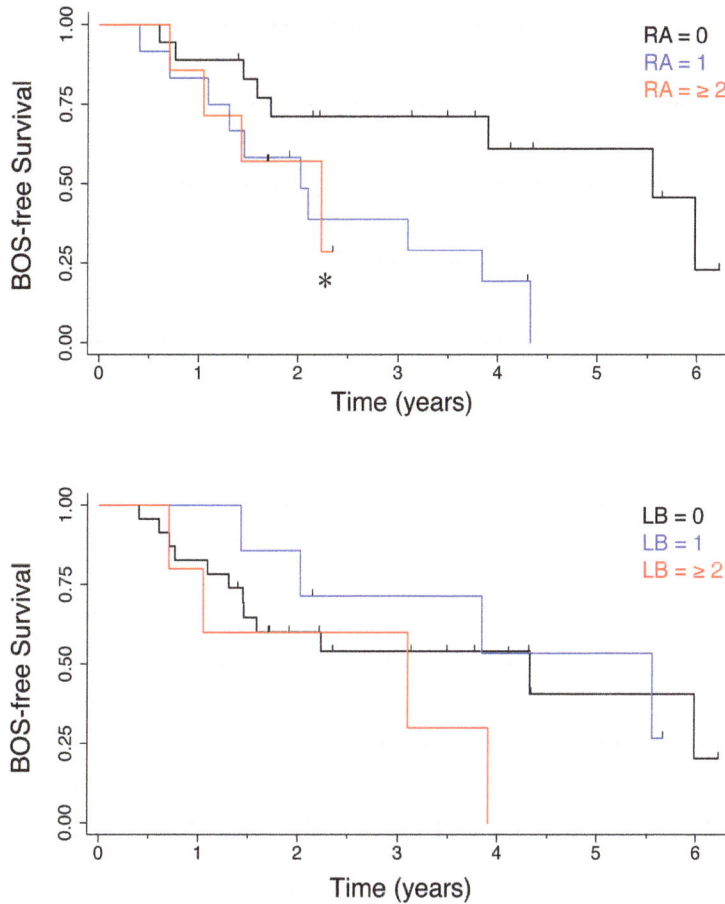

Figure 2. Kaplan-Meier analysis of BOS-free survival in 38 subjects based categorized by grade A rejection status (RA, top panel) or by grade of lymphocytic bronchiolitis (LB, bottom panel). *, P = 0.03 for RA by Mantel-Cox log rank test.

Table 2. Maximum grade A rejection (RA), lymphocytic bronchiolitis (LB), maximum HLA-G concentrations (U/ml), and presence of infection in 38 subjects prior to onset of BOS.

RA*, N (%)	
0	18 (48.6)
1	12 (32.4)
≥2	7 (18.9)
LB**, N (%)	
0	23 (65.7)
1	7 (20.0)
≥2	5 (14.3)
HLA-G, median (interquartile)	
Plasma	41.7 (10.6–74.0)
BAL	26.9 (6.8–49.2)
Number of infections, N (%)	
0	15 (39.5)
1	21 (55.3)
2	2 (5.3)

* 1 missing.
** 3 missing.

downward trend in serum HLA-G concentrations in patients with significant RA noted on transbronchial biopsy is not statistically significant but will need to be examined in the context of a larger study. Serum markers clearly are easier to obtain and, along with other serum markers, provide context for the overall status of the immune system. Correlations with circulating regulatory and effector T cell trafficking to the lung allograft will be needed to understand the potential role of serum sHLA-G in LT recipients.

In one recent single-center, retrospective study of 64 LT recipients within 1 year of transplant, HLA-G protein expression was seen in both bronchial and alveolar epithelial cells most frequently in stable patients but less so in patients with frequent AREs or in patients with BOS [19]. That study however did not evaluate the presence of either circulating sHLA-G in plasma or local sHLA-G in bronchoalveolar lavage. HLA-G also is found in lung macrophages [24], and evaluation of cell pellets by immunofluorescent staining collected from several LT recipients in our study demonstrated significant macrophage expression of sHLA-G (data not shown). Thus, sHLA-G found in bronchoalveolar lavage may represent the combined expression and secretion from both central and alveolar epithelial cells and from macrophages; changes in expression in either cell type might account for changes in the final presence in the lung. Understanding which cells contribute to final expression and presence after lung transplantation, and how that expression is

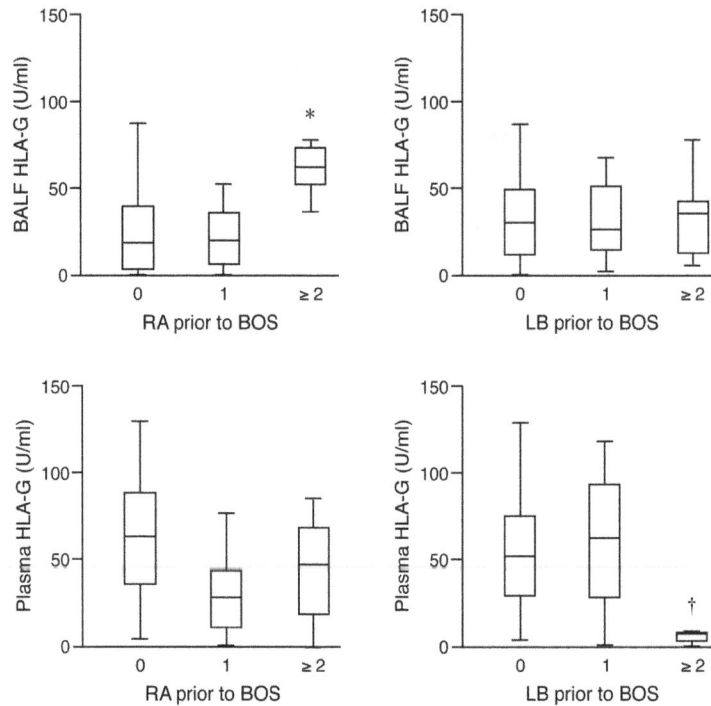

Figure 3. Concentrations of sHLA-G, in maximum U/ml prior to onset of BOS, in bronchoalveolar lavage fluid (BALF) (upper panels) and plasma (lower panels) in 38 subjects based categorized by grade A rejection status (RA, left panels) or by grade of lymphocytic bronchiolitis (LB, right panels). *, P = 0.006 by Kruskal-Wallis test, †, P = 0.044 by Kruskal-Wallis test.

modified by immunosuppressive drug treatment, infection and evolving chronic rejection, will require further study.

HLA-G induces expansion of CD4+FoxP3+ Treg cells [8] which may be important in allograft survival in transplantation. We have previously demonstrated that low numbers of lung FoxP3+ Treg cells are associated with accelerated rejection and the development of BOS in LT recipients [20]. Other investigators have demonstrated similar findings in stem cell [25] and bone marrow [26] transplantation, while increasing their number and function is associated with less alloreactivity in graft versus host disease [21]. Our new data raises the possibility that higher expression of *HLA-G* in the allograft may stimulate the presence and/or survival of lung Treg lymphocytes that then may modulate tolerance; this will need to be confirmed in future studies. In particular, our data do not make clear whether the change in allograft HLA-G expression is reactive, due to some rejection episode or stimulus from cells that ordinarily mediate rejection, or is innate and dependent more on a subject's (or allograft) genotype. HLA-G also inhibits both NK cell- and CD8+ T cell-mediated cytolysis [9], suppresses CD4+ T cell alloproliferative responses [10], and induces apoptosis of CD8+ T cells [11]. Likewise, HLA-G-bearing antigen-presenting cells not only inhibit CD4+ T cell proliferation but also induce the differentiation of CD4+ T cells into suppressor cells [12,13]. Each action may improve allograft outcome, and will require evaluation in the context of LT.

Our study was too small to detect whether either plasma or local lung (BAL) HLA-G concentrations were associated with survival or BOS-free survival. Similarly, given the few time points that were collected for each subject and the missing samples, we were unable to assess changes in sHLA-G concentrations in BAL and serum reliably over time. Both limitations are typical of single-center studies and suggests that a multi-center trial with a

significantly larger number of study subjects will be required to answer this question. Nevertheless our study does suggest that HLA-G is protective against LB; we predict that over a longer period of time and in larger studies that this will translate into improved BOS-free survival.

An additional issue is whether sHLA-G concentrations in BAL fluid reflect the local concentrations of sHLA-G at the tissue level. Previous studies in heart and lung transplant recipients have evaluated sHLA-G presence in endomyocardial and transbronchial biopsies, respectively [14,19]. In the peripheral lung, sHLA-G presence in BAL fluid may reflect the combined relative contributions of airway epithelial cells [19] and of alveolar macrophages [24]. We did not directly compare the BAL concentrations to tissue presence of sHLA-G in this study, and both the correlation and the assignment of the BAL contribution to epithelial cell and/or macrophage origin will need to be addressed in future studies.

Our study also was too small to examine the potential relation of genotype on lung allograft function and the development of BOS. The influence of *HLA-G* genotype of both the donor graft and recipient has been examined in small studies of other solid organ transplants. While alleles encoding polymorphisms in the coding region apparently have little effect in renal transplantation [27], the 14 bp in/del polymorphism in exon 8 in the 3' un-translated region of *HLA-G* may help predict renal [28] and bone marrow transplant [29] complications. Understanding how both donor and recipient genotypes influence tolerance will have important implications in matching donors to recipients in the future: as one example, if both genotypes predict low HLA-G expression, then clinicians may need to increase immunosuppressive therapy in terms of dosing or combinations of medications; and likewise, if either or both genotypes predict high expression, lower immuno-suppressive therapy may be sufficient. Multi-center studies of

HLA-G and its expression in lung allografts and in recipients will be needed to answer this question.

As may often happen in clinical studies with the collection of biological specimens, data were not available at each pre-specified time point because of the clinical condition (e.g., clinical instability during the bronchoscopy procedure) of the patient or logistics of specimen collection. However, the data remain useful despite these missing samples. In addition, we cannot exclude that different patient phenotypes or the variety of clinical events such as infection may bias our results. The putative use of lung sHLA-G as a biomarker for early allograft rejection clearly will require further study and confirmation in larger cohorts from different transplant centers.

In summary, we demonstrate the presence of sHLA-G in both the lung and serum of LT recipients. There is an association of high BAL sHLA-G presence and the development of grade A rejection within 2 years. While the mechanisms by which lung sHLA-G presence increases are not clear, this adaptive immunity mediator may be a marker of rejection in lung transplantation.

Acknowledgments

We thank Bharathi Laxman, Ph.D., Randi Stern, M.S., and Zhongping Xu, M.S. for assistance in sample analysis.

Author Contributions

Conceived and designed the experiments: SRW SMB. Performed the experiments: SRW SMB TF. Analyzed the data: SRW CL. Contributed reagents/materials/analysis tools: SRW CL. Wrote the paper: SRW CL SMB.

References

1. Christie JD, Edwards LB, Aurora P, Dobbels F, Kirk R, et al. (2008) Registry of the International Society for Heart and Lung Transplantation: twenty-fifth official adult lung and heart/lung transplantation report–2008. J Heart Lung Transplant 27: 957–969.
2. Bando K, Paradis IL, Similo S, Konishi H, Komatsu K, et al. (1995) Obliterative bronchiolitis after lung and heart-lung transplantation. An analysis of risk factors and management. J Thorac Cardiovasc Surg 110: 4–13; discussion 13-14.
3. Todd JL, Palmer SM (2011) Bronchiolitis obliterans syndrome: the final frontier for lung transplantation. Chest 140: 502–508.
4. Nicolae D, Cox NJ, Lester LA, Schneider D, Tan Z, et al. (2005) Fine mapping and positional candidate studies identify HLA-G as an asthma susceptibility gene on chromosome 6p21. Am J Hum Genet 76: 349–357.
5. Ishitani A, Geraghty DE (1992) Alternative splicing of HLA-G transcripts yields proteins with primary structures resembling both class I and class II antigens. Proc Natl Acad Sci U S A 89: 3947–3951.
6. Colonna M, Navarro F, Bellon T, Llano M, Garcia P, et al. (1997) A common inhibitory receptor for major histocompatibility complex class I molecules on human lymphoid and myelomonocytic cells. J Exp Med 186: 1809–1818.
7. Colonna M, Samaridis J, Cella M, Angman L, Allen RL, et al. (1998) Human myelomonocytic cells express an inhibitory receptor for classical and nonclassical MHC class I molecules. J Immunol 160: 3096–3100.
8. Selmani Z, Naji A, Zidi I, Favier B, Gaiffe E, et al. (2008) Human leukocyte antigen-G5 secretion by human mesenchymal stem cells is required to suppress T lymphocyte and natural killer function and to induce CD4+CD25high-FOXP3+ regulatory T cells. Stem Cells 26: 212–222.
9. Riteau B, Rouas-Freiss N, Menier C, Paul P, Dausset J, et al. (2001) HLA-G2, -G3, and -G4 isoforms expressed as nonmature cell surface glycoproteins inhibit NK and antigen-specific CTL cytolysis. J Immunol 166: 5018–5026.
10. Lila N, Rouas-Freiss N, Dausset J, Carpentier A, Carosella ED (2001) Soluble HLA-G protein secreted by allo-specific CD4+ T cells suppresses the allo-proliferative response: a CD4+ T cell regulatory mechanism. Proc Natl Acad Sci U S A 98: 12150–12155.
11. Contini P, Ghio M, Poggi A, Filaci G, Indiveri F, et al. (2003) Soluble HLA-A,-B,-C and -G molecules induce apoptosis in T and NK CD8+ cells and inhibit cytotoxic T cell activity through CD8 ligation. Eur J Immunol 33: 125–134.
12. LeMaoult J, Krawice-Radanne I, Dausset J, Carosella ED (2004) HLA-G1-expressing antigen-presenting cells induce immunosuppressive CD4+ T cells. Proc Natl Acad Sci U S A 101: 7064–7069.
13. Le Rond S, Azema C, Krawice-Radanne I, Durrbach A, Guettier C, et al. (2006) Evidence to support the role of HLA-G5 in allograft acceptance through induction of immunosuppressive/regulatory T cells. J Immunol 176: 3266–3276.
14. Lila N, Amrein C, Guillemain R, Chevalier P, Latremouille C, et al. (2002) Human leukocyte antigen-G expression after heart transplantation is associated with a reduced incidence of rejection. Circulation 105: 1949–1954.
15. Luque J, Torres MI, Aumente MD, Marin J, Garcia-Jurado G, et al. (2006) Soluble HLA-G in heart transplantation: their relationship to rejection episodes and immunosuppressive therapy. Hum Immunol 67: 257–263.
16. Basturk B, Karakayali F, Emiroglu R, Sozer O, Haberal A, et al. (2006) Human leukocyte antigen-G, a new parameter in the follow-up of liver transplantation. Transplant Proc 38: 571–574.
17. Qiu J, Terasaki PI, Miller J, Mizutani K, Cai J, et al. (2006) Soluble HLA-G expression and renal graft acceptance. Am J Transplant 6: 2152–2156.
18. Naji A, Le Rond S, Durrbach A, Krawice-Radanne I, Creput C, et al. (2007) CD3+CD4low and CD3+CD8low are induced by HLA-G: novel human peripheral blood suppressor T-cell subsets involved in transplant acceptance. Blood 110: 3936–3948.
19. Brugiere O, Thabut G, Pretolani M, Krawice-Radanne I, Dill C, et al. (2009) Immunohistochemical study of HLA-G expression in lung transplant recipients. Am J Transplant 9: 1427–1438.
20. Bhorade SM, Chen H, Molinero L, Liao C, Garrity ER, et al. (2010) Decreased percentage of CD4+FoxP3+ cells in bronchoalveolar lavage from lung transplant recipients correlates with development of bronchiolitis obliterans syndrome. Transplantation 90: 540–546.
21. Rezvani K, Mielke S, Ahmadzadeh M, Kilical Y, Savani BN, et al. (2006) High donor FOXP3-positive regulatory T-cell (Treg) content is associated with a low risk of GVHD following HLA-matched allogeneic SCT. Blood 108: 1291–1297.
22. Stewart S, Fishbein MC, Snell GI, Berry GJ, Boehler A, et al. (2007) Revision of the 1996 working formulation for the standardization of nomenclature in the diagnosis of lung rejection. J Heart Lung Transplant 26: 1229–1242.
23. Holtzman MJ, Patel DA, Zhang Y, Patel AC (2011) Host epithelial-viral interactions as cause and cure for asthma. Curr Opin Immunol 23: 487–494.
24. Pangault C, Le Friec G, Caulet-Maugendre S, Lena H, Amiot L, et al. (2002) Lung macrophages and dendritic cells express HLA-G molecules in pulmonary diseases. Hum Immunol 63: 83–90.
25. Hicheri Y, Bouchekioua A, Hamel Y, Henry A, Rouard H, et al. (2008) Donor regulatory T cells identified by FoxP3 expression but also by the membranous CD4+CD127low/neg phenotype influence graft-versus-tumor effect after donor lymphocyte infusion. J Immunother 31: 806–811.
26. Noel G, Bruniquel D, Birebent B, DeGuibert S, Grosset JM, et al. (2008) Patients suffering from acute graft-versus-host disease after bone-marrow transplantation have functional CD4+CD25hiFoxp3+ regulatory T cells. Clin Immunol 129: 241–248.
27. Pirri A, Contieri FC, Benvenutti R, Bicalho Mda G (2009) A study of HLA-G polymorphism and linkage disequilibrium in renal transplant patients and their donors. Transpl Immunol 20: 143–149.
28. Piancatelli D, Maccarone D, Liberatore G, Parzanese I, Clemente K, et al. (2009) HLA-G 14-bp insertion/deletion polymorphism in kidney transplant patients with metabolic complications. Transplant Proc 41: 1187–1188.
29. La Nasa G, Littera R, Locatelli F, Lai S, Alba F, et al. (2007) The human leucocyte antigen-G 14-basepair polymorphism correlates with graft-versus-host disease in unrelated bone marrow transplantation for thalassaemia. Br J Haematol 139: 284–288.

9

Impact of Commonly Used Transplant Immunosuppressive Drugs on Human NK Cell Function Is Dependent upon Stimulation Condition

Aislin C. Meehan[1,2], **Nicole A. Mifsud**[1,2], **Thi H. O. Nguyen**[1,2], **Bronwyn J. Levvey**[2], **Greg I. Snell**[2], **Tom C. Kotsimbos**[1,2], **Glen P. Westall**[1,2]*

1 Department of Medicine, Monash University, Melbourne, Victoria, Australia, **2** Department of Allergy, Immunology and Respiratory Medicine, The Alfred Hospital, Melbourne, Victoria, Australia

Abstract

Lung transplantation is a recognised treatment for patients with end stage pulmonary disease. Transplant recipients receive life-long administration of immunosuppressive drugs that target T cell mediated graft rejection. However little is known of the impact on NK cells, which have the potential to be alloreactive in response to HLA-mismatched ligands on the lung allograft and in doing so, may impact negatively on allograft survival. NK cells from 20 healthy controls were assessed in response to Cyclosporine A, Mycophenolic acid (MPA; active form of Mycophenolate mofetil) and Prednisolone at a range of concentrations. The impact of these clinically used immunosuppressive drugs on cytotoxicity (measured by CD107a expression), IFN-γ production and CFSE proliferation was assessed in response to various stimuli including MHC class-I negative cell lines, IL-2/IL-12 cytokines and PMA/Ionomycin. Treatment with MPA and Prednisolone revealed significantly reduced CD107a expression in response to cell line stimulation. In comparison, addition of MPA and Cyclosporine A displayed reduced CD107a expression and IFN-γ production following PMA/Ionomycin stimulation. Diminished proliferation was observed in response to treatment with each drug. Additional functional inhibitors (LY294002, PD98059, Rottlerin, Rapamycin) were used to elucidate intracellular pathways of NK cell activation in response to stimulation with K562 or PMA-I. CD107a expression was significantly decreased with the addition of PD98059 following K562 stimulation. Similarly, CD107a expression significantly decreased following PMA-I stimulation with the addition of LY294002, PD98059 and Rottlerin. Ten lung transplant patients, not receiving immunosuppressive drugs pre-transplant, were assessed for longitudinal changes post-transplant in relation to the administration of immunosuppressive drugs. Individual patient dynamics revealed different longitudinal patterns of NK cell function post-transplantation. These results provide mechanistic insights into pathways of NK cell activation and show commonly administered transplant immunosuppression agents and clinical rejection/infection events have differential effects on NK cell function that may impact the immune response following lung transplantation.

Editor: Antonio Perez-Martinez, Hospital Infantil Universitario Niño Jesús, Spain

Funding: This work has been supported by the National Health and Medical Research Council (NHMRC) with the provision of the Dora Lush Postgraduate Research Scholarship and the Margaret Pratt Foundation (http://www.mprattfoundation.com.au/). The funders had no role in study design, data collection and analysis, decision to publish, or preparation of the manuscript.

Competing Interests: The authors have declared that no competing interests exist.

* E-mail: G.Westall@alfred.org.au

Introduction

Lung transplantation is an established treatment for patients with end stage pulmonary disease. Whilst lung transplant recipients (LTR) require life-long administration of immunosuppressive drugs to minimize alloreactivity and maintain optimal lung allograft function, episodes of acute cellular rejection remain relatively common and complications of chronic rejection and decline in lung function continue to impact on long term survival. LTR receive immunosuppressive drugs that target alloreactive T cells, the primary driver of acute cellular rejection. However, human studies suggest that other effector cells of the immune system, such as NK cells, may also have alloreactive potential and influence clinical outcomes following transplantation [1].

NK cells are a key component of the innate immune system, mediating cell lysis without prior antigen stimulation and were initially described as providing the first line of defence against tumours and viral infections. Whilst the intrinsic role of NK cells relates to host defence, more recent attention has focused on their role in influencing adverse clinical outcomes following allogeneic transplantation in the setting of either hematopoietic stem cells or solid organs [2,3,4,5,6].

Activation of NK cells is regulated by the balance between expressed inhibitory and activating NK cell receptors and their respective ligands on target cells [7]. These ligands typically include self HLA molecules. NK cells responding to HLA-mismatched ligands on the lung allograft have the potential to, both directly via engagement of receptor ligands on the allograft and indirectly through release of cytokines, enhance effector T cell activation and contribute to alloreactivity [8].

Following lung transplantation, an immunosuppressive regimen consisting of a calcineurin inhibitor, an anti-proliferative agent and a corticosteroid are given to suppress the immune response to the non-self allograft thereby minimizing episodes of rejection. Calcineurin inhibitors, such as Cyclosporine A or Tacrolimus, block the calcineurin pathway by forming complexes with cyclophilin and FK-binding protein, respectively. These immunophilins prevent calcineurin from dephosphorylating the NFAT transcription factor thus inhibiting transcription of genes encoding IL-2 and leading to a dampened effector T cell response [9]. Antiproliferative agents including Azathioprine and Mycophenolate mofetil (MMF) impede lymphocyte growth and expansion. The anti-metabolite MMF is rapidly converted into its active form of Mycophenolic acid (MPA) after administration which then inhibits the enzyme, inosine monophosphate dehydrogenase, involved in *de novo* purine synthesis resulting in diminished lymphocyte proliferation [9,10,11]. Corticosteroids, such as Prednisolone, bind with glucocorticoid receptors, forming a complex which interacts with cellular DNA in the nucleus to modify gene transcription. Steroids impinge on various stages of antigen presentation, cytokine production and proliferation, all of which contribute to an anti-inflammatory and immunosuppressive effect [12,13].

Given that there is little reported evidence relating to the impact of lung transplantation immunosuppressive drugs on NK cell function in either immunocompetent individuals or immunosuppressed lung transplant recipients (LTR), we performed a detailed analysis of the impact of a series of functional inhibitors on NK cell activity in healthy controls. These included clinically used immunosuppressive drugs such as a calcineurin inhibitor (Cyclosporine A), an anti-proliferative agent (MPA) and a corticosteroid (Prednisolone), but also the additional intracellular signalling inhibitor drugs Rapamycin (inhibitor of mTOR), Rottlerin (inhibitor of PKC in the NFkB pathway), LY294002 (inhibitor of Pi3K activity) and PD98059 (inhibitor of MEK in MAPK pathway). In addition, we studied NK cell function longitudinally both pre- and post- lung transplantation in a cohort of patients receiving immunosuppressive drugs.

Materials and Methods

Ethics Statement

All patients and controls gave written informed consent and the study was approved by The Alfred Hospital ethics committee (Project 175/02).

LTR demographics and Controls

A group of 20 healthy volunteer controls, age and gender-matched to the LTR cohort, were recruited and analysed at a single time point. A cohort of 10 patients (mean age 41) who received HLA-mismatched bilateral lung transplants at The Alfred Hospital in 2009, were enrolled in a longitudinal analysis of NK cell function in response to immunosuppression. Individual LTR were identified based on disease status indicating the absence of immunosuppressive drugs prior to receiving a lung allograft. All LTR received a standard triple-therapy immunosuppression drug regime consisting of a calcineurin inhibitor (Tacrolimus), an anti-proliferative agent (Azathioprine) and a corticosteroid (Prednisolone). Induction therapy with the anti-thymocyte globulin (ATG) was given to two patients. LTR at-risk for CMV infection or reactivation (donor and/or recipient seropositive for CMV) were given intravenous ganciclovir (5 mg/kg) for 2 weeks followed by oral valganciclovir (900 mg/day) for a further 18 weeks. Surveillance bronchoscopy was performed at 1, 3, 6, 9 and 12 months post-transplantation or if clinically indicated, with bronchoalveolar lavage (BAL) and transbronchial biopsy sampling. Acute allograft

rejection was diagnosed on transbronchial biopsy according to the International Society of Heart and Lung Transplantation guidelines [14]. At the time of routine surveillance bronchoscopy, whole blood samples (9 mL in sodium heparin tubes) from LTR were collected for later analysis of NK cell function.

Cell preparation

Peripheral blood mononuclear cells (PBMC) were isolated from whole blood samples using Ficoll-Paque (GE Healthcare, NSW, Australia) and resuspended in RPMI-1640 containing 10% heat-inactivated FCS (SAFC, Sigma-Aldrich, NSW, Australia), 2 mM L-glutamine (GIBCO, NY, USA), 2 mM MEM non-essential amino acids (GIBCO), 100 mM HEPES (GIBCO), 50 μM 2-ME (GIBCO) and 1 U/ml penicillin/streptomycin (GIBCO); hereafter referred to as RF-10. PBMC thawed from cryopreserved LTR samples were rested overnight in 4 mL autologous plasma (diluted 1:2 in RPMI-1640) prior to use in functional assays. The HLA class I negative target cell lines K562 and 721.221 were maintained in RF-10 media (approx 2.5×10^5 cells/ml).

Functional assessment of NK cell cytotoxic potential and cytokine production

Monoclonal antibodies (mAb) anti-CD3-PerCPCy5.5 (clone SK7) and anti-CD56-APC (clone NCAM 16.2) were used to phenotype both NK cell (CD56$^+$CD3$^-$) and T cell (CD56$^-$CD3$^+$) subsets, detected on a FACS Calibur flow cytometer (Becton Dickinson [BD], CA, USA). PBMC were stimulated with K562 target cells at a 2:1 ratio for 6 h (37°C, 5% CO$_2$). PMA (40 ng/ml, Sigma) with Ionomycin (1 μg/ml, Sigma), hereafter referred to as PMA-I, stimulation of PBMC was used as the positive control and unstimulated PBMC as the negative control. Anti-CD107a FITC (1:20 dilution, clone H4A3) and Brefeldin A (10 μg/ml, Sigma) with monensin (2 μM, Sigma) were added to the cell culture at 0 and 1h, respectively. Cells were stained with anti-CD56 APC and anti-CD3 PerCPCy5.5 mAbs to differentiate NK cells and T cells, fixed (1% paraformaldehyde, ProSciTech, QLD, Australia), permeabilized (0.3% Saponin, Sigma) and stained with mAbs to detect production of intracellular IFN-γ PE (clone B27). All mAbs were purchased from BD Pharmingen and titrated to determine optimal staining. Samples were rested overnight at 4°C prior to performing flow cytometry. Lymphocytes were identified based on size and granularity. Both NK cell and T cell frequencies were then defined as a percentage of total lymphocytes and CD107a and IFN-γ positive expression defined as a percentage of total NK or T cells. Data was analysed using FlowJo software (TreeStar Inc, OR, USA).

Immunosuppressive drugs and NK cell intracellular pathway functional assays

The impact of the commonly administered lung transplant immunosuppressive drugs Cyclosporine A (Novartis, NSW, Australia), MMF (using the active metabolite MPA; Sigma) and Prednisolone (Pfizer, NSW, Australia) on NK cell function was determined. Whilst the LTR received Tacrolimus and Azathioprine, these drugs are relatively unstable following prolonged storage and were unsuitable for the *in vitro* cultures performed, thus the alternative calcineurin inhibitor, Cyclosporine A, and anti-proliferative drug, MPA, were used in the assays performed with the healthy controls. Administered concentrations of the drugs were consistent with previous studies [12,13,15,16,17,18] with each immunosuppressive drug being added to the NK cell and T cell functional assays at concentrations of 10 ng/ml, 100 ng/ml and 1000 ng/ml. These concentrations encompass physiologically equivalent standard therapeutic doses given to patients following transplantation. Drugs to inhibit intracellular signaling pathways were tested at a range of concentrations to determine toxicity to PBMC. Propidium iodide (PI) uptake by non-viable cells in response to inhibitor concentrations of LY294002 (Merck, VIC, Australia) and PD98059 (Merck) (each at 5 μM, 10 μM, 25 μM, 50 μM, 100 μM), Rapamycin (Merck; 10 nM, 50 nM, 100 nM, 200 nM, 500 nM) and Rottlerin (Merck; 1 μM, 2 μM, 5 μM, 10 μM, 50 μM) was used to determine the inhibitor drug concentrations to use in the subsequent NK cell functional assays. NK cells from six healthy controls were stimulated with K562 target cells and PMA-I (CD107a intracellular cytokine staining described previously) with or without the additional intracellular signalling inhibitors LY294002 (25 uM), PD98059 (25 uM), Rapamycin (100 nM) and Rottlerin (5 uM).

Chromium release cytotoxicity assay

A standard chromium release cytotoxicity assay was used to assess NK cells lysis of K562 target cells, as previously described [6]. Briefly, ^{51}Cr-labelled targets (2×10^3 cells/well) were incubated with PBMC at effector-to-target (E:T) ratios of 50:1, 100:1 and 200:1. Spontaneous-release and maximal-release controls were evaluated by incubating target cells with RF-10 and 1% Triton-X, respectively. Cytotoxicity was calculated as % specific lysis = [(experimental release − spontaneous release)/(maximal release − spontaneous release)] ×100.

NK cell purification from whole PBMC and proliferation assay

PBMC were depleted of monocytes by overnight culture in RF-10 media and subsequent retrieval of non-adherent cells. NK cells were then isolated from the PBMC by magnetic bead negative selection according to the manufacturer's instructions (Magnetic Activated Cell Sorting (MACS) NK cell isolation kit, Miltenyi Biotech, Teterow, Germany) to achieve a purity of greater than 98% $CD56^+$ $CD3^-$ NK cells. MACS enriched NK cells, from three of the 20 controls, were labelled with 1 μM CFSE (Sigma) at a cell density of 10^7/ml in PBS. After 5 min at 37°C, 5% CO_2, cells were washed once with PBS containing 1% FCS, washed once with PBS containing 0.1% FCS and resuspended in RF-10. CFSE labelled NK cells were plated in triplicate into 96 well U-bottom plates at 5×10^4 cells/well for three days of *in vitro* culture at 37°C, 5% CO_2. NK cells were stimulated to proliferate with the addition of the cell line 721.221 at a 1:1 ratio and a combination of IL-2 (250 U/ml; Peprotech, NJ, USA) and IL-12 (10 U/ml; Peprotech) cytokines in the presence or absence of immunosuppressive drugs. Both media and immunosuppressive drugs were replenished every second day. Cell staining, acquisition and analysis of NK cells was performed as described in the previous section.

Statistical analysis

Numerical data were expressed as means ± standard of error (SEM). Repeated one-way analysis of variance (ANOVA) was used to assess differences in NK cell CD107a and IFN-γ expression and proliferation at each concentration of drug used. One-way ANOVA was performed to assess differences between pre- and post-transplant NK cell function compared to healthy controls. Statistical significance was defined as $p<0.05$ using GraphPad Prism version 5.00 for Windows (GraphPad Software, San Diego, CA, USA).

Results

Differential effect of immunosuppressive drugs on NK cell cytotoxicity is stimulus dependent *in vitro*

To determine the cytotoxic potential of activated NK cells, cell surface expression of CD107a indicating recent degranulation of cytotoxic granules, was used as the surrogate marker (Figure 1A) [19,20]. Compared to baseline CD107a expression in the absence of immunosuppressive drugs (7.9%±1.0%), there was a dose-response decline with the addition of Prednisolone at 10 ng/ml (6.0%±0.9%), 100 ng/ml (5.7%±0.7%) and 1000 ng/ml (3.8%±0.5%). Whereas, only high dose MPA significantly reduced CD107a expression (1.8%±0.3%) and no effect was observed for Cyclosporine A treatment (Figure 1B).

To support these findings, a standard chromium release assay was used as an alternate measure of NK cell cytotoxicity. The kinetics mirrored those observed in the CD107a cell surface expression assay for treatment with MPA and Cyclosporine A. However, in this assay system only addition of high dose Prednisolone had a significant effect compared to the control (13.1%±2.9% vs 20.9%±3.3%) (Figure 1C). The chromium release assay system was found to be less sensitive than the flow cytometry based CD107a assay which was able to identify more subtle changes in NK cell cytotoxicity.

Stimulation of PBMC was also achieved using PMA-I. Surprisingly, inverse kinetic profiles for both Cyclosporine A and Prednisolone were shown, compared to that observed using K562 cell line as the stimulus. In contrast to baseline NK cell (9.6%±2.4%) and T cell (4.8%±0.7%) expression, Cyclosporine A significantly reduced CD107a expression at 10 ng/ml (6.0%±1.8% and 2.7%±0.5%), 100 ng/ml (3.6%±1.0% and 1.8%±0.4%) and 1000 ng/ml (2.9%±0.5% and 1.6%±0.3%), respectively. High dose MPA decreased CD107a expression on NK cells (2.5%±0.4%) and T cells (0.8%±0.2%) whilst Prednisolone demonstrated no change (Figures 1D, E).

When the whole NK cell population was analysed into the two main subsets of CD56bright and CD56dim NK cells, it was observed that the function of both NK cell subsets was influenced in the same way with the addition of immunosuppression, thus data was presented as whole CD56+ NK cells. Although following PMA-I stimulation, but not with K562 stimulation, the decline in positive expression of CD107a was more striking in the CD56bright subset compared to the CD56dim cells suggesting the CD56bright cells were more severely affected by the immunosuppressive drugs (Figure 1F).

Clear link between cytokine production and cytotoxicity profiles in NK cells

The impact of immunosuppression on NK cell activation was evaluated by quantitative measurement of IFN-γ cytokine production (Figure 1A). In the absence of immunosuppression the percentage of NK cells producing IFN-γ was 1.3%±0.2% and 9.9%±2.2% following stimulation with either K562 cell line or PMA-I, respectively (Figures 2A, B). Interestingly, IFN-γ cytokine profiles were similar to those of cytotoxicity with K562 stimulation, showing dose-response decreases were shown with addition of Cyclosporine A at 10 ng/ml (0.5%±0.08%), 100 ng/ml (0.2%±0.02%) and 1000 ng/ml (0.2%±0.02%) and Prednisolone at 10 ng/ml (0.9%±0.2%), 100 ng/ml (0.6%±0.1%) and 1000 ng/ml (0.3%±0.04%), whilst MPA significantly decreased IFN-γ production only at the highest concentration (0.3%±0.06%) (Figure 2A).

Stimulation of both NK cells and T cells with PMA-I emulated data obtained in the cytotoxicity assays. High dose MPA

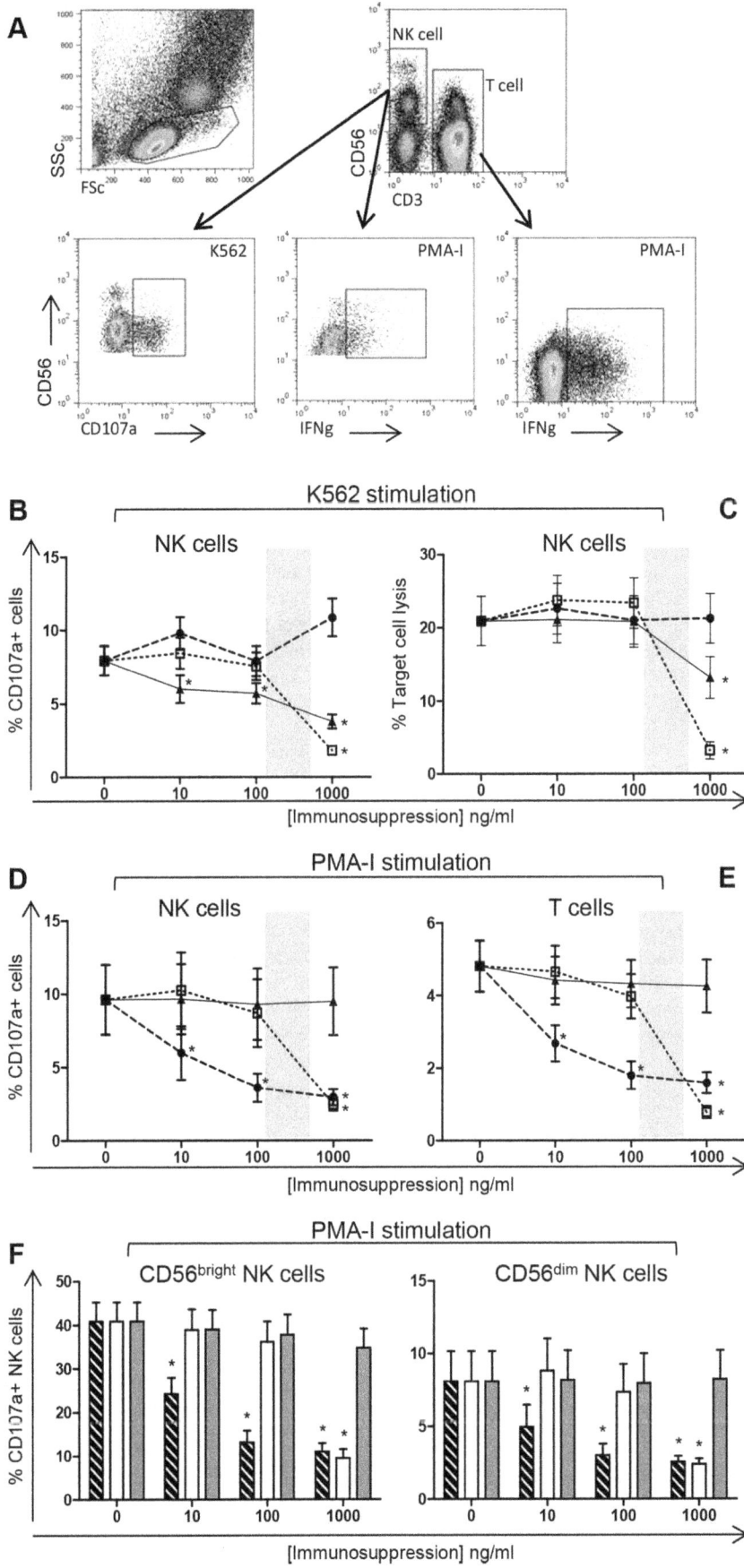

Figure 1. NK cell and T cell cytotoxicity in the presence of immunosuppressive drugs. PBMC from 20 healthy controls were stimulated in culture with the cell line K562 or PMA-I in the presence or absence of varying concentrations of immunosuppressive drugs. An example of the flow cytometry gating strategy for identification of positive expression is shown (A). NK cell cytotoxicity measured by CD107a surface expression (B) and chromium release assay, at a 50:1 effector-to-target ratio (C), in response to K562 stimulation. CD107a expression for whole CD56+ NK cells (D), T cells (E) and NK cell subsets CD56bright and CD56dim (F) measured following PMA-I stimulation. Statistical significance was defined as $p<0.001$. Graphed data are presented as mean ± SEM. Symbols represent immunosuppressive drugs: ●, dashed bars: Cyclosporine A; □, white bars: MPA; ▲, grey bars: Prednisolone. Shaded areas signify therapeutic range.

significantly reduced IFN-γ production by NK cells (0.54%±0.09%) and T cells (0.7%±0.1%). Cyclosporine A significantly reduced IFN-γ production by NK cells and T cells at 10 ng/ml (3.1%±1.0% and 4.3%±0.6%), 100 ng/ml (1.1% ±0.2% and 2.3%±0.3%) and 1000 ng/ml (1.2%±0.2% and 2.4%±0.3%), respectively (Figures 2B, C). The same effect, as that observed with CD107a, was also seen for IFN-γ expression by CD56bright and CD56dim NK cells (data not shown).

NK cell proliferation impeded by use of clinical immunosuppressive drugs

The ability of NK cells to proliferate *in vitro* following stimulation with the 721.221 cell line with IL-2 and IL-12 cytokines was measured by decreased CFSE intensity compared to the undivided parental population (Figure 3A). The dynamics of proliferating NK cells under immunosuppressive conditions matched those of cytokine production with a significant decline in proliferation from baseline (57.5%±14.5%) in the presence of Cyclosporine A at 100 ng/ml (6.6%±4.5%) and 1000 ng/ml (3.7%±1.8%), Prednisolone at 100 ng/ml (18.2%±6.7%) and 1000 ng/ml (6.3%±1.7%) and MPA at 1000 ng/ml (2.3%±0.8%) (Figure 3B).

Additional inhibition of intracellular signalling pathways

To help elucidate which intracellular signalling pathways the K562 cell line and PMA-I stimulation of NK cells were acting through, additional functional assays were performed with immune cell inhibitor drugs LY294002 (inhibitor of Pi3K activity), PD98059 (inhibitor of MEK in MAPK pathway), Rapamycin (inhibitor of mTOR) and Rottlerin (inhibitor of PKC in the NFkB pathway). The toxicity at five concentrations of each inhibitor was tested by determining PI uptake by non-viable cells as compared to the control. The percentage of PI+ non-viable cells was observed

to decide the optimal non-toxic concentration to proceed with in further assays (data not shown). NK cells were stimulated with K562 target cells and PMA-I, as described previously, with or without the addition of the inhibitors LY294002 (25 uM), PD98059 (25 uM), Rapamycin (100 nM) and Rottlerin (5 uM). It was observed that CD107a expression after K562 stimulation was significantly decreased with the addition of the inhibitor PD98059 at 25 uM (13.3%±3.5% vs 6.1%±2.0%), whilst there was a trend for a decline observed with LY294002 and Rottlerin (Figure 4Ai). Similarly, following PMA-I stimulation there was a significant decrease in CD107a expression compared to the control (27.0%±4.0%) with the addition of LY294002 (17.7%±3.8%), PD98059 (18.0%±2.8%) and Rottlerin (18.6%±3.0%) (Figure 4Aii). No effect was observed on IFNγ production following PMA-I stimulation (Figure 4B).

Lung transplantation affects NK cell function

Ten LTR, all of whom were not receiving immunosuppression pre-transplant, were included in a longitudinal analysis of NK cell function in response to immunosuppression. Demographic details of the LTR are shown in Table 1. The expression of both CD107a and IFN-γ on NK cells following PMA-I stimulation did not significantly differ between healthy controls (n = 20) or transplant recipients group analyses, either pre-transplant or within the first year post-transplant (data not shown). However individual patient dynamics revealing three different longitudinal patterns of NK cell function were observed (Figure 5). Stable NK cell function over time was seen in two of three patients who in the first year post-transplant had no evidence of either allograft rejection or viral infection (clinically stable). Four patients who developed viral infections early post-transplant demonstrated a transient increase in NK cell cytotoxicity contemporaneous to the viral infection. The observed changes in NK cell activity were not found to be

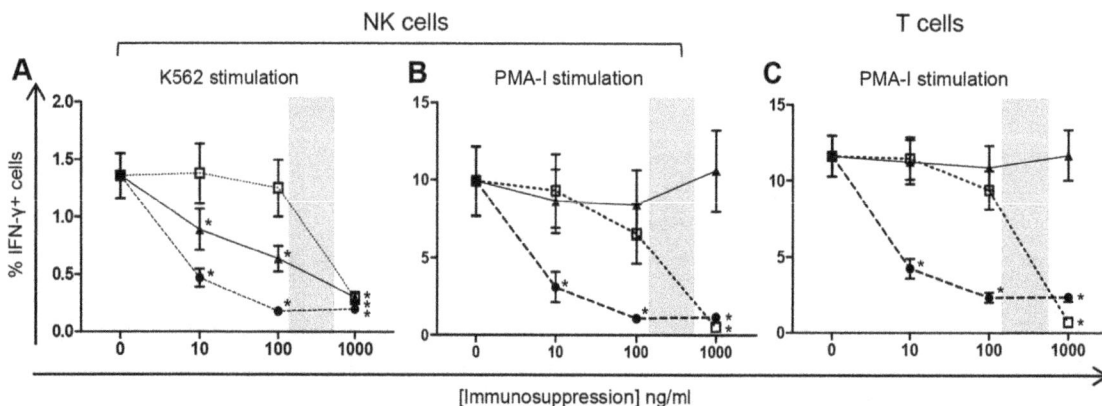

Figure 2. NK cell and T cell IFN-γ production in the presence of immunosuppressive drugs. PBMC from 20 healthy controls were stimulated in culture with the cell line K562 or PMA-I in the presence of varying concentrations of immunosuppressive drugs. NK cell IFN-γ production measured in response to stimulation with K562 cell line (A) and PMA-I (B). T cell IFN-γ production measured in response to PMA-I stimulation (C). Statistical significance was defined as $p<0.001$. Graphed data are presented as mean ± SEM. Symbols represent immunosuppressive drugs: ●, Cyclosporine A; □, MPA; ▲, Prednisolone. Shaded areas signify therapeutic range.

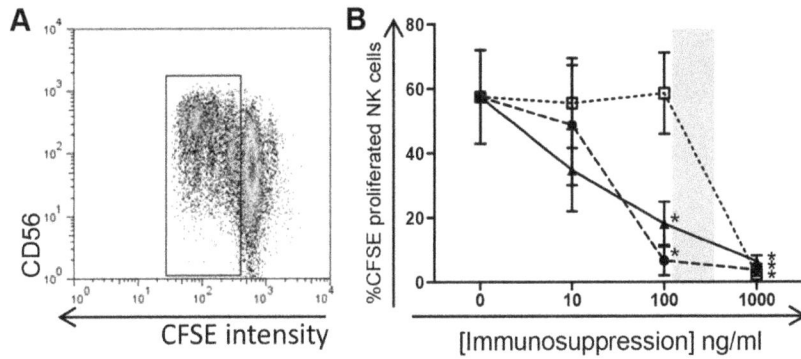

Figure 3. Proliferation of NK cells in the presence of immunosuppressive drugs. MACS enriched NK cells from three healthy controls were labelled with CFSE and stimulated in culture for three days with a combination of IL-2, IL-12 and 721.221 cell lines in the presence or absence of immunosuppressants Cyclosporine A, MPA and Prednisolone. An example of the change in CFSE intensity as the cells proliferate is shown (A). NK cell proliferation is displayed in response to treatment with varying concentrations of the immunosuppressive drugs (B, $p<0.05$ for all). Graphed data are presented as the mean $\pm$ SEM from three independent experiments. Symbols represent immunosuppressive drugs: ●, Cyclosporine A; □, MPA; ▲, Prednisolone. Shaded area signifies therapeutic range.

solely attributable to the induction therapy the patients (Tx#1 and Tx#8) received. Finally, increased NK cell cytotoxicity was seen in patients who developed histologically-confirmed acute cellular rejection between 9 and 12 months post-transplant. Compared to pre-transplant levels, the three patients who experienced acute cellular rejection demonstrated a 3.6 fold increase in NK cytotoxicity at the time of allograft rejection, whilst the four patients who developed viral infections demonstrated a 2.3 fold increase in NK cell cytotoxicity at the time of viral recrudescence compared to baseline values. Given that the study was limited to the first year post-transplant, we were unable to confirm that NK cell function decreased to basal levels following clinical intervention.

Discussion

In a cohort of healthy controls and LTR we performed a detailed analysis of NK cell function in the presence of differing stimulation conditions and following administration of the commonly used clinical immunosuppressants, calcineurin inhibitors, anti-proliferative agents and corticosteroids. We demonstrated using well-defined *in vitro* assays that the addition of specific immunosuppressive drugs differentially impacted on NK cell cytotoxicity, cytokine production and proliferation, which was dependent on the primary stimulus. Importantly, these immunosuppressive drugs were found to impair NK cell function at concentrations corresponding to the therapeutic range used in the management of lung transplant patients [9,10,21,22,23].

The absence of HLA class I molecules expressed on K562 means that there is no inhibitory signal provided when NK cell receptors engage with the target cells resulting in NK cell activation and the release of cytotoxic granules containing perforin and granzymes and subsequent target cell lysis [7]. Observation of the differential effects of each of the three immunosuppressive drugs (Cyclosporine A, MPA and Prednisolone) on inhibiting NK cell cytotoxity following K562 stimulation provides mechanistic

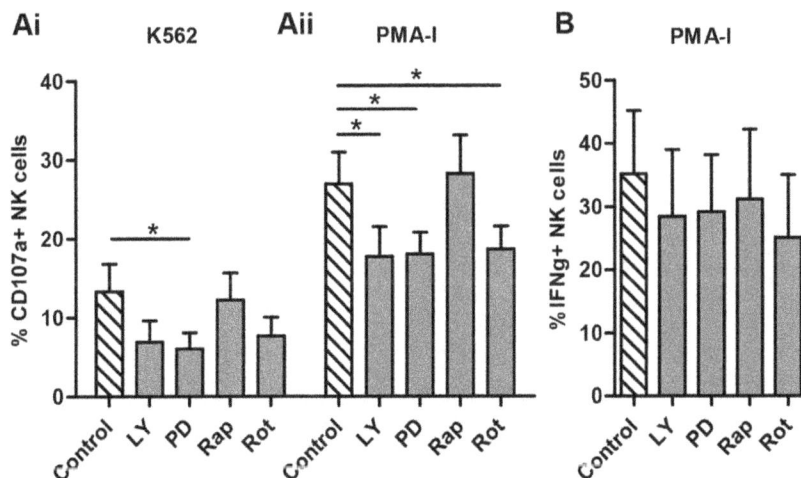

Figure 4. Inhibition of intracellular signaling pathways. NK cells from six controls were cultured with K562 and PMA-I alone (control) or in the presence of the inhibitor drugs LY294002 (25 μM), PD98059 (25 μM), Rapamycin (100 nM) and Rottlerin (5 μM). NK cell function was assessed for CD107a expression (A) and IFN-γ production (B) in response to addition of inhibitor drugs in culture. CD107a expression is shown to be reduced by addition of inhibitor drugs affecting pathways of cellular activation. Statistical significance was defined as $p<0.05$. Graphed data presented as mean $\pm$ SEM.

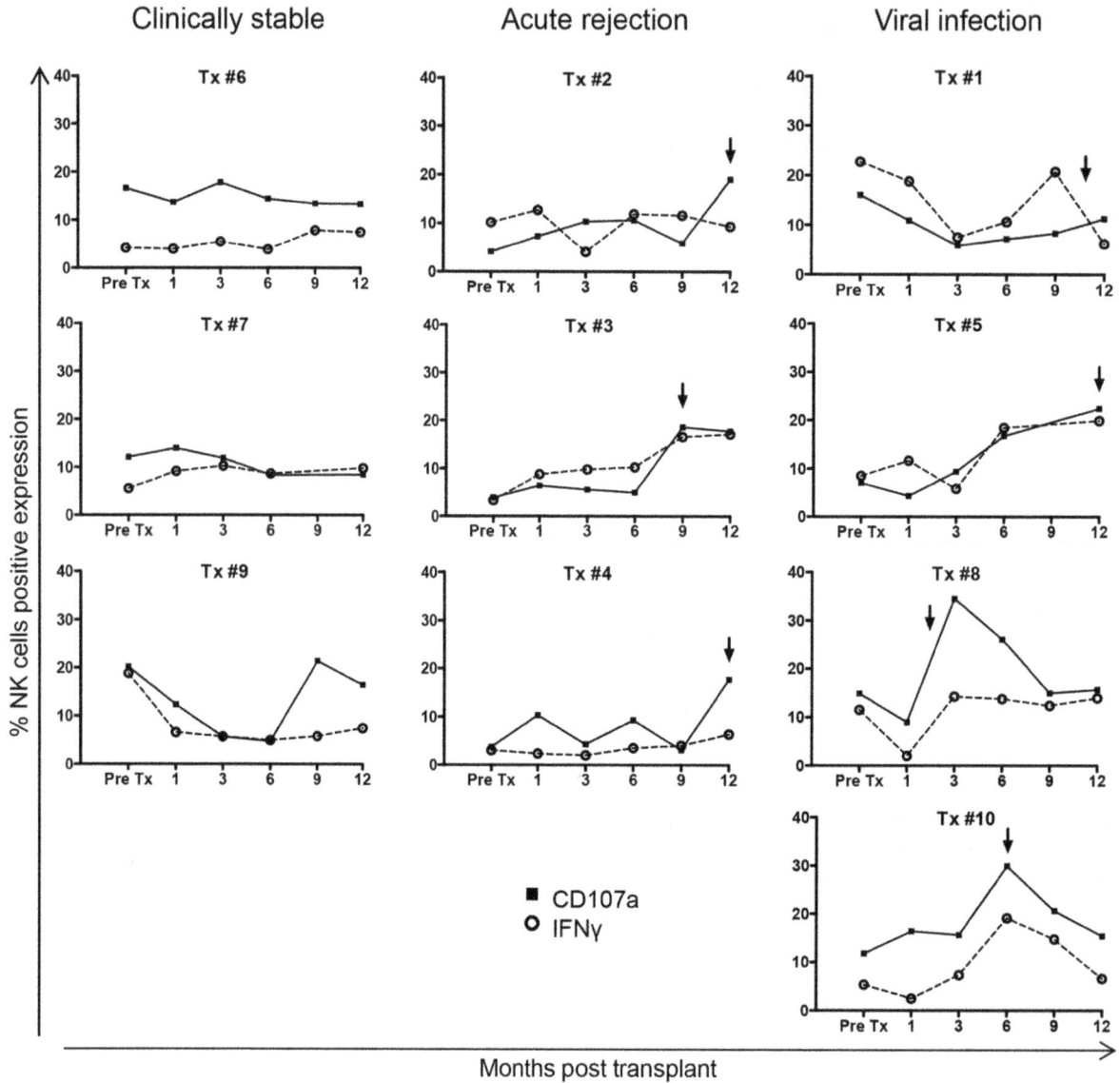

Figure 5. Functional changes in NK cells from lung transplant patients. PBMC from ten LTR, not receiving immunosuppression pre-transplant (Pre-Tx), were stimulated in culture with PMA-I. Individual graphs of NK cell CD107a expression (closed square) and IFN-γ production (open circle) from LTR with clinically stable post-transplantation follow-up (Tx #6, #7, #9), episodes of acute rejection (Tx #2, #3, #4) or viral infection (Tx #1, #5, #8, #10). The arrows represent the occurrence of each clinical event in the months post-transplant.

insights into how these drugs influence NK cell activation pathways. Unlike MPA and Prednisolone, Cyclosporine A, an inhibitor that effectively reduces IL-2 production by blocking the calcineurin pathway [9], failed to inhibit NK cell cytotoxicity following K562 stimulation, suggesting activation of NK cells by K562 occurs via a calcineurin-independent pathway. Given that Cyclosporine A prevents calcineurin from dephosphorylating the NFAT transcription factor thus inhibiting transcription of genes encoding IL-2 and leading to a dampened effector T cell response, it is likely that NK cells have a similar intracellular calcineurin pathway to T cells. This finding of ineffectual activity towards NK cell cytotoxicity corroborates previous reports demonstrating that NK cells cultured in the presence of Cyclosporine A retained their cytotoxic capabilities against various target cell lines, including K562 [16,18,24,25,26]. Similarly, the alternative calcineurin inhibitor Tacrolimus was also found to have no effect on NK

cell cytotoxicity against target cells [16,27,28]. However there are contradictory reports in the literature as to whether NK cell degranulation/cytotoxicity is affected by Cyclosporine [27,29,30]. The differences observed in these studies may be explained by the use of different experimental techniques used in these assays and pre-incubation of effector cells with immunosuppressive drugs in culture for an extended period of time which likely severely impairs the activity of the cells prior to testing in functional assays.

The effects of Prednisolone and MPA on decreasing NK cell cytotoxicity fits with published observations describing impaired NK cell lysis of K562 target cells in an *in vitro* environment [25,31] down regulation of NK cell activating receptors and inhibition of cytotoxic granule exocytosis [12,13]. With the inclusion of additional intracellular pathway inhibitors LY, PD and Rottlerin, NK cell function following K562 stimulation was shown to be decreased. However as this observation was only significantly

Table 1. Lung transplant patient and healthy control demographics.

Patient	Age at time of Tx	Gender	Transplantation Indication	CMV Serostatus D/R
Tx #1*	30	M	CF	−/−
Tx #2	58	M	EMP	+/+
Tx #3	30	F	CF	+/−
Tx #4	52	F	EMP	−/+
Tx #5	30	F	CF	−/−
Tx #6	30	M	CF	−/−
Tx #7	51	F	EMP	−/−
Tx #8*	59	M	COPD	+/+
Tx #9	52	M	EMP	−/−
Tx #10	19	M	BRON	−/+
Control #1–20	Mean: 42	10M/10F	NA	NA

Tx indicates transplant; D indicates donor; R indicates recipient; CF indicates cystic fibrosis; EMP indicates emphysema; COPD indicates chronic obstructive pulmonary disease; BRON indicates bronchiectasis; NA indicates not applicable.
*Patients who received Anti-thymocyte globulin.

affected with the addition of PD, it can be surmised that K562 stimulation of NK cell cytotoxicity has most influence acting through the MAP-kinase pathway of activation.

To determine whether the type of stimulus was a critical factor influencing the role of immunosuppressive drugs on NK cell function, PMA-I was used as an alternative stimulant. PMA is a phorbol ester that induces activation of Protein Kinase C (PKC), resulting in phosphorylation of activators of transcription leading to increased gene expression [32]. Ionomycin is an ionophore that raises the intracellular level of calcium and is commonly used in conjunction with PMA to stimulate intracellular production of various cytokines including interferons and IL-2 [32,33]. Interestingly following PMA-I stimulation, an inverse inhibition pattern was observed in NK cells following treatment with Prednisolone and Cyclosporine A, compared to K562 stimulation. Specifically, high dose MPA and Cyclosporine A significantly reduced NK cell cytotoxicity, whilst Prednisolone had no functional effect. Given the mechanism of inhibition by Cyclosporine A in this setting, it is likely that NK cell activation following PMA-I stimulation is directed via the calcineurin pathway of intracellular signalling possibly in response to increased levels of calcium (which activate calcineurin) due to inclusion of Ionomycin. Cytotoxicity inhibition kinetics were shown to be identical for both NK cell and T cell populations, suggesting that the same intracellular signalling pathways are used following PMA-I stimulation. As the addition of the inhibitors LY, PD and Rottlerin caused a significant reduction in NK cell cytotoxicity in a similar manner to that observed with Cyclosporine and MPA, it can be suggested that the point of action of PMA-I on NK cell stimulation occurs through multiple pathways of intracellular activation (including PKC and calcineurin pathways, as expected) or alternatively at a common point downstream of each pathway.

The production of immunomodulatory cytokines following stimulation is a hallmark feature associated with functionally activated cells. Following K562 stimulation, the ability of NK cells to produce IFN-γ was severely impaired by individual treatment with the three immunosuppressive drugs, with NK cells exhibiting a 100-fold increase in sensitivity in the presence of Cyclosporine A and Prednisolone compared to MPA. However, this inhibition was not mirrored following use of the alternate stimulus PMA-I. In this setting NK cells treated with high does Prednisolone did not show

impairment of IFN-γ production, which was also observed in the T cell population. Collectively, these observations convincingly demonstrated that immunosuppressive drugs have differential NK cell functional effects, which are dependent on the primary stimulus for the induction of independent intracellular signalling pathways. Cyclosporine A inhibits cytokine production via calcineurin inhibition. On the other hand, Prednisolone inhibition of NK cell function may be related to its action at the transcriptional level to regulate gene expression. Prednisolone has been shown to inhibit the expression of NK cell receptors necessary for activation and cytotoxicity [12,13]. Depending on the NK cell stimulus used in our culture setting, either receptor engagement with target cell or through the action of PMA-I, different transcription factors are likely to be involved to promote different gene expression for various aspects of NK cell function.

In addition to investigating the ability of NK cells to induce cytotoxicity and cytokine production in the presence of immunosuppressive drug treatment, the proliferative capacity following dual stimulation with cytokines (IL-2 and IL-12) and a HLA class-I deficient cell line (721.221) was also explored. A dose-dependent reduction in NK cell proliferation for both Prednisolone and Cyclosporine A was observed with a 10-fold increase in sensitivity compared to MPA treatment. Interestingly, although we expected that the anti-proliferative agent, MPA, would have dramatically reduced NK cell proliferation at all concentrations tested this was not the case. This observation may be explained by the presence of IL-2 at a high concentration of 250 U/ml, a prominent stimulator of lymphocyte activation and growth, in the assay culture used to stimulate the NK cells [34,35]. The addition of IL-2 may have provided an environment conducive to dampen down the immunosuppressive effects of MPA at lower concentrations but not influence the drug action of Cyclosporine A or Prednisolone. Cyclosporine A selectively blocks IL-2 transcription in activated cells and impairs both the synthesis and cell surface expression of the high affinity IL-2R [9]. Prednisolone, through its action of modifying gene transcription, may also act to reduce expression of the IL-2R thus causing NK cells to not become activated in response to the IL-2 in the culture medium. The absence of both IL-2 and the IL-2R would reduce the proliferative potential of NK cells following stimulation. The data generated in our in vitro assay system correlated with a previous report demonstrating reduced proliferation of the major blood population of CD56dim NK cells in response to Cyclosporine A [18] and impaired NK cell proliferation and survival with the addition of methylprednisolone following IL-2 stimulation [13]. As prolonged exposure to Cyclosporine A for 7 days and Prednisolone for 5 days has been shown to induce NK cell apoptosis [13,18], and activation-induced cell death occurs in a proportion of NK cells after they bind to a target cell and carry out 'natural cytotoxicity' [36]; the observed loss in proliferation after three days culture may be influenced by the death of some NK cells.

We have previously published work showing changes in the phenotype of NK cells corresponding to clinical episodes in the early months following lung transplantation [6]. However this work did not directly address NK cell functional changes post-transplantation.

This longitudinal study follows on from the phenotypic analysis, to assess NK cell function in LTR and has revealed a number of interesting findings. Surprisingly NK cell function (cytotoxicity and IFN-γ production), as a collective group, did not significantly vary between normal controls and LTR when analysed cross-sectionally. Whilst NK cells might be expected to become activated following a HLA-mismatched transplant, this may have been nullified by the addition of immunosuppressive drugs. The longitudinal analysis showed that even in the presence of immunosuppressive drugs, NK cells are capable of becoming transiently more active in the setting of self-limiting viral infections or acute rejection. While this study was not able to assess whether NK cells are primarily responsible for viral clearance following infection, it is worth noting that viral infections in immunosup-pressed individuals are associated with increased viral load suggesting that viral clearance mechanisms are impaired in this setting [37,38].

This study showed that NK cell function is impaired in the presence of therapeutic doses of immunosuppressive drugs that are commonly given to solid organ transplant recipients. Our findings confirm other published results demonstrating altered NK cell function in response to transplantation immunosuppression and support the view that this is an important area for future investigation in both the laboratory and in the clinic. We demonstrated that NK cell function changed with time from transplant and in parallel to clinical episodes of viral infection and acute rejection. Future studies are now being undertaken to formally assess NK cell alloreactivity against KIR-ligand mis-matched targets both in the presence and absence of commonly used immunosuppressive drugs, and as to whether NK cell profiles influence the long term survival of lung allografts following transplantation.

Acknowledgments

The authors would like to acknowledge all the clinicians, nurses and Allied Health professionals associated with the Lung Transplant Service at The Alfred Hospital, and the patients and controls recruited for this study.

Author Contributions

Conceived and designed the experiments: ACM NAM THON TCK GPW. Performed the experiments: ACM. Analyzed the data: ACM GPW. Wrote the paper: ACM GPW NAM THON BJL GIS TCK.

References

1. van der Touw W, Bromberg JS (2010) Natural killer cells and the immune response in solid organ transplantation. Am J Transplant 10: 1354–1358.

2. Fildes JE, Yonan N, Tunstall K, Walker AH, Griffiths-Davies L, et al. (2008) Natural killer cells in peripheral blood and lung tissue are associated with chronic rejection after lung transplantation. J Heart Lung Transplant 27: 203–207.

3. Kwakkel-van Erp JM, van de Graaf EA, Paantjens AWM, van Ginkel WGJ, Schellekens J, et al. (2008) The killer immunoglobulin-like receptor (KIR) group A haplotype is associated with bronchiolitis obliterans syndrome after lung transplantation. J Heart Lung Transplant 27: 995–1001.

4. Pratschke J, Stauch D, Kotsch K (2009) Role of NK and NKT cells in solid organ transplantation. Transpl Int 22: 859–868.

5. Ruggeri L, Capanni M, Urbani E, Perruccio K, Shlomchik WD, et al. (2002) Effectiveness of donor natural killer cell alloreactivity in mismatched hematopoietic transplants. Science 295: 2097–2100.

6. Meehan AC, Sullivan LC, Mifsud NA, Brooks AG, Snell GI, et al. (2010) Natural killer cell activation in the lung allograft early posttransplantation. Transplantation 89: 756–763.

7. Parham P (2005) MHC class I molecules and KIRs in human history, health and survival. Nat Rev Immunol 5: 201–214.

8. Fildes JE, Yonan N, Leonard CT (2008) Natural killer cells and lung transplantation, roles in rejection, infection, and tolerance. Transpl Immunol 19: 1–11.

9. Gummert JF, Ikonen T, Morris RE (1999) Newer immunosuppressive drugs: a review. J Am Soc Nephrol 10: 1366–1380.

10. Allen J (2004) Immunosuppression for lung transplantation. Thorac Cardiovasc Surg 16: 333–341.

11. Srinivas TR, Kaplan B, Meier-Kriesche HU (2003) Mycophenolate mofetil in solid-organ transplantation. Expert Opin Pharmacother 4: 2325–2345.

12. Vitale C, Chiossone L, Cantoni C, Morreale G, Cottalasso F, et al. (2004) The corticosteroid-induced inhibitory effect on NK cell function reflects down-regulation and/or dysfunction of triggering receptors involved in natural cytotoxicity. Eur J Immunol 34: 3028–3038.

13. Chiossone L, Vitale C, Cottalasso F, Moretti S, Azzarone B, et al. (2007) Molecular analysis of the methylprednisolone-mediated inhibition of NK-cell function: evidence for different susceptibility of IL-2- versus IL-15-activated NK cells. Blood 109: 3767–3775.

14. Stewart S, Fishbein MC, Snell GI, Berry GJ, Boehler A, et al. (2007) Revision of the 1996 working formulation for the standardization of nomenclature in the diagnosis of lung rejection. J Heart Lung Transplant 26: 1229–1242.

15. Barten MJ, Dhein S, Chang H, Bittner HB, Tarnok A, et al. (2003) Assessment of immunosuppressive drug interactions: inhibition of lymphocyte function in peripheral human blood. J Immunol Methods 283: 99–114.

16. Wai LE, Fujiki M, Takeda S, Martinez OM, Krams SM (2008) Rapamycin, but not cyclosporine or FK506, alters natural killer cell function. Transplantation 85: 145–149.

17. Gummert JF, Barten MJ, Sherwood SW, van Gelder T, Morris RE (1999) Pharmacodynamics of immunosuppression by mycophenolic acid: inhibition of both lymphocyte proliferation and activation correlates with pharmacokinetics. J Pharmacol Exp Ther 291: 1100–1112.

18. Wang H, Grzywacz B, Sukovich D, McCullar V, Cao Q, et al. (2007) The unexpected effect of cyclosporin A on CD56+CD16 and CD56+CD16+ natural killer cell subpopulations. Blood 110: 1530–1539.

19. Alter G, Malenfant JM, Altfeld M (2004) CD107a as a functional marker for the identification of natural killer cell activity. J Immunol Methods 294: 15–22.

20. Cooper MA, Fehniger TA, Caligiuri MA (2001) The biology of human natural killer-cell subsets. Trends Immunol 22: 633–640.

21. Morton JM, Williamson S, Kear LM, McWhinney BC, Potter J, et al. (2006) Therapeutic drug monitoring of prednisolone after lung transplantation. J Heart Lung Transplant 25: 557–563.

22. Oellerich M, Armstrong VW, Schutz E, Shaw LM (1998) Therapeutic drug monitoring of cyclosporine and tacrolimus. Update on Lake Louise Consensus Conference on cyclosporin and tacrolimus. Clin Biochem 31: 309–316.

23. Arns W, Cibrik DM, Walker RG, Mourad G, Budde K, et al. (2006) Therapeutic drug monitoring of mycophenolic acid in solid organ transplant patients treated with mycophenolate mofetil: review of the literature. Transplantation 82: 1004–1012.

24. Petersson E, Qi Z, Ekberg H, Ostraat O, Dohlsten M, et al. (1997) Activation of alloreactive natural killer cells is resistant to cyclosporine. Transplantation 63: 1138–1144.

25. Eissens DN, Van Der Meer A, Van Cranenbroek B, Preijers FW, Joosten I (2010) Rapamycin and MPA, but not CsA, impair human NK cell cytotoxicity due to differential effects on NK cell phenotype. Am J Transplant 10: 1981–1990.

26. Shao-Hsien C, Lang I, Gunn H, Lydyard P (1983) Effect of in vitro cyclosporin A treatment on human natural and antibody-dependent cell-mediated cytotoxicity. Transplantation 35: 127–129.

27. Wasik M, Gorski A, Stepien-Sopniewska B, Lagodzinski Z (1991) Effect of FK506 versus cyclosporine on human natural and antibody-dependent cytotoxicity reactions in vitro. Transplantation 51: 268–270.

28. Hoogduijn MJ, Roemeling-van Rhijn M, Korevaar SS, Engela AU, Weimar W, et al. (2011) Immunological aspects of allogeneic and autologous mesenchymal stem cell therapies. Hum Gene Ther 22: 1587–1591.

29. Introna M, Allavena P, Spreafico F, Mantovani A (1981) Inhibition of human natural killer activity by cyclosporin A. Transplantation 31: 113–116.

30. Morteau O, Blundell S, Chakera A, Bennett S, Christou CM, et al. (2010) Renal transplant immunosuppression impairs natural killer cell function in vitro and in vivo. PLoS One 5: e13294.

31. Thum MY, Bhaskaran S, Abdalla HI, Ford B, Sumar N, et al. (2008) Prednisolone suppresses NK cell cytotoxicity in vitro in women with a history of infertility and elevated NK cell cytotoxicity. Am J Reprod Immunol 59: 259–265.

32. Nishizuka Y (1992) Intracellular signaling by hydrolysis of phospholipids and activation of protein kinase C. Science 258: 607–614.

33. Baran J, Kowalczyk D, Ozog M, Zembala M (2001) Three-color flow cytometry detection of intracellular cytokines in peripheral blood mononuclear cells: comparative analysis of phorbol myristate acetate-ionomycin and phytohemagglutinin stimulation. Clin Diagn Lab Immunol 8: 303–313.

34. Lan RY, Selmi C, Gershwin ME (2008) The regulatory, inflammatory, and T cell programming roles of interleukin-2 (IL-2). J Autoimmun 31: 7–12.

35. Pillet AH, Bugault F, Theze J, Chakrabarti LA, Rose T (2009) A programmed switch from IL-15- to IL-2-dependent activation in human NK cells. J Immunol 182: 6267–6277.

36. Warren HS (2011) Target-induced natural killer cell loss as a measure of NK cell responses. J Immunol Methods 370: 86–92.

37. Yokoyama WM (2005) Specific and non-specific natural killer cell responses to viral infection. Adv Exp Med Biol 560: 57–61.

38. Engstrand M, Lidehall AK, Totterman TH, Herrman B, Eriksson BM, et al. (2003) Cellular responses to cytomegalovirus in immunosuppressed patients: circulating CD8+ T cells recognizing CMVpp65 are present but display functional impairment. Clin Exp Immunol 132: 96–104.

10

Herpes Virus Infection Is Associated with Vascular Remodeling and Pulmonary Hypertension in Idiopathic Pulmonary Fibrosis

Fiorella Calabrese[1]*, **Anja Kipar**[2,3,4], **Francesca Lunardi**[1], **Elisabetta Balestro**[1], **Egle Perissinotto**[1], **Emanuela Rossi**[1], **Nazarena Nannini**[1], **Giuseppe Marulli**[1], **James P. Stewart**[2,3], **Federico Rea**[1]

1 Department of Cardiac, Thoracic and Vascular Sciences, University of Padova, Padova, Italy, 2 Department of Infection Biology, University of Liverpool, Liverpool, United Kingdom, 3 School of Veterinary Science, University of Liverpool, Liverpool, United Kingdom, 4 Veterinary Pathology, Department of Basic Veterinary Science, Faculty of Veterinary Medicine, University of Helsinki, Helsinki, Finland

Abstract

Background: Pulmonary hypertension (PH) represents an important complication of idiopathic pulmonary fibrosis (IPF) with a negative impact on patient survival. Herpes viruses are thought to play an etiological role in the development and/or progression of IPF. The influence of viruses on PH associated with IPF is unknown. We aimed to investigate the influence of viruses in IPF patients focusing on aspects related to PH. A laboratory mouse model of gamma-herpesvirus (MHV-68) induced pulmonary fibrosis was also assessed.

Methods: Lung tissue samples from 55 IPF patients and 41 controls were studied by molecular analysis to detect various viral genomes. Viral molecular data obtained were correlated with mean pulmonary arterial pressure (mPAP) and arterial remodelling. Different clinical and morphological variables were studied by univariate and multivariate analyses at time of transplant and in the early post-transplant period. The same lung tissue analyses were performed in MHV-68 infected mice.

Results: A higher frequency of virus positive cases was found in IPF patients than in controls ($p = 0.0003$) and only herpes virus genomes were detected. Viral cases showed higher mPAP ($p = 0.01$), poorer performance in the six minute walking test (6MWT; $p = 0.002$) and higher frequency of primary graft (PGD) dysfunction after lung transplant ($p = 0.02$). Increased arterial thickening, particularly of the intimal layer ($p = 0.002$ and $p = 0.004$) and higher TGF-β expression ($p = 0.002$) were demonstrated in viral cases. The remodelled vessels showed increased vessel cell proliferation (Ki-67 positive cells) in the proximity to metaplastic epithelial cells and macrophages. Viral infection was associated with higher mPAP ($p = 0.03$), poorer performance in the 6MWT ($p = 0.008$) and PGD ($p = 0.02$) after adjusting for other covariates/intermediate factors. In MHV-68 infected mice, morphological features were similar to those of patients.

Conclusion: Herpesviral infections may contribute to the development of PH in IPF patients.

Editor: Martin R.J. Kolb, McMaster University, Canada

Funding: This study was supported by the Italian Ministry of Instruction, University and Research (prot. 60A07-0959/11). The funder had no role in study design, data collection and analysis, decision to publish, or preparation of the manuscript.

Competing Interests: The authors have declared that no competing interests exist.

* E-mail: fiorella.calabrese@unipd.it

Introduction

Idiopathic pulmonary fibrosis (IPF), morphologically usual interstitial pneumonia, is a chronic progressive disease of unknown aetiology with irreversible scarring in the lung [1]. No proven effective treatment is available other than lung transplantation. Survival time is estimated at 2.5 years after initial diagnosis, although disease progression is highly variable [2,3]. Acute exacerbation, lung cancer and pulmonary hypertension (PH) are the main complications which adversely affect the survival of IPF patients. Different from acute exacerbation which can occur at any stage of the disease, lung cancer and pulmonary hypertension (PH) are more likely in advanced disease. For the latter, a frequency of 20–90% has been reported and it carries severe consequences

including decreased exercise capacity and increased mortality before and after lung transplantation [4–7].

Recent studies have shown that PH measured with right-heart catheterization or transthoracic echocardiography in IPF patients is associated with low DLCO, shorter walk distances, and desaturation during exercise [5,6]. Similar relationships have been identified when brain natriuretic peptide was used as a surrogate marker for PH in IPF patients [8].

However to date no clinical or biohumoral parameters are available as predictive markers of PH in IPF patients. Several authors have shown that PH in IPF relates poorly to the degree of pulmonary function test and is not always confined to advanced disease [6]. Indeed even in end stage IPF cohorts, no association between the presence of PH and severity of the disease (both in terms of functional parameters and fibrosis extension) has been observed [6,9].

Pathogenic mechanisms of IPF and of its main complications are complex and still largely unknown although different hypotheses have been proposed, varying from previous chronic inflammation with subsequent widespread fibrosis to abnormal wound healing. Increasing evidence suggests that a key event in IPF is deregulated epithelial cell function with ongoing alveolar epithelial injury and an associated abnormal host repair response, leading to patchy and heterogeneous morphological changes [10]. The complex biological processes that underlie pulmonary fibrosis might directly contribute to the pathogenesis of vascular remodelling which is equally patchy and heterogeneous. Fibrotic areas have fewer blood vessels but adjacent, non fibrotic tissues seem highly vascularised [11]. Structural changes range from capillary loss to complex vascular lesions with intima, media thickening and adventitial fibrosis. Endothelial injury, usually occurring through apoptotic cell death is another crucial aspect in the pathogenesis of IPF-associated PH as reported in recent studies [12–14]. Different types of mediators, including those released by injured endothelial cells, may be involved in vascular remodelling by influencing vessel smooth muscle or adventitial cell proliferation. Several studies have implicated viral infection as a cause of epithelial injury and therefore an important factor in its pathogenesis [15–34]. Among viral agents herpes viruses, in particular Epstein Barr virus (EBV), have been suggested as principal cofactors (as initiating or exacerbating agents) of fibrotic lung disease and treatment with ganciclovir has been shown to attenuate disease progression in a subgroup of patients [35].

Alveolar epithelial cells, one of the most important targets of the virus, are then involved in the activation of different signalling pathways responsible for fibrotic lung remodelling. In viral animal and cell models several profibrogenic cytokines/chemokines have been shown to be over-expressed and among these transforming growth factor beta 1 (TGF-β1) plays a key role [27,32–34]. While many works, experimental and clinical, have highlighted the influence of EBV in promoting fibrotic parenchymal remodelling, its influence on endothelial injury and vessel remodelling and other related parameters of PH has not been yet assessed.

The aim of the study was to investigate the relevance of respiratory viruses in IPF patients, with special emphasis on cases complicated by PH. For this purpose a large number of IPF patients and control subjects including other non-IPF diffuse parenchymal lung diseases (DPLDs) were studied. Viral molecular data were correlated with mean pulmonary arterial pressure (mPAP) and arterial remodelling. Different clinical and morphological variables were studied by univariate and multivariate analysis at time of transplant and in the early post-transplant period.

A mouse model was used to examine whether murine gammaherpesvirus-68 (MHV-68), genetically and biologically similar to EBV, contributes to the development of vessel remodelling other than pulmonary fibrosis.

Materials and Methods

Study Population

Native lungs from 55 IPF patients who underwent lung transplantation (LT) between September 1998 and February 2010 in our Centre were studied (39 males and 16 females; mean age: 55.2±9.2 yrs, 33 single vs 22 bilateral LT). The control group consisted of 22 native lungs from other non-IPF -DPLDs- (8 males and 14 females; mean age: 44±11.4 yrs, 11 lymphangioleiomyomatosis, 4 Langerhans-cell histiocytosis, 2 sarcoidosis, 2 hypersen-

sitivity pneumonitis, 1 non-specific interstitial pneumonia, 1 desquamative interstitial pneumonia, 1 scleroderma lung fibrosis) and 19 normal lungs (13 non implanted donor lungs and 6 autopsy cases). Prior to LT after the diagnosis of IPF, the majority received oral prednisone while a minority were treated with prednisone and azathioprine.

Each patient underwent pulmonary function testing, high resolution computed tomography and right heart catheterization. These tests were performed in all patients at the time of waiting list inclusion and before LT. For the present study clinical/functional parameters collected at the time of LT were considered.

The diagnosis of interstitial lung disease was based on the diagnostic criteria of the American Thoracic Society/European Respiratory Society Consensus Classification System [1]. The clinical history was collected, with special emphasis on age at onset of symptoms, smoking history, occupational exposure, co-morbidities and therapy (medical and non medical).

Moreover, short term post-transplant follow-up (12 months after LT) was also considered in all IPF cases, mainly focusing on primary graft dysfunction (PGD) and acute rejection, both considered causes of early and late graft dysfunction. PGD and acute rejection were graded as proposed by the International Society for Heart and Lung Transplantation (ISHLT) Working Group [36,37]. Acute rejection was evaluated in 143 scheduled transbronchial biopsies collected in the first post-transplant year. These data have been presented at the 2010 ISHLT annual meeting.

Written informed consent was obtained from all subjects. The work was approved by the Institutional Ethics Committee. Relevant clinical data of the IPF and non-IPF DPLD population are summarized in Table 1.

Table 1. Study subjects (IPF patients and non-IPF DPLDs).

IPF patients (n = 55)		DPLDs (n = 22)
Age at transplantation (years)	55.1 (7.9)	44.1 (12.6)
Type of transplantation (bilateral)	22 (40.0%)	16 (72.7%)
Men	39 (70.9%)	9 (40.2%)
BMI	27.1 (4.0)	23.4 (5.2)
Smoking status		
never smoked	9 (16.4%)	10 (45.4%)
previous smoker	46 (83.6%)	7 (31.8%)
History of environmental exposure	3 (5.5%)	0
Co-morbidities		
Gastritis	5 (9.1%)	1 (4.5%)
Diabetes	6 (10.9%)	0
CHD	4 (7.3%)	0
Obesity	13 (23.6%)	2 (9.1%)
FEV1 (% of predicted value)	47.9 (16.2)	39.2 (25.3)
FVC (% of predicted value)	45.6 (14.5)	49.0 (22.4)
VC (% of predicted value)	43.4 (14.3)	51.0 (21.0)
TLC (% of predicted value)	53.4 (15.4)	71.4 (20.9)
DLco (% of predicted value)	26.0 (17.0)	23.5 (20.5)
mPAP	24.0 (8.9)	28.8 (15.4)

Data are number of patients (%) or mean (sd). IPF: idiopathic pulmonary fibrosis; DPLDs: Diffuse parenchymal lung diseases; BMI: body mass index; CHD: coronary heart disease.

Molecular Viral Detection

Nucleic acids were extracted from fresh lung tissues sampled from different areas (~1 mg of tissue) of all 96 cases (55 IPF patients and 41 control subjects) using a modified RNAzol method [38]. Reverse transcriptase (RT)-polymerase chain reaction (PCR), PCR or nested-PCR were used to detect principal respiratory viral genomes: adenovirus, cytomegalovirus (CMV), EBV, rhinovirus, influenzavirus A and B, metapneumovirus, herpes virus (HHV)-6, HHV-7, HHV-8, parvovirus (PV) B19, parainfluenzavirus 1 and 3 and respiratory syncytial virus (as heminested PCR) as previously reported [39]. The oligonucleotides used to ascertain the quality of extracted RNA or DNA were complementary to the mRNA glyceraldehyde-3-phosphate dehydrogenize (3GPDH) and β-globin gene, respectively [40,41,]. All samples were processed alongside negative controls (i.e. reaction mixture without DNA or RNA template) and positive (virally infected cells). Precautions were taken to avoid false positive results due to contamination by PCR product carry over, by strictly following guidelines for the general handling of the PCR procedure, such as separation of rooms, boards, and lab benches [42]. Sensitivity of PCR in our laboratory has beforehand been reported [43].

Samples were considered as true positive when the reproducibility of PCR analysis was verified a second time. Amplicon specificity was verified by direct cycle sequencing as previously described [39].

Since EBV was identified with high frequency in IPF patients, RNA-in situ hybridization-ISH (Epstein-Barr encoded RNAs, Biogenex, San Ramon, CA) was performed to identify the viral target cells. To quantify DNA viral genome copies real time PCR was also carried out in EBV positive cases whose additional DNA was available using artus® EBV TM PCR KIT [44].

Analysis of Fibrosis Extension, TGF-β Expression and Vessel Remodelling

The extent of fibrosis was evaluated in Masson's trichrome stained sections analyzing 10 random fields using computer-assisted morphometric software (Image ProPlus® 5.1), as previously reported [45]. The immunohistochemical detection and quantification of the profibrotic cytokine TGF-β (mouse monoclonal anti-TGF-β NovoCastra, Newcastle, UK), was performed as described before: immunostaining scores were based on the products of percentage positive cells multiplied by stain intensity (0 = negative, 1 = weak, 2 = moderate, 3 = strong) in three different high power fields. Control sections were stained without the primary antibody, without primary and secondary antibodies, or with normal sera to control for background reactivity [45].

Arterial thickening was quantified using computer-assisted morphometric software on elastic-Van Gieson (EVG) stained lung sections focusing on muscular arteries of an average diameter of 300 μm (range: 100–500 μm). In particular, medial thickening (MT) was evaluated as previously described in at least 5 arterial sections. The same approach was used to measure intimal thickening (IT): MT% = (2 × medial layer thickening/external diameter) × 100; IT% = (2 × intimal layer thickening/external diameter) × 100 [46]. The assessment of vascular remodelling also included an evaluation of apoptosis and proliferation of vessel cell components using the TUNEL technique and Ki-67 immunostaining respectively, as previously described [47]. Briefly, for TUNEL, after proteinase K (Boehringer, Mannheim, Germany) digestion at a concentration of 20 μg/ml, the slides were incubated with TdT/biotinylated dUTP diluted in buffer (Boehringer, Mannheim, Germany) and any labeling visualized with 3-3'-diaminobenzidine and 30 ml hydrogen peroxide. Slides incubated in buffer without TdT or biotinylated UTP served as

negative controls and slides incubated with 1 μg/ml DNAse (Sigma-Aldrich, Milan, Italy) served as positive controls.

For Ki-67 immunohistochemistry, after microwave antigen retrieval, the sections were treated with normal serum (Immunotech, Marseille, France) and incubated for 60 min with the primary monoclonal antibody anti-Ki67 (MIB-1, Gene Tex, Irvine, CA) at a dilution of 1:100. Sections were subsequently incubated with rabbit HRP polymer (Dako, Glostrup, Denmark) for 30 min. Immunoreactivity was visualized with 3-3'-diaminobenzidine (Dako). Negative controls processed omitting the primary antibody did not show any reaction. Ki-67 expression and TUNEL positivity were evaluated only in blood vessel cell components. All evaluations were performed blindly.

Animal Model

Female, 5 to 8 week old CD-1 mice [Hsd:ICR (CD1)] were purchased from Harlan Laboratories, UK and housed at the University of Liverpool under specific pathogen-free conditions. Mice were intranasally infected with 4×10^5 PFU MHV-68 and euthanized 7 days (n = 3), 14 days (n = 6) and 23 days (n = 3) post infection (post infection). Uninfected mice (n = 4) served as controls.

Immediately after death, lungs were collected and parts frozen at −80°C for RNA extraction: others were fixed in 10% buffered formalin and routinely embedded in paraffin wax. All experiments were performed in strict accordance with the recommendations in the Guide for the Care and Use of Laboratory Animals of The National Institutes of Health. The protocol was approved by UK Home Office regulations and under Project Licence number 40/2483 and Personal Licence number 60/6501. All infections were performed under light isoflorane anaesthesia. All experiments were carried out in manner to minimize suffering.

Analysis of Fibrosis Extension, TGF-β Expression and Vessel Remodelling

Consecutive paraffin-embedded sections were stained with haematoxylin and eosin for histology, with Masson's trichrome stain for fibrosis extension and with EVG for vessel remodelling, both morphometrically measured as above. The evaluation of arterial thickening focused on pulmonary arteries with an average diameter of 82 μm ranging from 43 to 100 μm. The assessment of vascular remodelling also included an evaluation of apoptosis and proliferation of vessel cell components using the TUNEL technique and Ki-67 immunostaining, as described above. Ki-67 antibody used for this analysis was rabbit polyclonal (Abcam, Cambridge, UK). Immunohistochemistry was also employed for the detection of MHV-68 antigen, to highlight lung macrophages (expression of lysozyme) and to demonstrate TGF-β expression (Genetex, Irvane, CA). Viral tRNA was demonstrated by RNA-ISH [48].

Statistical Analysis

Data were analyzed using the SAS statistical software version 9.1.3 (SAS Institute, Cary, NC, USA). For quantitative variables the results are expressed as mean values ± standard deviation if normally distributed, otherwise as median, Q1–Q3. The normality of distribution of quantitative variables was tested by means of Shapiro-Wilk statistics. For quantitative characteristics, differences between subjects with and without viral infection were evaluated by using the Mann-Whitney test. The prevalence of specific conditions was expressed as a percentage, and differences between groups were evaluated using the χ-squared test and exact Fisher's test, as adequate.

Unadjusted and adjusted relationships between virus and clinical/morphological features were tested with general linear models (GLM procedure). In all analyses, a two-tail level for significance was set at 0.05. Simple logistic regression models were applied to estimate odds ratios (ORs) for PGD using recipients' and donors' characteristics as predictors. A multivariate logistic model was used to estimate the adjusted OR of virus for PGD, controlling for PAP>25 mmHg. Considering that incidence was quite common in the study population, adjusted risk ratios (RRs) were approximated from adjusted ORs [49].

Results

Study Population

Viral data, tissue and vessel remodelling. Patients with IPF showed a higher frequency of viral infection than control cases (40% vs 7.3%; $p = 0.0003$). Normal lungs were all negative. Herpes viruses were the only detected genomes in IPF and EBV resulted as the most frequent, present in more than half of IPF patients. In 2 cases double infection was found. EBV was never detected in control cases (DPLDs and normal lungs). Gene sequencing of all amplicons showed a high homology (from 95% to 99%) with human viral genome sequences. RNA-ISH for EBV (EBER) identified viral RNA in 40% of EBV-PCR positive IPF cases. The positivity was detected in alveolar epithelial cells other than within monocytes/macrophages (Figure 1). Real time PCR showed a high number of EBV genome copies (mean±SD:1085000±120208 copies/μl DNA). The extent of fibrosis in IPF lungs showed a mean of 36.7±12.3% (range: 14.6%–65.3%) and was significantly higher than in the DPLD control group (36.7±12.3% vs 15.4±15.4%, p<0.0001). Normal lungs from donors showed no evidence of pathological remodelling.

TGF-β expression in IPF lungs was mainly detected in macrophages (median, Q1–Q3: 100, 20–210) and metaplastic alveolar epithelial cells (120, 70–210). Median TGF-β scores in the alveolar epithelium were significantly higher in IPF patients than in the DPLD group (120, 70–210 vs 0, 0–0, p<0.0001). In normal lungs, TGF-β expression was restricted to only scattered intraalveolar macrophages. Arterial remodelling in IPF cases showed a median total thickness score of 43.8% (Q1–Q3: 35.7–53.1%) with IT and MT scores of 17.7% (Q1–Q3: 13.5–24%) and 26.2% (Q1–Q3: 21.8–28.9%) respectively. These values were significantly lower in the DPLD group (total thickness: 37.9% vs 43.8%, $p = 0.03$; IT: 12.3% vs 17.7%, $p = 0.005$). Normal lungs did not show arterial remodelling (Table 2).

Correlation between viral molecular data and clinical/morphological parameters in IPF patients. Virus-positive IPF cases showed increased mPAP (28.6±10.9 mmHg vs 21.2±6.0 mmHg, $p = 0.01$) and worse performance in the 6MWT (175.2±100 vs 300.5±138.8, $p = 0.002$) than virus negative cases (Figure 2 A,B). The statistical value of these associations (mPAP and 6MWT) was still evident when EBV positive IPF patients were compared with both other virus positive and negative IPF cases (p<0.05 for both).

Virus positive IPF cases showed a higher total thickening of muscular arteries (50.3%, 43.8–58.8% vs 39.5%, 34.7–45.7%, $p = 0.002$) than virus negative cases. The intimal layer was most severely affected (21.8%, 17.2–26.8% vs 15.5%, 12.6–19.1%; $p = 0.004$) (Figure 3 A,B,C,D). TUNEL staining was mainly detected in the endothelial cells of the microvasculature (Figure S1) while cell proliferation was frequently seen in remodelled pulmonary arteries. Strong Ki-67 positivity was observed in both endothelial cells (CD31 positive, data not shown) and smooth muscle cells (smooth muscle actin positive, data not shown). Vessel cell proliferation was particularly seen in pulmonary arteries in proximity to metaplastic alveolar epithelial cells or macrophages (Figure 4 A and B). TGF-β scores were

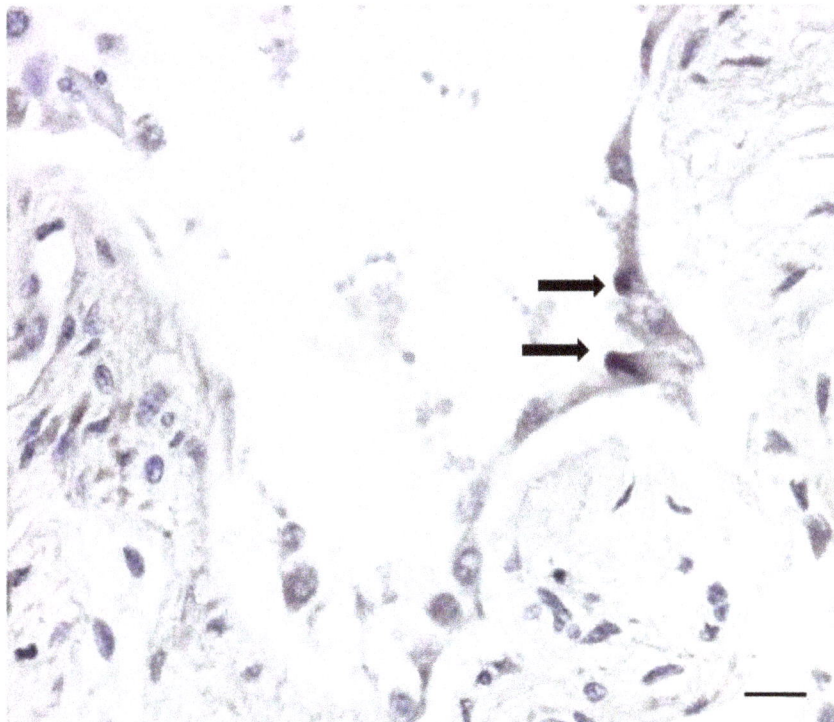

Figure 1. In situ hybridization for EBV. EBER transcripts well seen in the nuclei of two alveolar epithelial cells (arrows). Bar scale: 10 μm.

Table 2. Viral genome frequency and pathological data in IPF and control cases.

	IPF patients (55)	Control cases (41)*	p-values
Virus positive cases	22/55 (40%)	3/41 (7.3%)	0.0003
EBV	13/22 (59.1%)	0	
HHV-6	7/22 (31.8%)	1/3 (33.3%)**	
CMV	4/22 (18.2%)	2/3 (66.7%)**	
PVB19	0	1/3 (33.3%)**	
Fibrotic extension, mean % (SD)	36.7 (12.3)	15.4 (15.4)***	<0.0001
Medial arterial remodelling, median % (Q1–Q3)	26.2 (21.8–28.9)	22.4 (18.9–27.5)***	ns
Intimal arterial remodelling, median % (Q1–Q3)	17.7 (13.5–24.0)	12.3 (9.0–17.0) ***	0.005
Total arterial remodelling, median % (Q1–Q3)	43.8 (35.7–53.1)	37.9 (31.7–44.6) ***	0.03
Macrophagic TGF-ß score, median % (Q1–Q3)	100 (20–210)	50 (10–180) ***	ns
Alveolar epithelial TGF-β score, median % (Q1–Q3)	120 (70–210)	0 (0–0)***	<0.0001

IPF: idiopathic pulmonary fibrosis; EBV: Epstein Barr virus; HHV6: herpes virus 6; CMV: cytomegalovirus PV: parvovirus; TGF : transforming growth factor.
*All donor lungs were negative;
**these viruses were detected only in patients with LAM.
Double infections were detected in two IPF patients and 1 control case.
***These parameters were quantified only in DPLD patients, not in normal lungs.

higher in virus-positive cases, although this was only statistically significant when epithelial expression was considered (score: 195, 140–210 vs 100, 40–120; $p = 0.002$) (Figure 5 A,B,C,D). The statistical value of these parameters (vessel remodelling and TGF-β expression) was still evident when EBV positive IPF patients were compared with both other virus positive and negative IPF cases (p<0.05 for all). A summary of all main clinicopathological features in relation to virus infection among IPF patients is shown in the Table S1.

Viral presence was significantly associated with higher mPAP ($p = 0.03$) after adjusting for other related covariates and intermediate factors (i.e.; age, sex, duration of disease, smoking history, and fibrosis extension). Moreover, viral presence was an independent marker of significantly poorer performance in the 6MWT ($p = 0.008$) using the GLM adjusting for covariates (i.e. VC, FVC, DLCO and fibrosis extension). When we considered the short-term post-transplant follow-up we found a higher frequency of PGD (50% vs 14%, $p = 0.02$) and, although not

statistically significant, an increased rate of acute rejection (50% vs 25%, p: ns) in virus positive compared to negative IPF cases. A multivariate analysis identified an increased risk for PGD to be associated with viral infection independently of the major recipient/donor characteristics that are usually considered to influence PGD, including PH (adjusted RR: 5.43, 95% CI: 1.56–7.10, $p = 0.02$) (Table S2).

MHV-68 Infected CD1 Mice

Tissue and vessel remodelling. Analysis of MHV-68 DNA load showed, as previously demonstrated, that viral infection peaked on day 7 post infection [50].

The histological examination of uninfected control animals did not identify any pathological changes. On day 7 post infection, all infected animals exhibited increased, macrophage-dominated interstitial cellularity, mild type II pneumocyte hyperplasia and perivascular inflammatory infiltration. The latter infiltrates were associated with slight patchy collagen

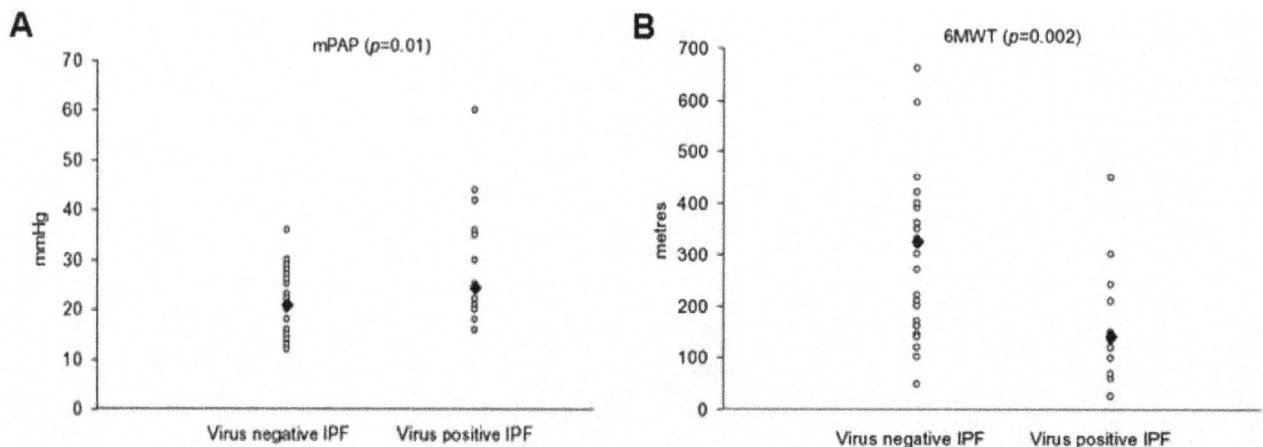

Figure 2. Mean pulmonary arterial pressure (mPAP) values. Significant higher values of mPAP (A) and worse 6MWT (B) in virus positive compared to virus negative cases.

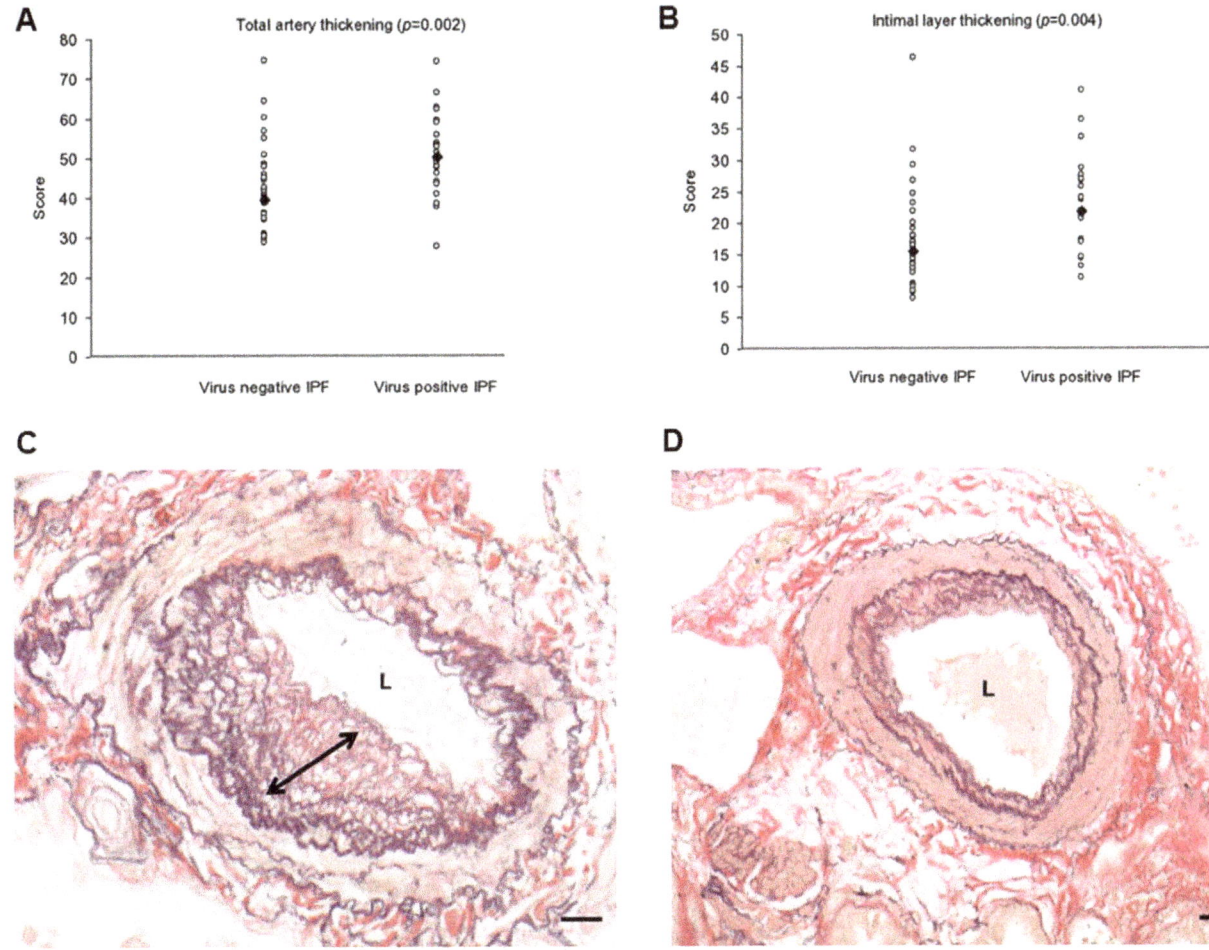

Figure 3. Vascular remodelling in IPF lung tissue. Significantly increased arterial thickening (A) particularly of the intimal layer (B) is seen in virus positive cases. Elastic Van Gieson stained sections showed increased wall thickening (increased elastic and collagen fibers) especially of the intimal layer (arrow) in virus positive (C) compared to virus negative cases (D). Bar scale: 100 μm. L = lumen.

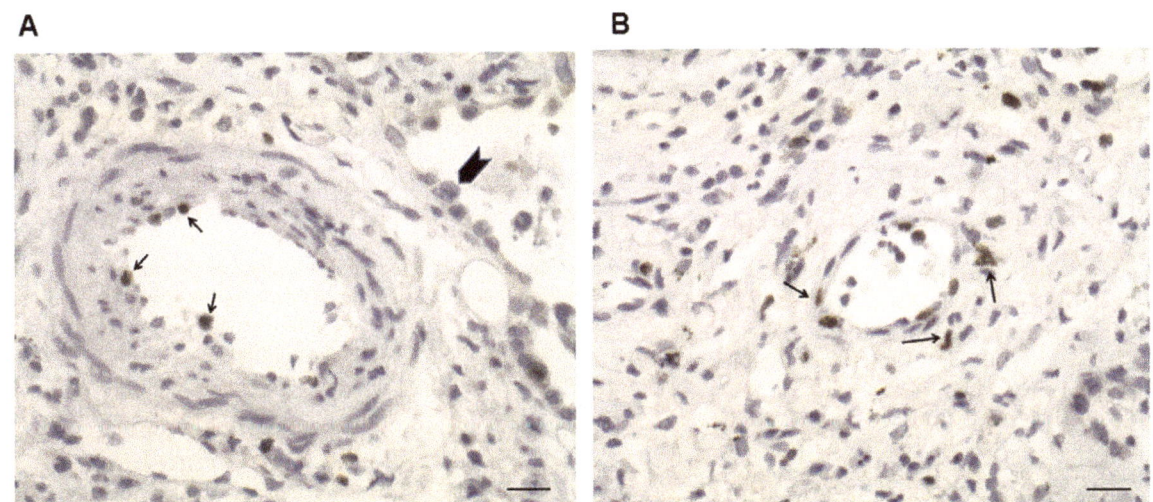

Figure 4. Vessel cell proliferation in IPF lung tissue. Strong Ki-67 immunostaining was observed both in endothelial (A, arrows) and in smooth muscle cells (B, arrows) of remodelled pulmonary arteries adjacent to metaplastic epithelial cells (well seen in A, arrowhead). Bar scale: 10 μm.

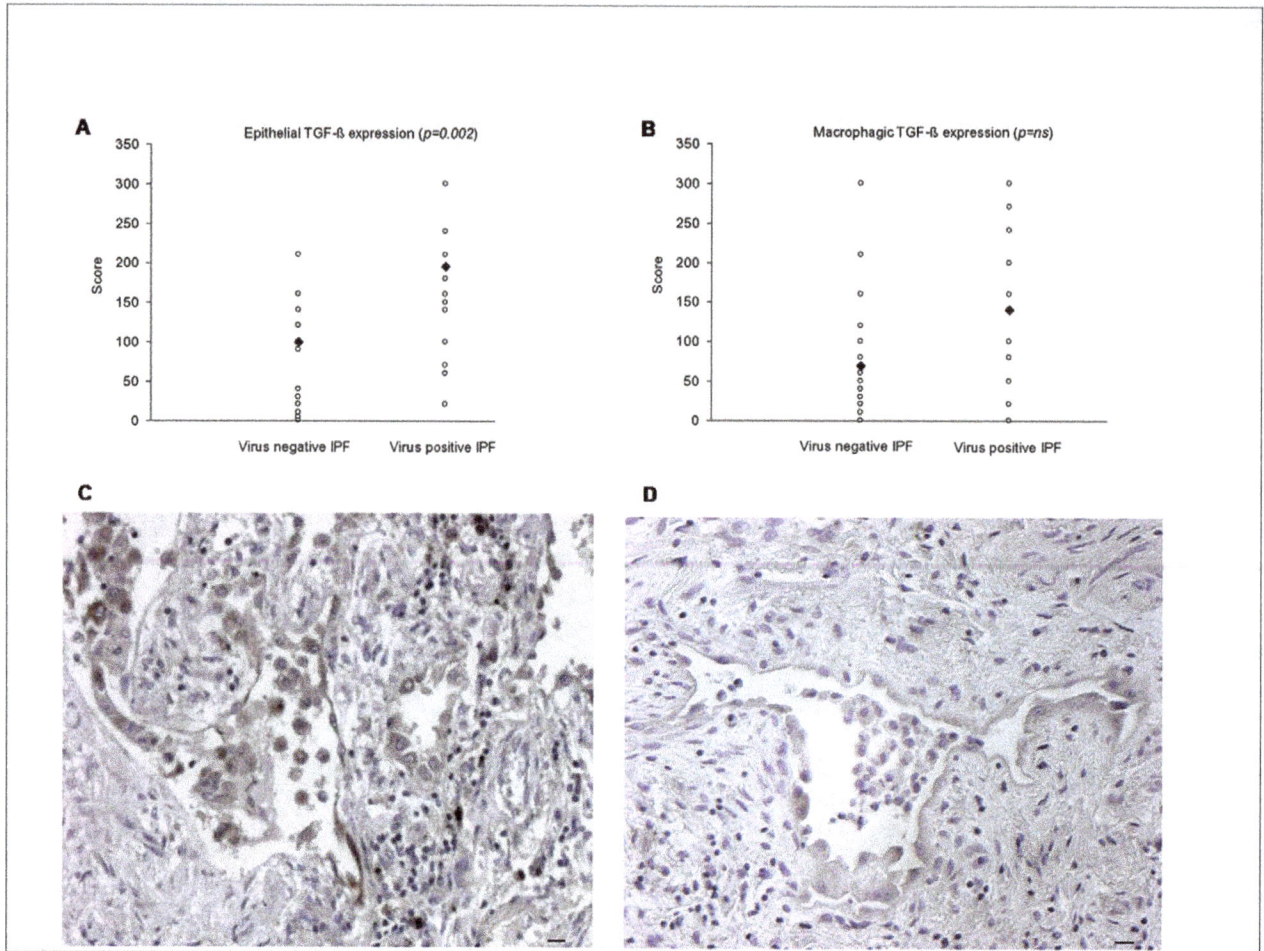

Figure 5. TGF-β expression in IPF lung tissue. A) Significantly increased TGF-β median score values of epithelial cells are seen in virus positive cases. B) TGF-β median score values of macrophages in virus positive and virus negative cases. Stronger and more extensive TGF-β immunostaining well seen in virus positive (C) than virus negative case (D). Bar scale: 5 μm.

deposition. Scattered individual macrophages and metaplastic alveolar epithelial cells were found to express MHV-68 antigen. Viral latency, represented by the expression of viral tRNA, was detected in type II pneumocytes and alveolar macrophages. On day 14 post infection, mild multifocal, almost diffuse fibrosis of alveolar septa was observed with a median of 26% (range: 17–38%). In some animals, this was associated with random patches of collagen deposition. Numerous macrophages were seen within the interstitium and often around arteries. In addition, some type II pneumocytes exhibited TGF-β expression (Figure 6 A, B).

Arteries were assessed for vessel remodelling and compared for the thickening scores. In uninfected control mice, the average score was 16.5. Seven and 14 days post infection, it was 18 and 24.5 respectively (Figure 7 A,B,C,D). The extent of fibrosis was slightly more marked in mice with vessel wall thickening. On day 23 post infection both the parenchymal and vessel remodelling were less evident. Similar to human cases TUNEL staining was mainly detected in endothelial cells of the microvasculature (Figure S2) while cell proliferation was frequently seen in endothelial cells and smooth muscle cells of pulmonary arteries, in particular in vessels surrounded by macrophages (Figure 8 A, B).

Discussion

In the present study different respiratory viruses were investigated in lungs from a large cohort of IPF patients and the control group (non IPF DPLDs and normal lungs) displaying the prevalent role of herpes viruses. The work highlights the broad impact of herpesviral infection, particularly EBV, in the disease emphasizing its association with a more severe disease phenotype as IPF with associated higher mPAP and worse 6MWT. A multiple logistic regression analysis demonstrated that herpesviral infection was independently associated with more marked vessel remodelling, higher value of PAP and worse performance in the 6MWT.Neither clinical data (smoking history, age at diagnosis and at transplant, duration of the disease, BMI, lung volumes and hypoxemic respiratory failure) nor morphological changes (fibrosis extension) had more significant impact than viral infection. Of particular note is that the presence of viral infection had also early-term negative influence on the graft function. IPF virus positive recipients showed a higher frequency of PGD, independent of other recipient and donor characteristics. Viral products and/or the activated immune system related to viral infection in native IPF lungs may potentiate the immune response to alloantigens after transplantation, thus resulting in early graft dysfunction. Only one previous study performed on 24 IPF patients reported

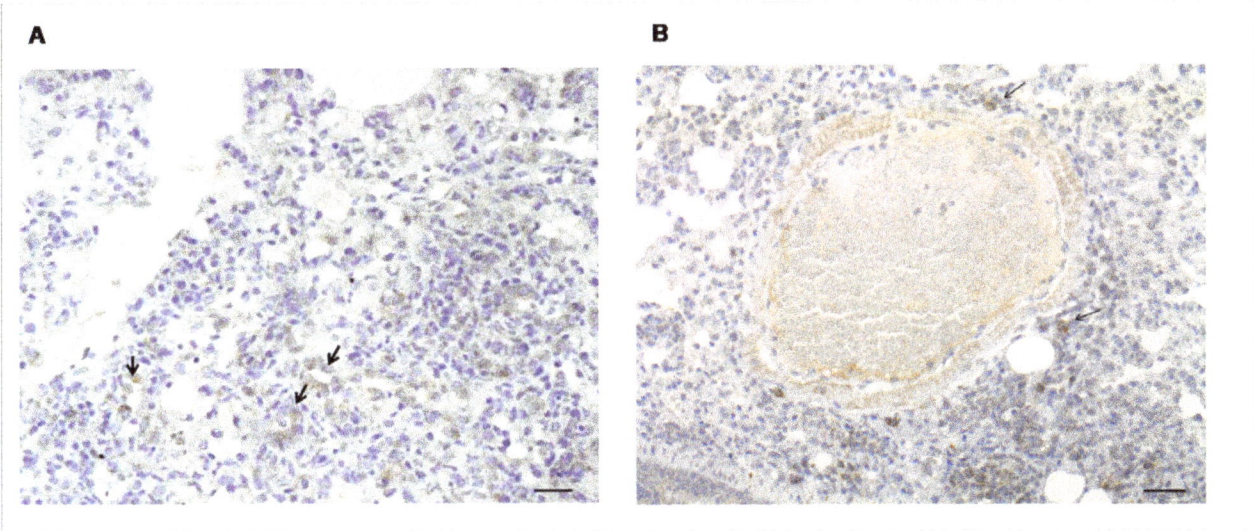

Figure 6. Immunohistochemistry for TGF-β in lung tissue of MHV-68 infected CD1 mice. Numerous metaplastic alveolar epithelial cells (arrows) are marked (A); positive macrophages (arrows) are seen around a remodelled artery (B). Bar scale: 40 μm.

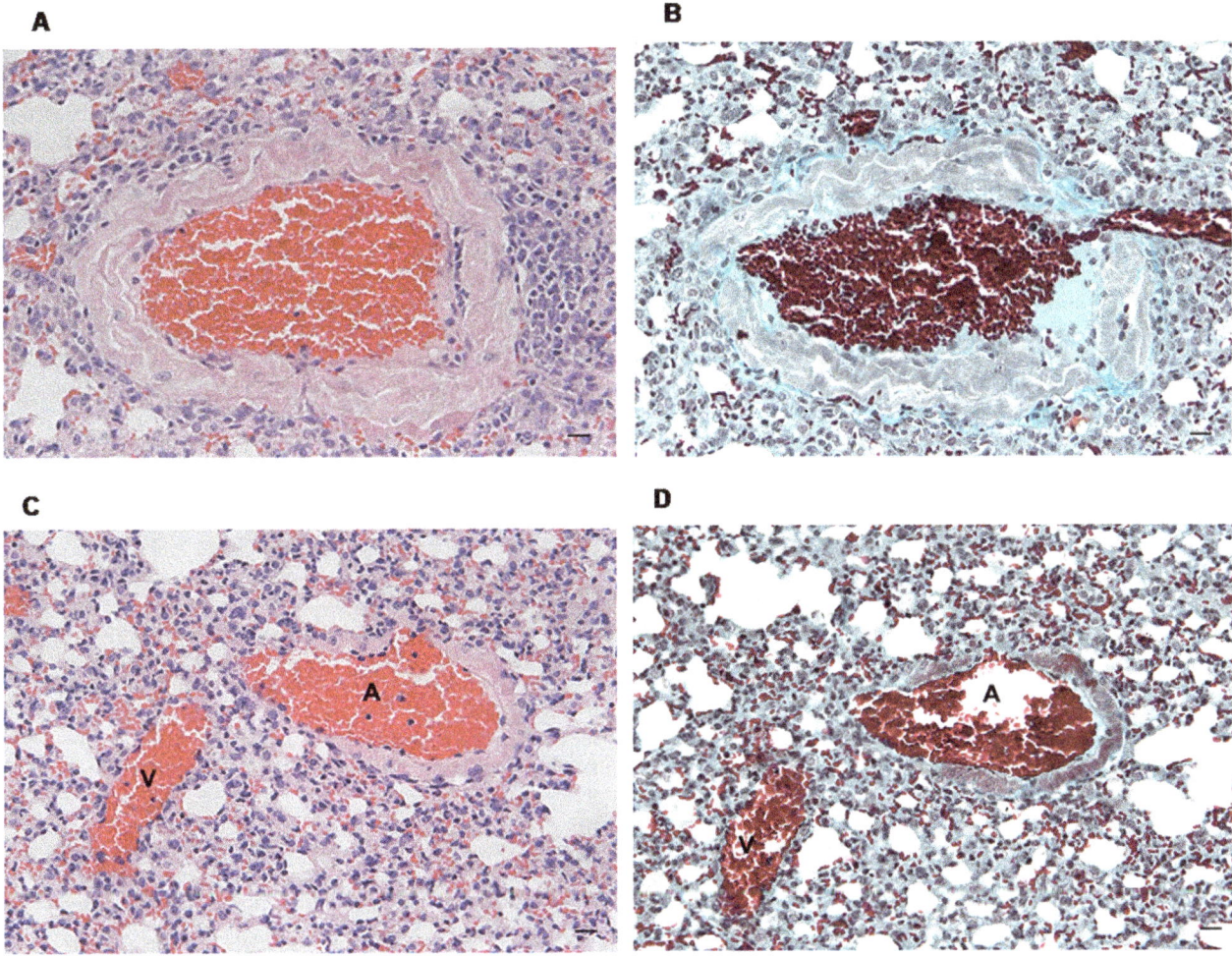

Figure 7. Vascular remodelling in lung tissue of MHV-68 infected CD1mice. Haematoxylin-Eosin (A, C) and Masson' trichrome (B, D) stained sections: marked arterial thickening is seen in a MHV-68 infected mouse (A and B, scale bars: 20 μm) in comparison to an uninfected mouse (C and D). Bar scale: 20 μm. A: small artery; V: venule.

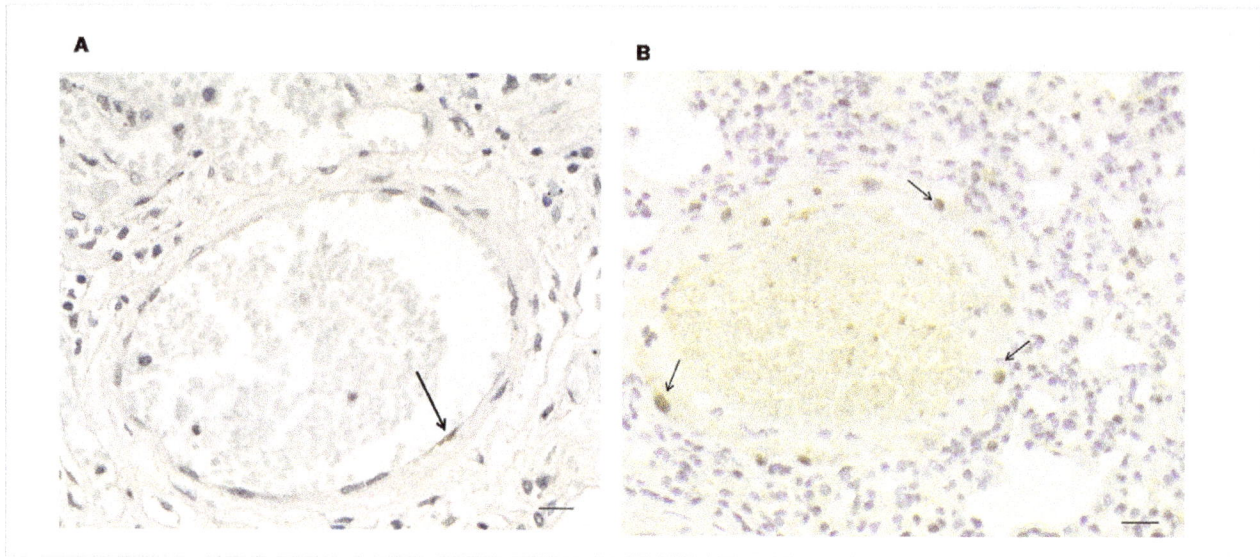

Figure 8. Vessel cell proliferation in lung tissue of MHV-68 infected CD1mice. Strong Ki-67 immunostaining was observed both in endothelial (A, arrow) and smooth muscle (B, arrows) cells adjacent to macrophages. Bar scale: 20 μm.

more rapid disease progression in EBV positive cases. The majority of viral cases died from respiratory failure at a mean of 41 month follow up. In the study PH was not specifically considered [51].

The reported frequency of herpes viruses in IPF lungs ranges from 30 to 100%. These differences may be related to technical sensitivity, disease heterogeneity or selection of patients. The presence of herpes viruses detected in our cases may even be underestimated due the fact that the molecular investigation was performed on tissue samples from end-stage diseases. Viral clearance, after initial injury, could occur in some cases with persistence and progression of lung injury due to activation of an immunological response, as it occurs in other chronic virus-related diseases, e.g. dilated-cardiomyopathy-post-myocarditis [52]. EBV, the most frequent herpes virus detected in IPF, has a well known epitheliotropism other than lymphotropism. Several works have detected EBV in alveolar epithelial cells of IPF lungs, thus confirming the concept that these cells represent the principal viral target in IPF [15,27,29,30,33,53]. The role of herpes viruses, important contributing factors for the development of pulmonary fibrosis, has been emphasized in different experimental models and the TGF–β signalling pathway seems to play a crucial role in the profibrogenetic action.

To the best of our knowledge no attempt has been made to specifically investigate the influence of herpes viruses on arterial remodelling and PH in IPF patients.

Several types of viruses, particularly those of the herpes family, have been found to be associated with vessel remodelling, development of atherosclerosis and clinical features of hypertension [54,55]. Vasculotropism of gamma herpes viruses (such as HHV-8, EHV-5 and MHV68) has been demonstrated in lung parenchyma of patients and animals (horses) with PH even if a causal relationship still remains quite debated [55–57]. Up to today, there is little evidence of a "direct" role of viral agents in the pathogenesis of PH. Even when more significant arterial intimal thickness could more convincingly suggest a direct viral endothelial injury, in our work EBV was never detected in endothelial cells of IPF cases. The presence of chemokines and cytokines, viral protein components, and increased expression of growth and

transcriptional factors released at the site of infection could contribute to further recruitment of inflammatory cells and proliferation of smooth muscle and endothelial cells. An interesting finding of our study was the most frequent distribution of remodelled vessels with proliferating components in proximity to metaplastic epithelial cells and/or macrophages, both cell types considered as principal targets of EBV. Injured epithelial or endothelial cells involved in tissue and vessel remodelling are considered an important source of growth factors and mediators, among which TGF-β plays a key role.

Although the function of TGF in vascular cell growth in *vivo* has not been well defined, in vitro and experimental studies have demonstrated an important influence of this cytokine in muscle/fibroblast proliferation, endothelial-mesenchymal transition, and extracellular matrix production of intimal and medial layers [58]. In our study significantly higher TGF-β levels detected in our viral IPF cases as well as in MHV-68 infected mice suggest an indirect influence of viral infection on vessel remodelling through this cytokine even if TGF-β expression was not significantly related to arterial thickening. Similar data were found by Farkas L. et al. in a different experimental model of pulmonary fibrosis [13]. The authors detected high levels of active TGF-β in areas with increased fibrogenesis and pulmonary artery remodelling. At day 14, this was significantly associated with pulmonary hypertension.

The demonstration of a direct causal relationship between herpesvirus infection and vessel remodelling/PH in IPF would require longitudinal studies of the same patients, an impossible task with lung tissue but attainable with bronchoalveolar lavage or peripheral blood samples. However this limitation has been partially overcome in the present study using a laboratory MHV-68 infected mouse model. Indeed, in these animals 2 weeks after infection significant arterial remodelling and increased TGF-β expression was seen, as those observed in clinical lung specimens from IPF patients with high mPAP.

Conclusion

In summary, our results demonstrated for the first time a different phenotype of virus-positive IPF patients. In particular virus-positive IPF cases showed more pronounced vessel remodelling and a higher mPAP and significantly higher PGD after transplantation. While there is large mechanistic evidence of epithelial herpesvirus-associated alveolar injury, the effect of these viruses on the pulmonary vasculature in IPF merits investigation. A deeper knowledge of viral-induced pathways in endothelial cells could give new insights for a targeted therapeutic approach of this important complication in the subgroup of patients (virus positive cases). In this context, the high degree of similarity between MHV-68 infection of CD-1 mice and virus positive IPF indicates that this is an excellent model with which to study pathogenesis and interventions.

Acknowledgments

The authors thank Luca Braghetto, Laura Vignato and Linda Tosetto for their excellent technical assistance and Judith Wilson for English revision. We are grateful to Valerie Tilston in the Histology Laboratory, Veterinary Laboratory Services, School of Veterinary Sciences, University of Liverpool, for excellent histology work.

Author Contributions

Conceived and designed the experiments: FC AK JPS FR. Performed the experiments: FL EB NN AK JPS GM. Analyzed the data: FC FL ER EP. Contributed reagents/materials/analysis tools: FC AK JPS EB GM FR. Wrote the paper: FC AK JPS.

References

1. American Thoracic Society, European Respiratory Society (2002) American Thoracic Society/European Respiratory Society International Multidisciplinary Consensus Classification of the Idiopathic Interstitial Pneumonias. This joint statement of the American Thoracic Society (ATS), and the European Respiratory Society (ERS) was adopted by the ATS board of directors, June 2001 and by the ERS Executive Committee, June 2001. Am J Respir Crit Care Med 165: 277–304.
2. Raghu G, Weycker D, Edelsberg J, Bradford WZ, Oster G (2006) Incidence and prevalence of idiopathic pulmonary fibrosis. Am J Respir Crit Care Med 174: 810–816.
3. King TE Jr, Pardo A, Selman M (2011) Idiopathic pulmonary fibrosis. Lancet 378: 1949–1961.
4. Whelan TP, Dunitz JM, Kelly RF, Edwards LB, Herrington CS, et al. (2005) Effect of preoperative pulmonary artery pressure on early survival after lung transplantation for idiopathic pulmonary fibrosis. J Heart Lung Transplant 24: 1269–1274.
5. Nadrous HF, Pellikka PA, Krowka MJ, Swanson KL, Chaowalit N, et al. (2005) The impact of pulmonary hypertension on survival in patients with idiopathic pulmonary fibrosis. Chest 128: 616S–617S.
6. Lettieri CJ, Nathan SD, Barnett SD, Ahmad S, Shorr AF (2006) Prevalence and outcomes of pulmonary arterial hypertension in advanced idiopathic pulmonary fibrosis. Chest 129: 746–752.
7. Patel NM, Lederer DJ, Borczuk AC, Kawut SM (2007) Pulmonary hypertension in idiopathic pulmonary fibrosis. Chest 132: 998–1006.
8. Leuchte HH, Neurohr C, Baumgartner R, Holzapfel M, Giehrl W, et al. (2004) Brain natriuretic peptide and exercise capacity in lung fibrosis and pulmonary hypertention. Am J Respir Crit Care Med 170: 360–365.
9. Zisman DA, Karlamangla AS, Ross DJ, Keane MP, Belperio JA, et al. (2007) High-resolution chest CT findings do not predict the presence of pulmonary hypertension in advanced idiopathic pulmonary fibrosis. Chest 132: 773–779.
10. Selman M, King TE, Pardo A, American Thoracic Society, European Respiratory Society, et al. (2001) American College of Chest Physicians. Idiopathic pulmonary fibrosis: prevailing and evolving hypotheses about its pathogenesis and implications for therapy. Ann Intern Med 134: 136–151.
11. Ebina M, Shimizukawa M, Shibata N, Kimura Y, Suzuki T, et al. (2004) Heterogeneous increase in CD34-positive alveolar capillaries in idiopathic pulmonary fibrosis. Am J Respir Crit Care Med 169: 1203–1208.
12. Nathan SD, Noble PW, Tuder RM (2007) Idiopathic pulmonary fibrosis and pulmonary hypertension: connecting the dots. Am J Respir Crit Care Med 175: 875–880.
13. Farkas L, Farkas D, Ask K, Möller A, Gauldie J, et al. (2009) VEGF ameliorates pulmonary hypertension through inhibition of endothelial apoptosis in experimental lung fibrosis in rats. J Clin Invest 119: 1298–1311.
14. Farkas L, Gauldie J, Voelkel NF, Kolb M (2011) Pulmonary hypertension and idiopathic pulmonary fibrosis: a tale of angiogenesis, apoptosis, and growth factors. Am J Respir Cell Mol Biol 45: 1–15.
15. Egan JJ, Stewart JP, Hasleton PS, Arrand JR, Carroll KB, et al. (1995) Epstein-Barr virus replication within pulmonary epithelial cells in cryptogenic fibrosing alveolitis. Thorax 50: 1234–1239.
16. Kuwano K, Nomoto Y, Kunitake R, Hagimoto N, Matsuba T, et al. (1997) Detection of adenovirus E1A DNA in pulmonary fibrosis using nested polymerase chain reaction. Eur Respir J 10: 1445–1449.
17. Stewart JP, Egan JJ, Ross AJ, Kelly BG, Lok SS, et al. (1999) The detection of Epstein-Barr virus DNA in lung tissue from patients with idiopathic pulmonary fibrosis. Am J Respir Crit Care Med 159: 1336–1341.
18. Kelly BG, Lok SS, Hasleton PS, Egan JJ, Stewart JP (2002) A rearranged form of Epstein-Barr virus DNA is associated with idiopathic pulmonary fibrosis. Am J Respir Crit Care Med 166: 510–513.
19. Lok SS, Haider Y, Howell D, Stewart JP, Hasleton PS, et al. (2002) Murine gammaherpcs virus as a cofactor in the development of pulmonary fibrosis in bleomycin resistant mice. Eur Respir J 20: 1228–1232.
20. Tang YW, Johnson JE, Browning PJ, Cruz-Gervis RA, Davis A, et al. (2003) Herpesvirus DNA is consistently detected in lungs of patients with idiopathic pulmonary fibrosis. J Clin Microbiol 41: 2633–2640.
21. Zamò A, Poletti V, Reghellin D, Montagna L, Pedron S, et al. (2005) HHV-8 and EBV are not commonly found in idiopathic pulmonary fibrosis. Sarcoidosis Vasc Diffuse Lung Dis 22: 123–128.
22. Mora AL, Woods CR, Garcia A, Xu J, Rojas M, et al. (2005) Lung infection with gamma-Herpes virus induces progressive pulmonary fibrosis in Th2-biased mice. Am J Physiol Lung Cell Mol Physiol 289: L711–721.
23. Mora AL, Torres-González E, Rojas M, Corredor C, Ritzenthaler J, et al. (2006) Activation of alveolar macrophages via the alternative pathway in Herpes virus-induced lung fibrosis. Am J Respir Cell Mol Biol 35: 466–473.
24. Mora AL, Torres-González E, Rojas M, Xu J, Ritzenthaler J, et al. (2007) Control of virus reactivation arrests pulmonary Herpes virus-induced fibrosis in IFN-gamma receptor-deficient mice. Am J Respir Crit Care Med 175: 1139–1150.
25. McMillan TR, Moore BB, Weinberg JB, Vannella KM, Fields WB, et al. (2008) Exacerbation of established pulmonary fibrosis in a murine model by gammaHerpes virus. Am J Respir Crit Care Med 177: 771–780.
26. Arase Y, Suzuki F, Suzuki Y, Akuta N, Kobayashi M, et al. (2008) Hepatitis C virus enhances incidence of idiopathic pulmonary fibrosis. World J Gastroenterol 14: 5880–5886.
27. Malizia AP, Keating DT, Smith SM, Walls D, Doran PP, et al. (2008) Alveolar epithelial cell injury with Epstein-Barr virus up-regulates TGFbeta1 expression. Am J Physiol Lung Cell Mol Physiol 295: L451–460.
28. Pozharskaya V, Torres-González E, Rojas M, Gal A, Amin M, et al. (2009) Twist: a regulator of epithelial-mesenchymal transition in lung fibrosis. PLoS One 4: e7559.
29. Malizia AP, Egan JJ, Doran PP (2009) IL-4 increases CD21-dependent infection of pulmonary alveolar epithelial type II cells by EBV. Mol Immunol 46: 1905–1910.
30. Malizia AP, Lacey N, Walls D, Egan JJ, Doran PP (2009) CUX1/Wnt signaling regulates epithelial mesenchymal transition in EBV infected epithelial cells. Exp Cell Res 315: 1819–1831.
31. Pulkkinen V, Bruce S, Rintahaka J, Hodgson U, Laitinen T, et al. (2010) ELMOD2, a candidate gene for idiopathic pulmonary fibrosis, regulates antiviral responses. FASEB J 24: 1167–1177.
32. Vannella KM, Luckhardt TR, Wilke CA, van Dyk LF, Toews GB, et al. (2010) Latent Herpes virus infection augments experimental pulmonary fibrosis. Am J Respir Crit Care Med 181: 465–477.
33. Sides MD, Klingsberg RC, Shan B, Gordon KA, Nguyen HT, et al. (2011) The Epstein-Barr virus latent membrane protein 1 and transforming growth factor-

β1 synergistically induce epithelial-mesenchymal transition in lung epithelial cells. Am J Respir Cell Mol Biol 44: 852–862.

34. Pulkkinen V, Salmenkivi K, Kinnula VL, Sutinen E, Halme M, et al. (2012) A novel screening method detects herpesviral DNA in the idiopathic pulmonary fibrosis lung. Ann Med 44: 178–186.

35. Egan JJ, Adamali HI, Lok SS, Stewart JP, Woodcock AA (2011) Ganciclovir antiviral therapy in advanced idiopathic pulmonary fibrosis: an open pilot study. Pulm Med 2011: 240805.

36. Christie JD, Carby M, Bag R, Corris P, Hertz M, et al. (2005). Report of the ISHLT working group on primary lung graft dysfunction: Part II. Definition. J Heart Lung Transplant 24: 1454–1459.

37. Stewart S, Fishbein MC, Snell GI, Berry GJ, Boehler A, et al. (2007) Revision of the 1996 working formulation for the standardization of nomenclature in the diagnosis of lung rejection. J Heart Lung Transplant 26: 1229–1242.

38. Chomczynski P, Sacchi N (2006) The single-step method of RNA isolation by acid guanidinium thiocyanate-phenol-chloroform extraction: twenty-something years on. Nat Protoc 1: 581–585.

39. Calabrese F, Rizzo S, Giacometti C, Panizzolo C, Turato G, et al. (2008) High viral frequency in children with gastroesophageal reflux-related chronic respiratory disorders. Pediatr Pulmonol 43: 690–696.

40. Ercolani L, Florence B, Denaro M, Alexander M (1988) Isolation and complete sequence of glyceraldehyde-3-phosphate dehydrogenase gene. J Biol Chem 263: 1535–1541.

41. Saiki RK, Scharf S, Faloona F, Mullis KB, Horn GT, et al. (1985) Enzymatic amplification of beta globin genomic sequence and restriction site analysis for diagnosis of sickle cell anemia. Science 230: 13450–13454.

42. Kwok S, Higuchi R (1989) Avoiding false positives with PCR. Nature 339: 237–238.

43. Calabrese F, Angelini A, Thiene G, Basso C, Nava A, et al. (2000) No detection of enteroviral genome in the myocardium of patients with arrhythmogenic right ventricular cardiomyopathy. J Clin Pathol 53: 382–387.

44. Lunardi F, Calabrese F, Furian L, Rigotti P, Valente M (2011) Epstein-Barr Virus-Associated Gastric Carcinoma Thirthy-Three Years After Kidney Transplantation. NDT Plus 4: 49–52.

45. Calabrese F, Lunardi F, Giacometti C, Marulli G, Gnoato M, et al. (2008) Overexpression of squamous cell carcinoma antigen in idiopathic pulmonary fibrosis: clinicopathological correlations. Thorax 63: 795–802.

46. Delgado JF, Conde E, Sánchez V, López-Ríos F, Gómez-Sánchez MA, et al. (2005) Pulmonary vascular remodeling in pulmonary hypertension due to chronic heart failure. Eur J Heart Fail 7: 1011–1016.

47. Calabrese F, Giacometti C, Beghe B, Rea F, Loy M, et al. (2005) Marked alveolar apoptosis/proliferation imbalance in end-stage emphysema. Respir Res. 6: 14.

48. Egan J, Stewart J, Yonan N, Arrand J, Woodcock A (1994) Non-Hodgkin lymphoma in heart/lung transplant recipients. Lancet 343: 481.

49. Zhang J, Yu KF (1998) What's the relative risk? A method of correcting the odds ratio in cohort studies of common outcomes. JAMA 280: 1690–1691.

50. Payne CM, Heggie CJ, Brownstein DG, Stewart JP, Quinn JP (2001) Role of Tachykinins in the Host Response to Murine GammaHerpes virus Infection. Journal of Virology 75: 10467–10471.

51. Tsukamoto K, Hayakawa H, Sato A, Chida K, Nakamura H, et al. (2000) Involvement of Epstein-Barr virus latent membrane protein 1 in disease progression in patients with idiopathic pulmonary fibrosis. Thorax 55: 958–961.

52. Cooper LT Jr (2009) Myocarditis. N Engl J Med 360: 1526–1538.

53. Lung ML, Lam WK, So SY, Lam WP, Chan KH, et al. (1985) Evidence that respiratory tract is major reservoir for Epstein-Barr virus. Lancet 1: 889–892.

54. Hansson GK, Robertson AK, Söderberg-Nauclér C (2006) Inflammation and atherosclerosis. Annu Rev Pathol 1: 297–329.

55. Cool CD, Rai PR, Yeager ME, Hernandez-Saavedra D, Serls AE, et al. (2003) Expression of human herpesvirus 8 in primary pulmonary hypertension. N Engl J Med 349: 1113–1122.

56. Williams KJ, Maes R, Del Piero F, Lim A, Wise A, et al. (2007) Equine Multinodular Pulmonary Fibrosis: A Newly Recognized Herpes virus-Associated Fibrotic Lung Disease. Vet Pathol 44: 849–862.

57. Suarez AL, van Dyk LF (2008) Endothelial Cells Support Persistent Gammaherpesvirus 68 Infection. PLoS Pathog 4: e1000152.

58. Mihira H, Suzuki HI, Akatsu Y, Yoshimatsu Y, Igarashi T, et al. (2012) TGF-{beta}-induced mesenchymal transition of MS-1 endothelial cells requires Smad-dependent cooperative activation of Rho signals and MRTF-A. J Biochem 151: 145–156.

11

Recipient-Related Clinical Risk Factors for Primary Graft Dysfunction after Lung Transplantation

Yao Liu, Yi Liu, Lili Su, Shu-juan Jiang*

Department of Respiratory Medicine, Provincial Hospital Affiliated to Shandong University, Jinan, Shandong, China

Abstract

Background: Primary graft dysfunction (PGD) is the main cause of early morbidity and mortality after lung transplantation. Previous studies have yielded conflicting results for PGD risk factors. Herein, we carried out a systematic review and meta-analysis of published literature to identify recipient-related clinical risk factors associated with PGD development.

Method: A systematic search of electronic databases (PubMed, Embase, Web of Science, Cochrane CENTRAL, and Scopus) for studies published from 1970 to 2013 was performed. Cohort, case-control, or cross-sectional studies that examined recipient-related risk factors of PGD were included. The odds ratios (ORs) or mean differences (MDs) were calculated using random-effects models

Result: Thirteen studies involving 10042 recipients met final inclusion criteria. From the pooled analyses, female gender (OR 1.38, 95% CI 1.09 to 1.75), African American (OR 1.82, 95%CI 1.36 to 2.45), idiopathic pulmonary fibrosis (IPF) (OR 1.78, 95% CI 1.49 to 2.13), sarcoidosis (OR 4.25, 95% CI 1.09 to 16.52), primary pulmonary hypertension (PPH) (OR 3.73, 95%CI 2.16 to 6.46), elevated BMI (BMI$\geq$25 kg/m^2) (OR 1.83, 95% CI 1.26 to 2.64), and use of cardiopulmonary bypass (CPB) (OR 2.29, 95%CI 1.43 to 3.65) were significantly associated with increased risk of PGD. Age, cystic fibrosis, secondary pulmonary hypertension (SPH), intra-operative inhaled nitric oxide (NO), or lung transplant type (single or bilateral) were not significantly associated with PGD development (all $P>0.05$). Moreover, a nearly 4 fold increased risk of short-term mortality was observed in patients with PGD (OR 3.95, 95% CI 2.80 to 5.57).

Conclusions: Our analysis identified several recipient related risk factors for development of PGD. The identification of higher-risk recipients and further research into the underlying mechanisms may lead to selective therapies aimed at reducing this reperfusion injury.

Editor: Mauricio Rojas, University of Pittsburgh, United States of America

Funding: This work was supported by the research grant from National Natural Science Foundation of China (No. 81301790). The funders had no role in study design, data collection and analysis, decision to publish, or preparation of the manuscript.

Competing Interests: The authors have declared that no competing interests exist.

* E-mail: doctorliuyao@126.com

Introduction

Although lung transplantation has become an increasingly common procedure in recent years, it has consistently lagged behind other organs in survival rates [1], and early postoperative allograft dysfunction remains a significant cause of post-transplantation morbidity and mortality [2]. Primary graft dysfunction (PGD) is a severe form of acute lung injury induced by ischemia-reperfusion injury that occurs in approximately 10–25% of lung graft recipients [2,3]. Reported 30-day mortality rates of patients with severe PGD are nearly 8 times as high as those for patients without PGD [4]. PGD leads to increased duration of mechanical ventilation and intensive care unit stay, poor functional outcomes, and increase rates of perioperative complications [5].

A number of previous studies have been designed to identify the clinical risk factors associated with PGD [6–23]. This field is of great clinical interest, since better understanding those transplant recipients most at risk might revolve around a concept of earlier detection for targeted therapy and aggressive support. In this regard, a number of clinical risk factors have been identified, including both organ donor and recipient characteristics. Donor characteristics previously identified include female gender, African American race, heavy smokers, older (>45 yr) or younger (<21 yr) donor age, and closed head injury as a cause of death [9,10,18,19,20]. Recipient characteristics previously linked to PGD include a diagnosis of primary pulmonary hypertension (PPH) [6,10,13,19], and elevated pulmonary artery pressures (PAP) [6,19]. In spite of this, there are several recipient-related risk factors that have been inconsistently reported in the literature.

Considering a single study may lack the power of providing a reliable conclusion, we carried out a rigorous systematic review and meta-analysis of published literature to gain more precise and quantitative estimates of recipient-related risk factors associated with development of PGD.

```
┌─────────────────────────────┐        ┌─────────────────────────────┐
│  Potential relevant studies │        │    Additional records       │
│  identified through database│        │  identified through other   │
│     searching (n=307)       │        │      sources (n=42)         │
└─────────────────────────────┘        └─────────────────────────────┘
              │                                        │
              ▼                                        ▼
┌──────────────────────────────────────────────────────────────────────┐
│            Records after duplicates removed (n=331)                    │
└──────────────────────────────────────────────────────────────────────┘
              │
              │              ┌──────────────────────────────────────────┐
              │              │ Excluded after screening for title       │
              │─────────────▶│ and abstract (n=289)                     │
              │              │   Not evaluating primary research        │
              │              │   question or irrelevant                 │
              │              └──────────────────────────────────────────┘
              ▼
┌──────────────────────────────────────────────────────────────────────┐
│         Full-text articles assessed for eligibility (n =42)            │
└──────────────────────────────────────────────────────────────────────┘
              │
              │              ┌──────────────────────────────────────────┐
              │              │ Full-text articles excluded (n=29)       │
              │              │   Not report relevant outcomes           │
              │              │   (n=16)                                 │
              │─────────────▶│   Reported the risk factors in an        │
              │              │   unusable format (n=3)                  │
              │              │   No objective diagnosis of PGD          │
              │              │   (n=4)                                  │
              │              │   Duplicate studies (same cohort         │
              │              │   of patients with different            │
              │              │   endpoints measured) (n=6)              │
              │              └──────────────────────────────────────────┘
              ▼
┌──────────────────────────────────────────────────────────────────────┐
│          Studies included in meta-analysis (n=13)                      │
└──────────────────────────────────────────────────────────────────────┘
```

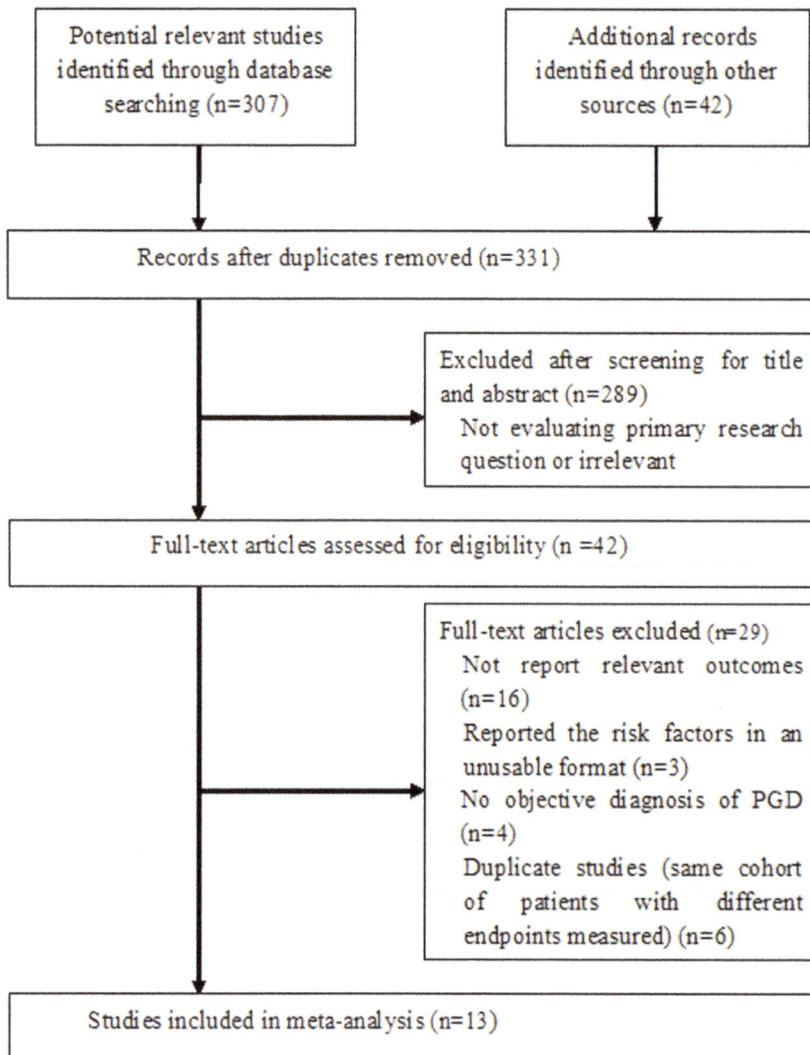

Figure 1. Flow of study identification, inclusion, and exclusion.

Methods

This meta-analysis followed the Meta-analysis of Observational Studies in Epidemiology (MOOSE) guidelines [24].

Search Strategy

Two reviewers (YL and SJJ) systematically searched PubMed, Embase, ISI Web of Science, Cochrane CENTRAL, and Scopus for articles published until October 2013. The following keywords were used in searching: "primary graft dysfunction" or "primary graft failure" or "ischemia-reperfusion injury" or "acute lung injury" or "early graft failure", combined with "lung transplantation". Language restrictions were not applied. From the title, abstract or descriptors, the literature search was reviewed independently to identify potentially relevant trials for full review. The "related articles" function was used to broaden the search. In addition, a manual review of references from primary or review articles was performed to identify any additional relevant studies.

Study selection

Cohort, case-control, and cross-sectional studies were included if they investigated which recipient-related factors directly influencing the development of PGD after lung transplantation. The potential variables assessed could be recipient demographics, co-morbidities, laboratory test, operative data, and postoperative complications. We did not address molecular or genetic markers as these require access to laboratory resources and genetic expertise. After obtaining full reports of candidate studies, the same reviewers independently assessed eligibility. Differences in data between the two reviewers were resolved by reviewing corresponding articles, and the final set was agreed on by consensus. When multiple articles for a single study had been published, we used the latest publication and supplemented it, if necessary, with data from the earlier publications. Attempts were also made to contact investigators for unpublished data.

Data Extraction

Two investigators (YL and SJJ) independently summarized the studies meeting the inclusion criteria, and performed data extraction using a standard data sheet [25]. Disagreement was

Table 1. Characteristics of Selected Studies.

Author	Date of study (Year)	Country	Study Design	No. of Subjects (M/F)	Mean age, %	Definition of PGD	Quality Assessment
King et al,[7] 2000	1990–1998	USA	Retrospective, single-center chart review	100(NA)	49	Patients with a chest x-ray film (CXR) score of ≥6 and a PaO2/FiO2 gradient of less than 200 mm Hg	Fair
Thabut et al,[8] 2002	1988–2000	France	Retrospective multicenter cohort study	257 (169/88)	48	The presence of reperfusion pulmonary edema with or without early hemodynamic failure.	Fair
Christie et al,[9] 2003	199–2000	USA	Retrospective single-center cohort study	252(123/129)	49	The presence of a diffuse alveolar infiltrate and a PaO2/FiO2 gradient of less than 200 mm Hg	Good
Whitson et al,[10] 2006	1992–2004	USA	Retrospective, single-center chart review	402 (185/217)	50	ISHLT PGD Grading System	Fair
Burton et al,[11] 2007	1999–2004	Denmark	Retrospective	180 (82/98)	56	The presence of a unilateral diffuse radiological infiltrate of the lung allograft.	Fair
Krenn et al,[12] 2007	2003–2006	Austria	Prospective single-center cohort study	150 (76/74)	38	ISHLT PGD Grading System	Good
Kuntz et al,[13] 2009	1994–2002	USA	Secondary analysis of multicenter registry (UNOS/ISHLT)	6984 (4315/2669)	—	A PaO2/FiO2 ratio less than 200, with evidence of radiographic infiltrates, and absence of secondary causes of allograft dysfunction.	Good
Felten et al,[14] 2011	2006–2008	France	Retrospective, multicenter cohort study	122 (63/59)	25	ISHLT PGD Grading System	Good
Fang et al,[15] 2011	2002–2007	USA	Prospective multicenter cohort study	126 (60/66)	56	ISHLT PGD Grading System	Good
Allen et al,[16] 2012	2002–2007	USA	Prospective, single-center cohort study	28 (12/16)	51	ISHLT PGD Grading System	Fair
Shah et al,[17] 2012	2006–2008	USA	Prospective multicenter cohort study	108(56/52)	37	ISHLT PGD Grading System	Good
Samano et al,[18] 2012	2003–2010	Brazil	Retrospective, single-center chart review	78 (46/32)	44	ISHLT PGD Grading System	Fair
Diamond et al,[19] 2013	2002–2010	USA	Prospective, multicenter cohort study (LTOG)	1255 (211/1044)	35	ISHLT PGD Grading System	Good

M, male; F, female; PGD, primary graft dysfunction; ISHLT, International Society for Heart and Lung Transplantation.

Table 2. The recipient-related risk factors examined in the original articles.

Author	Age	Gender	Race	Pulmonary Diagnosis	PAP	BLT vs SLT	BMI	CPB	Inhaled NO	Blood products transfusion	Mortality
King et al,[7]	√			√	√	√		√			√
Thabut et al,[8]	√	√		√		√		√			√
Christie et al,[9]	√	√	√	√	√	√			√		
Whitson et al,[10]		√		√		√	√				√
Burton et al,[11]	√	√		√			√	√			√
Krenn et al,[12]	√	√		√	√	√		√			√
Kuntz et al,[13]		√	√	√			√				
Felten et al,[14]	√	√					√	√	√	√	
Fang et al,[15]	√	√	√		√	√	√	√			
Allen et al,[16]	√	√		√	√	√		√	√		√
Shah et al,[17]	√	√	√	√	√	√	√				
Samano et al,[18]	√	√				√	√				√
Diamond et al,[19]		√		√	√	√	√	√		√	√

PAP, pulmonary artery pressure; BLT, bilateral lung transplant; SLT, single lung transplant; BMI, body mass index; CPB, cardiopulmonary bypass; NO, nitric oxide.

resolved by consensus or by a third party. For each study, the following data were extracted: first author's last name, publication year, study date, country, study design, sample size, patient characteristics (age and gender) and definition of PGD. Initially, we scrutinized in detail the literature about PGD after lung transplantation to identify all possible risk factors. The initial search yielded 18 possible risk factors. Following review by an expert panel (YL, LLS and SJJ), 10 factors that were considered to be easily measured in routine clinical practice and had been analyzed in at least 2 studies were selected for the full systematic review. These factors assessed including age, gender, race, pulmonary diagnosis, PAP, type of transplant (single lung transplant (SLT) vs bilateral lung transplant (BLT)), body mass index (BMI), cardiopulmonary bypass (CPB), intra-operative inhaled nitric oxide (NO), and blood products transfusion.

Study Quality Assessment

The Newcastle-Ottawa Scale was used to assess the quality of observational studies based on the following nine questions: (1) representativeness of the exposed cohort; (2) selection of the non-exposed cohort; (3) ascertainment of exposure; (4) demonstration that the outcome was not present at outset of study; (5) comparability; (6) assessment of outcome; (7) length of follow-up sufficient; (8) adequacy of participant follow-up; (9) total stars [26]. Maximum score on this scale is a total of 9. "Good" was defined as a total score of 7 to 9; "fair," a total score of 4–6; and "poor," defined as a total score of <4.

Statistical analyses

Our meta-analysis and statistical analyses were performed with Revman software (version 5.2; Cochrane Collaboration, Oxford, United Kingdom) and Stata software (version 11.0; Stata Corporation, College Station, TX, USA). The odds ratios (ORs)

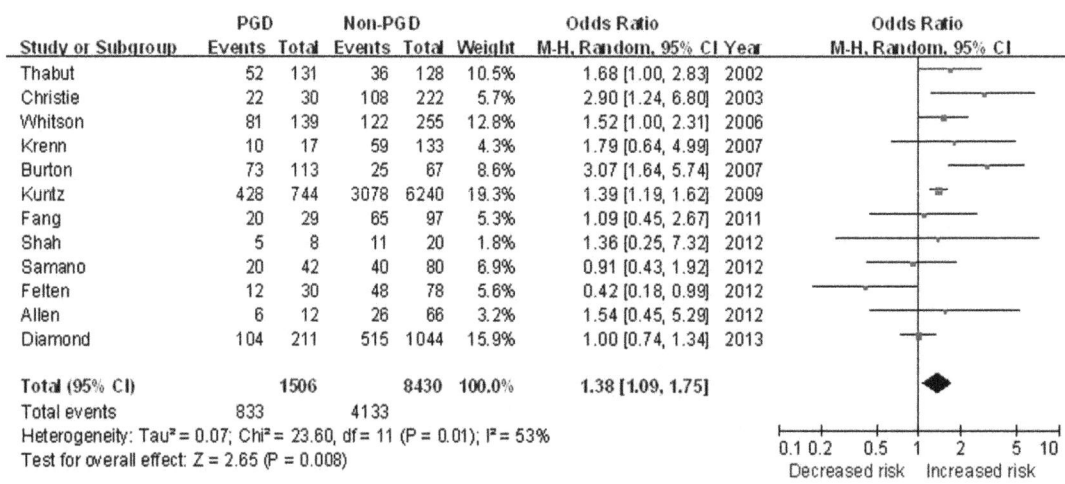

Study or Subgroup	PGD Events	PGD Total	Non-PGD Events	Non-PGD Total	Weight	Odds Ratio M-H, Random, 95% CI	Year
Thabut	52	131	36	128	10.5%	1.68 [1.00, 2.83]	2002
Christie	22	30	108	222	5.7%	2.90 [1.24, 6.80]	2003
Whitson	81	139	122	255	12.8%	1.52 [1.00, 2.31]	2006
Krenn	10	17	59	133	4.3%	1.79 [0.64, 4.99]	2007
Burton	73	113	25	67	8.6%	3.07 [1.64, 5.74]	2007
Kuntz	428	744	3078	6240	19.3%	1.39 [1.19, 1.62]	2009
Fang	20	29	65	97	5.3%	1.09 [0.45, 2.67]	2011
Shah	5	8	11	20	1.8%	1.36 [0.25, 7.32]	2012
Samano	20	42	40	80	6.9%	0.91 [0.43, 1.92]	2012
Felten	12	30	48	78	5.6%	0.42 [0.18, 0.99]	2012
Allen	6	12	26	66	3.2%	1.54 [0.45, 5.29]	2012
Diamond	104	211	515	1044	15.9%	1.00 [0.74, 1.34]	2013
Total (95% CI)		1506		8430	100.0%	1.38 [1.09, 1.75]	
Total events	833		4133				

Heterogeneity: Tau² = 0.07; Chi² = 23.60, df = 11 (P = 0.01); I² = 53%
Test for overall effect: Z = 2.65 (P = 0.008)

Figure 2. The influence of recipient gender on PGD.

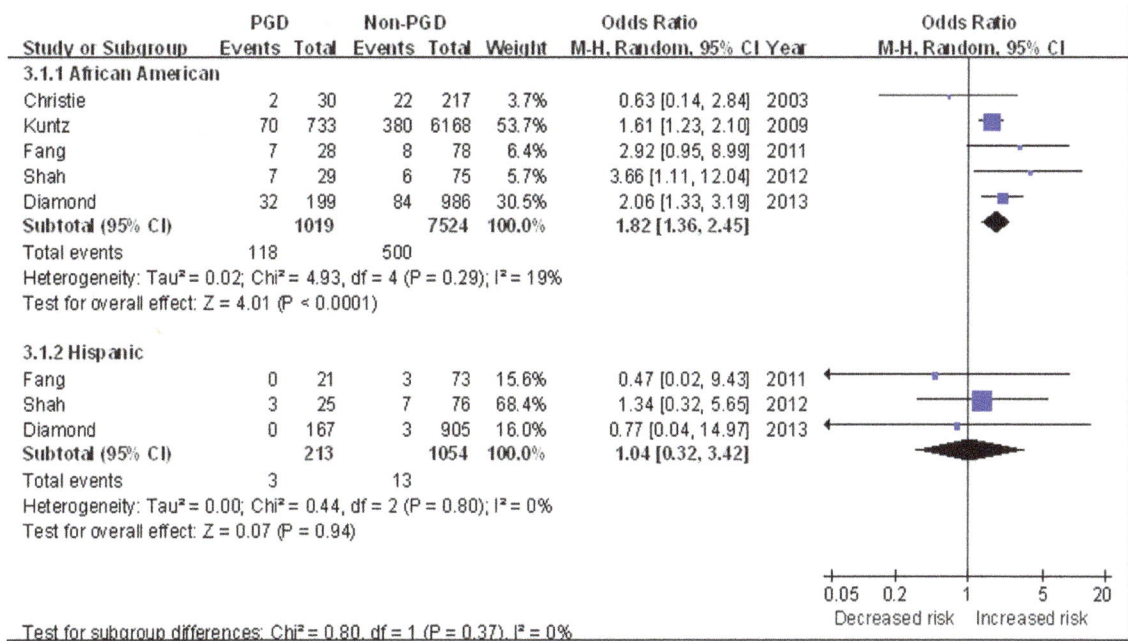

Figure 3. The influence of African American and Hispanic race on PGD compared with white race.

and 95% confidence intervals (CIs) were calculated to estimate the association between binary factors and development of PGD. When mean values and SDs for a certain risk factor were provided, we calculated the mean differences (MDs) between patients with and without PGD. The statistical estimates of effect were derived using a random-effects (DerSimonian and Laird) model, which assumes that the true underlying effect varies among included studies, because of the different characteristics of study population, transplantation procedure, and the PGD definitions that were involved in the original trials.

The definitions of PGD may be a potential source of heterogeneity. In order to analyze the heterogeneity associated with different definitions, we performed subgroup analyses by comparing summary results obtained from subsets of studies grouped by "the International Society for Heart and Lung Transplantation (ISHLT) PGD Grading System [28]" or other definitions. Statistical heterogeneity of treatment effects between studies was formally tested with Cochran's χ2 statistics and with significance set at $P < 0.10$. The I^2 statistic was used to quantify heterogeneity. Using accepted guidelines [27], an I^2 of 0% to 40% was considered to exclude heterogeneity, an I^2 of 30% to 60% to represent moderate heterogeneity, an I^2 of 50% to 90% to represent substantial heterogeneity, and an I^2 of 75% to 100% to represent considerable heterogeneity. Publication bias was assessed with funnel plots and the Begg's test.

Results

Literature search and study characteristics

The method used to select studies is shown in Figure 1. A total of 331 potentially eligible articles were initially identified, and 289 articles were excluded as they were not relevant to the purpose of the current meta-analysis. Therefore, 42 potentially relevant articles were selected for detailed evaluation. From the overall pool of full-text articles, 29 articles were excluded because they did not provide PGD data according to the risk factors we evaluated (n = 16), reported the risk factors in an unusable format (n = 3), did

not make any objective diagnosis of PGD (n = 4), or were duplicate studies (same cohort of patients with different endpoints measured) (n = 6). Thus, 13 studies were included in the meta-analysis with a total of 10042 patients [7–19]. Additional data were requested from the authors of three studies but didn't receive any reply.

Baseline characteristics of the studies included are shown in Table 1. The 13 included studies consisted of 5 prospective cohort studies [12,15–17,19], 7 retrospective analyses of cohort data or chart review [7–11,14,18], and 1 secondary analysis of multicenter registry [13]. Eight of the 13 studies involved American subjects [7,9,10,13,15–17,19], and the populations of the remaining five studies came from France [8,14], Denmark [11], Austria [12], and Brazil [18]. The studies varied in size from 28 to 6984 subjects, and the average age of the patients ranged from 25 to 56 years.

There were some variations in the definition of PGD. The ISHLT PGD grading schema was used in the majority of the studies. The other 5 studies also defined PGD based on the presence of infiltrates in the lung allograft on chest radiograph and/or the PaO2/FiO2 ratio [7–9,11,13]. PGD, as defined in the original articles, was present in 16.4% of the lung transplant patients. All studies were of high methodological quality (good or fair) as assessed by the Newcastle-Ottawa Scale [26] (Table 1). The risk factors examined in the 13 included studies are summarized in Table 2.

Outcomes and synthesis of results

Age. Ten studies investigated the influence of recipient age on the occurrence of PGD [7–9,11,12,14–18], including 434 patients with PGD and 969 controls. Findings from this analysis suggested no significant difference in mean age between patients with or without PGD (MD -0.75 y, 95% CI -2.12 to 0.63 y, $P = 0.29$). Statistical heterogeneity among the studies was significant ($I^2 = 61\%$, $P = 0.006$).

Gender. Twelve studies investigated the influence of recipient gender on the occurrence of PGD [8–19]. These studies included 1506 patients with PGD and 8430 controls. The proportion of

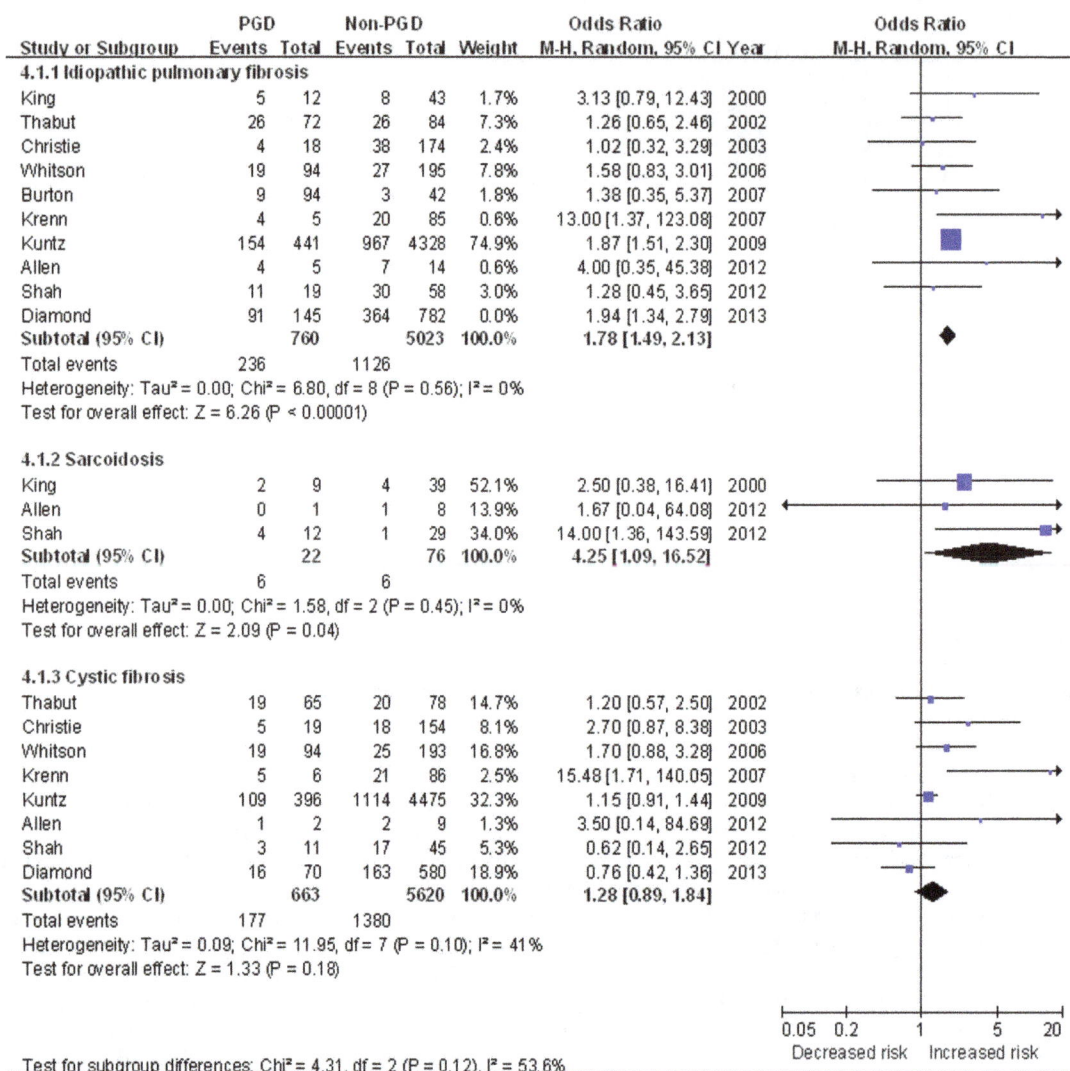

Figure 4. The influence of recipient pulmonary diagnosis on PGD. COPD was used as the reference group.

female recipients was 55.3% in patients with PGD compared with 49.0% in patients without. Analysis suggested female recipients had an increased risk of PGD (OR 1.38, 95% CI 1.09 to 1.75, $P = 0.008$) (Figure 2).

Race. Five studies reported the influence of recipient race [9,13,15,17,19]. PGD was found in 11.4% of patients with white race, 19.1% of African American patients, and 18.7% of Hispanic patients. White race was used as the reference group given the lowest incidence of PGD. Analysis of these studies showed compared with white race, African American was associated with a significantly increased risk of PGD (OR 1.82, 95%CI 1.36 to 2.45, $P<0.0001$), while Hispanic race did not appear to affect the risk of PGD (OR 1.04, 95%CI 0.32 to 3.42, $P = 0.94$) (Figure 3).

Pulmonary Diagnosis. The effect of recipient pulmonary diagnosis on PGD development was evaluated in 10 studies [7–13,16,17,19]. The incidence of PGD was 11.8% in patients with chronic obstructive pulmonary disease (COPD), 18.0% in patients with idiopathic pulmonary fibrosis (IPF), 50% in sarcoidosis and 12.4% in cystic fibrosis. For patients with pulmonary hypertension, PGD was observed in 30.3% of patients with PPH and 29.3% of secondary pulmonary hypertension (SPH).

Using COPD as the reference group (with the lowest incidence of PGD), IPF (OR 1.78, 95% CI 1.49 to 2.13, $P<0.0001$) [7–13,16,17,19] and sarcoidosis (OR 4.25, 95% CI 1.09 to 16.52, $P = 0.04$) [7,16–17] were both associated with increased risk of PGD; while cystic fibrosis was non-significantly associated with PGD development (OR 1.28, 95% CI 0.89 to 1.84, $P = 0.18$) [8–10,12,13,16,17,19] (Figure 4). PPH was also significantly associated with PGD, with a 3.73-fold increased risk of PGD was observed (OR 3.73, 95%CI 2.16 to 6.46, $P<0.001$) [7–10,12,13,16–17]; while unlike PPH, SPH did not confer an significantly increased risk of PGD (OR 2.23, 95%CI 0.65 to 7.69, $P = 0.20$) [10,13] (Figure 5).

PAP. There were 7 studies compared the mean PAP between patients with and without PGD (325 PGD patients and 1093 controls) [7,9,12,15–17,19]. Findings from the meta-analysis showed a significant higher PAP was observed in the PGD patients as compared with the controls (MD 6.00 mmHg, 95% CI 3.91 to 8.09 mmHg, $P<0.0001$). Statistical heterogeneity was observed among the studies ($I^2 = 77\%$, $P = 0.0003$) (Figure 6).

BLT vs. SLT. Eleven studies evaluated the impact of BLT vs. SLT on PGD development, including 4554 patients undergoing

Study or Subgroup	PGD Events	PGD Total	Non-PGD Events	Non-PGD Total	Weight	Odds Ratio M-H, Random, 95% CI	Year	Odds Ratio M-H, Random, 95% CI
4.2.1 Primary pulmonary hypertension								
King	5	6	6	13	3.4%	5.83 [0.52, 64.82]	2000	
Thabut	9	55	4	62	8.8%	2.84 [0.82, 9.80]	2002	
Christie	6	20	12	148	9.8%	4.86 [1.58, 14.94]	2003	
Whitson	19	94	27	195	15.4%	1.58 [0.83, 3.01]	2006	
Krenn	3	4	3	68	3.1%	65.00 [5.12, 825.79]	2007	
Kuntz	84	371	243	3604	20.0%	4.05 [3.07, 5.33]	2009	
Allen	1	2	1	8	1.8%	7.00 [0.22, 226.00]	2012	
Shah	2	10	1	29	3.1%	7.00 [0.56, 87.50]	2012	
Subtotal (95% CI)		562		4127	65.3%	3.73 [2.16, 6.46]		
Total events	129		297					
Heterogeneity: Tau² = 0.21; Chi² = 12.99, df = 7 (P = 0.07); I² = 46%								
Test for overall effect: Z = 4.71 (P < 0.00001)								
4.2.2 Secondary pulmonary hypertension								
Whitson	25	100	47	215	16.6%	1.19 [0.68, 2.08]	2006	
Kuntz	29	316	83	3444	18.1%	4.09 [2.64, 6.35]	2009	
Subtotal (95% CI)		416		3659	34.7%	2.23 [0.65, 7.69]		
Total events	54		130					
Heterogeneity: Tau² = 0.73; Chi² = 12.16, df = 1 (P = 0.0005); I² = 92%								
Test for overall effect: Z = 1.27 (P = 0.20)								
Total (95% CI)		978		7786	100.0%	3.20 [1.98, 5.17]		
Total events	183		427					
Heterogeneity: Tau² = 0.28; Chi² = 27.97, df = 9 (P = 0.0010); I² = 68%								
Test for overall effect: Z = 4.74 (P < 0.00001)								
Test for subgroup differences: Chi² = 0.55, df = 1 (P = 0.46), I² = 0%								

Odds Ratio scale: 0.01 0.1 1 10 100 — Decreased risk / Increased risk

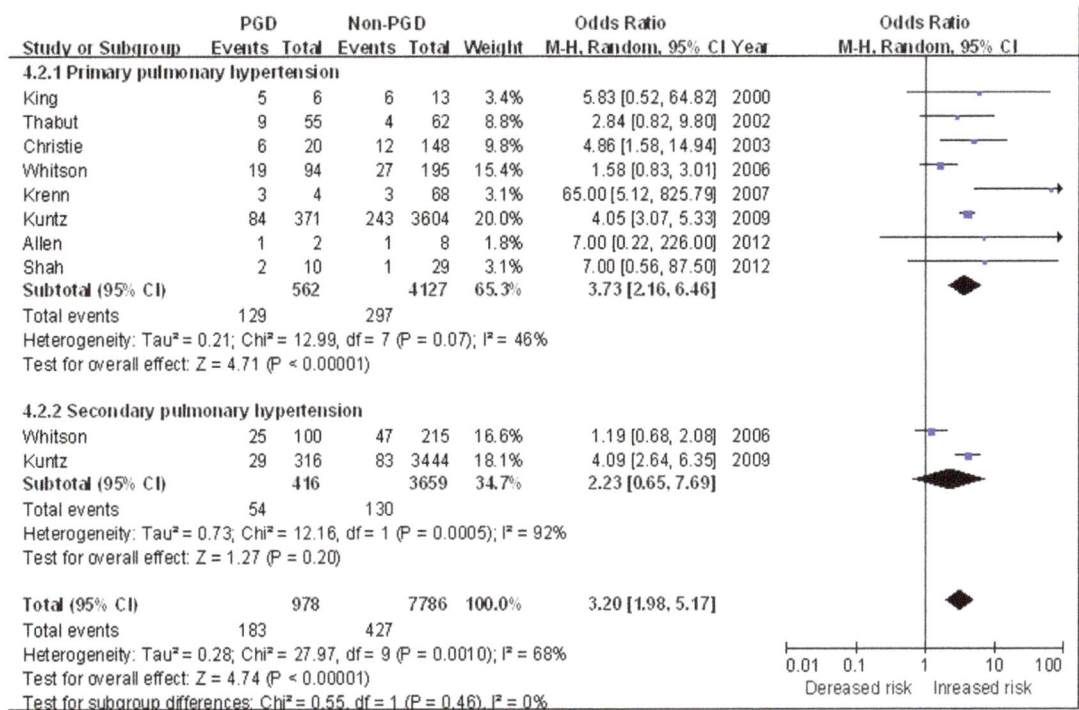

Figure 5. The influence of recipient pulmonary hypertension on PGD. COPD was used as the reference group.

BLT and 5190 patients undergoing SLT [7–10,12,13,15–19]. The pooled analysis showed the incidence of PGD was 14.5% in BLT recipients, compared to 13.8% in SLT recipients. Findings from the meta-analysis showed an insignificant association between the transplant type (SLT or BLT) and PGD (OR 1.10, 95% CI 0.97 to 1.24, P = 0.14). No statistically significant heterogeneity was observed between studies (I² = 0%, P = 0.65).

BMI. Two studies evaluated the effect of BMI (as a continuous variable) on PGD [11,14], including 155 patients with PGD and 147 controls. The pooled analysis of the 2 studies showed patients with PGD had a higher mean BMI level than controls (MD 1.20 kg/m², 95% CI 0.13 to 2.27 kg/m², P = 0.03). Other 2 studies investigated the impact of elevated BMI (BMI ≥ 25 kg/m²) on PGD development [13,19]. The incidence of PGD was 15.2% in the 3105 patients with elevated BMI, compared to 9.4% in the 5091 patients with normal BMI. Analysis

of these studies showed a significant association between elevated BMI level and PGD (OR 1.83, 95% CI 1.26 to 2.64, P = 0.001).

CPB. Eleven studies evaluated the effect of CPB for PGD [7,8,10–12,14–19]. PGD was found in 263 of 813 patients (32.3%) use of CPB compared to 490 of 1984 patients (24.7%) without CPB. The pooled analysis of these studies showed a 2.29-fold increased risk of PGD was present for patients requiring CPB (OR 2.29, 95% CI 1.43 to 3.65, P = 0.0005), with statistical heterogeneity among the studies (I² = 69%, P = 0.0004).

Inhaled NO. Four studies investigated the influence of intra-operative use of inhaled NO on the occurrence of PGD [9,14–16]. The incidence of PGD was 23.4% (50 of 214 patients) and 18.8% (59 of 314 patients) in patients with and without use of inhaled NO, respectively. Findings from this analysis suggested there was no significant association between intra-operative inhaled NO use and development of PGD (OR 1.09, 95% CI 0.68 to 1.74,

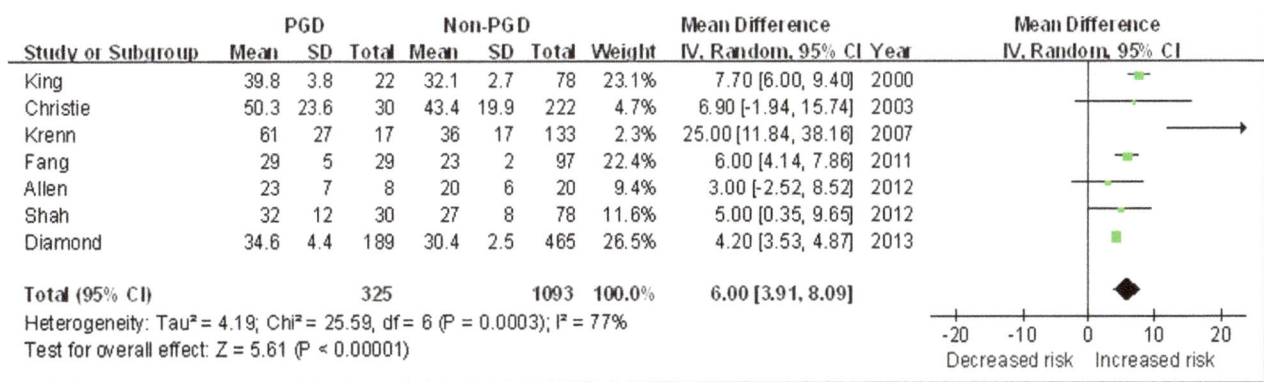

Study or Subgroup	PGD Mean	PGD SD	PGD Total	Non-PGD Mean	Non-PGD SD	Non-PGD Total	Weight	Mean Difference IV, Random, 95% CI	Year	Mean Difference IV, Random, 95% CI
King	39.8	3.8	22	32.1	2.7	78	23.1%	7.70 [6.00, 9.40]	2000	
Christie	50.3	23.6	30	43.4	19.9	222	4.7%	6.90 [-1.94, 15.74]	2003	
Krenn	61	27	17	36	17	133	2.3%	25.00 [11.84, 38.16]	2007	
Fang	29	5	29	23	2	97	22.4%	6.00 [4.14, 7.86]	2011	
Allen	23	7	8	20	6	20	9.4%	3.00 [-2.52, 8.52]	2012	
Shah	32	12	30	27	8	78	11.6%	5.00 [0.35, 9.65]	2012	
Diamond	34.6	4.4	189	30.4	2.5	465	26.5%	4.20 [3.53, 4.87]	2013	
Total (95% CI)			325			1093	100.0%	6.00 [3.91, 8.09]		
Heterogeneity: Tau² = 4.19; Chi² = 25.59, df = 6 (P = 0.0003); I² = 77%										
Test for overall effect: Z = 5.61 (P < 0.00001)										

Mean Difference scale: -20 -10 0 10 20 — Decreased risk / Increased risk

Figure 6. The influence of mean pulmonary artery pressures (PAP) on PGD.

Study or Subgroup	PGD Events	Total	Non-PGD Events	Total	Weight	Odds Ratio M-H, Random, 95% CI	Year	Odds Ratio M-H, Random, 95% CI
King	9	22	9	78	8.6%	5.31 [1.77, 15.91]	2000	
Thabut	38	131	14	128	18.9%	3.33 [1.70, 6.51]	2002	
Whitson	24	139	23	255	21.4%	2.11 [1.14, 3.89]	2006	
Krenn	2	17	8	133	4.1%	2.08 [0.40, 10.73]	2007	
Burton	16	113	2	67	4.9%	5.36 [1.19, 24.10]	2007	
Allen	3	8	2	20	2.7%	5.40 [0.70, 41.75]	2012	
Samano	8	12	18	66	6.2%	5.33 [1.43, 19.90]	2012	
Diamond	49	211	52	1044	33.3%	5.77 [3.78, 8.82]	2013	
Total (95% CI)		653		1791	100.0%	3.95 [2.80, 5.57]		
Total events	149		128					

Heterogeneity: Tau² = 0.05; Chi² = 8.66, df = 7 (P = 0.28); I² = 19%
Test for overall effect: Z = 7.83 (P < 0.00001)

0.05   0.2   1   5   20
Decreased risk   Increased risk

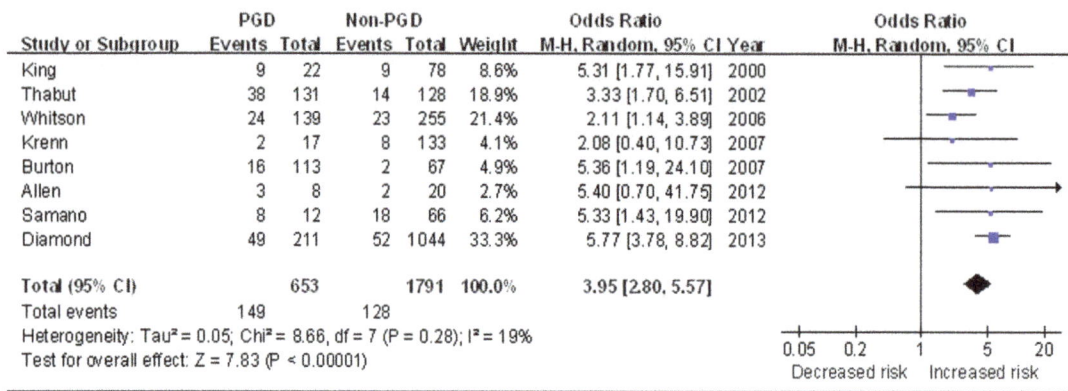

Figure 7. The influence of PGD on short-term mortality (mortality within 90 days).

$P = 0.72$). No statistical heterogeneity was observed between studies ($I^2 = 0\%$, $P = 0.95$).

Blood products transfusion. Three studies reported the amount of packed red blood cells (RBCs) and plasma used during the lung transplant procedure to evaluate the effect of intra-operative transfusion on PGD [14,15,19]. Findings from the meta-analysis showed a greater amount of packed RBCs and plasma transfused in patients with PGD compared with those without (RBCs: MD 341 ml, 95% CI 254 to 427 ml, $P < 0.001$; plasma: MD 131 ml, 95% CI 71 to 191 ml, $P < 0.001$). The χ^2 test for heterogeneities were also non-significant ($I^2 = 0\%$, $P = 0.84$ and $I^2 = 44\%$, $P = 0.17$).

Mortality risk for PGD. The impact of PGD on mortality (within 90 days) was reported in 8 studies [7,8,10–12,16,18,19]. All-cause mortality within 90 days was 22.8% for patients with PGD versus 7.1% for patients without. The pooled analysis suggested patients with PGD was associated with a nearly 4 fold increased risk of short-term mortality (OR 3.95, 95% CI 2.80 to 5.57, $P < 0.001$) compared with those without PGD. There was no statistical heterogeneity among the studies ($I^2 = 19\%$, $P = 0.28$) (Figure 7).

Subgroup analysis according to the definitions for PGD. In the subgroup meta-analysis, we compared the associations between above risk factors and PGD in subsets of studies grouped by ISHLT PGD grade or other definitions (Table 3). The results showed no matter which definition was used in the original studies, no significant difference was observed in the effects of age, gender, race, pulmonary diagnosis, mPAP, BLT vs SLT, use of CPB, or inhaled NO in PGD development (P for subgroup difference > 0.05).

Publication Bias

We performed funnel plot analysis and Begg's test to assess publication bias. Funnel plot analysis was performed using the recipient gender as an index, the funnel plot of the 12 studies appeared to be symmetrical (Figure 8), and the Begg's test of funnel plot suggested no publication bias ($P = 0.87$). Also no publication bias was detected by Begg's test for other outcomes analysis (all $P > 0.05$).

Discussion

Despite the significant morbidity and mortality in patients with PGD after lung transplantation, the recipient related risk factors contributing to this devastating syndrome remain controversial. Our meta-analysis comprehensively reviewed 13 studies involving

10042 lung transplantation recipients which addressed the clinical risk factors for PGD. The results showed recipient female gender, African American race, preoperative diagnosis of IPF, sarcoidosis, or PPH, elevated mean PAP and BMI, use of CPB and blood products transfusion were significantly and consistently associated with development of PGD. All of these factors are likely to be measured and monitored in the primary care setting. To the best of our knowledge, this is the first systematic review on this topic.

Among baseline variables, we have demonstrated that female gender and African-American race had increased risk of PGD, which have not been validated in previous studies. Female gender has been associated with a higher risk of development of acute respiratory distress syndrome (ARDS) in the Ibuprofen in Sepsis Study Group [29], as well as in a cohort study of trauma patients [30]. Similarly, donor female gender was also shown to have an independent impact on PGD [9]. Possible mechanisms for these findings are unclear. Some theories for the differential outcome based on gender differences have been advocated, including immunity and tolerance theories [31] and the influence of gender hormones [32]. However, as of now few data have been published that evaluate the effect of gender on graft function and survival. Similarly, mechanisms for the observed worse outcome of African-American race remain speculative, but may reflect differences in vascular endothelium (such as expression of angiotensin-converting enzyme) [33,34], which could potentially predispose African Americans to more severe ischemia reperfusion injury.

Elevated BMI was another risk factor for PGD in our meta-analysis. Prior studies have identified obesity as a risk factor for early mortality and increased intensive care unit stay after lung transplant [35,36]. Technical difficulties of performing a lung transplant operation in obese recipients may increase risk of PGD. Other possible explanations may be obesity affects the milieu of cytokines produced by adipose tissue during ischemia-reperfusion, such as leptin [37], which has been shown to be increased in patients with acute lung injury and play a role in the development of acute lung injury in animal model [38]. In the study by Lederer et al, higher plasma leptin levels were associated with PGD after lung transplantation [39]. In addition, modulation of lung inflammation by other adipokines, such as resistin, adiponectin, which produced by macrophages recruited to hypertrophic and hypoxic adipose tissue, could also be responsible [39–41]. Future studies of adipokines in lung tissue or bronchoalveolar lavage fluid and examination of their roles in the development of PGD should be pursued.

Table 3. Subgroup analysis according to the definitions for PGD.

	No.of studies	Test for association		Test for subgroup difference	
		OR (95% CI)	P	I²	P
Age				0%	0.72
ISHLT	5	−1.33 (−5.09 to 2.43)	0.49		
Othe definitions	5	−0.58 (−2.17 to 1.10)	0.48		
Female				0%	0.33
ISHLT	8	1.21 (0.82 to 1.77)	0.33		
Othe definitions	4	1.50 (1.23 to 1.83)	<0.001		
Race					
African-American				36%	0.21
ISPGS	3	2.28 (1.55 to 3.36)	<0.001		
Othe definitions	3	1.37 (0.68 to 2.74)	0.38		
Diagnosis					
IPF				0%	0.58
ISHLT	5	1.88 (1.40 to 2.54)	<0.001		
Othe definitions	5	1.65 (1.14 to 2.38)	0.0009		
Cystic fibrosis				0%	0.71
ISHLT	5	1.41 (0.63 to 3.18)	0.41		
Othe definitions	3	1.20 (0.93 to 1.55)	0.16		
PPH				0%	0.61
ISHLT	5	6.58 (1.04 to 41.59)	<0.001		
Othe definitions	3	4.04 (3.12 to 5.24)	0.05		
Mean PAP				0%	0.61
ISHLT	4	5.80 (1.65 to 9.94)	0.006		
Othe definitions	3	6.93 (5.69 to 8.17)	<0.001		
BLT vs SLT				0%	0.73
ISHLT	6	1.06 (0.84 to 1.33)	0.63		
Othe definitions	5	1.11 (0.96 to 1.28)	0.15		
CPB				0%	0.77
ISHLT	7	2.31 (1.23 to 4.33)	0.009		
Othe definitions	4	2.62 (1.47 to 4.66)	0.001		
Use of inhaled NO				0%	0.69
ISHLT	2	1.22 (0.59 to 2.51)	0.60		
Othe definitions	2	1.00 (0.54 to 1.85)	0.99		

PGD, primary graft dysfunction; ISHLT, International Society for Heart and Lung Transplantation; IPF, idiopathic pulmonary fibrosis; PPH, primary pulmonary hypertension; PAP, pulmonary artery pressure; BLT, bilateral lung transplant; SLT, single lung transplant; CPB, cardiopulmonary bypass; NO, nitric oxide.

In nearly all previous studies, diagnosis of PPH was the most significant risk factor for PGD [6,10,13,19], and our findings further support this, showing both PPH and elevated mPAP were strongly associated with PGD after lung transplant. Possible explanations are not fully understood. In PPH, right ventricular dysfunction is universally present, and the hypertrophied, failing right ventricle is acutely afterload reduced at transplantation, resulting in increased shear stress on the formerly hypoxic pulmonary vascular endothelium. Shear stress leads to capillary leak and worse graft function [42,43]. Christie et al showed diagnosis of PPH was even more strongly associated with an increased risk of PGD after adjustment for recipient PAP (adjusted RR = 9.24, P = 0.009) [9]. This implies it is the disease state of PPH that increases the risk, rather than just the presence or severity of pulmonary hypertension. Unlike PPH, our study suggested SPH did not confer an increased risk of PGD. In prior studies, the association between SPH and PGD was controversial and the conclusions were inconsistent [10,13,15,18]. Fang et al demonstrated SPH in patients with IPF was independently associated with the development of PGD [15]. While for patients with CF, based on data from the ISHLT registry, no significant difference was observed in PGD incidence for patients with and without pulmonary hypertension [6]. These findings suggested that the association between pulmonary hypertension and PGD might depend on the underlying diagnoses to some extent. For studies included in this meta-analysis, SPH has been all-inclusive, regardless of cause [10,13,18]. Therefore, for further discussion, it is better to focus on the primary disease of SPH.

IPF was also identified as a risk factor with intermediate risk of PGD in our analysis. Previous observational studies reported patients undergoing transplantation for IPF had somewhat worse survival than for other indications, when matched on multiple

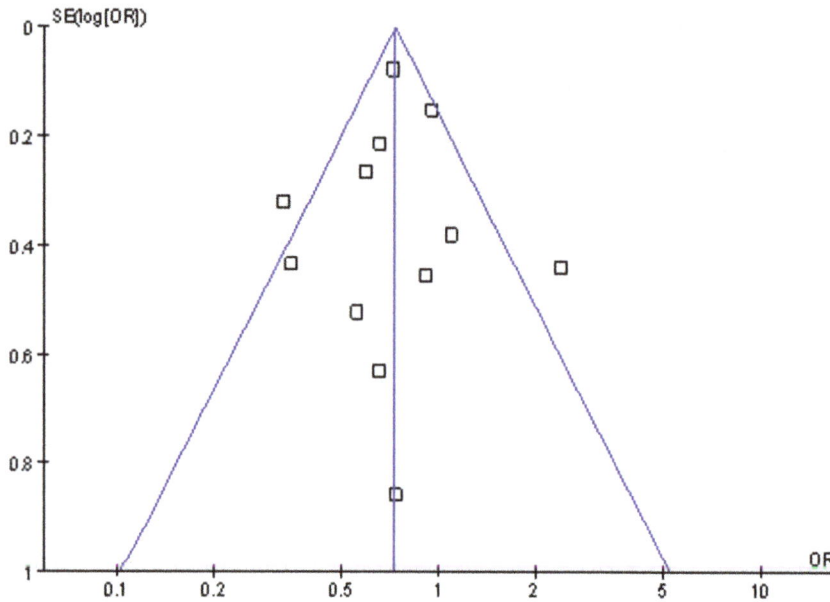

Figure 8. Funnel plot of the 12 studies evaluated the effect of the recipient gender on PGD.

variables [44,45]. Possible explanations may be related to the pathogenesis of IPF. IPF carries a progressive course of pulmonary dysfunction that is inhibited, but not eliminated, by transplantation. Vasoactive mediators such as endothelin-1, platelet-derived growth factor, transforming growth factor-β, and fibroblast growth factor have all been implicated in the pathogenesis of IPF, and also contribute to the development of lung injury [46]. Moreover, IPF patients have a restrictive pattern of pulmonary disease with smaller-than-predicted total lung capacity. Shrinking lung volume may have caused irreversible damage to pulmonary mechanics by contracting the chest wall (remodeling). This relative "oversize" donor lung within smaller chest may lead to worse graft function [45,47]. Nevertheless, at this point, reasons for the poor outcomes of IPF after transplantation remain elusive and warrant focused investigation.

The intra-operative use of CPB was another potential contributor to PGD in our meta-analysis. CPB causes a systemic, pro-inflammatory response with activation of cytokines, leukocytes and the complement cascade [48,49]. Patients requiring CPB have been shown to have more radiographic infiltrates, worse immediate graft function, longer intubation, and ultimately, decreased survival [50,51]. However, a notable difficulty in interpreting the data is the overall severity of the patient's illness or operative difficulty requiring the use of CPB. It is not possible to accurately differentiate planned use of CPB from emergent initiation intra-operatively because of deterioration in patient hemodynamics or oxygenation. As a result, independent of indication for CPB use, the association between PGD and CPB is still debatable. The type of transplant procedure (bilateral vs. single) was not identified as a significant risk factor for PGD in our study. Although the reported incidence of PGD was somewhat higher in BLT recipients, higher pre-transplant PAP and CPB use in BLT recipients likely confounded these results [5,10].

The finding of blood products transfusion as a risk factor for PGD has been shown in recent multicenter studies and our meta-analysis confirmed this tendency [19,52], but the exact relationship between the two processes is not yet clear. Blood products transfusion in-and-of-itself is associated with transfusion-related

lung injury, which results in an ARDS-like picture similar to that seen with PGD [53]. The transfusion-related lung injury might accentuate any underlying mild ischemia/reperfusion injury, resulting in the onset of clinically significant PGD [53]. Nonetheless, the need for blood products administration has been shown to collinear with other PGD risk factors, including PPH and the use of CPB, and unmeasured operative characteristics may also lead to transfusion requirements [54]. Therefore dissecting the independence of the relationship between blood transfusion and PGD is difficult.

Inhaled NO has been investigated as a potential agent for the prevention of PGD, given its effects on pulmonary vasodilation and capillary integrity. Although our analysis did not support use of inhaled NO to be effective in PGD prevention, it may be beneficial in clinical settings of established PGD. Several reports and case series have shown improved outcomes with inhaled NO administration [55,56]. However, there have also been studies that do not show efficacy in the setting of PGD [57]. Lack of randomized clinical trials showing survival benefit precludes widespread recommendation of inhaled NO for the treatment of PGD. Again, extrapolating from inhaled NO use in studies with ARDS, the beneficial effects of inhaled NO may be real, but also appear to be transient [58].

Limitations of the review

Although we believe that the current meta-analysis provided useful information, some potential limitations should be addressed. Firstly, heterogeneity in our study is substantial and may be attributed to differences in type of patients, study era, operative practice, and definition of PGD. Definition of PGD is a major cause of heterogeneity, and with potential for misclassification bias. As the ISHLT PGD criteria were first published in 2005, studies performed before 2005 did not use standard defining criteria; even for the studies defined PGD based on the ISHLT guidelines, the PGD grades were retrospectively assigned to those patients enrolled before 2005. To clarify the heterogeneity, subgroup analyses were performed by dividing studies according to ISHLT or other definitions, and the results suggested our findings were not significantly affected by varying definitions. Secondly, our analysis was by necessity restricted to individual risk factors. Therefore, the distinct possibility exists that the strength of association may be weaker with a multi-factorial regression analysis; for instance, the individual effects of CPB, use of blood products, and elevated PAP cannot be delineated since they are often apparent in the same patients. In the present meta-analysis, it was not possible to adjust or stratify for potential confounders, which restricted us doing more detailed relevant analysis and obtaining more comprehensive results. Finally, given that a proportion of studies included are retrospective, a possibility of residual confounding variables by unmeasured factors cannot be eliminated. This provided associative, not causal, evidence and mandates caution when interpreting these results.

Conclusion

Our systematic review and meta-analysis have identified several recipient-related risk factors for development of PGD, all of which are readily available in clinical settings. The identification of

higher-risk recipients has great clinical relevance with respect to individual screening, risk factor modification, selective management aimed at prevention of PGD, and ultimately improves the outcomes of patients undergoing lung transplantation. Further research into the underlying mechanisms responsible for these associations should be advocated.

Author Contributions

Conceived and designed the experiments: Yao Liu Yi Liu LS SJJ. Performed the experiments: Yao Liu Yi Liu SJJ. Analyzed the data: Yao Liu LS SJJ. Contributed reagents/materials/analysis tools: Yao Liu Yi Liu LS SJJ. Wrote the paper: Yao Liu SJJ.

References

1. Arcasoy SM, Kotloff RM (1999) Lung transplantation. N Engl J Med 340:1081–1091.
2. Christie JD, Van Raemdonck D, de Perrot M, Barr M, Keshavjee S, et al; ISHLT Working Group on Primary Lung Graft Dysfunction (2005) Report of the ISHLT Working Group on Primary Lung Graft Dysfunction part I: introduction and methods. J Heart Lung Transplant 24:1451–1453.
3. King RC, Binns OA, Rodriguez F, Kanithanon RC, Daniel TM, et al. (2000) Reperfusion injury significantly impacts clinical outcome after pulmonary transplantation. Ann Thorac Surg 69:1681–1685.
4. Christie JD, Kotloff RM, Ahya VN, Tino G, Pochettino A, et al. (2005) The effect of primary graft dysfunction on survival after lung transplantation. Am J Respir Crit Care Med 171:1312–131.
5. Lee JC, Christie JD, Keshavjee S (2010) Primary graft dysfunction: definition, risk factors, short- and long-term outcomes. Semin Resp Crit Care Med 31:161–71.
6. Barr ML, Kawut SM, Whelan TP, Girgis R, Bottcher H, et al. (2005) Report of the ISHLT Working Group on Primary Lung Graft Dysfunction part IV: recipient-related risk factors and markers. J Heart Lung Transplant 24:1468–1482.
7. King RC, Binns OA, Rodriguez F, Kanithanon RC, Daniel TM, et al. (2000) Reperfusion injury significantly impacts clinical outcome after pulmonary transplantation. Ann Thorac Surg 69:1681–5.
8. Thabut G, Vinatier I, Stern JB, Lesèche G, Loirat P, et al. (2002) Primary graft failure following lung transplantation: predictive factors of mortality. Chest 121:1876–82.
9. Christie JD, Kotloff RM, Pochettino A, Arcasoy SM, Rosengard BR, et al. (2003) Clinical risk factors for primary graft failure following lung transplantation. Chest 124:1232–1241.
10. Whitson BA, Nath DS, Johnson AC, Walker AR, Prekker ME, et al. (2006) Risk factors for primary graft dysfunction after lung transplantation. J Thorac Cardiovasc Surg 131:73–80.
11. Burton CM, Iversen M, Milman N, Zemtsovski M, Carlsen J, et al. (2007) Outcome of lung transplanted patients with primary graft dysfunction. Eur J Cardiothorac Surg 31:75–82.
12. Krenn K, Klepetko W, Taghavi S, Lang G, Schneider B, et al. (2007) Recipient vascular endothelial growth factor serum levels predict primary lung graft dysfunction. Am J Transplant 7:700–6.
13. Kuntz CL, Hadjiliadis D, Ahya VN, Kotloff RM, Pochettino A, et al. (2009) Risk factors for early primary graft dysfunction after lung transplantation: a registry study. Clin Transplant 23:819–30.
14. Felten ML, Sinaceur M, Treilhaud M, Roze H, Mornex JF, et al. (2012) Factors associated with early graft dysfunction in cystic fibrosis patients receiving primary bilateral lung transplantation. Eur J Cardiothorac Surg 41:686–90.
15. Fang A, Studer S, Kawut SM, Ahya VN, Lee J, et al; Lung Transplant Outcomes Group (2011) Elevated pulmonary artery pressure is a risk factor for primary graft dysfunction following lung transplantation for idiopathic pulmonary fibrosis. Chest 139:782–7.
16. Allen JG, Lee MT, Weiss ES, Arnaoutakis GJ, Shah AS, et al (2012) Preoperative recipient cytokine levels are associated with early lung allograft dysfunction. Ann Thorac Surg 93:1843–9.
17. Shah RJ, Diamond JM, Lederer DJ, Arcasoy SM, Cantu EM, et al. (2012) Plasma monocyte chemotactic protein-1 levels at 24 hours are a biomarker of primary graft dysfunction after lung transplantation. Transl Res 160:435–42.
18. Samano MN, Fernandes LM, Baranauskas JC, Correia AT, Afonso JE Jr, et al. (2012) Risk factors and survival impact of primary graft dysfunction after lung transplantation in a single institution. Transplant Proc 44:2462–8.
19. Diamond JM, Lee JC, Kawut SM, Shah RJ, Localio AR, et al. (2013) Clinical risk factors for primary graft dysfunction after lung transplantation. Am J Respir Crit Care Med 187:527–34.
20. de Perrot M, Bonser RS, Dark J, Kelly RF, McGiffin D, et al. (2005) Report of the ISHLT Working Group on Primary Lung Graft Dysfunction part III: donor-related risk factors and markers. J Heart Lung Transplant 24:1460–1467.
21. Aeba R, Griffith BP, Kormos RL, Armitage JM, Gasior TA, et al. (1994) Effect of cardiopulmonary bypass on early graft dysfunction in clinical lung transplantation. Ann Thorac Surg 57: 715–22.
22. Shigemura N, Toyoda Y, Bhama JK, Gries CJ, Crespo M, et al. (2013) Donor smoking history and age in lung transplantation: a revisit. Transplantation 95:513–8.
23. Alvarez A, Moreno P, Illana J, Espinosa D, Baamonde C, et al. (2013) Influence of donor-recipient gender mismatch on graft function and survival following lung transplantation. Interact Cardiovasc Thorac Surg 16:426–35.
24. Stroup DF, Berlin JA, Morton SC, Olkin I, Williamson GD, et al. (2000) Meta-analysis of observational studies in epidemiology: a proposal for reporting. Meta-analysis Of Observational Studies In Epidemiology (MOOSE) group. JAMA 283: 2008–2012.
25. Moher D, Cook DJ, Eastwood S (1999) Improving the quality of reports of meta-analyses of randomized controlled trials: the QUOROM statement. Quality of reporting of meta-analyses. Lancet 354: 1896.
26. Wells G, Shea B, O'Connell D, Guyatt G, Peterson J, et al. (2006) The Newcastle-Ottawa Scale (NOS) for assessing the quality of nonrandomized studies in meta-analysis. Ottawa Health Research Institute (OHRI).
27. Higgins JPT, Green S, eds (2009) Cochrane handbook for systematic reviews of interventions. Version 5.0.2. New York, NY: Wiley. The Cochrane Collaboration. Available: www.cochrane-handbook.org. Accessed: 2008 June.
28. Christie JD, Carby M, Bag R, Corris P, Hertz M, et al. (2005) Report of the ISHLT working group on primary lung graft dysfunction, part II: definition. A consensus statement of the International Society for Heart and Lung Transplantation. J Heart Lung Transplant 24: 1454–9.
29. Mangialardi RJ, Martin GS, Bernard GR, Wheeler AP, Christman BW, et al. (2000) Hypoproteinemia predicts acute respiratory distress syndrome development, weight gain, and death in patients with sepsis: Ibuprofen in Sepsis Study Group. Crit Care Med 28:3137–3145.
30. Hudson LD, Milberg JA, Anardi D, Maunder RJ (1995) Clinical risks for development of the acute respiratory distress syndrome. Am J Respir Crit Care Med 151:293–301.
31. Simpson E, Scott D, Chandler P (1997) The male-specific histocompatibility antigen. Ann Rev Immunol 15:39–61.
32. Sweezey N, Tchepichev S, Cagnon S, Fertuck K, O'Brodovich H (1998) Female gender hormones regulate mRNA levels and function of the rat lung epithelial Na channel. Am J Physiol 274:379–86.
33. Hooper WC, Lally C, Austin H, Benson J, Dilley A, et al. (1999) The relationship between polymorphisms in the endothelial cell nitric oxide synthase gene and the platelet GPIIIa gene with myocardial infarction and venous thromboembolism in African Americans. Chest 116:880–886.
34. Jones DS, Andrawis NS, Abernethy DR (1999) Impaired endothelial dependent forearm vascular relaxation in black Americans. Clin Pharmacol Ther 65:408–412.

35. Kanasky WF Jr, Anton SD, Rodrigue JR, Perri MG, Szwed T, et al. (2002) Impact of body weight on long-term survival after lung transplantation. Chest 121:401–6.

36. Madill J, Gutierrez C, Grossman J, Allard J, Chan C, et al. (2001) Nutritional assessment of the lung transplant patient: body mass index as a predictor of 90-day mortality following transplantation. J Heart Lung Transplant 20:288–96.

37. Jain M, Budinger GS, Lo A, Urich D, Rivera SE, et al. (2011) Leptin promotes fibroproliferative ARDS by inhibiting peroxisome proliferator-activated receptor-γ. Am J Respir Crit Care Med 183:1490–1498.

38. Bellmeyer A, Martino JM, Chandel NS, Scott Budinger GR, Dean DA, et al. (2007) Leptin resistance protects mice from hyperoxia-induced acute lung injury. Am J Respir Crit Care Med 175:587–594.

39. Lederer DJ, Kawut SM, Wickersham N, Winterbottom C, Bhorade S, et al. (2011) Obesity and primary graft dysfunction after lung transplantation: the Lung Transplant Outcomes Group Obesity Study. Am J Respir Crit Care Med 184:1055–1061.

40. Medoff BD, Okamoto Y, Leyton P, Weng M, Sandall BP, et al. (2009) Adiponectin deficiency increases allergic airway inflammation and pulmonary vascular remodeling. Am J Respir Cell Mol Biol 41:397–406.

41. Summer R, Little FF, Ouchi N, Takemura Y, Aprahamian T, et al. (2008) Alveolar macrophage activation and an emphysema-like phenotype in adiponectin-deficient mice. Am J Physiol Lung Cell Mol Physiol 294:L1035–L1042.

42. Pierre AF, DeCampos KN, Liu M, Edwards V, Cutz E, et al. (1998) Rapid reperfusion causes stress failure in ischemic rat lungs. J Thorac Cardiovasc Surg 116:932–42.

43. Halldorsson AO, Kronon MT, Allen BS, Rahman S, Wang T (2000) Lowering reperfusion pressure reduces the injury after pulmonary ischemia. Ann Thorac Surg 69: 198–203.

44. Thabut G, Mal H, Castier Y, Groussard O, Brugière O, et al. (2003) Survival benefit of lung transplantation for patients with idiopathic pulmonary fibrosis. J Thorac Cardiovasc Surg 126:469–75.

45. Mason DP, Brizzio ME, Alster JM, McNeill AM, Murthy SC, et al. (2007) Lung transplantation for idiopathic pulmonary fibrosis. Ann Thorac Surg 84:1121–8.

46. Wahidi MM, Ravenel J, Palmer SM, McAdams HP (2002) Progression of idiopathic pulmonary fibrosis in native lungs after single lung transplantation. Chest 121:2072–6.

47. Khalil N, O'Connor R (2004) Idiopathic pulmonary fibrosis: current understanding of the pathogenesis and the status of treatment. CMAJ 171:153–60.

48. Wan S, LeClerc JL, Vincent JL (1997) Inflammatory response to cardiopulmonary bypass: mechanisms involved and possible therapeutic strategies. Chest 112:676–92.

49. Butler J, Rocker GM, Westaby S (1993) Inflammatory response to cardiopulmonary bypass. Ann Thorac Surg 55: 552–9.

50. Aeba R, Griffith BP, Kormos RL, Armitage JM, Gasior TA, et al. (1994) Effect of cardiopulmonary bypass on early graft dysfunction in clinical lung transplantation. Ann Thorac Surg 57:715–22.

51. Gammie JS, Cheul Lee J, Pham SM, Keenan RJ, Weyant RJ, et al. (1998) Cardiopulmonary bypass is associated with early allograft dysfunction but not death after double-lung transplantation. J Thorac Cardiovasc Surg 115:990–7.

52. Christie JD, Shah CV, Kawut SM, Mangalmurti N, Lederer DJ, et al.(2009) Plasma levels of receptor for advanced glycation end products, blood transfusion, and risk of primary graft dysfunction. Am J Respir Crit Care Med 180: 1010–1015.

53. Webert KE, Blajchman MA (2003) Transfusion-related acute lung injury. Transfus Med Rev 17:252–262.

54. Wang Y, Kurichi JE, Blumenthal NP, Ahya VN, Christie JD, et al. (2006) Multiple variables affecting blood usage in lung transplantation. J Heart Lung Transplant 25:533–538.

55. Adatia I, Lillehei C, Arnold JH, Thompson JE, Palazzo R, et al. (1994) Inhaled nitric oxide in the treatment of postoperative graft dysfunction after lung transplantation. Ann Thorac Surg 57:1311–1318.

56. Macdonald P, Mundy J, Rogers P, Harrison G, Branch J, et al. (1995) Successful treatment of life-threatening acute reperfusion injury after lung transplantation with inhaled nitric oxide. J Thorac Cardiovasc Surg 110:861–863.

57. Garat C, Jayr C, Eddahibi S, Laffon M, Meignan M, et al. (1997) Effects of inhaled nitric oxide or inhibition of endogenous nitric oxide formation on hyperoxic lung injury. Am J Respir Crit Care Med 155: 1957–1964.

58. Shargall Y, Guenther G, Ahya VN, Ardehali A, Singhal A, et al. (2005) Report of the ISHLT working group on primary lung graft dysfunction: Part VI. Treatment. J Heart Lung Transplant 24:1489–1500.

12

High Variability in Oral Glucose Tolerance among 1,128 Patients with Cystic Fibrosis: A Multicenter Screening Study

Nicole Scheuing[1][*][¶]**, Reinhard W. Holl**[1][¶]**, Gerd Dockter**[2]**, Julia M. Hermann**[1]**, Sibylle Junge**[3]**,
Cordula Koerner-Rettberg[4]**, Lutz Naehrlich**[5]**, Christina Smaczny**[6]**, Doris Staab**[7]**, Gabriela Thalhammer**[8]**,
Silke van Koningsbruggen-Rietschel[9]**, Manfred Ballmann**[4]

1 Institute of Epidemiology and Medical Biometry, Central Institute for Biomedical Technology, University of Ulm, Ulm, Germany, 2 Cystic Fibrosis Centre, Saarland University Hospital for Pediatric and Adolescent Medicine, Homburg/Saar, Germany, 3 Clinic for Pediatric Pneumology and Neonatology, Hannover Medical School, Hannover, Germany, 4 Department of Pediatric Pulmonology, St. Josef Hospital Pediatric Clinic, Ruhr University Bochum, Bochum, Germany, 5 Department of Pediatrics, Justus-Liebig University Giessen, Giessen, Germany, 6 Medical Clinic I, Pneumology and Allergology, University Hospital Frankfurt/Main, Goethe University, Frankfurt/Main, Germany, 7 Division of Pulmonology and Immunology, Department of Pediatrics, Charité Berlin, Berlin, Germany, 8 Department for Pediatric Pulmonology and Allergology, Medical University of Graz, Graz, Austria, 9 Cystic Fibrosis Centre Cologne, Childrens Hospital, University of Cologne, Cologne, Germany

Abstract

Background: In cystic fibrosis, highly variable glucose tolerance is suspected. However, no study provided within-patient coefficients of variation. The main objective of this short report was to evaluate within-patient variability of oral glucose tolerance.

Methods: In total, 4,643 standardized oral glucose tolerance tests of 1,128 cystic fibrosis patients (median age at first test: 15.5 [11.5; 21.5] years, 48.8% females) were studied. Patients included were clinically stable, non-pregnant, and had at least two oral glucose tolerance tests, with no prior lung transplantation or systemic steroid therapy. Transition frequency from any one test to the subsequent test was analyzed and within-patient coefficients of variation were calculated for fasting and two hour blood glucose values. All statistical analysis was implemented with SAS 9.4.

Results: A diabetic glucose tolerance was confirmed in 41.2% by the subsequent test. A regression to normal glucose tolerance at the subsequent test was observed in 21.7% and to impaired fasting glucose, impaired glucose tolerance or both in 15.2%, 12.0% or 9.9%. The average within-patient coefficient of variation for fasting blood glucose was 11.1% and for two hour blood glucose 25.3%.

Conclusion: In the cystic fibrosis patients studied, a highly variable glucose tolerance was observed. Compared to the general population, variability of two hour blood glucose was 1.5 to 1.8-fold higher.

Editor: Dominik Hartl, University of Tübingen, Germany

Funding: The study was funded by the German and French CF associations (Mukoviszidose e.V. and its regional group Saarland-Pfalz, Vaincre de la Mucoviszidose), and by Novo Nordisk. The funders had no role in study design, data collection and analysis, decision to publish, or preparation of the manuscript.

Competing Interests: The study was partly funded by Novo Nordisk. There are no patents, products in development or marketed products to declare. Mukoviszidose e.V. - the German CF association - is a registered not-for-profit charity with tax-exempt status under German tax law. It is by no means a "commercial funder".

* Email: nicole.scheuing@uni-ulm.de

¶ Shared first authorship.

Introduction

Cystic fibrosis (CF) is a life-limiting autosomal recessive illness occurring in about one of 2,500 newborns in Europe. As the life expectancy for CF patients has increased due to earlier diagnosis and improved care, CF-related comorbidities became more frequent over the last decades. A growing comorbidity with

impact on the course of CF is cystic fibrosis-related diabetes (CFRD). The latest comprehensive guidelines for CFRD recommend yearly screening for abnormal glucose metabolism by oral glucose tolerance test (OGTT) in CF patients aged ≥10 years [1]. A small study suspected that CF patients have a high variation in glucose tolerance over time [2].

Therefore, we aimed to investigate in this short report the variability of glucose tolerance in a large cohort of CF patients. For the first time, a within-patient coefficient of variation (CV) for 2-hour blood glucose was calculated in CF.

Materials and Methods

Ethics statement

The ethical committees of Ulm University and Hannover Medical School approved the study, and patients or their parents provided written informed consent.

Study subjects

Between 2001 and 2010, 1,778 CF patients aged 10 years or older were screened serially by OGTT in a multicenter screening program carried out by 43 German/Austrian specialized centers (Trial No. NCT00662714). All patients had a physician-based diagnosis of CF according to the latest German guidelines [3]. OGTTs were performed and interpreted in line with recommendations of the World Health Organization modified by the American Diabetes Association as described in detail previously [4,5].

In total, 5,765 OGTTs among clinically stable CF patients were carried out until the end of the study (Figure 1). As mentioned in reference [4], all patients screened had to be without symptoms of acute infections or exacerbations of chronic infections and should not have a reduced carbohydrate intake. Moreover, patients with respiratory failure (FEV1<40%) or with enteral tube feeding were excluded. In case of a confirmed diagnosis of CFRD or the use of anti-hyperglycemic treatment, patients were also excluded from screening.

For the present analysis, only OGTTs of non-pregnant patients with no prior systemic steroid therapy or lung transplantation were considered (Figure 1). If patients awaited lung transplantation, OGTTs were also excluded. Furthermore, at least two OGTTs had to be performed per patient (Figure 1). The final study population comprised 4,643 OGTTs of 1,128 CF patients. For each patient included, test results were classified as normal glucose tolerance (NGT), impaired fasting glucose (IFG), impaired glucose tolerance (IGT), IFG and IGT combined, or diabetic glucose tolerance (DGT). The detailed cut-offs are described in reference [4]. As there are some CF patients with isolated IFG [4] and the pathophysiology between IFG and IGT is at least in part different [6], we introduced an IFG group in this analysis. CFRD was defined as a diabetic OGTT confirmed by a consecutive OGTT in the DGT range [1]. Body mass index standard deviation score (BMI-SDS) was calculated using data from the German Health Interview and Examination Survey for Children and Adolescents (KiGGS study, [7]) as national reference. The KiGGS study was used as a reference in a number of previous publications by our group to calculate BMI-SDS in CF patients [4,8,9] and is the best currently available reference data for healthy German children. Data to calculate BMI-SDS on the basis of CF-specific anthropometric reference percentiles are currently not available.

Statistical analysis

To analyze the variation in glucose tolerance, transition frequency from any one test to the subsequent test was studied. As there is no subsequent test for the last test in each patient, 3,515 pairs of consecutive OGTTs were available in the study population (the number of OGTT pairs therefore equals the total number of OGTTs minus the number of patients). For each pair of OGTTs, the first test was categorized in one of the five glucose

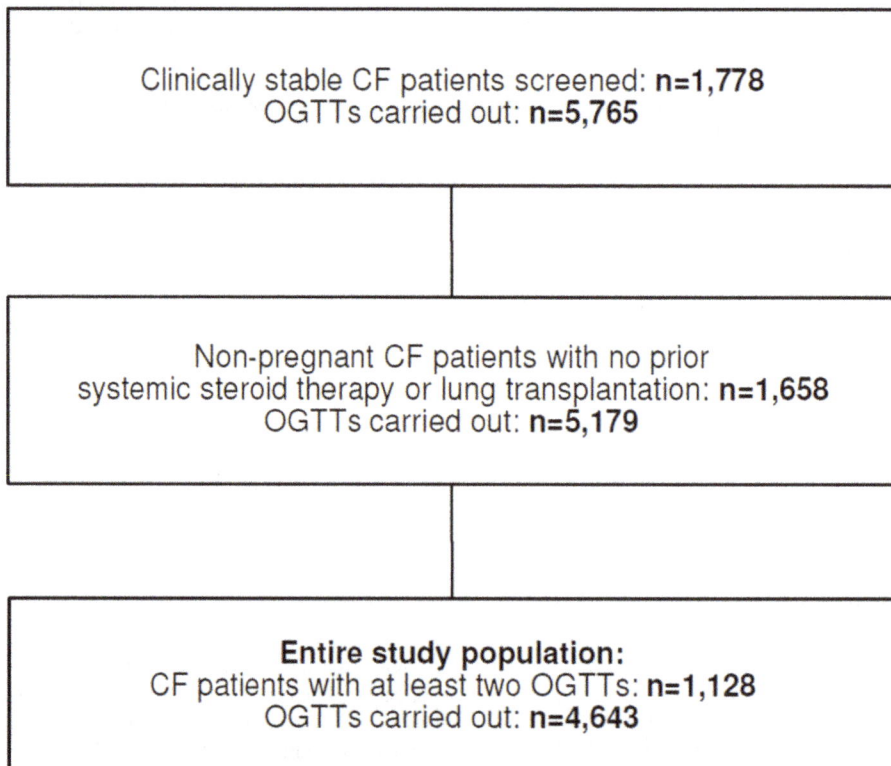

Figure 1. Selection of study population. Abbreviations: *CF* cystic fibrosis, *OGTT* oral glucose tolerance test.

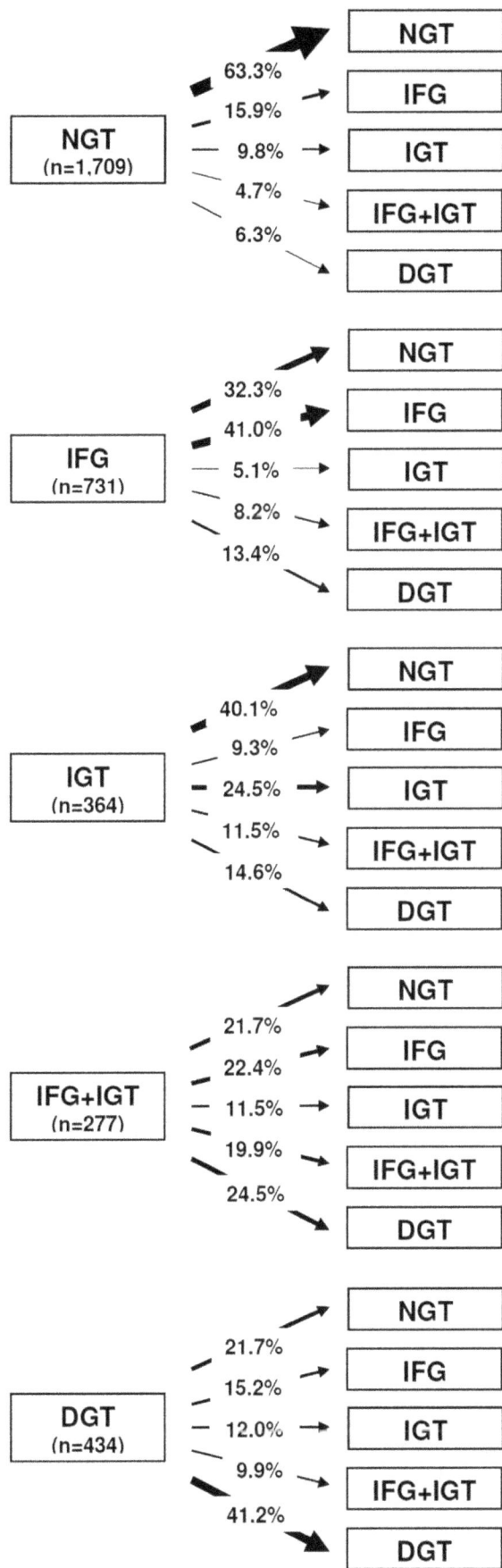

Figure 2. Transition from any one test to a subsequent test. In total, 3,515 pairs of consecutive OGTTs are summarized. For each pair, the first test was categorized in one of the five glucose tolerance classes (NGT, IFG only, IGT only, IFG+IGT, DGT). The figure shows the percentage of subsequent test results for each glucose tolerance category. The number in parentheses indicates the number of OGTTs available for analysis. Abbreviations: *NGT* normal glucose tolerance, *IFG* impaired fasting glucose, *IGT* impaired glucose tolerance, *DGT* diabetic glucose tolerance, *OGTT* oral glucose tolerance test.

tolerance classes (NGT, IFG only, IGT only, IFG+IGT, DGT) and the percentage of subsequent test results was calculated. Moreover, the variation in glucose tolerance is depicted in three individual patients who had seven consecutive OGTTs with at least one diabetic result. To assess the degree of variability of serially measured fasting and 2-hour blood glucose values in CF patients, within-patient CVs (defined as ratio between within-subject standard deviation and mean) were calculated and compared to the general population. CVs were calculated as they are normalized measures of the variability and independent of the mean level.

To evaluate gender or age differences in the deterioration of glucose tolerance from test to test, a logistic mixed regression model was applied. Deterioration of glucose metabolism was defined as worsening of glucose tolerance in a subsequent test compared to the pretest or as confirmation of a diabetic OGTT. Sex and age were entered as independent fixed effects. Age was categorized as 10–<15 years, 15–<20 years and ≥20 years. To account for repeated OGTTs per patient, random effects with first-order autoregressive covariance structure were used. Results are given as odds ratios (OR) with lower and upper confidence limit (CL).

Statistical analyses were performed with SAS 9.4. The level of significance was set at 0.05. To compare demographics between patients included and excluded, Kruskal-Wallis test was applied for continuous parameters and χ^2-test for dichotomous parameters.

Results

48.8% of patients included were female and 28.9% were >20 years. Median [Q_1;Q_3] (mean±SD) age at first OGTT was 15.5 [11.5; 21.5] (18.0±8.4) years and at last OGTT 18.6 [15.3; 25.4] (21.3±8.5) years. At baseline OGTT, the youngest patient aged 10.0 years and the oldest patient 63.9 years. On average, median (mean) duration between two consecutive OGTTs was 1.0 [0.7; 1.2] (1.1±0.7) year. A diabetic OGTT was repeated within a median (mean) time of 6.9 [4.9; 12.9] (9.1±6.2) weeks. As published previously [4], the median duration between two consecutive OGTTs in the DGT range (confirmed diagnosis of CFRD) was 8.1 [5.1; 27.9] weeks. All patients with suspected CFRD (i.e. one OGTT in the DGT range) at the end of the study were followed-up outside the context of the screening study. Each patient with a confirmed diagnosis of CFRD was invited to participate in a randomized controlled trial investigating the use of repaglinide in comparison to insulin therapy. CFRD patients not participating in the clinical trial received insulin therapy and CF-specific nutritional counseling as recommended by guidelines.

Baseline characteristics of the 650 patients excluded are depicted in table 1. Excluded patients were older and had on average a lower BMI-SDS.

Figure 2 displays the transition frequency from any one test to a subsequent test. For example, an OGTT in the DGT range was confirmed in 41.2% by the subsequent test.

Table 1. Demographics of patients included and patients excluded at baseline OGTT.

	Patients included	Patients excluded	p-value
Number, n	1,128	650	-
Age, years	15.5 [11.5; 21.5] (18.0±8.4)	17.4 [12.3; 25.2] (20.0±9.3)	<0.001
Female sex, %	48.8	45.1	NS
Weight, kg	47.8 [34.5; 57.8] (47.8±15.4)	50.2 [35.5; 59.0] (49.0±15.2)	0.04
Height, cm	160.0 [145.6; 170.0] (157.8±15.6)	162.0 [147.0; 172.0] (159.8±15.9)	0.008
BMI, kg/m^2	18.4 [16.2; 20.4] (18.6±3.3)	18.6 [16.2; 20.7] (18.7±3.3)	NS
BMI-SDS	−0.76 [−1.42;−0.11] (−0.80±1.08)	−0.87 [−1.65;−0.18] (−0.99±1.26)	0.005

Data are given as median with quartiles (mean with standard deviation) or as percentage. Abbreviations: *BMI* body mass index, *SDS* standard deviation score, *NS* not significant.

Until the end of the screening study, a total of 136 CF patients revealed a confirmed diagnosis of CFRD i.e. two consecutive OGTTs revealing DGT. Despite the fact that two consecutive OGTTs in the DGT range are sufficient to diagnose CFRD, 54 out of the 136 patients had additional OGTTs. In 42.6% (n = 23) of patients, all subsequent tests were diabetic. In 20.4% (n = 11) of cases, at least one of the subsequent tests revealed NGT.

Figure 3 indicates that independent of age, glucose tolerance varied highly from test to test in three individual patients.

Overall, in CF patients the average within-patient CV for fasting blood glucose values was 11.1% and for 2-hour blood glucose 25.3%. Analyzing patients with (n = 339) and without (n = 789) at least one OGTT in the DGT range separately, patients without an OGTT in the diabetic range had lower CVs for both fasting and 2-hour blood glucose values (fasting: 8.9 vs. 16.1%, p<0.001; 2-hour: 22.2 vs. 32.4%, p<0.001).

Logistic regression analysis revealed for girls a 1.18-fold [lower CL: 1.03; upper CL: 1.36] higher risk for the deterioration of

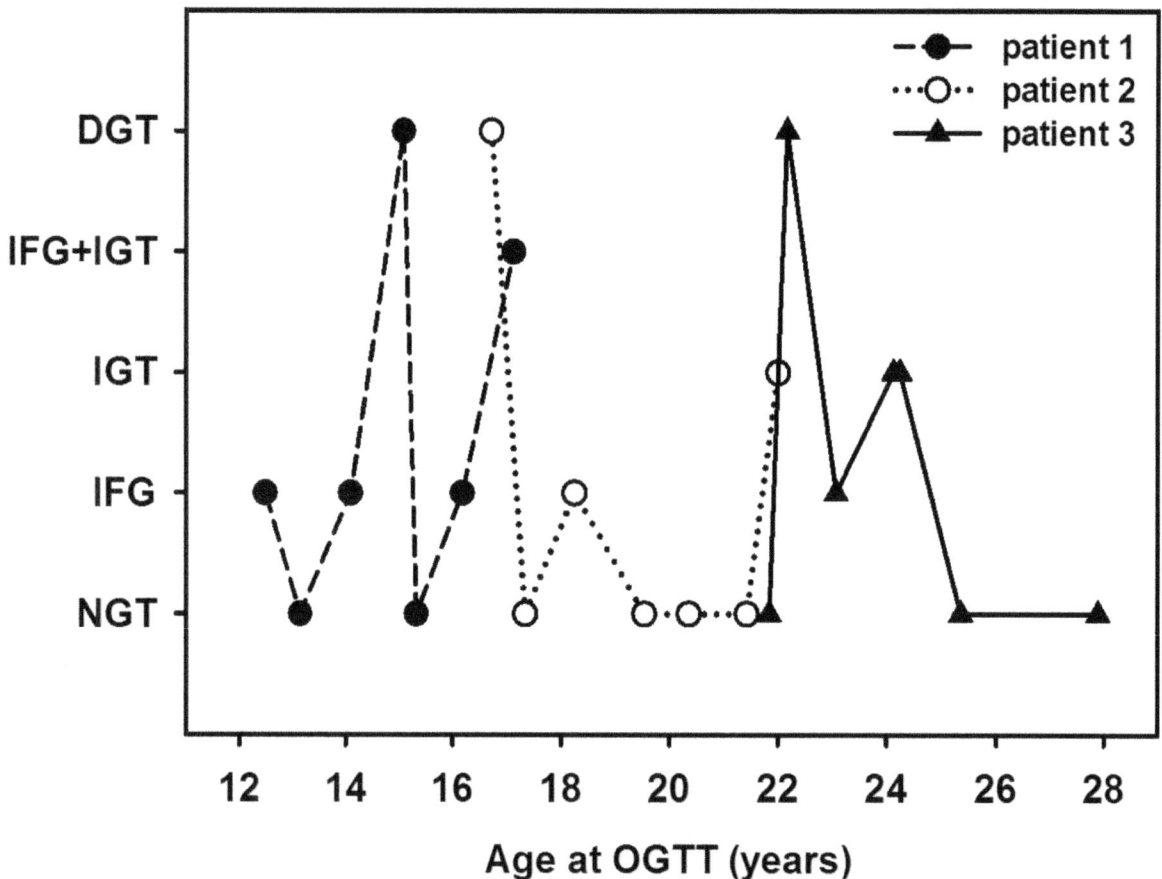

Figure 3. Variation of glucose tolerance in three patients of different age. Each patient had seven consecutive OGTTs with at least one diabetic result. Abbreviations: *DGT* diabetic glucose tolerance, *IFG* impaired fasting glucose, *IGT* impaired glucose tolerance, *NGT* normal glucose tolerance, *OGTT* oral glucose tolerance test.

glucose tolerance compared to boys (p = 0.015). In addition, patients aged 15–<20 years (OR: 1.23 [1.04; 1.47], p = 0.019) or ≥20 years (OR: 1.22 [1.03; 1.44], p = 0.024) had a higher risk than patients aged 10–<15 years. In 15 to <20 year old patients, risk was comparable to patients aged ≥20 years (OR: 1.01 [0.86; 1.19], p = 0.867).

Analyzing the influence of sex in the subgroup of older patients (>20 years at baseline OGTT; n = 326 patients with 1,276 OGTTs), revealed also an increased risk in females compared to males, even though the influence was no longer significant due to the lower number of patients studied (OR: 1.23 [0.92; 1.63], p = 0.162).

Discussion

Our analysis among asymptomatic CF patients revealed a high variability in glucose tolerance over time, even though patients without DGT seem to be more stable with respect to glucose tolerance. Compared to the general population [10–12], overall within-patient variability of 2-hour blood glucose is 1.5 to 1.8-fold higher in CF. The NHANES III Second Examination revealed a within-patient CV of 16.6% for 2-hour blood glucose [12] and the Hoorn study of 16.7% [11]. In a general practice [10], a within-patient CV of 14.3% was observed. Fluctuating levels of insulin resistance due to acute and chronic infections or CF-related inflammatory cytokines may explain the highly variable glucose tolerance in CF.

The fluctuation in glucose tolerance observed in this study implicates regular control of glucose metabolism in CF. Future guidelines should provide recommendations regarding an adequate time frame for repeating OGTTs in patients with abnormal glucose tolerance as well as for the confirmation interval of a diabetic test result. As outlined by the study protocol and described previously [4], a diabetic OGTT had to be repeated within 4 to 6 weeks in the present study and an OGTT revealing IFG or IGT after 6 months. According to guidelines, all patients with a confirmed CFRD diagnosis or with a diabetic OGTT and classical symptoms of diabetes should receive insulin treatment immediately [1]. Oral antidiabetic agents are not advised until sufficient data become available regarding their efficiency.

Reasons for performing additional OGTTs in patients with already confirmed CFRD are unknown. Maybe patients requested an additional OGTT in the context of intensifying therapy. Especially, asymptomatic CF patients often have problems starting insulin treatment besides numerous CF-related therapies. Another possibility might be that patients with a confirmed CFRD diagnosis were not totally clinically stable at the time of the confirmation test and the medical team therefore decided to repeat the test at a later time point. As OGTT results depend also on the supplementation of pancreatic enzymes, the medical team may have repeated the confirmation test after adjusting pancreatic enzyme substitution.

Although the OGTT revealed a high degree of within-patient variance in CF, it is the best screening tool for abnormalities in glucose tolerance currently available. Fasting plasma glucose, hemoglobin A1c or other classical methods applicable for type 1 or type 2 diabetes are not recommended in CF [1]. In the future, continuous glucose monitoring or standardized test meals might be a useful alternative to OGTT. However, there are no reference values for continuous glucose monitoring so far. To minimize the variability of OGTTs in CF patients, CF-adapted standardization

might be one possibility. At the moment, criteria for the performance and interpretation of OGTT are identical to other diabetes types. However, pancreatic enzyme substitution and the grade of inflammation (e.g. C-reactive protein measurement) should be considered before performing an OGTT in CF, and when interpreting OGTT results. More advanced interpretation criteria that take into account dynamics in oral glucose challenge in CF patients might be appropriate. As CFRD is less common compared to the more frequent type 1 or type 2 diabetes, other measures of ß-cell function (e.g. C-peptide) or calculation of indices for insulin secretion and sensitivity might be practicable in clinical settings that may result in better assessment of glucose tolerance in CF patients.

The higher risk for deterioration of glucose tolerance in girls confirms previous studies indicating an earlier onset and a higher prevalence of CFRD in females [4,13,14]. The lower risk in patients younger than 15 years compared to older patients might be explained by the rare occurrence of CFRD in patients <10 years and the increasing prevalence of abnormal glucose tolerance with age [4,15,16].

Selection biases might be one limitation of the present study. Not all centers or CF patients participated, although all German/Austrian medical facilities providing care for CF patients were invited for participation in written form. Moreover, some CF-related therapies (e.g. steroids, lung transplantation) led to exclusion of patients and the complexity of CF itself made study participation often difficult. The higher age and the lower BMI-SDS of patients excluded may point to a more severe progression of the disease compared to patients included. Exclusion criterion for the majority of the 650 patients not analyzed was the availability of solely one OGTT. This might be due to termination of the study or occurrence of exclusion criteria after the first OGTT. Moreover, each patient could withdraw from the study at any time.

In summary, in the asymptomatic CF patients studied, one diabetic OGTT seems not sufficient to diagnose CFRD due to the existing high variability of glucose tolerance. A normal glucose tolerance after a confirmed CFRD diagnosis (i.e. two consecutive OGTTs revealing DGT) cannot be excluded. Despite improvement of glucose tolerance, these patients are classified as diabetic [1], although this labelling may be contra-intuitive for patients and physicians. It is still a debate whether solely a persistently diabetic glucose tolerance is associated with an increased risk of clinical decline in CF or even a pre-diabetic condition.

Acknowledgments

The authors thank all participating centers for performing OGTTs and providing data for the present analysis. A detailed list of centers was recently published [4].

Author Contributions

Conceived and designed the experiments: RWH MB. Performed the experiments: GD SJ CKR LN CS DS GT SVKR MB. Analyzed the data: NS JMH RWH. Contributed reagents/materials/analysis tools: GD SJ CKR LN CS DS GT SVKR MB. Contributed to the writing of the manuscript: NS. Revision of manuscript: RWH GD JMH SJ CKR LN CS DS GT SVKR MB. Final approval of the version to be published: NS RWH GD JMH SJ CKR LN CS DS GT SVKR MB.

References

1. Moran A, Brunzell C, Cohen RC, Katz M, Marshall BC, et al. (2010) Clinical care guidelines for cystic fibrosis-related diabetes: A position statement of the American Diabetes Association and a clinical practice guideline of the Cystic Fibrosis Foundation, endorsed by the Pediatric Endocrine Society. Diabetes Care 33: 2697–2708.

2. Sterescu AE, Rhodes B, Jackson R, Dupuis A, Hanna A, et al. (2010) Natural history of glucose intolerance in patients with cystic fibrosis: Ten-year prospective observation program. J Pediatr 156: 613–617.

3. Naehrlich L, Stuhrmann-Spangenberg M, Barben J, Bargon J, Blankenstein O, et al. (June 2013) S2 consensus-guideline: diagnostic of mucoviscidosis. AWMF 026–023.Available: www.awmf.org/uploads/tx_szleitlinien/026-023 m_S2k_Diagnostik_der_Mukoviszidose_ 2013-07.pdf. Accessed 2014 June 4.

4. Scheuing N, Holl RW, Dockter G, Fink K, Junge S, et al. (2013) Diabetes in cystic fibrosis: Multicenter screening results based on current guidelines. PLoS One 8: e81545.

5. Schmid K, Fink K, Holl RW, Hebestreit H, Ballmann M (2014) Predictors for future cystic fibrosis-related diabetes by oral glucose tolerance test. J Cyst Fibros 13: 80–85.

6. Nathan DM, Davidson MB, DeFronzo RA, Heine RJ, Henry RR, et al. (2007) Impaired fasting glucose and impaired glucose tolerance: implications for care. Diabetes Care 30: 753–759.

7. Rosario AS, Kurth BM, Stolzenberg H, Ellert U, Neuhauser H (2010) Body mass index percentiles for children and adolescents in Germany based on a nationally representative sample (KiGGS 2003–2006). Eur J Clin Nutr 64: 341–349.

8. Scheuing N, Berger G, Bergis D, Gohlke B, Konrad K, et al. (2014) Adherence to clinical care guidelines for cystic fibrosis-related diabetes in 659 German/Austrian patients. J Cyst Fibros [Epub]. DOI:10.1016/j.jcf.2014.05.006.

9. Scheuing N, Badenhoop K, Borkenstein M, Konrad K, Lilienthal E, et al. (2014) Why is insulin pump treatment rarely used in adolescents and young adults with cystic fibrosis-related diabetes? Pediatr Diabetes [Epub]. DOI:10.1111/pedi.12158.

10. Feskens EJ, Bowles CH, Kromhout D (1991) Intra- and interindividual variability of glucose tolerance in an elderly population. J Clin Epidemiol 44: 947–953.

11. Mooy JM, Grootenhuis PA, de Vries H, Kostense PJ, Popp-Snijders C, et al. (1996) Intra-individual variation of glucose, specific insulin and proinsulin concentrations measured by two oral glucose tolerance tests in a general Caucasian population: The Hoorn study. Diabetologia 39: 298–305.

12. Selvin E, Crainiceanu CM, Brancati FL, Coresh J (2007) Short-term variability in measures of glycemia and implications for the classification of diabetes. Arch Intern Med 167: 1545–1551.

13. Ode KL, Frohnert B, Laguna T, Phillips J, Holme B, et al. (2010) Oral glucose tolerance testing in children with cystic fibrosis. Pediatr Diabetes 11: 487–492.

14. Konrad K, Thon A, Fritsch M, Fröhlich-Reiterer E, Lilienthal E, et al. (2013) Comparison of cystic fibrosis-related diabetes with type 1 diabetes based on a German/Austrian pediatric diabetes registry. Diabetes Care 36: 879–886.

15. Lanng S, Thorsteinsson B, Lund-Andersen C, Nerup J, Schiøtz PO, et al. (1994) Diabetes mellitus in Danish cystic fibrosis patients: prevalence and late diabetic complications. Acta Paediatr 83: 72–77.

16. Moran A, Dunitz J, Nathan B, Saeed A, Holme B, et al. (2009) Cystic fibrosis-related diabetes: current trends in prevalence, incidence, and mortality. Diabetes Care 32: 1626–1631.

13

Local and Systemic RAGE Axis Changes in Pulmonary Hypertension: CTEPH and iPAH

Bernhard Moser[1]*, Anna Megerle[1], Christine Bekos[1,2], Stefan Janik[1], Tamás Szerafin[3], Peter Birner[4], Ana-Iris Schiefer[4], Michael Mildner[5], Irene Lang[6], Nika Skoro-Sajer[6], Roela Sadushi-Kolici[6], Shahrokh Taghavi[1], Walter Klepetko[1], Hendrik Jan Ankersmit[1,2]

1 Department of Thoracic Surgery, Division of Surgery, Medical University Vienna, Vienna, Austria, 2 Christian Doppler Laboratory for the Diagnosis and Regeneration of Cardiac and Thoracic Diseases, Medical University Vienna, Vienna, Austria, 3 Department of Cardiac Surgery, University of Debrecen, Debrecen, Hungary, 4 Department of Pathology, Medical University Vienna, Vienna, Austria, 5 Department of Dermatology, Medical University Vienna, Vienna, Austria, 6 Department of Internal Medicine II, Division of Cardiology, Medical University Vienna, Vienna, Austria

Abstract

Objective: The molecular determinants of chronic thromboembolic pulmonary hypertension (CTEPH) and idiopathic pulmonary arterial hypertension (iPAH) remain poorly understood. The receptor for advanced glycation endproducts (RAGE) and its ligands: HMGB1 and S100A9 are involved in inflammatory disorders. We sought to investigate the role of the RAGE axis in patients with CTEPH undergoing pulmonary endarterectomy (PEA), iPAH undergoing lung transplantation (LuTX). The high pulmonary vascular resistance in CTEPH/iPAH results in pressure overload of the right ventricle. We compared sRAGE measurements to that of patients with aortic valve stenosis (AVS) – pressure overload of the left ventricle.

Methods: We enrolled patients with CTEPH(26), iPAH(15), AVS(15) and volunteers(33). Immunohistochemistry with antibodies to RAGE and HMGB1 was performed on PEA specimens and lung tissues. We employed enzyme-linked immunosorbent assays to determine the concentrations of sRAGE, esRAGE, HMGB1 and S100A9 in serum of volunteers and patients with CTEPH, iPAH, AVS before and after PEA, LuTX and aortic valve replacement (AVR).

Results: In endarterectomised tissues from patients with CTEPH RAGE and HMGB1 were identified in myofibroblasts (α-SMA$^+$vimentin$^+$CD34$^-$), recanalizing vessel-like structures of distal myofibrotic tissues and endothelium of neointima. RAGE was differentially expressed in prototypical Heath Edwards lesions in iPAH. We found significantly increased serum concentrations of sRAGE, esRAGE and HMGB1 in CTEPH. In iPAH, sRAGE and esRAGE were significantly higher than in controls. Serum concentrations of sRAGE were significantly elevated in iPAH($p<0.001$) and CTEPH($p=0.001$) compared to AVS. Serum sRAGE was significantly higher in iPAH compared to CTEPH($p=0.042$) and significantly reduced in AVS compared to controls($p=0.001$). There were no significant differences in sRAGE serum concentrations before and after surgical therapy for CTEPH, iPAH or AVS.

Conclusions: Our data suggest a role for the RAGE pathway in the pathophysiology of CTEPH and iPAH. PEA improves the local control of disease but may not influence the systemic inflammatory mechanisms in CTEPH patients through the RAGE pathway.

Editor: James West, Vanderbilt University Medical Center, United States of America

Funding: The study was funded by the Research laboratories of the Department of Surgery (FOLAB ARGE Moser) of the Medical University Vienna and the Christian Doppler laboratory for the Diagnosis and Regeneration of Cardiac and Thoracic Diseases. The funders had no role in study design, data collection and analysis, decision to publish, or preparation of the manuscript.

Competing Interests: The authors have declared that no competing interests exist.

* Email: bernhard.moser@meduniwien.ac.at

Introduction

Pulmonary hypertension (PH) is currently defined as a hemodynamic and pathophysiological condition with a mean pulmonary artery pressure (PAP*mean*) of $\geq$25 mmHg at rest. The European Society of Cardiology (ESC) and European Respiratory Society (ERS) have classified these conditions into six groups. Pulmonary arterial hypertension (PAH, group 1) can be the result of a wide array of underlying diseases. The entity idiopathic pulmonary arterial hypertension (iPAH, group 1.1) is used if no

underlying causative disease can be diagnosed. The increase in pulmonary vascular resistance (PVR) is related to different mechanisms, including vasoconstriction, proliferative and obstructive remodeling of the pulmonary vessel wall, inflammation and thrombosis. The pathology of idiopathic pulmonary arterial hypertension affects the small distal pulmonary arteries (PAs) with a diameter less than 500 μm. Typical findings are hypertrophy of the media, intimal proliferative and fibrotic changes, thickening of the adventitia with perivascular inflammatory infiltrates, complex

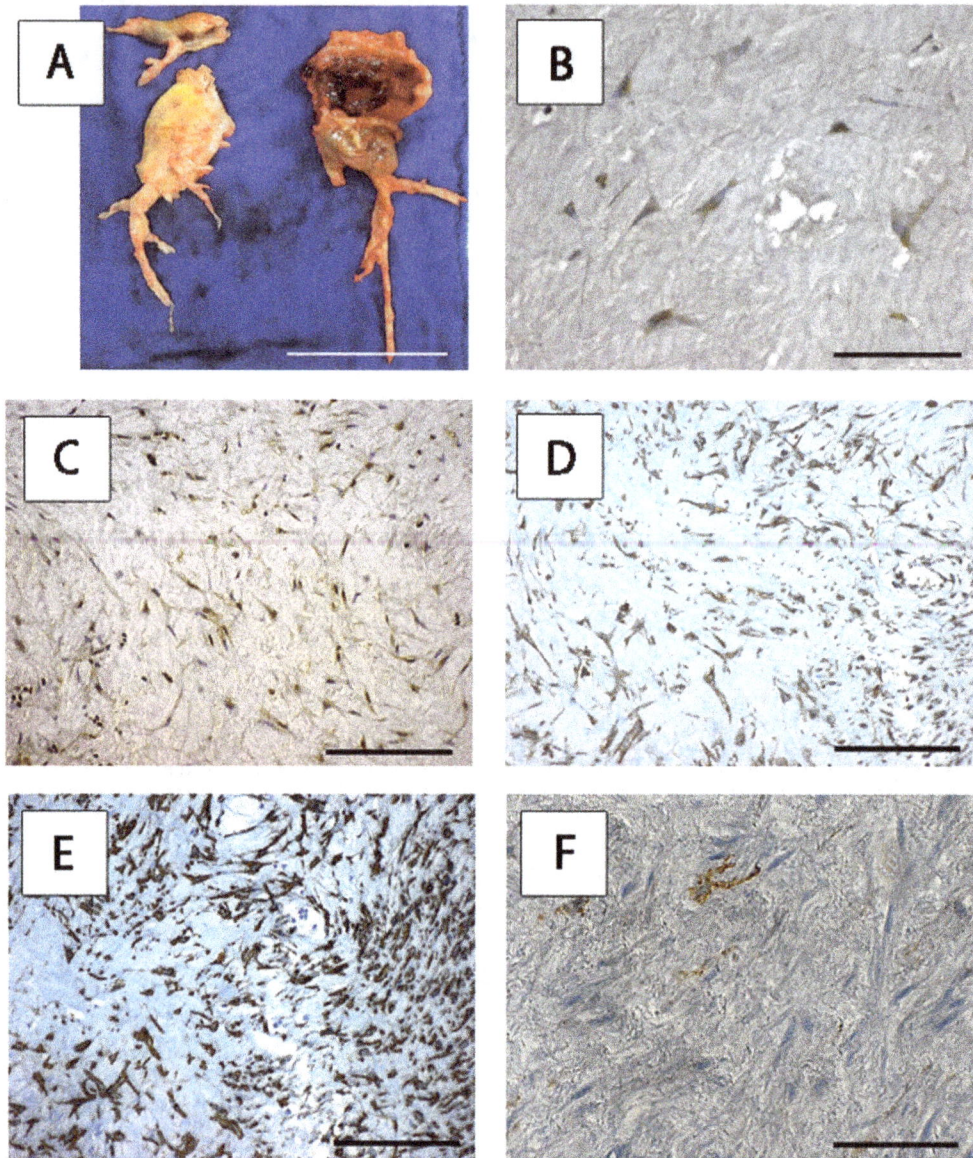

Figure 1. RAGE and HMGB1 are expressed in myofibroblasts of endarterectomised chronic thromboembolic tissues of CTEPH patients. One representative patient is shown (12 out of 15 patients (80%) displayed analogous staining patterns. Photograph showing the macroscopic aspect of a representative PEA specimen (A). Scale bar: 6 cm. Immunohistochemical expression of RAGE (B, scale bar: 20 μm), HMGB1 (C), vimentin (D), alpha-smooth muscle actin (E) and CD34 (F) on adjacent tissue sections of the PEA specimen shown in (A). Scale bar: 40 μm. *RAGE* receptor for advanced glycation endproducts, *HMGB1* high mobility group box 1, *CTEPH chronic thromboembolic pulmonary hypertension, PEA* pulmonary endarterectomy.

and thrombotic lesions [1]. A widely used pathological grading system for pulmonary arterial changes in hypertensive pulmonary vascular disease was published by Heath and Edwards in 1958 [2,3].

In stark contrast to iPAH, the characteristic pathology of chronic thromboembolic pulmonary hypertension (CTEPH, group 4) is remodeled central and proximal PAs. Organized thrombotic formations build the luminal lining of the PA vessel wall replacing physiological intima [1]. Endarterectomized tissues from patients with CTEPH show vessel-like structures in material obtained from distal areas, whereas proximal material is charac-

terized by lower cell density and sometimes the accumulation of fresh thrombotic material [4].

As described above, iPAH and CTEPH are progressive diseases of the distal (iPAH) and proximal (CTEPH) pulmonary vessels leading to increased PVR and PAP. In the further course of these diseases right ventricular dysfunction and ultimately right ventricular failure is the leading cause of death. The prognosis of patients is associated to right ventricular performance measures, such as cardiac index and right atrial pressure. Right heart failure is caused by pressure overload of the right ventricle. The increase in wall stress leads to increased wall thickness by muscular hypertrophy (increase in cell size by addition of sarcomeres).

Table 1. The basic characteristics of patients with CTEPH and controls (healthy volunteers) are listed.

	CTEPH (n = 26)	Controls (n = 33)	p value
Age *in years*	51.9 (56.2) ±14.7 (2.9), [31–75]	54.2 (54.0) ±15.2 (2.6), [30–83]	0.828
F:M ratio *n (%)*	9:17 (34.6:65.4)	12:21 (36.4:63.6)	0.985
PAP$_{mean}$ *[mmHg]*	52.9 (52.0) ±14.6 (2.9), [32–90]		
PVR *[dynes·s^{-1}·cm^{-5}]*	787.2 (757.0) ±386.6 (75.8), [281–1646]		
CI *[l/min/m^2]*	4.4 (4.5) ±0.99 (0.19), [2.2–5.4]		
sRAGE *[pg/ml]*	467.2 (331.8) ±370.4 (72.6), [105.0–1461.6]	198.6 (142.8) ±162.9 (28.3), [6.4–807.6]	0.001
esRAGE *[pg/ml]*	703.7 (610.8) ±309.3 (63.1), [170.0–1370.0]	414.5 (378.8) ±177.1 (31.8), [180.0–790.0]	<0.001
S100A9 *[µg/ml]*	2.1 (0.7) ±3.9 (0.8), [0.3–18.2]	0.7 (0.6) ±0.5 (0.09), [0.2–2.1]	0.064
HMGB1 *[pg/ml]*	1141.1 (865.8) ±865.6 (173.1), [226.5–3584.8]	464.3 (411.3) ±371.1 (66.6), [0–1818.4]	0.001

Reported is mean (median) ± standard deviation (standard error mean), [range].
CTEPH chronic thromboembolic pulmonary hypertension, n number of patients, F:M ratio female to male ratio, PAP$_{mean}$ mean pulmonary artery pressure, PVR pulmonary vascular resistance; CI cardiac index, sRAGE soluble receptor for advanced glycation endproducts, esRAGE endogenous secretory receptor for advanced glycation endproducts, S100A9 member of S100 family of Ca$^+$ binding proteins, HMGB1 high mobility group box1.

However, the chronic exposure to high RV pressures results in RV dilation with a decrease in contractile forces. Pathological inflammatory responses, oxidative stress and humoral responses may further promote right heart failure [5]. The consequences of RV failure are intractable ascites, renal impairment, malnutrition and immobility [5,6]. Pharmacological therapy effective in PAH did not prove to benefit patients with CTEPH [7]. Surgical therapy for selected patients with CTEPH is pulmonary endarterectomy (PEA) [8]. Patients with CTEPH who are not amenable to PEA and patients with iPAH are possible candidates for lung transplantation (LuTX).

The overexpression of cytokine cascades may contribute to the progression of heart failure - "cytokine hypothesis" for heart failure [9]. Most of our knowledge on neurohormonal and cytokine signaling, oxidative stress, inflammation, ischemia, and cell death which may contribute to RV dilatation and failure is inferred from research on left sided heart failure [10]. In patients with chronic left-sided heart failure increased serum concentrations of proinflammatory cytokines, such as tumor necrosis factor-alpha (TNF-alpha), interleukin(IL)-1, and IL-6 correlate with clinical and hemodynamic parameters of disease severity [11,12]. A S100 protein family member, S100A8/A9, has recently been shown to activate cardiac fibroblasts to initiate angiotensin II-induced hypertension cardiac injury [13]. Recently, increased left ventricular hypertrophy (LVH) and diastolic dysfunction was demonstrated in chronic uremic mice with transgenic expression of the human S100/Calgranulin gene cluster containing the genes and regulatory elements for S100A8, S100A9, and S100A12. S100/calgranulin-mediated inflammation induced fibroblast growth factor 23 (FGF23) in cardiac fibroblasts which in a paracrine manner may mediate LVH and diastolic dysfunction [14]. The role of biomarkers in pulmonary hypertension has been reviewed recently [15].

The Receptor for Advanced Glycation Endproducts (RAGE), a transmembrane receptor, is a member of the immunoglobulin superfamily of receptors that interacts with different ligands. Since its first characterization in 1992 where a high basal expression in the lung was shown [16] a vast literature around this receptor, its lung and vascular biology and pathology has evolved [17,18,19,20]. First, advanced glycation endproducts (AGEs) were identified as ligands [16]. Next, RAGE was identified as a cell surface receptor for S100/Calgranulins amplifying chronic cellular activation and tissue injury [21]. Further ligands were detected

later: high-mobility group box 1 (HMGB1) - also known as amphoterin [22], Mac-1 and others. The current view that RAGE - RAGE-ligand interaction augments pro-inflammatory pathways is supported by the detection of RAGE and RAGE ligands in tissues of various disease processes, such as arteriosclerosis [18], diabetes [23], glomerulosclerosis [24], periodontal disease [25], arthritis [26], transplantation [27] and other chronic inflammatory disorders.

The extracellular soluble form of the receptor (sRAGE) can be detected in serum of patients [28]. Proteolytic shedding of RAGE by metalloproteinases has been described [29,30]. It functions to bind ligands and thereby blocks interaction with and activation of cell surface RAGE. An increased concentration of RAGE-ligands leads to the formation of circulating sRAGE-ligand complexes. An increasing occupation of sRAGE leads to lower concentration of free sRAGE in serum and therefore directs to increased surface RAGE-ligand interaction and possibly to a boost in inflammation. Nevertheless, it is currently unknown if high plasma/serum concentrations of sRAGE can be interpreted as protection against chronic inflammation or correlated with high levels of ongoing inflammation [29]. Currently available tools to measure sRAGE don't separate between sRAGE-ligand complexes and free sRAGE. There is an alternative splice variant of the RAGE gene, called endogenous secretory RAGE (esRAGE) that is actively secreted. [31,32]. In conclusion, neither the function nor the source of sRAGE in human physiology is known. Expression profiling for esRAGE in multiple human organs and RAGE in human thymus has recently been performed [33,34]. Plasma/serum concentrations of sRAGE in diabetes mellitus type 2 and coronary artery disease have been studied with conflicting findings [35,36].

The RAGE ligand HMGB1 is a non-histone chromosomal protein which functions as a DNA chaperone. The molecule is composed of two homologous DNA binding domains and an acidic tail. Different binding domains for its receptors: RAGE, Toll-like receptor 4 (TLR4) and a p53 transactivation domain have been identified. Once HMGB1 is released from the cell it acts as a signaling molecule, namely a damage-associated molecular pattern molecule (DAMP) [37,38].

There is a myriad of studies (mostly animal models) implicating a role for RAGE and its ligands in the pathogenesis of vascular disease. Most of these studies have investigated the systemic vessels. Studies in mice with diabetic atherosclerosis showed that

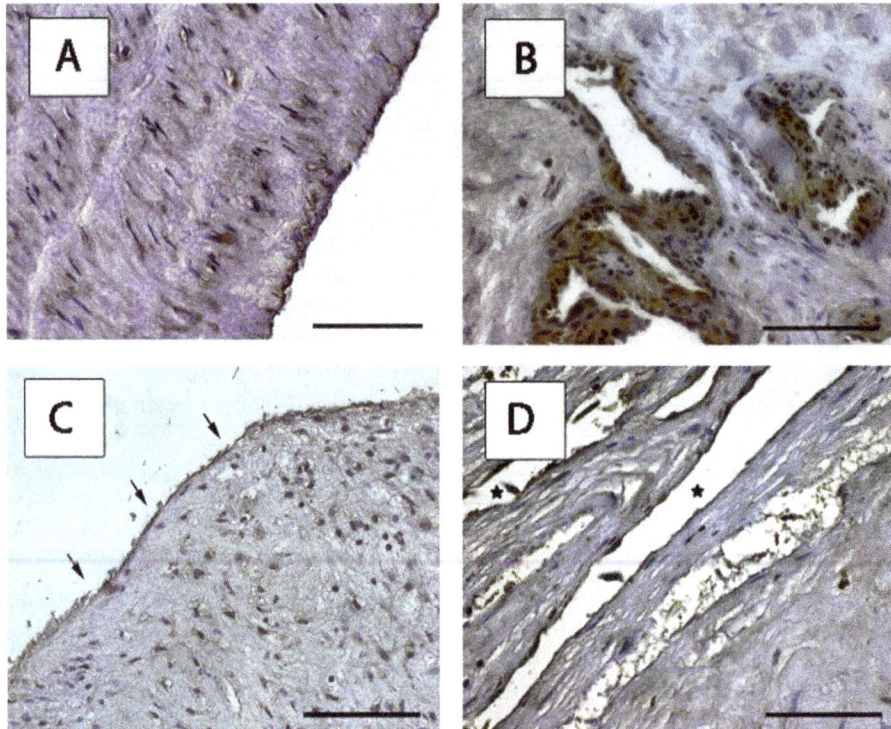

Figure 2. RAGE and HMGB1 expression on endothelial cells of regular PA and endarterectomised tissues. Representative examples of 12 examined patients are shown. Immunohistochemical analysis of regular main pulmonary artery with RAGE expression on endothelium and smooth muscle cells is shown (A). Scale bar: 40 μm. RAGE expressing endothelial cells in vessel-like structures recanalizing the matrix of distal PEA material (B). Endothelial cells expressing RAGE in proximal PEA tissue (arrows point at neointima, C) and HMGB1 (* in recanalizing vessel-like structures, D) in distal PEA specimen are displayed. Scale bar: 20 μm. *RAGE* receptor for advanced glycation endproducts, *HMGB1* high mobility group box 1, *PA* pulmonary artery, *PEA* pulmonary endarterectomy.

treatment with murine sRAGE suppressed the development of accelerated diabetic atherosclerosis in a dose-dependent manner [39,40].

The hypothesis that RAGE could be a key player in pulmonary hypertension was inferred from evidenced based reviews of the scientific literature [41]. The RAGE – RAGE-ligand axis might drive the inflammatory changes in the walls of pulmonary vessels (macro- and microangiopathy) in a similar way as has been shown for the systemic vasculature. A role for RAGE in human pulmonary artery smooth muscle cells (hPASMCs) of patients with idiopathic pulmonary arterial hypertension (iPAH) and in *in vivo* animal models of monocrotaline- and Sugen-induced PAH was recently described [42]. Further, HMGB1 was shown to contribute to PH via a Toll-like receptor 4 (TLR4)-dependent mechanism in a murine model of chronic hypoxia (CH)-induced PH [43].

In a mouse model of hypobaric hypoxia (10% O_2)-induced PH treatment with sRAGE was protective against increases in RV pressure but did not affect distal pulmonary vascular remodeling. In vitro the administration of sRAGE modulated vasoreactivity of intralobar pulmonary arteries from hypobaric hypoxic mice and further enhanced hypoxia-induced proliferation of Chinese hamster lung fibroblasts [44].

We sought to investigate a possible role of RAGE and HMGB1 in diseased main to segmental pulmonary arteries of patients with CTEPH undergoing PEA and small PAs (<500 μm) in iPAH patients undergoing lung transplantation. Moreover, we hypothesized that systemic inflammatory changes pertaining to RAGE and RAGE ligands (HMGB1, S100A9) can be measured in

patients with CTEPH and iPAH. We compared systemic measurements of CTEPH and iPAH patients to those of patients with aortic valve stenosis (AVS). We aimed to filter out changes specific to PH, a disease characterized by pressure overload of the right ventricle in comparison to a disease that inflicts pressure overload on the left ventricle, such as AVS. Lastly, we sought to investigate the effects of surgical therapy, such as PEA, LuTX and AVR on systemic inflammation.

Materials and Methods

Ethics Statement

Ethical approval was obtained from the Medical University Vienna review board on human research. Written informed consent was obtained from all patients and volunteers participating in this study.

Definitions

PH is defined as an increase in mean pulmonary arterial pressure (PAP) ≥25 mmHg at rest as assessed by right heart catheterization [1]. CTEPH is defined by the following observations after ≥3 months of effective anticoagulation: (1) mean PAP≥ 25 mmHg with a pulmonary capillary wedge pressure (PCWP) ≤ 15 mmHg; and (2) at least one (segmental) perfusion defect detected by lung scanning, multi-detector computed tomography angiography or pulmonary angiography [45].

iPAH is a clinical condition characterized by the presence of precapillary PH in the absence of other causes of precapillary PH [1].

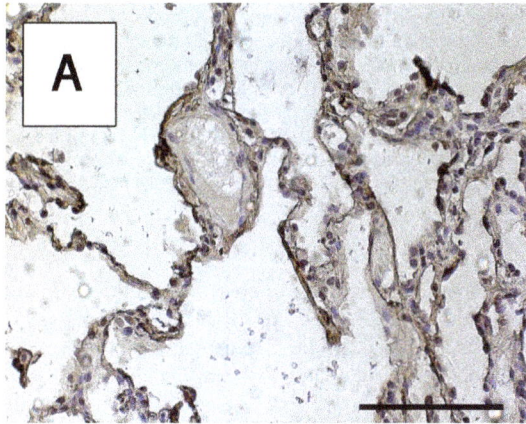
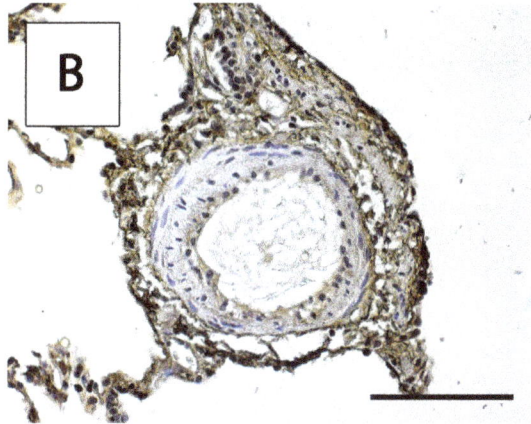
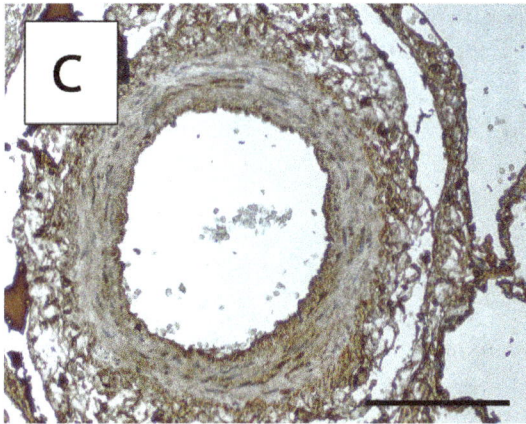
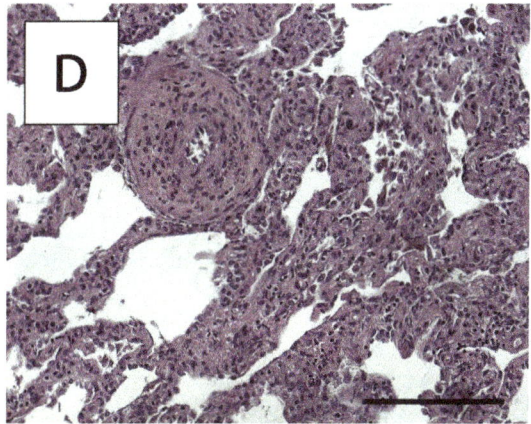
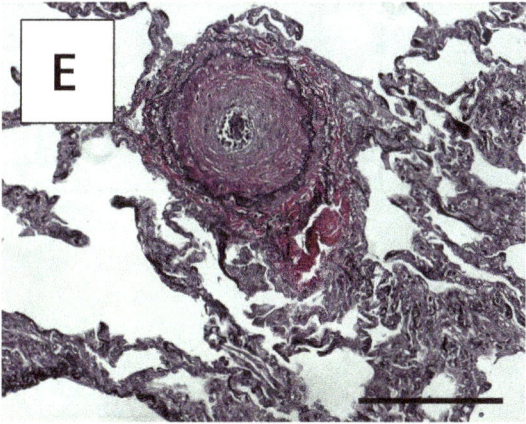
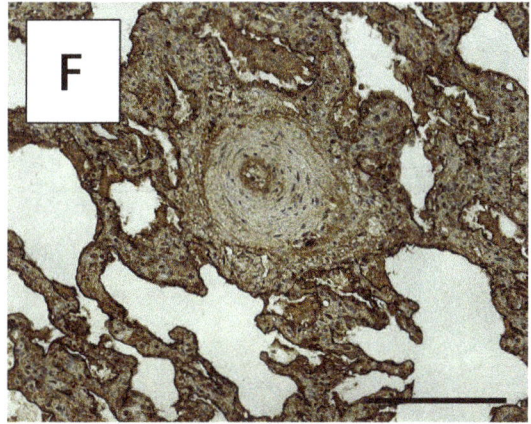
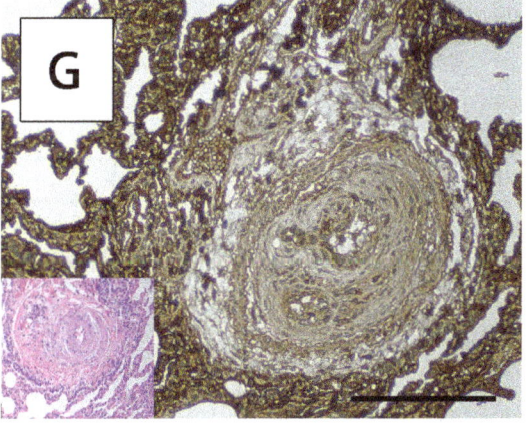
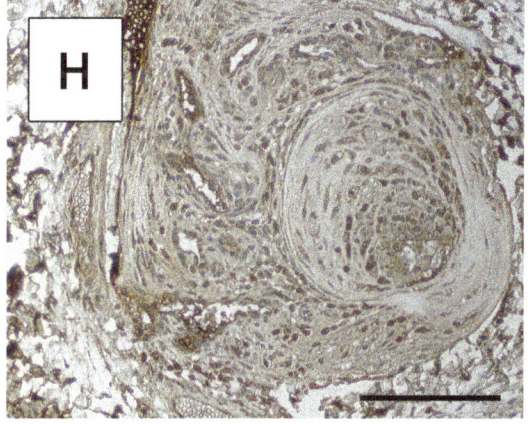

Figure 3. RAGE expression in pulmonary vascular changes of patients with iPAH. Representative examples of immunohistochemical analyses of pathognomonic lesions in lung of patients with iPAH according to the modified Heath Edwards classification in PA vessels smaller than 500 μm in diameter are shown (3 patients per every Heath Edwards group were analysed). RAGE expression in (A) a morphologically regular small PA - stage 0 and (B) a stage 1 histological change in lung of a patient operated for pneumothorax (COPD 0, centriacinar emphysematous changes). RAGE expression in characteristic stage 2 changes in a lung of a patient with iPAH (C). Scale bar in A, B and C: 80 μm. Adjacent sections of H&E (D) and EvG (E) and RAGE staining (F) for stage 3 changes in iPAH. Scale bar in D, E and F: 40 μm. Stage 4, angiomatoid (insert with adjacent H&E section, G), and stage 5, plexiform (H) PA vessel changes are shown. Scale bar in G and H: 80 μm. *iPAH* idiopathic pulmonary arterial hypertension, *PA* pulmonary artery, *RAGE* receptor for advanced glycation endproducts, *COPD* chronic obstructive pulmonary disease, *H&E* hematoxylin and eosin staining, *EvG* Elastica van Gieson staining.

Subjects

We prospectively enrolled 26 patients with CTEPH undergoing PEA, 15 patients with iPAH undergoing lung transplantation, 15 patients with severe aortic stenosis undergoing aortic valve replacement and 33 healthy control subjects between 2010 and 2014. PEA and LuTX surgery were carried out at the department of thoracic surgery, Medical University Vienna, aortic valve replacement (AVR) surgery at the department of cardiac surgery, University Debrecen. The diagnosis of CTEPH and indication for PEA surgery was established by teams of specialists in the diagnosis and treatment of patients with pulmonary hypertension, CTEPH and lung transplantation in every case. All patients with CTEPH were classified to have type 2 disease, intimal thickening and fibrosis proximal to the segmental arteries, according to the intraoperative classification system [8]. The diagnosis of AVS and indication for AVR surgery was established by teams of specialists in cardiology and cardiac surgery in every case. Patient characteristics are given in Tables 1–3.

None of the control subjects studied had any evidence or suspicion of any form of pulmonary hypertension, autoimmune disease, malignancies or infectious conditions at the time of entry into this study. None of the volunteers received anticoagulants,

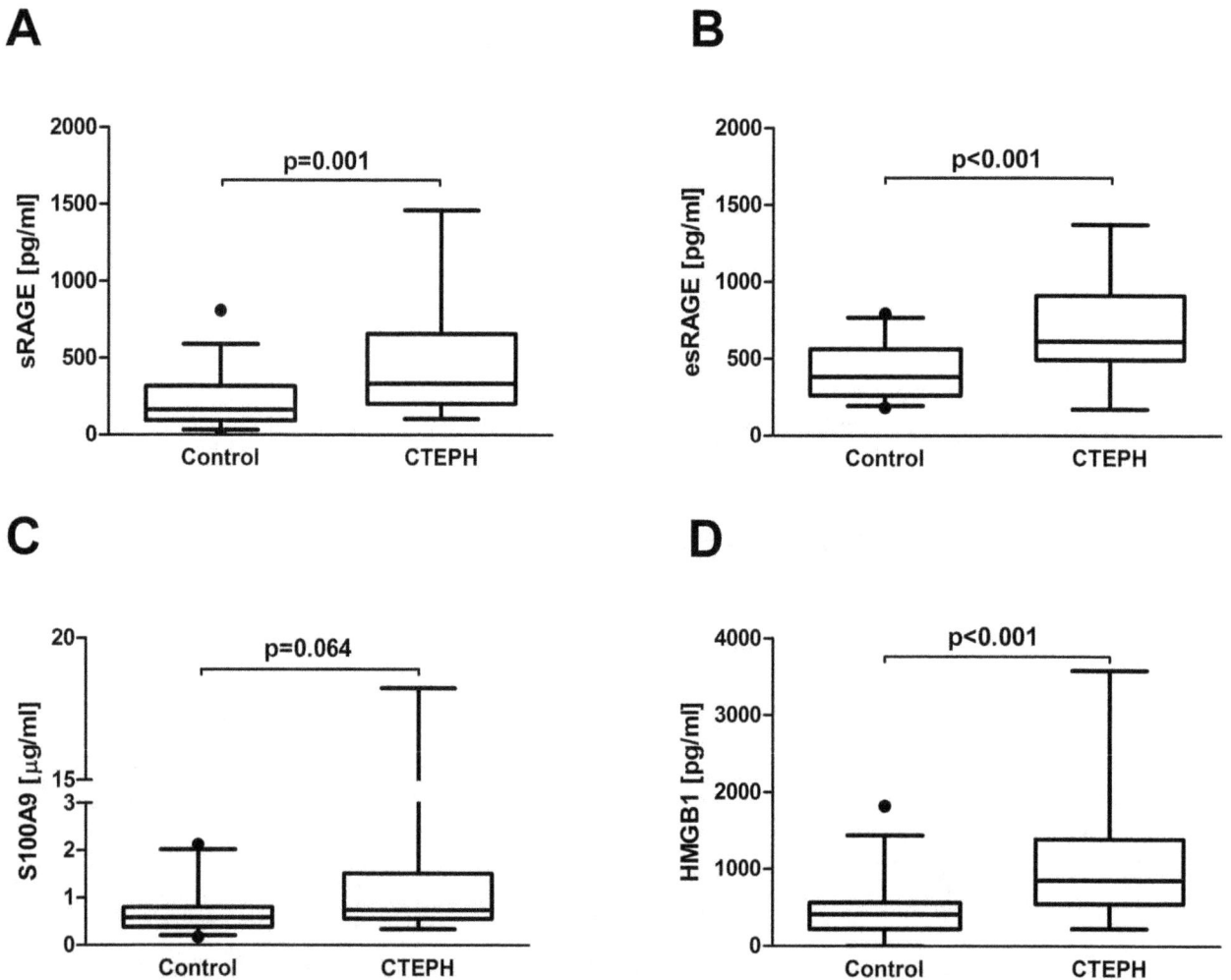

Figure 4. Serum concentrations of RAGE axis molecules in patients with CTEPH. Box plot analysis of serum concentrations of sRAGE (A), esRAGE (B), S100A9 (C) and HMGB1 (D) in patients with CTEPH (n = 26) and controls (n = 33). Independent Student's t-test was used to compare groups. *RAGE* receptor for advanced glycation endproducts, *sRAGE* soluble RAGE, *esRAGE* endogenous secretory RAGE, *S100A9* member of S100 family of Ca+ binding proteins, *HMGB1* high mobility group box1, *CTEPH* chronic thromboembolic pulmonary hypertension.

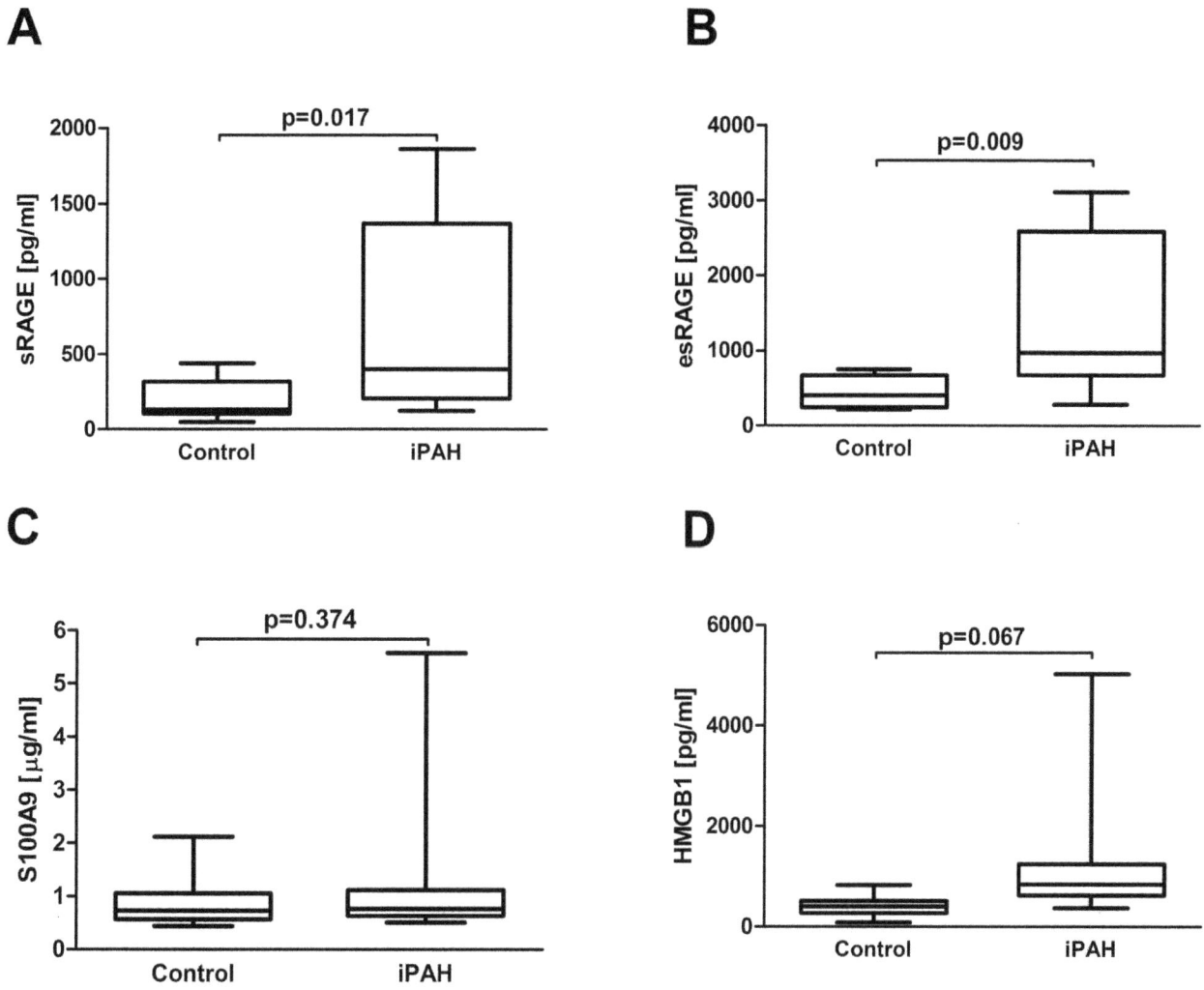

Figure 5. Serum concentrations of RAGE axis molecules in patients with iPAH. Box plot analysis of serum concentrations of sRAGE (A), esRAGE (B), S100A9 (C) and HMGB1 (D) in patients with iPAH (n = 8) and controls (n = 11). Independent Student's t-test was used to compare groups. *RAGE* receptor for advanced glycation endproducts, *sRAGE* soluble RAGE, *esRAGE* endogenous secretory RAGE, *S100A9* member of S100 family of Ca+ binding proteins, *HMGB1* high mobility group box1, *iPAH* idiopathic pulmonary arterial hypertension.

Table 2. The basic characteristics of patients with iPAH and controls (healthy volunteers) are listed.

	iPAH (n = 8)	Controls (n = 11)	p value
Age *in years*	36.6 (37.4) ±9.9 (3.5), [21–50]	36. 4(33.0) ±12.3 (3.7), [22–62]	0.963
F:M ratio *n (%)*	8:0 (100:0)	10:1 (90.9:9.1)	0.381
PAP$_{mean}$ *[mmHg]*	54.5 (57.5) ±20.0 (10.0), [28–75]		
PVR *[dynes·s^{-1}·cm^{-5}]*	1425.0 (1505.0) ±582.1 (291.0), [706–1984]		
CI *[l/min/m^2]*	3.7 (3.8) ±0.4 (0.1)		
sRAGE *[pg/ml]*	743.7 (401.9) ±672.9 (254.3), [123.9–1861.7]	195.5 (130.8) ±130.9 (39.5), [51.0–441.1]	0.017
esRAGE *[pg/ml]*	1391.1 (972.9) ±1073.2 (379.4), [280.0–3110.0]	423.2 (399.4) ±197.1 (59.4), [210.0–750.0]	0.009
S100A9 *[µg/ml]*	1.4 (0.8) ±1.7 (0.6), [0.5–5.6]	0.9 (0.7) ±0.5 (0.1), [0.4–2.1]	0.374
HMGB1 *[pg/ml]*	1419.4 (845.2) ±1614 (610.1), [381.5–5020.9]	415.1 (410.6) ±207.0 (65.5), [80.6–833.3]	0.067

Reported is mean (median) ± standard deviation (standard error mean), [range].
iPAH idiopathic pulmonary arterial hypertension, *n* number of patients, *F:M ratio* female to male ratio, *PAP$_{mean}$* mean pulmonary artery pressure, *PVR* pulmonary vascular resistance; *CI* cardiac index, *sRAGE* soluble receptor for advanced glycation endproducts, *esRAGE* endogenous secretory receptor for advanced glycation endproducts, *S100A9* member of S100 family of Ca$^+$ binding proteins, *HMGB1* high mobility group box1.

A

B

C

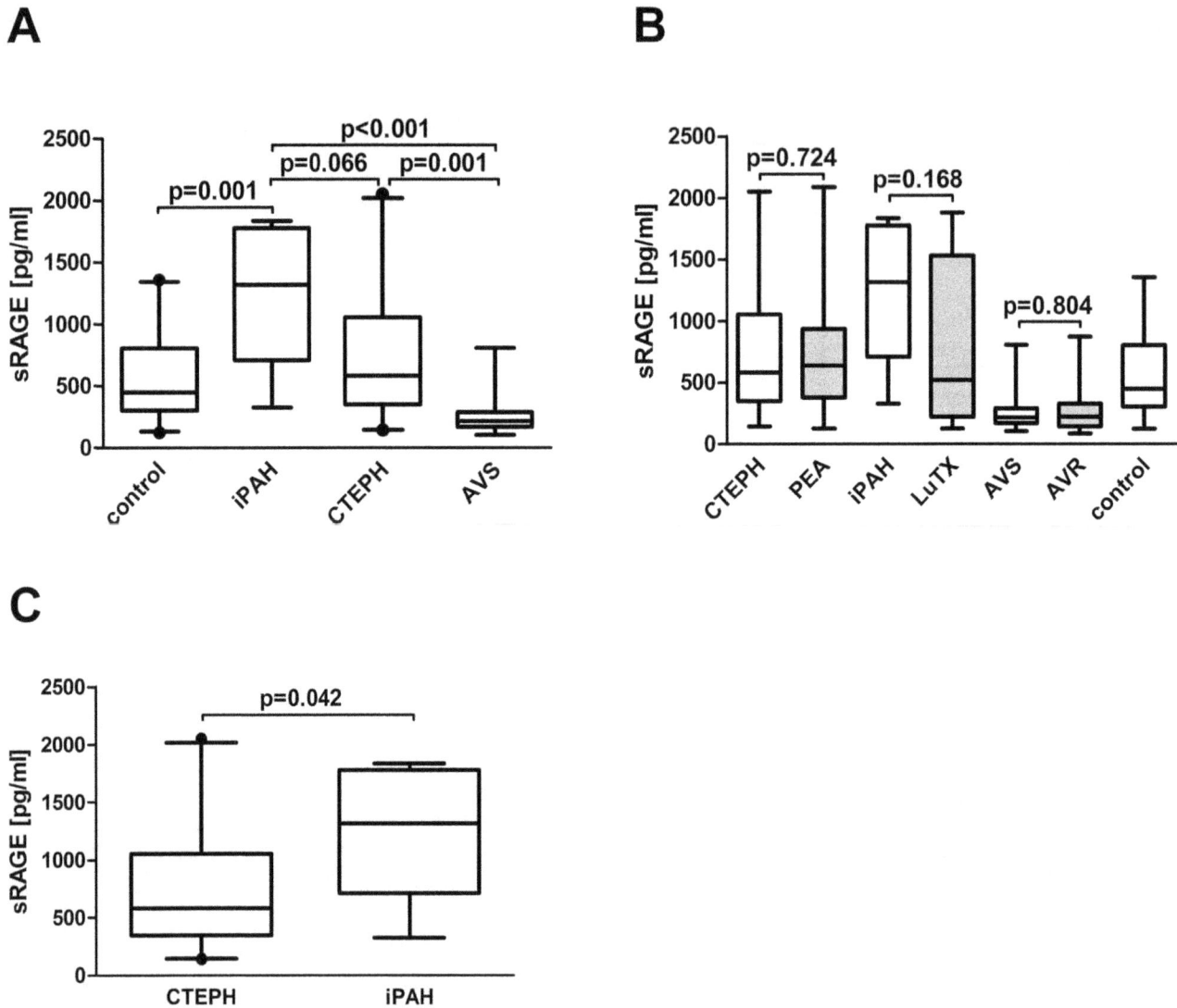

Figure 6. Serum concentrations of sRAGE in patients before and after surgery for CTEPH, iPAH and AVS. Box plot analysis of serum concentrations of sRAGE in patients with CTEPH (n = 20), iPAH (n = 7), AVS (n = 15) and controls (n = 28, A). Box plot analysis of sRAGE in serum of patients with CTEPH before and after PEA, in patients with iPAH before and after double lung transplantation and in patients with AVS before and after AVR (B). Box plot analysis of serum concentrations of sRAGE in patients with CTEPH and iPAH (C). One-way ANOVA was used to compare groups. Post hoc comparisons were computed with the Tukey correction. *RAGE* receptor for advanced glycation endproducts, *sRAGE* soluble RAGE, *CTEPH* chronic thromboembolic pulmonary hypertension, *PEA* pulmonary endarterectomy, *iPAH* idiopathic pulmonary arterial hypertension, *AVS* aortic valve stenosis, *AVR* aortic valve replacement.

prostaglandins, immunosuppressant therapy or any other type of prescribed medication.

Human tissue and serum sample collection

Fresh tissues (PEA specimens, pulmonary arteries and lung tissues) were harvested at the time of PEA (from patients with CTEPH), lung transplantation (from patients with iPAH, CF and COPD) and video-assisted thoracoscopic surgery for recurrent primary spontaneous pneumothorax (otherwise healthy individuals). Histological diagnoses and classification of iPAH in this study was routinely performed at the clinical institute of pathology at the Medical University Vienna.

Serum samples were centrifuged within 60 minutes of collection and stored at −80°C until analysis. In CTEPH the first results from serum analysis were obtained in 26 patients compared to 33 controls (table 1). For the next step we collected serum samples 10 days after (12 patients) and 1 year after PEA (9 different patients; summarized in table 3). Similarly, in iPAH the first result was obtained in serum of 8 patients compared to controls (table 2). In the next step we collected serum samples of 7 different patients with iPAH before and 3 weeks after lung transplantation (table 3). A total of 15 patients with iPAH were included in the study. Age- and sex-matched controls used for subset analysis are part of the whole control pool. Serum samples were collected before and 10 days after AVR (table 3). All postoperatively collected serum samples stem from patients with an uneventful postoperative course.

Table 3. Clinical characteristics of patients with CTEPH before and after PEA, iPAH before and LuTX, AVS before and after AVR.

CTEPH (n = 20)	Before PEA	After PEA	p value
sRAGE *[pg/ml]*	743.29 (582.90) ±117.62 (26.98), [125.33–2085.55]	688.70 (609.14) ±396.60 (88.68), [141.84–1712.88]	0.724
Age *in years*	60.24 (63.99) ±12.99 (2.91), [31–78]		
F:M ratio *n (%)*	5:15		
PAP$_{mean}$ *[mmHg]*	53.53 (53.00) ±15.26 (3.50), [28.00–90.00]	27.42 (27.00) ±6.05 (1.39), [18.00–39.00]	<0.001
PVR *[dynes·s^{-1}·cm^{-5}]*	701.27 (690.00) ±277.95 (67.41), [329.00–1257.00]	265.37 (248.00) ±117.62 (26.98), [88.00–539.00]	<0.001
CI *[l/min/m^2]*	1.92 (2.12) ±1.13 (0.25), [0.00–4.20]	2.08 (2.20) ±1.42 (0.33), [0.00–3.86]	0.542
iPAH (n = 7)	Before LuTX	After LuTX	
sRAGE *[pg/ml]*	1216.05 (1315.27) ±564.95 (213.53), [326.47–1835.31]	772.83 (519.91) ±694.85 (262.63), [125.95–1880.66]	0.168
Age *in years*	33.43 (34.00) ±6.23 (2.35), [21–40]		
F:M ratio *n (%)*	5:2		
PAP$_{mean}$ *[mmHg]*	82.57 (77.00) ±17.63 (6.66), [54.00–103.00]	22.57 (22.00) ±3.41 (1.29), [19.00–29.00]	<0.001
PVR *[dynes·s^{-1}·cm^{-5}]*	1733.60 (1800.00) ±200.71 (89.76), [1452.00–1984.00]		
CI *[l/min/m^2]*	1.99 (2.00) ±0.27 (0.11), [1.70–2.30]	4.27 (4.50) ±0.59 (0.34), [3.60–4.70]	0.074
AVS (n = 15)	Before AVR	After AVR	
sRAGE *[pg/ml]*	260.26 (216.04) ±171.40 (44.26), [104.01–808.26]	274.45 (221.26) ±199.24 (51.44), [83.91–874.58]	0.804
Age *in years*	65.23 (64.50) ±10.31 (2.66), [44–86]		
F:M ratio *n (%)*	6:9		
PAP$_{mean}$ *[mmHg]*	18.87 (19.00) ±4.94 (1.28), [9.00–28.00]		
Mean grad	47.47 (43.00) ±16.22 (4.19), [29.00–84.00]		
Vmax *m/s*	4.47 (4.30) ±0.73 (0.19), [3.80–6.20]		
AVA	0.76 (0.80) ±0.21 (0.06), [0.30–1.00]		
Controls (n = 28)			
sRAGE *[pg/ml]*	567.80 (446.78) ±329.09 (62.19) [122.48–1355.13]		
Age *in years*	58.50 (62.00) ±20.72 (3.92) [30–91]		
F:M ratio *n (%)*	12:16		

Reported is mean (median) ± standard deviation (standard error mean), [range].
CTEPH chronic thromboembolic pulmonary hypertension *PEA* pulmonary endarterectomy, *iPAH* idiopathic pulmonary arterial hypertension, *LuTX* double lung transplantation, *AVS* aortic valve stenosis; *AVR* aortic valve replacement, *Mean grad* mean transvalvular pressure gradient, *Vmax* maximum aortic stenosis jet velocity, *AVA* aortic valve area, *F:M* ratio female to male ratio, *PAP$_{mean}$* mean pulmonary artery pressure, *PVR* pulmonary vascular resistance; *CI* cardiac index, *sRAGE* soluble receptor for advanced glycation endproducts, *n* number of patients.

Immunohistochemistry

Formaldehyde-fixed and paraffin-embedded human PEA specimens, lung tissues and PAs were prepared according to routine protocols of the clinical institute of pathology. Briefly, sections 2 μm in thickness, were baked for 1 hour at 55°C, deparaffinized in three xylenes and rehydrated in ethanol as follows: 2×100%, 1×95%, 1×90%, and 1×70%, followed by PBS. Antigen retrieval was performed by boiling slides at 600 watt (3×5 min) in a microwave oven using citrate buffer at pH 6.0 (Target Retrieval Solution, Dako, USA). Endogenous peroxidase activity was blocked by applying hydrogen peroxide 0.3%. Sections were incubated with 2% bovine serum albumin or blocking serum of the same species as the biotinylated secondary antibody to deplete unspecific protein-protein interactions. Sections were stained using affinity-purified polyclonal goat anti-human RAGE IgG (R&D Systems, Minneapolis, MN, USA) or monoclonal mouse anti-human HMGB1 IgG2b (R&D Systems) and biotinylated anti-goat IgG or anti-mouse IgG secondary antibodies (Vector Laboratories, Burlingame, CA, USA). Immunoreactivity was amplified using biotin-avidin peroxidase conjugates (Vectastain ABC kit, Vector Laboratories). 3,3'-diaminobenzidine was used as chromogen (DAB Peroxidase substrate kit, Vector Laboratories). Counterstaining was performed using Mayer's hematoxylin. Slides were dehydrated with ethanol: 1×95% for 1 min, 1×100% for 6 min and cleared in n-Butanol before mounting (Pertex Mounting Media, Leica Microsystems, Germany).

Immunohistochemistry for representative markers of hematopoietic precursor cells CD34, the intermediate filament vimentin and smooth muscle α-actin (α-SMA) were performed on adjacent sections of PEA specimens using the automated Ventana Benchmark platform (Ventana Medical Systems, Tucson, AZ, USA) according to routine protocols of the clinical institute of pathology. Sections were stained with monoclonal mouse anti-human α-SMA (Clone1A4; Dako, Denmark, Europe), monoclonal mouse anti-human CD34 IgG$_1$ (Clone QBEnd/10; Novocastra, Leica Biosystems Newcastle, UK, Europe) and monoclonal rabbit anti-human vimentin IgG (clone SP20; Thermo Fisher Scientific, Fremont, USA). Heat pre-treatment was conducted in Ultra cell conditioner number 1 buffer (Ultra CC1; pH 6). Color was developed with Ultraview Universal Detection DAB-kit (Ventana Medical Systems). Immunohistochemical staining for RAGE and HMGB1 was reproduced with the described automated system.

Omission of primary antibody served as negative control. Hematoxylin and eosin (H&E) staining was performed according to routine protocols. Analysis and image documentation was done with Axio Imager 2 microscope and AxioVision software (Carl Zeiss International, Germany).

Grading of pulmonary vascular lesions

Specimens of explanted lungs from patients undergoing lung transplantation for iPAH were harvested at the time of transplantation. Sections were stained for hematoxylin and eosin (H&E) and Elastica van Gieson (EvG) to visualize elastin and analyzed according to a modified Heath Edwards classification system changes in small pulmonary arteries. Grade 1 is characterized by extension of muscle cells into distal arterioles and thickening of the media of muscular arteries. Grade 2 is defined as hypertrophy of the media with intimal proliferation in small muscular arteries. Grade 3 shows progressive fibrous vascular occlusion and concentric intimal fibrosis. Grade 4 is characterized by progressive arterial dilatation with plexiform lesions, grade 5 by chronic dilatation with fibrosis of intima and media, prominent plexiform and angiomatoid lesions and pulmonary hemosiderosis.

Evaluation of immunoreactivity

Analysis of immunoreactivity was performed by two observers blinded to the type of antibodies used for staining. Two to four slides per patient were assessed. We assigned a score from 0 to 3 to assess staining intensity for RAGE or HMGB1 cytoplasmic or nuclear expression in PEA specimens, PA and small PA in lungs of patients with pneumothorax, iPAH and COPD (0, no staining; 1, weak; 2, moderate; 3, strong).

Detection of serum proteins

To test the hypothesis that RAGE and HMGB1 are involved systemically in patients with pulmonary hypertension, we employed enzyme-linked immunosorbent assays (ELISA) for the detection of sRAGE, esRAGE, S100A9 and HMGB1 in serum of patients with CTEPH, iPAH, AVS and healthy volunteers. All ELISA tests were performed according to the manufacturers' instructions: sRAGE (RAGE Duoset Elisa, RnD Systems, Minneapolis, MN, USA), esRAGE (B-Bridge International Inc., CA, USA), S100A9 (Abnova, Taipei City, Taiwan) and HMGB1 (IBL International GmbH, Hamburg, Germany). Researchers performing the assays and data analyses were blinded to the groups associated with each sample.

Statistical methods

We performed an observational study with longitudinal (cohort study: measurements before and after PEA, LuTX and AVR) and cross-sectional design (e.g. serum sRAGE concentration in CTEPH/iPAH compared to controls). Statistical analysis of data was performed using SPSS software (version 20; IBM SPSS Inc., IL, USA). Data were reported as mean (median) ± standard deviation (and standard error mean) in tables and as mean ± standard error mean in the abstract and results section. The concentrations of proteins in serum of patients with CTEPH, iPAH and AVS were compared to those of healthy volunteers using independent Student's t test or One-way ANOVA for normal (Gaussian) distributions. Kruskal-Wallis rank test or Mann-Whitney U test was used to evaluate non-normal distributions. Post hoc comparisons were computed with the Tukey correction. The paired t-test was applied to before and after measurements made on the same group of subjects, such as sRAGE serum concentrations before and after PEA. Pearson's $\chi2$ test for independence was used for analysis of categorical data, such as sex differences. Spearman's rank correlation test was used to assess possible correlations of sRAGE and mean pulmonary artery pressure. The level of statistical significance was set at < 0.05 (two-tailed p-values).

Results

Expression of RAGE and HMGB1 in endarterectomized tissue from CTEPH patients, regular PA morphology and diseased small PAs in patients with iPAH

Expression of RAGE and HMGB1 in endarterectomized tissues of patients with CTEPH. Diseased central, lobar and segmental PAs in CTEPH patients undergoing PEA showed thromboembolic material incorporated into the remodeled vessel wall in the form of intimal thickening and formation of neointima. The macroscopic aspect of a representative PEA specimen is shown (Fig. 1A). Hematoxylin and eosin stained sections revealed the prototypic morphology of fibroblasts/fibrocytes forming a honeycomb-like network. To test the hypothesis that RAGE and HMGB1 are involved in CTEPH, we employed immunohistochemical analysis for the detection of RAGE and HMGB1 in PEA specimens (fig. 1B+C). We found cytoplasmic staining for RAGE and cytoplasmic and nuclear staining for HMGB1 in the majority of patients examined (12 out of 15 patients, 80.0%). The specimens of the same 12 patients stained for RAGE and HMGB1. Nuclear staining for RAGE was not detected. In positive specimens 70.9±4.2% of cells showed RAGE and 72.8±4.6% showed HMGB1 expression.

Identification of RAGE and HMGB1 expressing cells as myofibroblasts. We performed analysis on adjacent sections to further characterize RAGE$^+$ and HMGB1$^+$ cells in endarterectomized tissues. We found that RAGE$^+$ and HMGB1$^+$ cells were also expressing the intermediate filament vimentin and α-SMA. CD34, a representative marker of hematopoietic precursor cells, did not correlate with the expression pattern seen for RAGE$^+$ HMGB1$^+$ vimentin$^+$ α-SMA$^+$ cells. The expression of CD34 expressing cells can rather be described as sporadic nests in 30.0% of tissues, a homogeneous distribution throughout any of the specimens was not found (fig. 1).

RAGE and HMGB1 expression in neointima and small vessel-like structures recanalizing distal "myofibrotic" clots. RAGE cytoplasmic staining was detected in endothelium of the intimal vessel wall (100% of endothelial cells) and smooth muscle cells of the media (64.8%) of regular main PAs. Vessel-like structures in distal areas of endarterectomized tissues showed RAGE and HMGB1 expression. Neointima (cell layer outlining the luminal surface) covering the organized thromboembolic material of diseased PAs displayed RAGE and HMGB1 expression (fig. 2). These staining patterns were analogous in all 12 patients examined.

Differentiated expression of RAGE in small PAs (<500 μm in diameter). In order to quantify the expression of RAGE in PA changes prototypical for PH we employed immunohistochemical analysis for the detection of RAGE in lung tissue specimens of patients with iPAH, COPD and pneumothorax (fig. 3). Prototypical Heath Edwards lesions were identified by H&E and EvG staining. We investigated lesions from three patients for every Heath Edwards group. Cytoplasmic RAGE expression was found in endothelium of Heath Edwards stages 0–5. The staining intensity in endothelial cells was as follows: stages 0–1: weak, stages 2–5: moderate. In smooth muscle cells of small muscular PAs RAGE was detectable with the following staining intensities: stages 0–1 (absent to weak), stages 2–5 (weak to moderate). Nuclear staining for RAGE was not detected. The described staining patterns and intensities were uniform throughout all patients examined.

Systemic measurements: Concentration of sRAGE, esRAGE and RAGE ligands: HMGB1 and S100A9 in serum of patients with PH and AVS

Increased levels of sRAGE, esRAGE and HMGB1 in serum of patients with CTEPH. Basic demographic and hemodynamic data of patients with CTEPH and volunteers are detailed in table 1. There was no statistically significant difference in age (p = 0.828) and sex (p = 0.985) between patients with CTEPH (n = 26) and controls (n = 33). We found significantly elevated serum concentrations of sRAGE in patients with CTEPH compared to controls (sRAGE [pg/ml] 467.2±72.6 vs.198.6±28.3; p = 0.001). Similarly, serum concentrations of the splice variant esRAGE were significantly higher than those of controls (esRAGE [pg/ml] 703.7±63.1 vs. 414.5±31.8; p< 0.001). The RAGE ligand S100A9 was not significantly different (S100A9 [μg/ml] 2.1±0.8 vs. 0.7±0.09; p = 0.064) whereas HMGB1 was significantly elevated in serum of patients with CTEPH (HMGB1 [pg/ml] 1141.1±173.1 vs. 464.3±66.6; p = 0.001; fig. 4, table 1). There was no significant correlation of serum sRAGE concentrations with mean pulmonary artery pressure in patients with CTEPH (correlation coefficient 0.116, p = 0.646).

Higher concentrations of sRAGE and esRAGE, but not HMGB1 and S100A9 in patients with iPAH. Basic demographic and hemodynamic data of patients with iPAH and volunteers are detailed in table 2. There was no significant difference in age (p = 0.963) and sex (p = 0.381) between patients with iPAH and controls. We found significantly elevated concentrations of sRAGE and esRAGE in patients with iPAH (sRAGE [pg/ml]: 743.7±254.3 vs. 195.5±39.5; p = 0.017; esRAGE [pg/ml] 1391.1±379.4 vs. 423.2±59.4; p = 0.009). Conversely, the measured RAGE ligands: serum S100A9 and HMGB1 in patients with iPAH did not differ from controls (S100A9 [μg/ml] 1.4±0.6 vs. 0.9±0.1, p = 0.374; and HMGB1 [pg/ml] 1419.4±610.1 vs. 415.1±65.5, p = 0.067; fig. 5, table 2). There was no significant correlation of serum sRAGE concentrations with mean pulmonary artery pressure in patients with iPAH (correlation coefficient −0.144, p = 0.734).

Serum concentrations of sRAGE were significantly higher in iPAH and CTEPH (iPAH>CTEPH) in relation to reduced concentrations in AVS patients. We wanted to test the hypothesis that sRAGE serum concentrations are only elevated in diseases of the pulmonary circulation leading to pressure overload of the right ventricle compared to disease leading to pressure overload of the left ventricle, such as AVS. Basic demographic and hemodynamic data of patients with CTEPH undergoing PEA, iPAH undergoing lung transplantation, AVS undergoing AVR and volunteers are detailed in table 3. *ANOVA* analysis of sRAGE concentrations from patients with CTEPH, iPAH, AVS and healthy volunteers revealed significant differences (p<0.001). *Post-hoc* comparisons showed significantly higher serum concentrations of sRAGE in patients with iPAH (p< 0.001) and CTEPH (p = 0.001) compared to AVS (fig. 6). Further *post-hoc* comparisons revealed no difference in serum sRAGE concentration between patients with CTEPH and iPAH (p = 0.066). Separate analysis of patients with CTEPH and iPAH showed significantly higher serum sRAGE concentrations in patients with iPAH compared to CTEPH (independent samples t-test: p = 0.042). Serum sRAGE concentrations were significantly reduced in patients with AVS compared to controls (p = 0.001).

Influence of surgical therapy on serum sRAGE concentrations. There were no significant differences in sRAGE serum concentrations before and after surgical therapy for CTEPH, iPAH or AVS. Basic demographic and hemodynamic data are detailed in table 3. The results were as follows: CTEPH patients before and after PEA (sRAGE [pg/ml] 743.29±26.98 vs. 688.70±88.68, p = 0.724), iPAH patients before and after lung transplantation (sRAGE [pg/ml] 1216.0±213.5 vs. 772.8±262.6, p = 0.168) and patients with AVS before and after AVR (sRAGE [pg/ml] 260.2±44.2 vs. 274.4±51.4, p = 0.804; table 3, fig. 6).

For patients undergoing PEA, early (10 days after PEA) and late (one year after PEA) postoperative serum samples were available: There was no difference in sRAGE concentrations when measurements were stratified between early and late: before and early after PEA (n = 12): (sRAGE [pg/ml]: 692.8±168.3 vs. 534.1±59.8, p = 0.451; before and one year after PEA (n = 9): 804.9±214.7 vs. 877.6±167.1, p = 0.767; in comparison to all patients (n = 21) together: as above: p = 0.724.

Discussion

The results of this study describe for the first time the expression of RAGE and HMGB1 in myofibroblasts of patients with CTEPH. Prior studies have shown the majority of cells in endarterectomised tissues from patients with CTEPH to be myofibroblasts [46,47]. The presence of multipotent mesenchymal progenitor cells (capable of adipogenic and osteogenic differentiation) was described [46]. Further, endothelial progenitor cells (CD34+CD133+Flk-1+) were identified in neointima of proximal thromboembolic material as well as distal regions (downstream of the thromboembolic material) [47]. Myofibroblast-like cells were described as hyperproliferative, anchorage-independent, invasive and serum-independent [48]. These myofibroblast-like cells were later termed sarcoma-like cells as the injection into the tail veins of C.B-17/lcr-scid/scidJcl mice led to the development of tumors growing along the intimal surface of the pulmonary vessels (a mouse model for pulmonary artery intimal sarcoma) [49]. A possible functional role of RAGE and HMGB1 in myofibroblasts of remodeled PA vessels in patients with CTEPH may be inferred from recent studies describing a role for RAGE in iPAH. In PASMCs of patients with PAH, RAGE was 6-fold upregulated, induced STAT3 activation and decreased the expression of BMPR2 and PPARγ. The described cell phenotype could be induced by RAGE agonist 100A4 in control PASMCs and reversed by RAGE blockade with RAGE small interfering RNA (siRNA) in both cell types. RAGE blockade reduced PA pressures and right ventricular remodeling associated with improved lung perfusion and vascular remodeling in *in vivo* animal models of monocrotaline- and Sugen-induced PAH. Immunofluorescence staining revealed a correlation of RAGE protein expression with disease severity in patients with PAH [42]. Disease severity was classified as mild, moderate and severe. As increased sRAGE concentrations in our study did not correlate with PAP*mean*, we chose to investigate RAGE expression in prototypical vessel changes according to the modified Heath and Edwards classification that was routinely applied during the diagnostic workup of lungs with iPAH at our institution. We found a greater staining intensity in endothelial cells as well as smooth muscle cells of higher Heath Edwards grades.

Recently, a role of the damage-associated molecular pattern molecule (DAMP) HMGB1 was shown to contribute to PH via a TLR4-dependent mechanism in a mouse model of CH-induced PH. In patients with iPAH extra-nuclear HMGB1 in pulmonary vascular lesions was identified. Increased concentrations of serum HMGB1 correlated with PAP*mean*. In C57BL6/J mice exposed to CH-induced PH a statistically not significant nearly two-fold increase in RAGE mRNA was observed. Also of interest are the observations in RAGE knockout (RAGE−/−) compared to wildtype mice exposed to CH: there was the same increase in right ventricular (RV) systolic pressure, but decreased RV hypertrophy in RAGE$^{-/-}$ mice. In the same model RAGE$^{-/-}$ mice neither showed significantly different vascular changes nor did the levels of mouse endothelin -1 (ET-1) or mouse soluble intracellular adhesion molecule 1 (sICAM-1) differ [43]. Our data on human patients support a role of the RAGE axis, namely RAGE and HMGB1, in iPAH. The lack of significant differences in pulmonary vascular changes and circulating cytokines in RAGE$^{-/-}$ mice is puzzling and does not parallel our data – stronger expression of RAGE in higher Heath Edwards stages - or the above described data by Meloche et al - 6-fold upregulation of RAGE in PASMCs of patients with PAH [42]. With the current limited evidence we can only attribute the differences between mice and men to intrinsic mechanisms of the mouse model of CH-induced PH.

The migration of human pulmonary artery endothelial cells (huPAEC) in vitro could be inhibited by HMGB1 via TLR4 and IRF3-dependent mechanisms [50]. If this HMGB1 effect can also be reversed by blockade of RAGE still has to be tested. In our study we demonstrated RAGE expression in endothelial cells of large and small (<500 μm) regular PAs, neointima of proximal remodeled PAs and recanalizing vessel-like structures of distal endarterectomised tissue of patients with CTEPH, as well as prototypical Heath Edwards lesions in patients with PH. Endothelial RAGE was present in health and disease. The behavior of endothelial cells from diseased and healthy tissues could reveal further information.

In patients with chronic heart failure and impaired left ventricular function activation of the immune system as measured by increased levels of proinflammatory cytokines is associated with poor prognosis [51,52]. No differences in serum concentrations of the measured cytokines: TNF-alpha, its soluble receptors 1 and 2 (sTNFR1 and 2), IL-10, high sensitivity C-reactive protein (hsCRP) and N-terminal-pro-B-type natriuretic peptide (NT-proBNP was measured in plasma) were found when right ventricular dysfunction due to CTEPH and left ventricular dysfunction due to chronic heart failure were compared [51]. In order to help untangle the possible sources by which sRAGE serum concentrations increased in patients with CTEPH and iPAH we compared serum measurements in patients with CTEPH before and after PEA and in patients with iPAH before and after lung transplantation to those of patients with AVS before and after AVR. In this experiment right ventricular remodeling with pressure overload resulting from pulmonary vascular disease (CTEPH and iPAH) is compared to left ventricular remodeling as a consequence of the pressure-overloaded left ventricle observed in patients with aortic stenosis. The results of our experiment point to a pulmonary source of sRAGE as there was no elevation in serum of patients with AVS. A normalization of sRAGE in serum after PEA or lung transplantation can probably not be expected regarding the neurohumoral and immunological disturbances occurring in these patients [10]. Possible pitfalls of our model are two emerging conceptual differences between right and left ventricular adaptation and remodeling: (1) right ventricular enlargement occurs earlier in the course of PAH when compared to pressure-overloaded left ventricles, probably because of the smaller thickness of the right ventricle that will experience greater wall stress for comparable increases in pressure. And second, there is much less myocardial fibrosis in patients with RV pressure overload compared to patients with AVS which explains the high rate of recovery of right ventricular function after lung transplantation, even when right ventricular ejection fraction was severely reduced at the time of transplantation [53,54,55]. Regarding these

differences, we cannot exclude the possibility that sRAGE is derived (in part) from a myocardial source. Concerning the myocardium, the intra-coronary administration of sRAGE attenuated cardiac remodeling and fibrosis in minipigs with ischemia-reperfusion injury [56].

Our results on patients with AVS are in line with a previous study that showed that plasma sRAGE levels were significantly lower in patients with AVS than in controls and independently associated with the risk for AVS. In that study there was an inverse correlation with age, cholesterol levels and coronary calcification [57].

In lung transplant recipients elevated plasma sRAGE concentrations measured four hours after reperfusion of the lung allograft were associated with longer duration of mechanical ventilation and longer intensive care unit length of stay [58]. Increased plasma levels of sRAGE were associated with primary graft dysfunction at six and 24 hours after lung transplantation [59]. Elevated plasma sRAGE measured 24 hours postoperatively was associated with the development of bronchiolitis obliterans syndrome [60]. No data exist on RAGE and lung transplantation for iPAH. In our study there was a non-significant reduction in serum sRAGE concentrations in stable lung transplant recipients 3 weeks post transplantation.

Multivariate logistic regression analysis revealed plasma sRAGE concentrations immediately after cardiopulmonary bypass surgery to be an independent predictor for postoperative acute lung injury after cardiac surgery in children [61]. Similarly, S100A12 and sRAGE were associated with increased length of hospitalization after non-urgent coronary artery bypass grafting surgery [62]. The comparison of early (ten days) and late (one year) sRAGE measurement in our study did not show significant differences which infers that the high serum concentrations also after surgery may not only be influenced by the trauma of the surgical intervention alone but also by disease specific alterations in the RAGE axis that may not be influenced by current treatment modalities.

Current standard preoperative evaluation of PEA candidates is unreliable in predicting patients at risk for persistent pulmonary hypertension because of surgically inaccessible thromboembolic material or coexistent small vessel disease which are major reasons for poor outcome [63]. Attempts to identify high risk patients are currently investigated. In a recent study, the preoperative assessment of upstream resistance correlated with postoperative pulmonary resistance index and PAP*mean* [64]. In our study, preoperative sRAGE serum concentrations were significantly higher in patients with iPAH compared to CTEPH and did not correlate with the height of pulmonary artery pressures. This could have implications on the decision to perform pulmonary endarterectomy on patients with CTEPH. The question that has to be answered in future studies is: can high serum concentrations of sRAGE, such as measured in iPAH in this study, unmask distal disease that is not accessible to PEA and thus be of value in preoperative decision making regarding operability of CTEPH patients with high pulmonary vascular resistance (PVR>1200 dynes.cm/s^5) [65]?

As sRAGE serum concentrations did not correlate with their corresponding pulmonary artery pressures in this study we can only hypothesize about an on/off-phenomenon of chronic inflammation in iPAH and CTEPH patients. The current information raises new questions. What pathophysiologic threshold has to be reached to turn on chronic inflammation through the RAGE axis? Is the RAGE axis involved in the primary events of remodeling of the thromboembolic material into the PA vessel wall or is it turned on at later stages of CTEPH and iPAH? Could

RAGE blockade terminate chronic inflammation in these diseases and be of clinical value in patients as an adjunct to current therapies?

We are not suggesting that our absolute concentration values can be used to make any judgments about the diagnosis of, for example CTEPH. While comparative results (e.g. control vs. CTEPH) gained during one experiment could be repeated in separate ELISA experiments, the absolute values for the individual serum samples vary in our experienced hands with the recommended additional reagents from the manufacturer. So we never compare absolute values from samples measured with the RAGE Duoset from different experiments. The intraassay coefficient of variation was 2.3%. We run control serum samples on each ELISA. The RAGE Duoset has quite some interassay variability. The commercially available ELISA is sold for research use only and not for diagnostic purposes. We don't see this interassay variability with the other ELISA assays used in this manuscript.

Soluble RAGE was measured in serum/plasma of other pulmonary diseases with different methods. In stable COPD patients plasma sRAGE was significantly lower compared to healthy control subjects: 400.2 pg/ml vs. 783.3 pg/ml, $p<0.001$; measured by ELISA, R&D systems, Minneapolis, MN, USA [66]. Another study used two different multiplex platforms (Luminex multi-analyte profiling at Rules Based Medicine, RBM, Austin, TX and Searchlight at Aushon Biosystems, Bellaria, MA) to find significant differences in serum sRAGE concentrations in non-smokers, smokers, COPD I/II and COPD III/IV: median sRAGE values [ng/ml] 4.2, 3.2, 2.7 and 2.2, $p = 0.003$ [67]. A study using Quanitkine human RAGE ELISA kit (R&D systems, Minneapolis, MN, USA) found significantly different lower sRAGE concentrations in patients with COPD compared to smoking and nonsmoking controls subjects: sRAGE values [pg/ml]: 1351.1 vs. 1736.6 and 1797.3, $p<0.001$ [68]. There are 2.8-to 10.5-fold differences between the controls or COPD patients when the three studies with different analytical methods and different population samples are compared. Regarding the different absolute concentrations reported for sRAGE as exemplified with three studies for COPD as another pulmonary disease, it is too vague for us to draw conclusions from the comparison of absolute sRAGE measurements between our and other studies.

In summary, we have shown the expression of RAGE and HMGB1 in myofibroblasts of endarterectomised tissues from patients with CTEPH and increased expression of RAGE in prototypical lesions in lung of patients with iPAH. Our immunohistochemical results were corroborated by alterations in the serum concentration of soluble RAGE variants and HMGB1. The results may have substantial implications for diagnosis and/or treatment of patients with pulmonary hypertension. PEA improves the local control of disease with the resultant decrease in pulmonary artery pressure but may not influence the systemic inflammatory mechanisms in CTEPH patients through the RAGE pathway. A more detailed understanding of the RAGE-HMGB1 axis and related molecules in diseases associated with pulmonary hypertension is needed and warrants future study.

Acknowledgments

We thank Andrea Alvarez Hernandez for technical help with immunohistochemical techniques.

Author Contributions

Conceived and designed the experiments: BM. Performed the experiments: BM AM SJ TS CB PB AIS MM. Analyzed the data: BM AM CB SJ TS PB AIS MM IL RSK NSS ST WK HJA. Contributed reagents/materials/analysis tools: BM TS PB AIS IL NSS ST WK HJA. Contributed to the writing of the manuscript: BM AM CB SJ HJA.

References

1. Galiè N, Hoeper MM, Humbert M, Torbicki A, Vachiery JL, et al. (2009) Guidelines for the diagnosis and treatment of pulmonary hypertension. Eur Respir J 34(6): 1219–63.

2. Heath D, Edwards JE (1958) The pathology of hypertensive pulmonary vascular disease; a description of six grades of structural changes in the pulmonary arteries with special reference to congenital cardiac septal defects. Circulation 18(4 Part 1): 533–47.

3. Carlsen J, Hasseriis Andersen K, Boesgaard S, Iversen M, Steinbrüchel D, et al. (2013) Pulmonary arterial lesions in explanted lungs after transplantation correlate with severity of pulmonary hypertension in chronic obstructive pulmonary disease. J Heart Lung Transplant 32(3): 347–54.

4. Zabini D, Nagaraj C, Stacher E, Lang IM, Nierlich P, et al. (2012) Angiostatic factors in the pulmonary endarterectomy material from chronic thromboembolic pulmonary hypertension patients cause endothelial dysfunction. PLoS One 7(8): e43793. doi: 10.1371/journal.pone.0043793.

5. Delcroix M, Vonk Noordegraaf A, Fadel E, Lang I, Simonneau G, et al. (2013) Vascular and right ventricular remodelling in chronic thromboembolic pulmonary hypertension. Eur Respir J 41(1): 224–32.

6. van de Veerdonk MC, Kind T, Marcus JT, Mauritz GJ, Heymans MW, et al. (2011) Progressive right ventricular dysfunction in patients with pulmonary arterial hypertension responding to therapy. J Am Coll Cardiol 58(24): 2511–9.

7. Kim NH, Lang IM (2012) Risk factors for chronic thromboembolic pulmonary hypertension. Eur Respir Rev 21(123): 27–31.

8. Thistlethwaite PA, Mo M, Madani MM, Deutsch R, Blanchard D, et al. (2002) Operative classification of thromboembolic disease determines outcome after pulmonary endarterectomy. J Thorac Cardiovasc Surg 124(6): 1203–11.

9. Seta Y, Shan K, Bozkurt B, Oral H, Mann DL (1996) Basic mechanisms in heart failure: the cytokine hypothesis. J Card Fail 2(3): 243–9. Review.

10. Bogaard HJ, Abe K, Vonk Noordegraaf A, Voelkel NF (2009) The right ventricle under pressure: cellular and molecular mechanisms of right-heart failure in pulmonary hypertension. Chest 135(3): 794–804.

11. Mann DL (2002) Inflammatory mediators and the failing heart: past, present, and the foreseeable future. Circ Res 91(11): 988–98. Review.

12. Hartupee J, Mann DL (2013) Positioning of inflammatory biomarkers in the heart failure landscape. J Cardiovasc Transl Res 6(4): 485–92. Review.

13. Wu Y, Li Y, Zhang C, A X, Wang Y, et al. (2014) S100a8/a9 Released by CD11b+Gr1+ Neutrophils Activates Cardiac Fibroblasts to Initiate Angiotensin II-Induced Cardiac Inflammation and Injury. Hypertension. 2014 Apr 7. [Epub ahead of print] PMID: 24711518.

14. Yan L, Mathew L, Chellan B, Gardner B, Earley J, et al. (2014) S100/Calgranulin-mediated inflammation accelerates left ventricular hypertrophy and aortic valve sclerosis in chronic kidney disease in a receptor for advanced glycation end products-dependent manner. Arterioscler Thromb Vasc Biol 34(7): 1399–411.

15. Foris V, Kovacs G, Tscherner M, Olschewski A, Olschewski H (2013) Biomarkers in pulmonary hypertension: what do we know? Chest 144(1): 274–83. Review.

16. Neeper M, Schmidt AM, Brett J, Yan SD, Wang F, et al. (1992) Cloning and expression of a cell surface receptor for advanced glycosylation end products of proteins. J Biol Chem 267(21): 14998–5004.

17. Morbini P, Villa C, Campo I, Zorzetto M, Inghilleri S, et al. (2006) The receptor for advanced glycation end products and its ligands: a new inflammatory pathway in lung disease? Mod Pathol 19(11): 1437–45.

18. Bucciarelli LG, Wendt T, Qu W, Lu Y, Lalla E, et al. (2002) RAGE blockade stabilizes established atherosclerosis in diabetic apolipoprotein E-null mice. Circulation 106(22): 2827–35.

19. Ramasamy R, Yan SF, Herold K, Clynes R, Schmidt AM (2008) Receptor for advanced glycation end products: fundamental roles in the inflammatory response: winding the way to the pathogenesis of endothelial dysfunction and atherosclerosis. Ann N Y Acad Sci 1126: 7–13.

20. Yan SF, Ramasamy R, Naka Y, Schmidt AM (2003) Glycation, Inflammation, and RAGE: A Scaffold for the Macrovascular Complications of Diabetes and Beyond. Circ. Res 93;1159–1169.

21. Hofmann MA, Drury S, Fu C, Qu W, Taguchi A, et al. (1999) RAGE mediates a novel proinflammatory axis: a central cell surface receptor for S100/calgranulin polypeptides. Cell 97(7): 889–901.

22. Hori O, Brett J, Slattery T, Cao R, Zhang J, et al. (1995) The receptor for advanced glycation end products (RAGE) is a cellular binding site for amphoterin. Mediation of neurite outgrowth and co-expression of rage and amphoterin in the developing nervous system. J Biol Chem 270(43): 25752–61.

23. Yan SF, Ramasamy R, Bucciarelli LG, Wendt T, Lee LK, et al. (2004) RAGE and its ligands: a lasting memory in diabetic complications? Diab Vasc Dis Res 1(1): 10–20.

24. Wendt TM, Tanji N, Guo J, Kislinger TR, Qu W, et al. (2003) RAGE drives the development of glomerulosclerosis and impli-cates podocyte activation in the pathogenesis of diabetic nephropathy. Am J Pathol 162(4): 1123–37.

25. Lalla E, Lamster IB, Stern DM, Schmidt AM (2001) Receptor for advanced glycation end products, inflammation, and accelerated periodontal disease in diabetes: mechanisms and insights into therapeutic modalities. Ann Periodontol 6(1): 113–8. Review.

26. Hofmann MA, Drury S, Hudson BI, Gleason MR, Qu W, et al. (2002) RAGE and arthritis: the G82S polymorphism amplifies the inflammatory response. Genes Immun 3(3): 123–35.

27. Moser B, Szabolcs MJ, Ankersmit HJ, Lu Y, Qu W, et al. (2007) Blockade of RAGE suppresses alloimmune reactions in vitro and delays allograft rejection in murine heart transplantation. Am J Transplant 7(2): 293–302.

28. Maillard-Lefebvre H, Boulanger E, Daroux M, Gaxatte C, Hudson BI, et al. (2009) Soluble receptor for advanced glycation end products: a new biomarker in diagnosis and prognosis of chronic inflammatory diseases. Rheumatology (Oxford) 48(10): 1190–6.

29. Raucci A, Cugusi S, Antonelli A, Barabino SM, Monti L, et al. (2008) A soluble form of the receptor for advanced glycation endproducts (RAGE) is produced by proteolytic cleavage of the membrane-bound form by the sheddase a disintegrin and metalloprotease 10 (ADAM10). FASEB J 22(10): 3716–27.

30. Zhang L, Bukulin M, Kojro E, Roth A, Metz VV, et al. (2008) Receptor for advanced glycation end products is subjected to protein ectodomain shedding by metalloproteinases. J Biol Chem 283(51): 35507–16.

31. Kalea AZ, Schmidt AM, Hudson BI (2011) Alternative splicing of RAGE: roles in biology and disease. Front Biosci 1(17): 2756–2770.

32. Hudson BI, Carter AM, Harja E, Kalea AZ, Arriero M, et al. (2008) Identification, classification, and expression of RAGE gene splice variants. FASEB J 22(5): 1572–80.

33. Cheng C, Tsuneyama K, Kominami R, Shinohara H, Sakurai S, et al. (2005) Expression profiling of endogenous secretory receptor for advanced glycation end products in human organs. Mod Pathol 18(10): 1385–96.

34. Moser B, Janik S, Schiefer AI, Müllauer L, Bekos C, et al. (2014) Expression of RAGE and HMGB1 in thymic epithelial tumors, thymic hyperplasia and regular thymic morphology. PLoS One 9(4): e94118. doi: 10.1371/journal.-pone.0094118. eCollection 2014.

35. Prasad K (2014) Low levels of serum soluble receptors for advanced glycation end products, biomarkers for disease state: myth or reality. Int J Angiol 23(1): 11–6.

36. Koyama H, Yamamoto H, Nishizawa Y (2007) Endogenous Secretory RAGE as a Novel Biomarker for Metabolic Syndrome and Cardiovascular Diseases. Biomark Insights 2: 331–9.

37. Kang R, Zhang Q, Zeh HJ 3rd, Lotze MT, Tang D (2013) HMGB1 in Cancer: Good, Bad, or Both? Clin Cancer Res 19(15): 4046–57.

38. Sims GP, Rowe DC, Rietdijk ST, Herbst R, Coyle AJ (2010) HMGB1 and RAGE in inflammation and cancer. Annu Rev Immunol 28: 367–88. Review.

39. Park HY, Yun KH, Park DS (2009) Levels of Soluble Receptor for Advanced Glycation End Products in Acute Ischemic Stroke without a Source of Cardioembolism. J Clin Neurol 5(3): 126–32.

40. Naka Y, Bucciarelli LG, Wendt T, Lee LK, Rong LL, et al. (2004) RAGE axis: Animal models and novel insights into the vascular complications of diabe-tes. Arterioscler Thromb Vasc Biol 24(8): 1342–9.

41. Farmer DG, Kennedy S (2009) RAGE, vascular tone and vascular disease. Pharmacol Ther 124(2): 185–94. Review.

42. Meloche J, Courchesne A, Barrier M, Carter S, Bisserier M, et al. (2013) Critical role for the advanced glycation end-products receptor in pulmonary arterial hypertension etiology. J Am Heart Assoc 16;2(1): e005157.

43. Bauer EM, Shapiro R, Zheng H, Ahmad F, Ishizawa D, et al. (2013) High Mobility Group Box 1 Contributes to the Pathogenesis of Experimental Pulmonary Hypertension via Activation of Toll-like Receptor 4. Mol Med 18: 1509–18.

44. Farmer DG, Ewart MA, Mair KM, Kennedy S (2014) Soluble receptor for advanced glycation end products (sRAGE) attenuates haemodynamic changes to chronic hypoxia in the mouse. Pulm Pharmacol Ther 2014 Jan 10. pii: S1094–5539(14)00003–0. doi: 10.1016/j.pupt.2014.01.002. [Epub ahead of print].

45. Lang IM, Pesavento R, Bonderman D, Yuan JX (2013) Risk factors and basic mechanisms of chronic thromboembolic pulmonary hypertension: a current understanding. Eur Respir J 41(2): 462–8.

46. Firth AL, Yao W, Ogawa A, Madani MM, Lin GY, et al. (2010) Multipotent mesenchymal progenitor cells are present in endarterectomized tissues from patients with chronic thromboembolic pulmonary hypertension. Am J Physiol Cell Physiol 298(5): C1217–25.

47. Yao W, Firth AL, Sacks RS, Ogawa A, Auger WR, et al. (2009) Identification of putative endothelial progenitor cells (CD34+CD133+Flk-1+) in endarterecto-

48. mized tissue of patients with chronic thromboembolic pulmonary hypertension. Am J Physiol Lung Cell Mol Physiol 296(6): L870–8.

48. Maruoka M, Sakao S, Kantake M, Tanabe N, Kasahara Y, et al. (2012) Characterization of myofibroblasts in chronic thromboembolic pulmonary hypertension. Int J Cardiol 159(2): 119–27.

49. Jujo T, Sakao S, Kantake M, Maruoka M, Tanabe N, et al. (2012) Characterization of sarcoma-like cells derived from endarterectomized tissues from patients with CTEPH and establishment of a mouse model of pulmonary artery intimal sarcoma. Int J Oncol 41(2): 701–11.

50. Bauer EM, Shapiro R, Billiar TR, Bauer PM (2013) High mobility group Box 1 inhibits human pulmonary artery endothelial cell migration via a Toll-like receptor 4- and interferon response factor 3-dependent mechanism(s). J Biol Chem 288(2): 1365–73.

51. von Haehling S, von Bardeleben RS, Kramm T, Thiermann Y, Niethammer M, et al. (2010) Inflammation in right ventricular dysfunction due to thromboembolic pulmonary hypertension. Int J Cardiol 144(2): 206–11.

52. Anker SD, von Haehling S (2004) Inflammatory mediators in chronic heart failure: an overview. Heart 90(4): 464–70.

53. Vonk-Noordegraaf A, Haddad F, Chin KM, Forfia PR, Kawut SM, et al. (2013) Right heart adaptation to pulmonary arterial hypertension: physiology and pathobiology. J Am Coll Cardiol 62(25 Suppl): D22–33.

54. Sanz J, Dellegrottaglie S, Kariisa M, Sulica R, Poon M, et al. (2007) Prevalence and correlates of septal delayed contrast enhancement in patients with pulmonary hypertension. Am J Cardiol 100(4): 731–5.

55. Kasimir MT, Seebacher G, Jaksch P, Winkler G, Schmid K, et al. (2004) Reverse cardiac remodelling in patients with primary pulmonary hypertension after isolated lung transplantation. Eur J Cardiothorac Surg 26(4): 776–81.

56. Lu L, Zhang Q, Xu Y, Zhu ZB, Geng L, et al. (2010) Intra-coronary administration of soluble receptor for advanced glycation endproducts attenuates cardiac remodeling with decreased myocardial transforming growth factor-beta1 expression and fibrosis in minipigs with ischemia-reperfusion injury. Chin Med J (Engl) 123(5): 594–8.

57. Basta G, Corciu AI, Vianello A, Del Turco S, Foffa I, et al. (2010) Circulating soluble receptor for advanced glycation endproduct levels are decreased in patients with calcific aortic valve stenosis. Atherosclerosis 210(2): 614–8.

58. Calfee CS, Budev MM, Matthay MA, Church G, Brady S, et al. (2007) Plasma receptor for advanced glycation end-products predicts duration of ICU stay and mechanical ventilation in patients after lung transplantation. J Heart Lung Transplant 26(7): 675–80.

59. Christie JD, Shah CV, Kawut SM, Mangalmurti N, Lederer DJ, et al. (2009) Plasma levels of receptor for advanced glycation end products, blood transfusion, and risk of primary graft dysfunction. Am J Respir Crit Care Med. 2009 Nov 15;180(10): 1010–5.

60. Shah RJ, Bellamy SL, Lee JC, Cantu E, Diamond JM, et al. (2013) Early plasma soluble receptor for advanced glycation end-product levels are associated with bronchiolitis obliterans syndrome. Am J Transplant 13(3): 754–9.

61. Liu X, Chen Q, Shi S, Shi Z, Lin R, et al. (2012) Plasma sRAGE enables prediction of acute lung injury after cardiac surgery in children. Crit Care 16(3): R91.

62. Scheiber-Camoretti R, Mehrotra A, Yan L, Raman J, Beshai JF, et al. (2013) Elevated S100A12 and sRAGE are associated with increased length of hospitalization after non-urgent coronary artery bypass grafting surgery. Am J Cardiovasc Dis 3(2): 85–90.

63. Moser KM, Bloor CM (1993) Pulmonary vascular lesions occurring in patients with chronic major vessel thromboembolic pulmonary hypertension. Chest 103(3): 685–92.

64. Kim NH, Fesler P, Channick RN, Knowlton KU, Ben-Yehuda O, et al. (2004) Preoperative partitioning of pulmonary vascular resistance correlates with early outcome after thromboendarterectomy for chronic thromboembolic pulmonary hypertension. Circulation 109(1): 18–22.

65. Lang IM, Klepetko W (2008) Chronic thromboembolic pulmonary hyperten-sion: an updated review. Curr Opin Cardiol. 2008 Nov;23(6): 555–9.

66. Smith DJ, Yerkovich ST, Towers MA, Carroll ML, Thomas R, et al. (2011) Reduced soluble receptor for advanced glycation end-products in COPD. Eur Respir J 37(3): 516–22.

67. Cockayne DA, Cheng DT, Waschki B, Sridhar S, Ravindran P, et al. (2012) Systemic biomarkers of neutrophilic inflammation, tissue injury and repair in COPD patients with differing levels of disease severity. PLoS One 7(6): e38629. doi: 10.1371/journal.pone.0038629.

68. Cheng DT, Kim DK, Cockayne DA, Belousov A, Bitter H, et al. (2013) Systemic soluble receptor for advanced glycation endproducts is a biomarker of emphysema and associated with AGER genetic variants in patients with chronic obstructive pulmonary disease. Am J Respir Crit Care Med 188(8): 948–57.

14

MSC Therapy Attenuates Obliterative Bronchiolitis after Murine Bone Marrow Transplant

Kashif Raza[1¤a], **Trevor Larsen**[2ᕲ], **Nath Samaratunga**[2ᕲ], **Andrew P. Price**[3], **Carolyn Meyer**[3], **Amy Matson**[3¤b], **Michael J. Ehrhardt**[3], **Samuel Fogas**[3], **Jakub Tolar**[3], **Marshall I. Hertz**[1], **Angela Panoskaltsis-Mortari**[1,3]*

1 Pulmonary, Allergy, Critical Care and Sleep Medicine, University of Minnesota, Minneapolis, Minnesota, United States of America, 2 Breck High School, Edina, Minnesota, United States of America, 3 Pediatric Blood and Bone Marrow Transplant Program, University of Minnesota Cancer Center, Minneapolis, Minnesota, United States of America

Abstract

Rationale: Obliterative bronchiolitis (OB) is a significant cause of morbidity and mortality after lung transplant and hematopoietic cell transplant. Mesenchymal stromal cells (MSCs) have been shown to possess immunomodulatory properties in chronic inflammatory disease.

Objective: Administration of MSCs was evaluated for the ability to ameliorate OB in mice using our established allogeneic bone marrow transplant (BMT) model.

Methods: Mice were lethally conditioned and received allogeneic bone marrow without (BM) or with spleen cells (BMS), as a source of OB-causing T-cells. Cell therapy was started at 2 weeks post-transplant, or delayed to 4 weeks when mice developed airway injury, defined as increased airway resistance measured by pulmonary function test (PFT). BM-derived MSC or control cells [mouse pulmonary vein endothelial cells (PVECs) or lung fibroblasts (LFs)] were administered. Route of administration [intratracheally (IT) and IV] and frequency (every 1, 2 or 3 weeks) were compared. Mice were evaluated at 3 months post-BMT.

Measurements and Main Results: No ectopic tissue formation was identified in any mice. When compared to BMS mice receiving control cells or no cells, those receiving MSCs showed improved resistance, compliance and inspiratory capacity. Interim PFT analysis showed no difference in route of administration. Improvements in PFTs were found regardless of dose frequency; but once per week worked best even when administration began late. Mice given MSC also had decreased peribronchiolar inflammation, lower levels of hydroxyproline (collagen) and higher frequencies of macrophages staining for the alternatively activated macrophage (AAM) marker CD206.

Conclusions: These results warrant study of MSCs as a potential management option for OB in lung transplant and BMT recipients.

Editor: Peter Chen, Cedars-Sinai Medical Center, United States of America

Funding: This work was supported by National Heart, Lung and Blood Institute R01HL55209 (APM), National Institute of Arthritis and Musculoskeletal and Skin Diseases R01 AR063070 (JT), R01 AR059947 (JT), and T32 HL07741 ("Training in Lung Science" training grant support of KR). The confocal microscope was purchased through an NCRR Shared instrumentation grant (National Center for Research Resources grant 1S10RR16851). The funders had no role in study design, data collection and analysis, decision to publish, or preparation of the manuscript.

Competing Interests: The authors have declared that no competing interests exist.

* Email: panos001@umn.edu

ᕲ These authors contributed equally to this work.

¤a Current address: Department of Medicine, Columbia University, New York, New York, United States of America
¤b Current address: Georgetown Medical School, Washington, D.C., United States of America

Introduction

Obliterative bronchiolitis (OB) is a significant problem in lung transplant and BMT recipients. OB is directly or indirectly responsible for almost 40% of lung transplant related deaths [1]. This is mainly due to chronic allograft dysfunction, manifesting as OB, characterized histologically by inflammation and fibrosis of small airways. In BMT recipients, the incidence of OB has been reported to be as high as 29% with increased risk of mortality and is associated with chronic graft-versus-host disease (GVHD) [2,3].

After transplant, the host immune system is activated by exposure to allogeneic tissue antigens, resulting in an inflammatory cascade with alloimmune and non-alloimmune dependent factors contributing to the response. The cumulative end result of this cascade is OB [4]. Current management strategies involving immunosuppressive medications have not been very successful.

Lack of suitable animal models has limited efforts to understand and develop therapeutic strategies for OB. We have previously reported a new murine BMT model, in which chronic GVHD leads to OB similar to the chronic rejection seen in lung transplantation [5].

MSCs provide a promising management option for this population. They have immunomodulatory properties, among which is their ability to suppress T-lymphocyte activation and proliferation, key events in allograft rejection [6]. MSCs have been shown to inhibit maturation of dendritic cells and promote secretion of anti-inflammatory cytokines, resulting in generation of Tregs(reviewed in [7]). Tregs can suppress effector FoxP3[negative] cells and antigen presenting cells (APCs) thereby inhibiting inflammatory responses. MSCs and MSC-induced Tregs are capable of generating alternatively activated macrophages (AAMs), which are immunosuppressive and inhibit the proliferation of activated CD4[+] T cells [8].

MSCs have been used successfully to prolong allograft survival in other animal models of organ transplantation [9,10,11]. Donor human lungs (rejected for transplant) infused with MSCs have improved alveolar fluid clearance compared to the current state of the art technique [12]. In the context of BMT, MSCs have shown efficacy in ameliorating graft-versus-host-disease (GVHD) [13,14,15] and have been approved for steroid-refractory acute GVHD. They have been used safely as a co-infusion in patients undergoing unrelated allogeneic bone marrow transplant [16]. MSCs have not been previously evaluated as a cell therapy for OB post-BMT although they have been studied many times in other lung injury models where they are given as either a pretreatment or concomitantly with injury induction (reviewed in [17,18,19]. A number of clinical trials in a variety of lung diseases are underway using these cells to further establish their safety and efficacy [20]. In the present study, we tested the hypothesis that exogenous MSCs will reduce the occurrence and severity of OB in our murine model. We found that administration of MSCs attenuated injury and airway lumen obliteration and led to improvement of lung function even if given after lung function had declined.

Methods

Ethics Statement

All experiments were approved by the University of Minnesota Institutional Animal Care and Use Committee (assurance #A3456-01, IACUC # 0906A67041).

Bone marrow transplantation

Our BMT protocol has been described [5]. Recipient female B10.BR mice [lethally conditioned with cyclophosphamide 120 mg/kg/d on days -3,-2 (Bristol Myers Squibb, Seattle, WA) and 7.5 Gy irradiation on day -1] were given male C57BL/6J (B6) donor BM (15×10^6, T-cell depleted) without or with 2×10^6 B6 spleen cells via caudal vein. All experiments were approved by the University of Minnesota Institutional Animal Care and Use Committee (assurance #A3456-01, IACUC # 0906A67041). The results of 5 transplant experiments were used for this study, with each experiment consisting of at least 5 mice per group.

Isolation of MSCs

MSCs were isolated from male B6 GFP transgenic mice as described [21]. After 4 weeks of initial culture, adherent cells were plated at 50 cells/cm^2 in Iscove's modified Dulbecco medium (Invitrogen), 9% FCS, 9% horse serum, pen-strep, and 2 μM L-glutamine. Cells were expanded at low density (50–100 cells/cm^2) with medium replaced every 3–4 days. Consistent with the reported results of the Prockop lab [21], the MSCs demonstrated high expression of CD106 (86%), Sca-1 & CD44 (both 98%), low/very low expression of CD45 (3–4%), CD31 (<2%), CD117 (2%), CD90 (<2%) and MHC I (13%) (Figure S1). They were negative for MHC II. MSCs displayed osteocyte, chondrocyte and adipocyte trilineage differentiation as we have previously shown [22].

Control cells

Since many cell types can produce beneficial mediators, control cells were used to demonstrate the specificity of the cell therapy effect to MSCs.

PVECs were isolated in the lab of Dr. Robert Hebbel (UMN). Briefly, pulmonary vein from B6 mice was cut into pieces and treated with collagenase II. PVECs were grown using the method developed for microvascular endothelial cells [23]. The resulting cells were identified as endothelial by positive staining for CD31, von Willebrand factor, VE-cadherin, VCAM-1, and flk-1; and negative staining for vimentin and smooth-muscle actin.

Mouse lung fibroblasts (LFs) were isolated as described [24] from B6 mice. Fibroblasts were maintained in DMEM, 10% FBS, L-glutamine and pen-strep until time of administration.

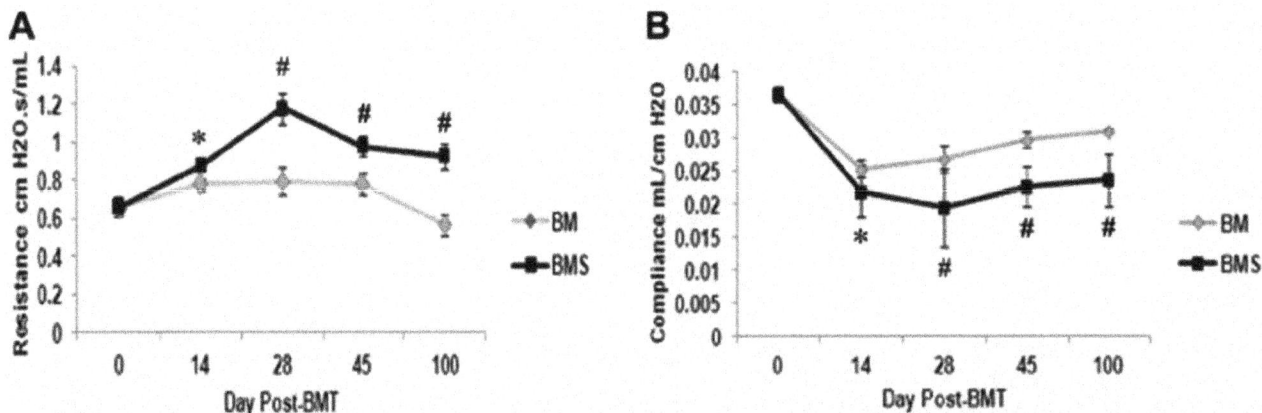

Figure 1. Kinetics of pulmonary function parameters post-BMT show that OB manifestations begin as early as 2 weeks. Lethally conditioned B10.BR mice were given B6 BM with (■BMS) or without (◇BM) spleen cells. PFTs were done on the days indicated sequentially on the same mice. **A**. Resistance; **B**. Compliance. *$p<0.05$ vs day 0 for BMS (OB) group. #$p<0.05$ BMS vs BM group. N = 5–40/group/time point pooled from 4 experiments.

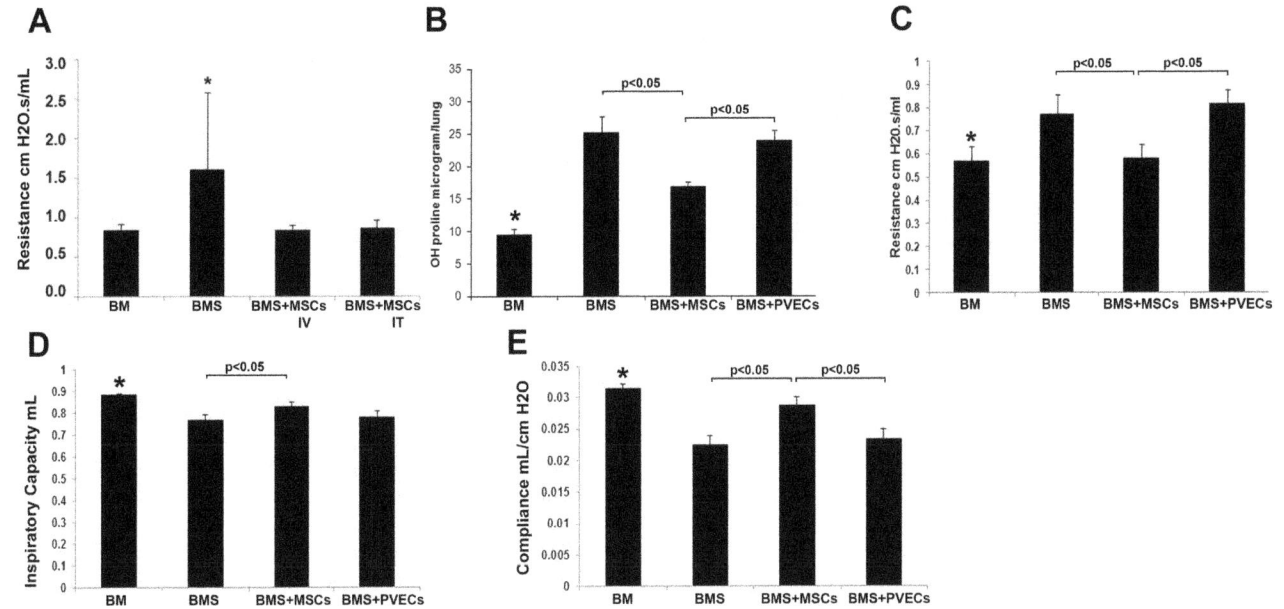

Figure 2. Early administration of MSC reduces post BMT manifestations of OB. Starting at 2 weeks post-BMT, MSCs or PVECs were administered IV or IT weekly and evaluated on day 90 post-BMT. **A.** Interim analysis at day 60 post-BMT shows equivalent efficacy of MSCs administered by either the IV or IT route as assessed by improved (reduced) airway resistance. N = 4–6/group, *p = 0.03 vs all other groups. **B.** Day 90 post-BMT hydroxyproline levels indicating degree of fibrosis is significantly reduced by administration of MSCs. *p<0.05 vs all other groups; other significant differences indicated on graph. N = 4–7/group, IV and IT combined) **C, D, E.** Improved day 90 post-BMT airway resistance, inspiratory capacity and compliance, respectively, by administration of MSCs. *p<0.05 vs BMS and BMS+PVECs; other significant differences indicated on graph. N = 4–7/group, IV and IT combined. PVECs = pulmonary vein endothelial cells used as control cells. All data are pooled from 2 experiments.

Administration of experimental and control cells

Cohorts of mice receiving BMS received either 10^4 passage 2–5 MSCs or control cells in a 50 µL aliquot of culture medium intra-tracheally (IT, under anesthesia with intubation under direct visualization) or IV starting at either 2 weeks or IV starting at 4 weeks post-BMT and continued up to 14 weeks post-BMT (given every 1, 2 or 3 weeks). BMS mice not receiving cell therapy were given non-conditioned medium alone.

Pulmonary Function Tests

PFTs were assessed by whole body plethysmography using the Flexivent system (Scireq, Montreal, PQ, Canada) as described previously [5]. The maximum pressure was set to 30 cmH$_2$O. The positive end-expiratory pressure remained constant at 2.5 cm H$_2$O.

Histopathology and OH-proline Quantification

Tissue preparation was done as described [5]. Cryosections (6 µm) were stained by H&E for pathological analysis. Lung pathology was assessed using a semi-quantitative (0–4 grade) scoring system [5]. Four sections from each lung were evaluated. OH-proline levels were determined by oxidation of 4-OH-L-proline to pyrrole and reaction with p-dimethylaminobenzalde-hyde (absorbance read at 560 nm).

Immunofluorescence

Immunofluorescence staining was used to detect AAMs and Tregs on serial sections as described [25]. Tregs were detected using biotinylated anti-FoxP3 (FJK16s; eBioscience) with strepta-vidin-cyanin 3 (Jackson ImmunoResearch) and FITC-anti-CD4. Macrophages were stained with CD11c (BDPharmingen) for conventional M1 macrophages and polyclonal rabbit IgG anti-

CD206 (Santa Cruz) followed by cyanin 3-labeled anti-rabbit antibody (Jackson) to identify AAMs (M2 macrophages). Images were acquired on an Olympus FluoView 500 BX51 confocal microscope and FluoView software version 4.3.

Flow Cytometry

Antibodies with specificity for CD4, FoxP3, CD 206 and F4/80 were obtained from eBioscience. For cell number quantification, PE, PerCP and APC labeled counting beads (Invitrogen) were used. Explanted lungs were digested in collagenase containing PBS for 60 minutes at 37C. Single cell suspension was obtained by passing the cells through 40 um cell strainer (BD). For intracellular cytokine staining, cells were stained for CD4, fixed, and permeabilized using the Fix&Perm kit (BD) and stained with antibody to FoxP3. Cells were analyzed on a 4-color FACS Calibur instrument (BD) with FlowJo version 8.8.

qRT-PCR

Total RNA was extracted from lungs on day 90 post-BMT using Trizol (Life Technologies, Grand Island, NY), purified using the PureLink RNA MiniKit (Life Technologies), and cDNA generated by reverse transcription with the Superscript III kit (Invitrogen) following manufacturer's instructions. Quantitative real-time PCR was performed on an ABI 7500 Real Time PCR System using TaqMan Gene Expression Master Mix (Applied Biosystems). Mouse probes for GAPDH (Mm99999915_g1), IL-10 (Mm00439615_g1) and CD206 (Mm01329362_m1) were purchased from Life Technologies (Grand Island, NY).

Cytokine Analysis

Cell culture supernatants (48-hours) were analyzed in duplicate by ELISA using kits: PGE2 (multi-species), rat IL-1RA, rat IL-10

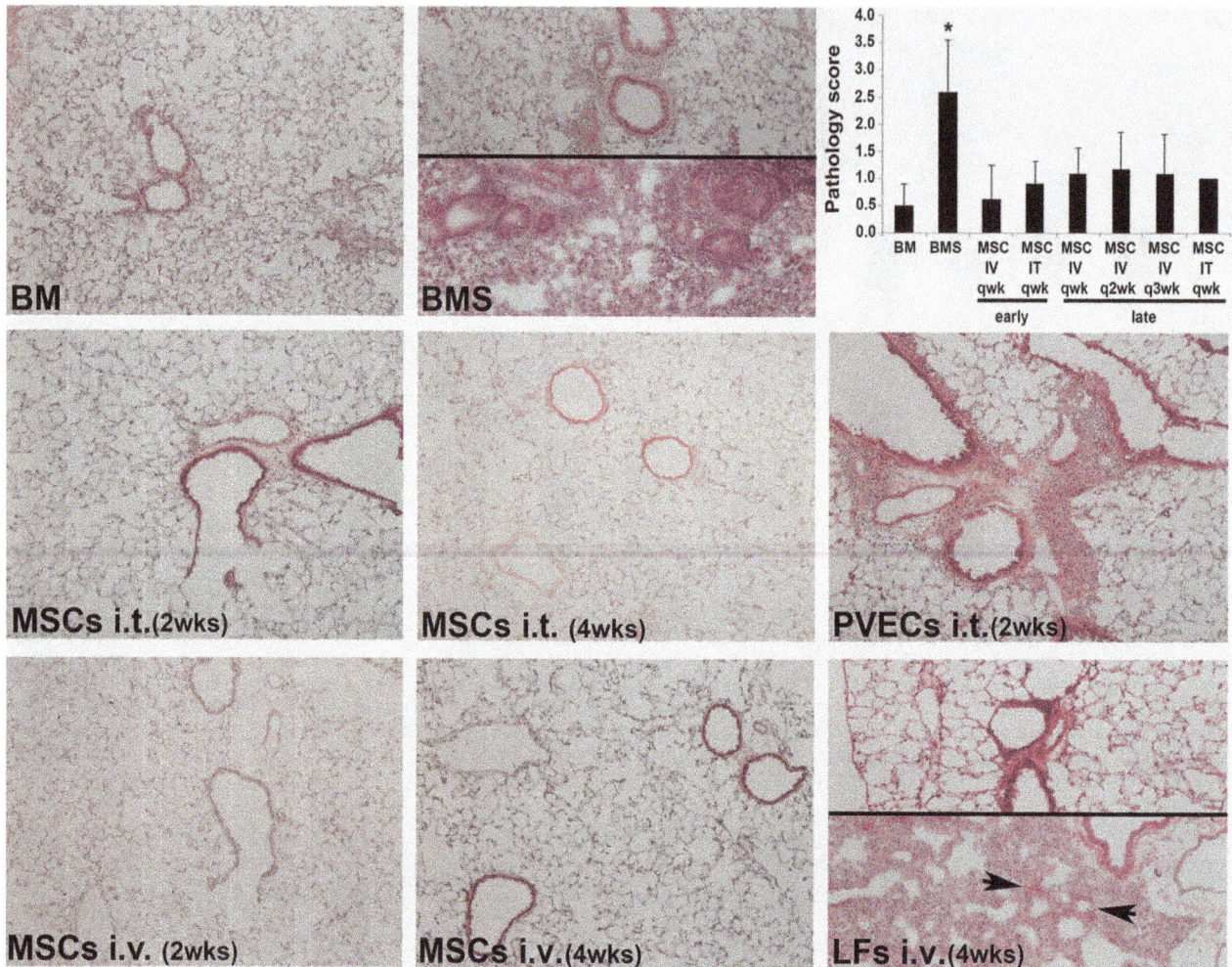

Figure 3. Administration of MSC post-BMT reduces OB histopathology. Representative H&E stained lung cryosections of day 90 post-BMT shown for mice receiving T cell-depleted bone marrow only (**BM**); BM and allogeneic splenocytes (**BMS**; OB group). The split panels show the range of injury in this model. **MSCs IV** or **IT** as indicated, beginning at 2 or 4 weeks and given weekly; **PVECs IT** beginning at 2 weeks and given weekly; **LFs IV** beginning at 4 weeks and given weekly until day 90. The split panels show the range of injury seen in this group similar to the BMS group. Original magnification 200× (20× objective lens). The top right corner panel shows semiquantitative pathology scores; n = 4–6/group pooled from 4 experiments.

(R&D Systems, Minneapolis, MN); FGF7/KGF (BlueGene, Shanghai); MPO (RayBioTech, Norcross, GA); TSG6 (MyBiosource, San Diego, CA). Other cytokines were evaluated on a Luminex (Austin, TX) using rat-specific bead sets: FasL, G-CSF, GM-CSF, IFNγ, IL-4, IL-12p40&p70, LIX, RANTES (Millipore, Billerica, MA); PAI-1, CXCL1, TNFα, IL1α, IL-2, IL-4, IL-6 (R&D Systems).

Statistical Analysis

Data were analyzed by analysis of variance or t test with significance at $P \leq 0.05$. Numerical data are shown as the mean ± standard error.

Results

Determination of time points for cell therapy intervention for OB

To understand the kinetics of OB development, and to define time points for intervention in each experiment, PFTs were done in individual mice sequentially at defined time points post-BMT.

(**Figure 1**) In the BMS mice (OB group), lung resistance and compliance deteriorated from 2 weeks post-BMT and diverged from the BM group at 4 weeks post-BMT. All mice, including those receiving BM only, have some reduction in lung function early after BMT; i.e. BMS mice were not statistically different from BM mice at 2 weeks. This resolves in BM mice as they recover and are hematopoietically rescued. Thus, an intervention would be more meaningful if it could be done when the beginning of OB manifestations can be clearly identified. In subsequent experiments, we considered these two times as points of intervention, with the 2 week point as "early" and the 4 week time point as "late" cell therapy. The initial decline in lung function by PFTs was confirmed for every mouse prior to cell therapy.

Early administration of MSCs resolves OB after BMT

Mice receiving BMS were given either MSCs or PVECs weekly starting at 2 weeks post-BMT (i.e. early). Interim analysis at day 60 post-BMT demonstrated that MSCs were equally as effective when administered via either the IV or IT route as shown by

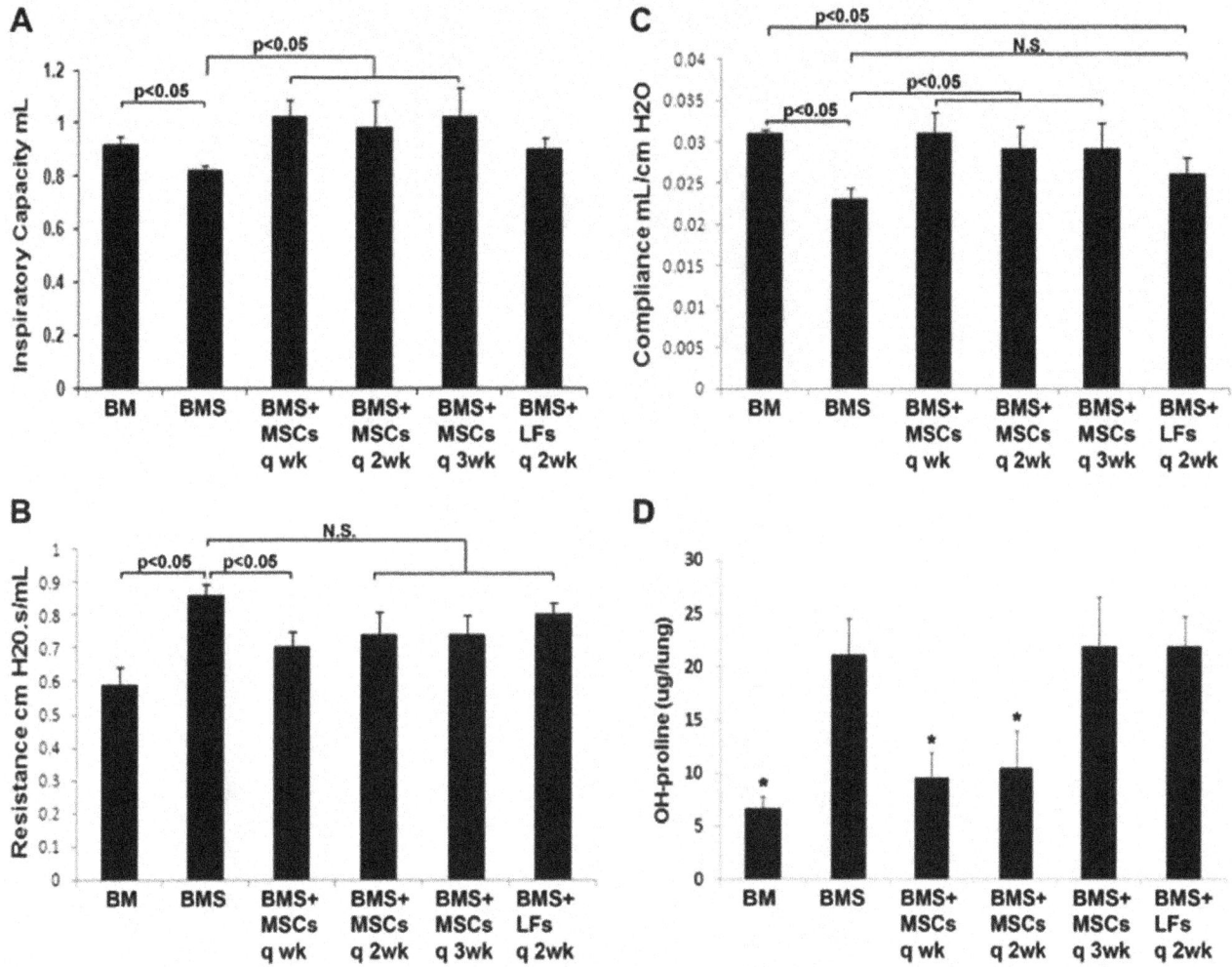

Figure 4. Late administration of MSC post-BMT reduces manifestations of OB. Starting at 4 weeks post-BMT, MSCs were administered IV every 1, 2 or 3 weeks until day 90. A. Inspiratory Capacity; B. Resistance; C. Compliance; D. OH-proline. Significant differences are indicated on graph. N = 6–14/group pooled from 2 experiments. LFs = mouse lung fibroblasts used as control cells.

reduced airways resistance in **Figure 2A**. However, repeated anesthesia for the IT administration took a toll on survival and subsequent data were combined. At day 90 post-BMT, consistent with our documented published mouse model, OB (BMS) mice exhibited increased levels of OH-proline, increased airways resistance, decreased inspiratory capacity and compliance (**Figure 2B, C, D&E**). Mice receiving MSCs had reduced levels of lung OH-proline, reduced airways resistance, increased inspiratory capacity and compliance compared to mice receiving control cells (PVECs) or medium only (BMS mice). Histopathologic examination showed extensive peribronchiolar inflammation in groups receiving BMS or PVECs after BMT (**Figure 3**); inflammation was not seen in mice given MSCs. Semi-quantitative pathologic scores were consistent with the above biochemical and physiologic parameters (graph in **Figure 3**). No ectopic tissue formation was found. Therefore, early administration of MSCs at a point when lung function begins to decline had a significant beneficial impact and led to reduction of OB manifestations.

Late administration of MSCs attenuates airway injury and improves PFT parameters after BMT

Mice receiving BMS were given either MSCs or LFs IV starting at 4 weeks post-BMT (i.e. late). To determine how frequently cells needed to be administered for benefit to be achieved, cell therapy was compared for administration every 1, 2 or 3 weeks. Mice receiving MSCs exhibited improved inspiratory capacity and lung compliance compared to BMS mice and those receiving control cells, even if cells were given only every 3 weeks (**Figure 4A and C**). The increase in resistance and OH-proline was attenuated in mice given MSCs every week (**Figure 4B & D**); q2week and q3week MSC groups also had lower resistance but it was not statistically significant compared to BMS mice. Mice given late administration of MSCs had histologically normal lungs (**Figure 3**). Therefore, late administration of MSCs at a point when lung function begins to decline had a significant beneficial impact and led to reduction of OB manifestations.

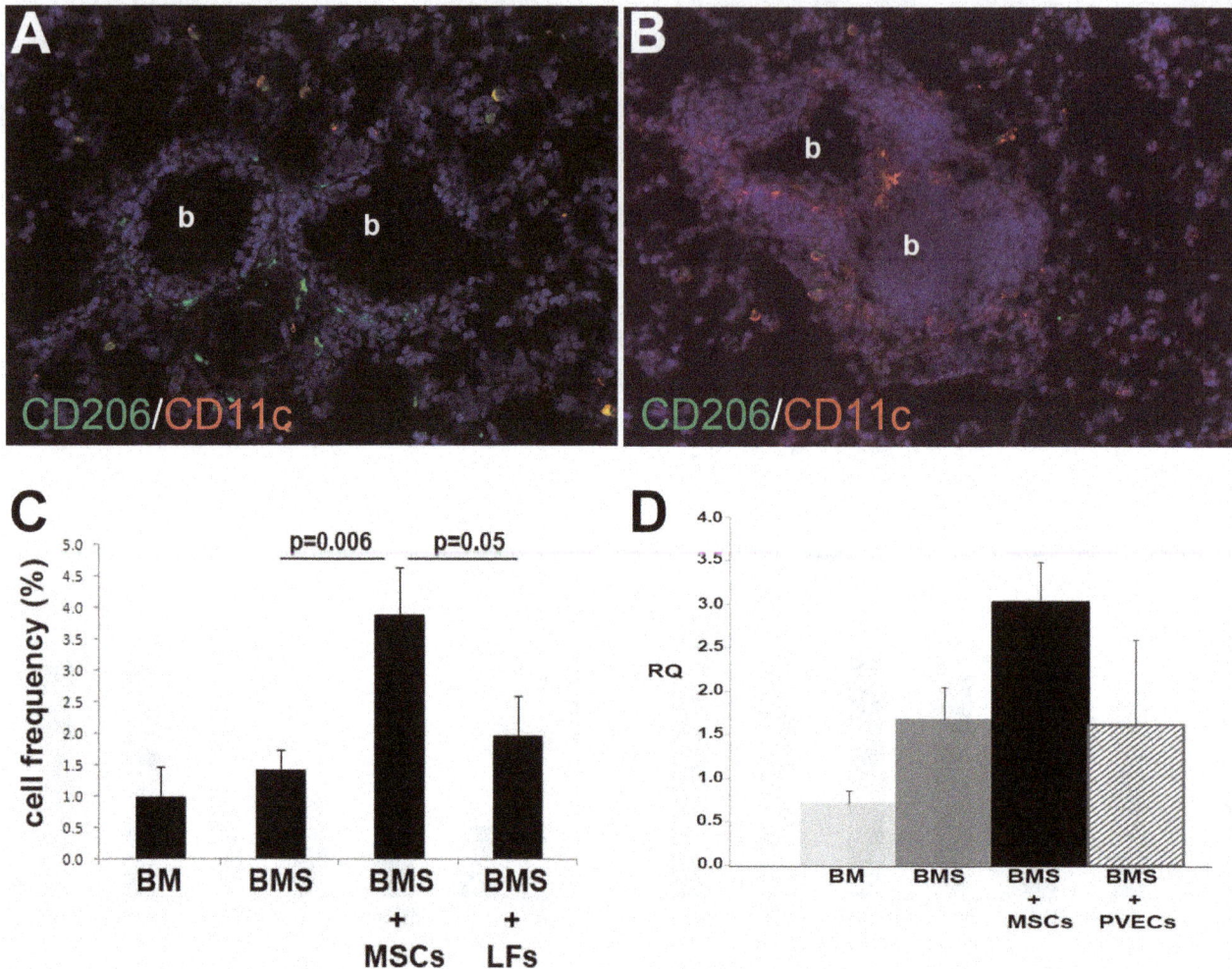

Figure 5. Increased expression of markers of AAMs in lungs of mice given MSC post-BMT. Starting at 4 weeks post-BMT, MSCs (**A**) or LFs (**B**) were administered IV weekly and evaluated on day 90 post-BMT. Lung cryosections were immunofluorescently stained for CD11c with CD206 (**A, B**) and frequency of CD206$^+$ cells was determined as a percent of total nucleated cells (data in **C** shown as mean ± SE, n = 5–7/group pooled from 2 experiments). Images are at 400X total magnification; "b" indicates bronchiolar airway. In **D**, cell therapy (IT, weekly) was started at 2 weeks and lungs examined on day 90 post-BMT by qRT-PCR for CD206 (n = 3/group).

Increased frequencies of AAMs in lungs of mice receiving MSCs

In order to determine the possible mechanism by which MSCs were ameliorating OB after BMT, lungs were examined for presence of AAMs. Immunofluorescence staining showed increased frequencies of CD206+ cells, indicative of AAMs, in the mice receiving MSCs (**Figure 5 A**) compared to those receiving control LFs (**Figure 5B**) or no cell therapy (compiled data shown in **Figure 5C**). **Figure 5D** shows that qRT-PCR analysis for CD206 expression in the lungs was also consistent with the increased presence of AAMs in MSC-treated mice. Flow cytometric analysis of lungs from a small cohort of mice also showed increased CD206$^+$ macrophages as well as an increase in CD4$^+$/FoxP3$^+$ cells albeit not reaching statistical significance due to small sample size (**Figure S2**).

Differential expression of cytokines identify TSG-6, FGF-7 and IL-1ra as potential mediators of anti-OB activity

In order to demonstrate that the beneficial effect of MSCs on OB was MSC-related, we compared the cytokine secretion profile

of MSCs with PVECs and LFs that were used as control cells. **Table 1** shows the mediators that were detected among the many cytokines we were able to test for (listed in methods). As shown in Table 1, several mediators were produced by all 3 cell types, namely, IL-6, CXCL1, and PAI-1. PGE2 was produced by both MSCs and LFs at equivalent levels. IL-1ra was also found in MSCs and LFs but to a higher level in MSCs. The only mediators found to be exclusively secreted by the MSCs were TSG6, FGF7 (KGF) and GM-CSF. Although IL-10 secretion by the MSCs was not detected in vitro, it does not negate their ability to secrete it in vivo after infusion. Analysis of IL-10 expression in lungs of mice given MSCs weekly starting at 2 weeks post-BMT, as assessed by qRT-PCR, revealed no increase (in fact it was lower) compared to mice given control, or no, cell therapy (**Figure S3**). Thus, potential effectors of the immunomodulatory activity of MSCs are TSG6, FGF7, GM-CSF and possibly IL-1ra.

Discussion

In this study, we have shown that cell therapy with MSCs can ameliorate OB in a murine BMT model. To our knowledge, this is

Table 1. Comparison of cytokine secretion.

Cells	PGE2	IL-1RA	TSG6	FGF7	GM-CSF	IL-6	CXCL1	PAI-1	G-CSF	LIX
MSC	++	++	++	+	+	+	++	+++	-	-
PVEC	-	-	-	-	-	+	++	+++	++	+
LF	++	+	-	-	-	+	++	+	+/-	-

Key: +++ = >1,000 pg/mL; ++ = 100–1000 pg/mL; + = 10–99 pg/mL; +/- = <10pg/mL; - = not detectable.

the first report to explore the impact of delayed administration of MSCs on development of OB in an experimental model system. Our intent was not to prove the mechanism of action but to demonstrate the potential of MSCs to treat OB and to determine some parameters of cell administration. In our study, we have shown the beneficial impact of MSCs not only when administered early but also when administered late, after the onset of OB has been confirmed by decline in PFTs.

In our current study, the MSCs used were syngeneic to the donor (i.e. autologous to the new immune system, but allogeneic to the recipient). In the clinical experience of MSCs for HSCT, the MSCs have been third party [26]. They are considered to be relatively immunoprivileged and their allogenicity has not been an issue in several studies [27,28]. However, many studies have shown allogeneic MSCs to be immunogenic, especially when pretreated with IFNγ ([29] and reviewed in [30]). IFNγγ pretreatment increases expression of immunosuppressive molecules by MSCs but also induces MHC Class II expression, enhancing their rejection [30]. There are certainly pros and cons in using either auto- or allogeneic MSCs, with or without IFNγ induction, encompassing their engraftment, immunosuppressive abilities and unwanted accelerated organ rejection, especially in the presence of donor-specific alloantibodies. The choice of optimal MSC preparation may depend on whether the disease indication is acute or chronic. It is also not resolved whether it is desirable to have MSCs persist long term at the site of injury.

MSCs in our study were administered in small doses at regular intervals to achieve the desired effect. This allows the possibility to achieve a favorable response by using smaller numbers of cells in a patient population using a strategy that can be very helpful in the clinical setting [10,31] where MSCs are more easily administered via an intravenous versus an intra-tracheal route. IV administration was used in recently reported early phase clinical trials for idiopathic pulmonary fibrosis and COPD and was shown to be safe [32,33]. IT administration was also safe [34]. We compared the IT to the IV route of administration and found in interim analysis that there was no difference when administration began early (i.e. at 2 weeks). However, we found that the mice did not tolerate the multiple anesthesias well in the context of the IT procedure, regardless of cell type given, at the late time points when lung function had declined significantly. Therefore, the IV route was considered the best option for late administration.

The administration of exogenous MSCs resulted in improved lung histology and pulmonary function tests. Administration of MSCs also resulted in increases of cells with morphology consistent with alternatively activated macrophages (AAMs) which have immunosuppressive properties [35]. In addition, MSC-treated mice had a statistical trend toward increased CD4+Foxp3+ cells, consistent with Tregs, as has been described earlier [36], including in a tracheal transplant model [37]. Generation of AAMs under the influence of MSCs has been reported [38,39]. It is interesting that CD11c expression was low in the lungs of MSC-treated mice. CD11c is expressed by lung macrophages, in contrast to macrophages from other organs and tissues. To our knowledge, it has not been described that AAM (M2) macrophages in the lung lose CD11c expression. However, it is known that the lung environment affects CD11c expression/upregulation and that GM-CSF is one of the factors that stimulates CD11c expression by lung macrophages (or of macrophages from other areas that are exposed to the lung environment) [40]. Indeed, our cytokine analysis did show that the MSCs produced GM-CSF in culture. We hypothesize that MSC-derived GM-CSF has affected the phenotype of the recruited macrophages.

A recent study has shown the beneficial effect of MSCs in the orthotopic tracheal transplant OB model being due to MSC-derived PGE2 leading to increased IL-10 levels in the tracheal graft [41]. Increased IL-10 was also found in MSC-treated mice with a heterotopic tracheal transplant [42]. However, our cytokine analysis indicated that PGE2-mediated IL-10 increase was not likely the mechanism responsible since LFs also produced PGE2 but did not ameliorate OB. Furthermore, we found no increase in IL-10 in the recipient lungs of MSC-treated mice compared to controls. Future studies using neutralizing antibodies to PGE2 and/or IL-10 (or IL-10$^{-/-}$ MSCs) are required to eliminate these mediators as effectors of donor MSCs in this model. Despite this, the in vitro production of PGE2 by our MSCs classifies them as anti-inflammatory MSC2 cells [43].

The beneficial effect of MSCs could be due to the immuno-regulatory properties of the MSCs directly by virtue of the mediators they produce, or indirectly by the generation of Tregs and AAMs. Other possible mechanisms include mitochondrial transfer to rescue stressed cells and improve cellular bioenergetics and function to allow for more efficient repair, as has been elegantly demonstrated previously [44]. Oxidative stress of lung epithelium has been demonstrated in humans with OB after lung transplant and in mice with induced alloimmune activation [45,46,47]. In addition, we have previously shown that the lungs are under oxidative stress after BMT in our mouse model and that this could be normalized by treatment with KGF, a factor typically secreted by MSCs [48]. In our current study, we never found engraftment of MSCs in the lungs consistent with the findings of many other groups in acute lung injury models. We did not find any effect on donor BM engraftment as demonstrated by others (albeit in a non-myeloablative setting) [49], as all recipient mice were found to be >95% donor engrafted (data not shown). Perhaps this is due to the administration of cells at a time sufficiently removed from the peri-BMT period in our study.

Our cytokine analysis comparing MSCs to the control cells identified TSG6, FGF7, GM-CSF and possibly IL-1ra as potential mediators of the MSC effect, although neutralizing antibodies or knockout approaches would be required to confirm this. The Prockop group has identified TSG6 as an anti-inflammatory mediator produced by MSCs that can ameliorate LPS- and bleomycin-induced lung injury in mice when given systemically in the early stages of inflammation [50,51]. MSCs injected into skin wounds controlled macrophage activation and limited fibrosis through a TSG6 mechanism in a murine model [52]. FGF7, also known as KGF, has been shown to be effective in preclinical models of lung injury including acute lung injury [53] and post-BMT-induced idiopathic pneumonia syndrome when given as a pretreatment [54]. In a recent study, human MSCs improved alveolar fluid clearance in human donor lungs (rejected for transplant), most likely by a KGF-mediated mechanism since anti-KGF neutralizing antibody abrogated the effect [12]. This demonstrated benefit could lead to an increase in the number of donor lungs suitable for transplantation. However, it has been demonstrated many times that KGF has little beneficial effect when given after injury, making its usefulness for OB less likely, although it is possible that it aids in preventing further injury, thus enabling repair. A recent study of repeated bleomycin-induced

lung injury did demonstrate that a slight (3-day) delay in administering MSCs could ameliorate inflammation and fibrosis, possibly through secretion of IL-1RA [55]. IL-1ra has also been shown to mediate beneficial effects of MSCs in murine lung injury models, but, again, only when given as a pre-treatment [56]. Notwithstanding the non-exhaustive list of analytes we were able to assay for, TSG6 stands out as the most likely candidate for the MSC effect, although adjunct activity of the aforementioned cytokines cannot be ruled out.

Further studies will be needed to determine the impact of MSC administration in combination with immunosuppressive medications to further evaluate their potential application in lung transplant recipients. More studies on the minimal effective dose and the need for cells versus cell-derived factors are also needed. MSCs have also been shown to have antimicrobial properties against a variety of pathogens [57]. As lung transplant and HCT recipients are at increased risk of opportunistic infections due to immunosuppressive medications, this may provide an additional advantage. All these characteristics make MSCs an attractive management option for lung transplant recipients which merits further evaluation and will hopefully show some promising results in an ongoing clinical trial led by the Chambers group in Australia (trial #NCT01175655).

Acknowledgments

We thank Julia Nguyen in Dr. Bob Hebbel's lab (UMN) for providing PVECs and Mrs. Lily Xia for isolating mouse BM-MSCs. We also thank the UMN Cytokine Reference Laboratory. The confocal microscope was purchased through a NCRR Shared Instrumentation Grant (1S10RR16851).

Author Contributions

Conceived and designed the experiments: KR APP JT MIH AP-M. Performed the experiments: KR TL NS APP AM CM MJE SF. Analyzed the data: KR TL NS APP AM CM AP-M. Contributed reagents/materials/analysis tools: JT. Wrote the paper: KR APP JT MIH AP-M.

References

1. Christie JD, Edwards LB, Kucheryavaya AY, Aurora P, Dobbels F, et al. (2010) The Registry of the International Society for Heart and Lung Transplantation: twenty-seventh official adult lung and heart-lung transplant report–2010. J Heart Lung Transplant 29: 1104–1118.

2. Panoskaltsis-Mortari A, Griese M, Madtes DK, Belperio JA, Haddad IY, et al. (2011) An official American Thoracic Society research statement: noninfectious lung injury after hematopoietic stem cell transplantation: idiopathic pneumonia syndrome. Am J Respir Crit Care Med 183: 1262–1279.

3. Williams KM, Hnatiuk O, Mitchell SA, Baird K, Gadalla SM, et al. (2014) NHANES III equations enhance early detection and mortality prediction of bronchiolitis obliterans syndrome after hematopoietic SCT. Bone Marrow Transplant 49: 561–566.

4. Belperio JA, Weigt SS, Fishbein MC, Lynch JP 3rd (2009) Chronic lung allograft rejection: mechanisms and therapy. Proc Am Thorac Soc 6: 108–121.

5. Panoskaltsis-Mortari A, Tram KV, Price AP, Wendt CH, Blazar BR (2007) A new murine model for bronchiolitis obliterans post-bone marrow transplant. Am J Respir Crit Care Med 176: 713–723.

6. Di Nicola M, Carlo-Stella C, Magni M, Milanesi M, Longoni PD, et al. (2002) Human bone marrow stromal cells suppress T-lymphocyte proliferation induced by cellular or nonspecific mitogenic stimuli. Blood 99: 3838–3843.

7. Burr SP, Dazzi F, Garden OA (2013) Mesenchymal stromal cells and regulatory T cells: the Yin and Yang of peripheral tolerance. Immunol Cell Biol 91: 12–18.

8. Tiemessen MM, Jagger AL, Evans HG, van Herwijnen MJ, John S, et al. (2007) CD4+CD25+Foxp3+ regulatory T cells induce alternative activation of human monocytes/macrophages. Proc Natl Acad Sci U S A 104: 19446–19451.

9. Casiraghi F, Azzollini N, Cassis P, Imberti B, Morigi M, et al. (2008) Pretransplant infusion of mesenchymal stem cells prolongs the survival of a semiallogeneic heart transplant through the generation of regulatory T cells. J Immunol 181: 3933–3946.

10. Ge W, Jiang J, Baroja ML, Arp J, Zassoko R, et al. (2009) Infusion of mesenchymal stem cells and rapamycin synergize to attenuate alloimmune responses and promote cardiac allograft tolerance. Am J Transplant 9: 1760–1772.

11. Madec AM, Mallone R, Afonso G, Abou Mrad E, Mesnier A, et al. (2009) Mesenchymal stem cells protect NOD mice from diabetes by inducing regulatory T cells. Diabetologia 52: 1391–1399.

12. McAuley DF, Curley GF, Hamid UI, Laffey JG, Abbott J, et al. (2014) Clinical grade allogeneic human mesenchymal stem cells restore alveolar fluid clearance in human lungs rejected for transplantation. Am J Physiol Lung Cell Mol Physiol 306: L809–815.

13. Le Blanc K, Rasmusson I, Sundberg B, Gotherstrom C, Hassan M, et al. (2004) Treatment of severe acute graft-versus-host disease with third party haploidentical mesenchymal stem cells. Lancet 363: 1439–1441.

14. Le Blanc K, Frassoni F, Ball L, Locatelli F, Roelofs H, et al. (2008) Mesenchymal stem cells for treatment of steroid-resistant, severe, acute graft-versus-host disease: a phase II study. Lancet 371: 1579–1586.

15. Yin F, Battiwalla M, Ito S, Feng X, Chinian F, et al. (2014) Bone marrow mesenchymal stromal cells to treat tissue damage in allogeneic stem cell transplant recipients: correlation of biological markers with clinical responses. Stem Cells 32: 1278–1288.

16. Moermans C, Lechanteur C, Baudoux E, Giet O, Henket M, et al. (2014) Impact of Cotransplantation of Mesenchymal Stem Cells on Lung Function After Unrelated Allogeneic Hematopoietic Stem Cell Transplantation Following Non-Myeloablative Conditioning. Transplantation.

17. Sinclair K, Yerkovich ST, Chambers DC (2013) Mesenchymal stem cells and the lung. Respirology 18: 397–411.

18. Weiss DJ, Kolls JK, Ortiz LA, Panoskaltsis-Mortari A, Prockop DJ (2008) Stem cells and cell therapies in lung biology and lung diseases. Proc Am Thorac Soc 5: 637–667.

19. Weiss DJ, Bates JH, Gilbert T, Liles WC, Lutzko C, et al. (2013) Stem cells and cell therapies in lung biology and diseases: conference report. Ann Am Thorac Soc 10: S25–44.

20. Antunes MA, Laffey JG, Pelosi P, Rocco PR (2014) Mesenchymal stem cell trials for pulmonary diseases. J Cell Biochem 115: 1023–1032.

21. Peister A, Mellad JA, Larson BL, Hall BM, Gibson LF, et al. (2004) Adult stem cells from bone marrow (MSCs) isolated from different strains of inbred mice vary in surface epitopes, rates of proliferation, and differentiation potential. Blood 103: 1662–1668.

22. Tolar J, Nauta AJ, Osborn MJ, Panoskaltsis Mortari A, McElmurry RT, et al. (2007) Sarcoma derived from cultured mesenchymal stem cells. Stem Cells 25: 371–379.

23. Hebbel RP, Vercellotti GM, Pace BS, Solovey AN, Kollander R, et al. (2010) The HDAC inhibitors trichostatin A and suberoylanilide hydroxamic acid exhibit multiple modalities of benefit for the vascular pathobiology of sickle transgenic mice. Blood 115: 2483–2490.

24. Baglole CJ, Reddy SY, Pollock SJ, Feldon SE, Sime PJ, et al. (2005) Isolation and Phenotypic Characterization of Lung Fibroblasts. Methods in Molecular Medicine 117: 115–127.

25. Bucher C, Koch L, Vogtenhuber C, Goren E, Munger M, et al. (2009) IL-21 blockade reduces graft-versus-host disease mortality by supporting inducible T regulatory cell generation. Blood 114: 5375–5384.

26. Kebriaei P, Robinson S (2011) Mesenchymal stem cell therapy in the treatment of acute and chronic graft versus host disease. Front Oncol 1: 16.

27. Sundin M, Barrett AJ, Ringden O, Uzunel M, Lonnies H, et al. (2009) HSCT recipients have specific tolerance to MSC but not to the MSC donor. J Immunother 32: 755–764.

28. Vaes B, Van't Hof W, Deans R, Pinxteren J (2012) Application of MultiStem((R)) Allogeneic Cells for Immunomodulatory Therapy: Clinical Progress and Pre-Clinical Challenges in Prophylaxis for Graft Versus Host Disease. Front Immunol 3: 345.

29. Isakova IA, Lanclos C, Bruhn J, Kuroda MJ, Baker KC, et al. (2014) Allo-reactivity of mesenchymal stem cells in rhesus macaques is dose and haplotype dependent and limits durable cell engraftment in vivo. PLoS One 9: e87238.

30. Sivanathan KN, Gronthos S, Rojas-Canales D, Thierry B, Coates PT (2014) Interferon-gamma modification of mesenchymal stem cells: implications of autologous and allogeneic mesenchymal stem cell therapy in allotransplantation. Stem Cell Rev 10: 351–375.

31. Perico N, Casiraghi F, Introna M, Gotti E, Todeschini M, et al. (2011) Autologous mesenchymal stromal cells and kidney transplantation: a pilot study of safety and clinical feasibility. Clin J Am Soc Nephrol 6: 412–422.

32. Chambers DC, Enever D, Ilic N, Sparks L, Whitelaw K, et al. (2014) A phase 1b study of placenta-derived mesenchymal stromal cells in patients with idiopathic pulmonary fibrosis. Respirology.

33. Weiss DJ, Casaburi R, Flannery R, LeRoux-Williams M, Tashkin DP (2013) A placebo-controlled, randomized trial of mesenchymal stem cells in COPD. Chest 143: 1590–1598.

34. Tzouvelekis A, Paspaliaris V, Koliakos G, Ntolios P, Bouros E, et al. (2013) A prospective, non-randomized, no placebo-controlled, phase Ib clinical trial to study the safety of the adipose derived stromal cells-stromal vascular fraction in idiopathic pulmonary fibrosis. J Transl Med 11: 171.

35. Goerdt S, Orfanos CE (1999) Other functions, other genes: alternative activation of antigen-presenting cells. Immunity 10: 137–142.

36. Workman CJ, Szymczak-Workman AL, Collison LW, Pillai MR, Vignali DA (2009) The development and function of regulatory T cells. Cell Mol Life Sci 66: 2603–2622.

37. Zhao Y, Gillen JR, Harris DA, Kron IL, Murphy MP, et al. (2014) Treatment with placenta-derived mesenchymal stem cells mitigates development of bronchiolitis obliterans in a murine model. J Thorac Cardiovasc Surg 147: 1668–1677 e1665.

38. Kim J, Hematti P (2009) Mesenchymal stem cell-educated macrophages: a novel type of alternatively activated macrophages. Exp Hematol 37: 1445–1453.

39. Maggini J, Mirkin G, Bognanni I, Holmberg J, Piazzon IM, et al. (2010) Mouse bone marrow-derived mesenchymal stromal cells turn activated macrophages into a regulatory-like profile. PLoS One 5: e9252.

40. Guth AM, Janssen WJ, Bosio CM, Crouch EC, Henson PM, et al. (2009) Lung environment determines unique phenotype of alveolar macrophages. Am J - Physiol Lung Cell Mol Physiol 296: L936–946.

41. Guo Z, Zhou X, Li J, Meng Q, Cao H, et al. (2013) Mesenchymal stem cells reprogram host macrophages to attenuate obliterative bronchiolitis in murine orthotopic tracheal transplantation. Int Immunopharmacol 15: 726–734.

42. Grove DA, Xu J, Joodi R, Torres-Gonzales E, Neujahr D, et al. (2011) Attenuation of early airway obstruction by mesenchymal stem cells in a murine model of heterotopic tracheal transplantation. J Heart Lung Transplant 30: 341–350.

43. Betancourt AM (2013) New Cell-Based Therapy Paradigm: Induction of Bone Marrow-Derived Multipotent Mesenchymal Stromal Cells into Pro-Inflammatory MSC1 and Anti-inflammatory MSC2 Phenotypes. Adv Biochem Eng Biotechnol 130: 163–197.

44. Islam MN, Das SR, Emin MT, Wei M, Sun L, et al. (2012) Mitochondrial transfer from bone-marrow-derived stromal cells to pulmonary alveoli protects against acute lung injury. Nat Med 18: 759–765.

45. Behr J, Maier K, Braun B, Schwaiblmair M, Vogelmeier C (2000) Evidence for oxidative stress in bronchiolitis obliterans syndrome after lung and heart-lung transplantation. The Munich Lung Transplant Group. Transplantation 69: 1856–1860.

46. Madill J, Aghdassi E, Arendt B, Hartman-Craven B, Gutierrez C, et al. (2009) Lung transplantation: does oxidative stress contribute to the development of bronchiolitis obliterans syndrome? Transplant Rev (Orlando) 23: 103–110.

47. Stober VP, Szczesniak C, Childress Q, Heise RL, Bortner C, et al. (2014) Bronchial epithelial injury in the context of alloimmunity promotes lymphocytic bronchiolitis through hyaluronan expression. Am J Physiol Lung Cell Mol Physiol 306: L1045–1055.

48. Ziegler TR, Panoskaltsus-Mortari A, Gu LH, Jonas CR, Farrell CL, et al. (2001) Regulation of glutathione redox status in lung and liver by conditioning regimens and keratinocyte growth factor in murine allogeneic bone marrow transplantation. Transplantation 72: 1354–1362.

49. Nauta AJ, Westerhuis G, Kruisselbrink AB, Lurvink EG, Willemze R, et al. (2006) Donor-derived mesenchymal stem cells are immunogenic in an allogeneic host and stimulate donor graft rejection in a nonmyeloablative setting. Blood 108: 2114–2120.

50. Foskett AM, Bazhanov N, Ti X, Tiblow A, Bartosh TJ, et al. (2014) Phase-directed therapy: TSG-6 targeted to early inflammation improves bleomycin-injured lungs. Am J Physiol Lung Cell Mol Physiol 306: L120–131.

51. Danchuk S, Ylostalo JH, Hossain F, Sorge R, Ramsey A, et al. (2011) Human multipotent stromal cells attenuate lipopolysaccharide-induced acute lung injury in mice via secretion of tumor necrosis factor-alpha-induced protein 6. Stem Cell Res Ther 2: 27.

52. Qi Y, Jiang D, Sindrilaru A, Stegemann A, Schatz S, et al. (2014) TSG-6 released from intradermally injected mesenchymal stem cells accelerates wound healing and reduces tissue fibrosis in murine full-thickness skin wounds. J Invest Dermatol 134: 526–537.

53. Ware LB, Matthay MA (2002) Keratinocyte and hepatocyte growth factors in the lung: roles in lung development, inflammation, and repair. Am J Physiol Lung Cell Mol Physiol 282: L924–940.

54. Panoskaltsis-Mortari A, Ingbar DH, Jung P, Haddad IY, Bitterman PB, et al. (2000) KGF pretreatment decreases B7 and granzyme B expression and hastens repair in lungs of mice after allogeneic BMT. Am J Physiol Lung Cell Mol Physiol 278: L988–999.

55. Moodley Y, Vaghjiani V, Chan J, Baltic S, Ryan M, et al. (2013) Anti-inflammatory effects of adult stem cells in sustained lung injury: a comparative study. PLoS One 8: e69299.

56. Ortiz LA, Dutreil M, Fattman C, Pandey AC, Torres G, et al. (2007) Interleukin 1 receptor antagonist mediates the antiinflammatory and antifibrotic effect of mesenchymal stem cells during lung injury. Proc Natl Acad Sci U S A 104: 11002–11007.

57. Meisel R, Brockers S, Heseler K, Degistirici O, Bulle H, et al. (2011) Human but not murine multipotent mesenchymal stromal cells exhibit broad-spectrum antimicrobial effector function mediated by indoleamine 2,3-dioxygenase. Leukemia 25: 648–654.

15

Timing of Umbilical Cord Blood Derived Mesenchymal Stem Cells Transplantation Determines Therapeutic Efficacy in the Neonatal Hyperoxic Lung Injury

Yun Sil Chang[1,2,9], Soo Jin Choi[3,9], So Yoon Ahn[1], Dong Kyung Sung[2], Se In Sung[1], Hye Soo Yoo[1], Won Il Oh[3], Won Soon Park[1,2]*

1 Department of Pediatrics, Samsung Medical Center, Sungkyunkwan University School of Medicine, Seoul, Korea, 2 Samsung Biomedical Research Institute, Sungkyunkwan University School of Medicine, Seoul, Korea, 3 Biomedical Research Institute, MEDIPOST Co., Ltd., Seoul, Korea

Abstract

Intratracheal transplantation of human umbilical cord blood (UCB)-derived mesenchymal stem cells (MSCs) attenuates the hyperoxia-induced neonatal lung injury. The aim of this study was to optimize the timing of MSCs transplantation. Newborn Sprague-Dawley rats were randomly exposed to hyperoxia (90% for 2 weeks and 60% for 1 week) or normoxia after birth for 21 days. Human UCB-derived MSCs (5×10^5 cells) were delivered intratracheally early at postnatal day (P) 3 (HT3), late at P10 (HT10) or combined early+late at P3+10 (HT3+10). Hyperoxia-induced increase in mortality, TUNEL positive cells, ED1 positive alveolar macrophages, myeloperoxidase activity and collagen levels, retarded growth and reduced alveolarization as evidenced by increased mean linear intercept and mean alveolar volume were significantly better attenuated in both HT3 and HT3+10 than in HT10. Hyperoxia-induced up-regulation of both cytosolic and membrane $p47^{phox}$ indicative of oxidative stress, and increased inflammatory markers such as tumor necrosis factor-α, interleukin (IL) -1α, IL-1β, IL-6, and transforming growth factor-β measured by ELISA, and tissue inhibitor of metalloproteinase-1, CXCL7, RANTES, L-selectin and soluble intercellular adhesion molecule-1 measured by protein array were consistently more attenuated in both HT3 and HT3+10 than in HT10. Hyperoxia-induced decrease in hepatocyte growth factor and vascular endothelial growth factor was significantly up-regulated in both HT3 and HT3+10, but not in HT10. In summary, intratracheal transplantation of human UCB derived MSCs time-dependently attenuated hyperoxia-induced lung injury in neonatal rats, showing significant protection only in the early but not in the late phase of inflammation. There were no synergies with combined early+late MSCs transplantation.

Editor: Dimas Tadeu Covas, University of Sao Paulo – USP, Brazil

Funding: This work was supported by a grant from the Korea Healthcare technology R&D Project, Ministry for Health, Welfare & Family Affairs, Republic of Korea (A102136), by the Basic Science Research Program through the National Research Foundation of Korea (NRF) funded by the Ministry of Education, Science, and Technology (S-2011-0317-000), and by a Samsung Biomedical Research Institute Grant (#SBRI CB11271). The funders had no role in study design, data collection and analysis, decision to publish, or preparation of the manuscript.

Competing Interests: The authors have the following interests: co-authors Soo Jin Choi and Won-il Oh are employed by MEDIPOST Co., Ltd. Co-author Won-il Oh is a board member and holds stocks in MEDIPOST Co., Ltd. Samsung Medical Center and MEDIPOST Co., Ltd. have issued or filed patents for "Method of treating lung diseases using cells separated or proliferated from umbilical cord blood" under the name of Yun Sil Chang, Won Soon Park and Yoon Sun Yang. The relevent application number is: PCT/KR2007/000535. There are no further patents, products in development or marketed products to declare.

* E-mail: wonspark@skku.edu

9 These authors contributed equally to this work.

Introduction

Recent improvements in neonatal intensive care medicine have resulted in marked improvements in the survival of the premature infants [1]. However, bronchopulmonary dysplasia (BPD), a chronic lung disease that follows ventilator and oxygen therapy in the premature infants, still remains a major cause of mortality and morbidity with few effective treatments [2,3].

Although the pathogenesis of BPD has not been clearly elucidate yet, oxidative stress and the ensuing inflammation mediated by neutrophils [4] and pro-inflammatory cytokines [5] is believed to play a seminal role in the lung injury process leading to the development of BPD [6]. Recently, we have shown that local intratracheal but not systemic intraperitoneal xenotransplantation of human umbilical cord blood (UCB)-derived mesenchymal stem

cells (MSCs) attenuates hyperoxia induced lung injuries such as impaired alveolarization, increased apoptosis and fibrosis in the immunocompetent neonatal rats [7]. Furthermore, these protective effects of stem cell transplantation were dose dependent [8]. Overall, these findings suggest that human UCB derived MSCs transplantation could be a novel therapeutic modality for BPD. However, while the administration of human UCB-derived MSCs at postnatal day (P) 5 was effective in our previous studies [7,8], the optimal timing for their administration has not been determined yet.

Previously, we have shown that the protective effects of human UCB-derived MSCs transplantation are primarily mediated by their anti-inflammatory effects rather than by their regenerative capabilities [7,8]. These findings suggest that the therapeutic time window of stem cell transplantation could be narrow, i.e., only during the early but not the late phase of inflammatory responses. In the present study, we thus tried to determine the optimal timing at which intratracheally delivered human UCB-derived MSCs could attenuate the hyperoxia-induced lung injuries in the newborn rat pups. We firstly conducted time course experiments of inflammatory responses by measuring inflammatory cytokines such as tumor necrosis factor (TNF)-α, interleukin (IL)-1α, 1β and 6 levels at P 0, 3, 5, 7, 10 and 14 in the hyperoxia-induced neonatal lung tissue. After then, we tried to determine the optimal timing by comparing the therapeutic efficacy of early (P3) versus late (P10) intratracheal administration of human UCB derived MSCs in attenuating the hyperoxia-induced lung injuries in the newborn rat pups. We also tried to determine whether combined early (P3)+late (P10) stem cell transplantation has any synergistic effects.

Materials and Methods

Cell Preparation

This study was approved by Institutional Review Board of Samsung Medical Center and by Medipost, Co., Ltd, Seoul, Korea. As previously reported, UCB was collected from umbilical veins after neonatal delivery with informed consent from pregnant mothers, and MSCs were isolated and cultivated from human UCB [9,10]. The cells expressed CD105 (99.6%) and CD73 (96.3%), but not CD34 (0.1%), CD45 (0.2%) and CD14 (0.1%) [7]. They were positive for HLA-AB (96.8%), but generally not for HLA-DR (0.1%). The cells also expressed pluripotency markers such as octamer-binding transcription factor 4 (Oct 4; 30.5%) [11] and stage-specific embryonic antigen 4 (SSEA-4; 67.7%) [12]. Human UCB-derived MSCs differentiated into various cell types such as respiratory epithelium, osteoblasts, chondrocytes and adipocytes with specific *in vitro* induction stimuli [7,10,12,13]. We confirmed the differentiation potential and karyotypic stability of the human UCB-derived MSCs up to the 11th passage.

Animal model

The experimental protocols described herein were reviewed and approved by the Animal Care and Use Committee of Samsung Biomedical Research Institute, Seoul, Korea. This study was also performed in accordance with the institutional and National Institutes of Health guidelines for laboratory animal care. Timed pregnant Sprague-Dawley rats (Orient Co., Seoul, Korea) were housed in individual cages with free access to water and laboratory chow. The rat pups were delivered spontaneously and reared with their dams. The experiment began within 10 h after birth, and continued through P21. Rat pups were randomly divided into four experimental groups; normoxia control group (NC), hyperoxia control group (HC), hyperoxia with early at P3 (HT3), late at P10 (HT10), or combined early+late at P3+10 (HT3+10) human UCB-derived MSCs transplantation group. Rat pups of NC were kept with a nursing mother rat in the standard cage at room air throughout the experiment. Rat pups of hyperoxia groups were maintained with a nursing mother in the standard cage within a 50 liter Plexiglas chambers in which the hyperoxia (oxygen concentration of 90%) was maintained until P14, and after then oxygen concentration was reduced to 60% until P21. Humidity and environmental temperature were maintained at 50% and 24°C, respectively. Nursing mother rats were rotated daily between litters in the normoxia and hyperoxia groups to avoid oxygen toxicity. Survival and body weight of rat pups in each group were checked daily throughout the experiment. The rat pups of NC and HC were sacrificed at P 1, 3, 5, 7, 10 and 14 for time course

experiments and at P21 for group comparison under deep pentobarbital anesthesia (60 mg/kg, intraperitoneal), and the whole lung tissue was obtained for morphometric and biochemical analyses. Six to eight animals were used in each subgroup of analysis.

Transplantation of human UCB-derived MSCs

The human UCB-derived MSCs from the 5th passage from a single donor were labeled using a PKH26GL Red Fluorescent Cell Membrane Labeling Kit (Sigma-Aldrich, St. Louis, MO, USA) for transplantation according to the manufacturer's protocol in the present study, as previously reported [7,8]. For donor cell transplantation, 5×10^5 cells in 0.05 ml phosphate buffered saline (PBS, pH 7.4) were administered intratracheally at P 3, P 10 or P 3+10. For NC and HC, equal volume of PBS was given intratracheally at P3 and P10. For intratracheal transplantation, the rats were anesthetized with an intraperitoneal injection of ketamine and xylazine mixture (45 mg/kg and 8 mg/kg, respectively), and restricted on a board at a fixed angle. MSCs were administered into the trachea through a 30-gauge needle syringe. After the procedure, the animals were allowed to recover from anesthesia, and were returned to their dams. There was no mortality associated with the transplantation procedure.

Tissue preparation

The lungs were resected after transcardiac perfusion with ice-cold phosphate buffered saline (PBS), snap-frozen in liquid nitrogen, and stored at −80°C for later biochemical analyses.

For morphometric analyses, lungs were fixed in situ by tracheal instillation of 10% buffered formalin at a constant inflation pressure of 20 cm H_2O, and then fixed overnight at room temperature in the same fixative. The fixed right lungs were embedded in paraffin, and the left lungs were embedded in an optimal cutting temperature (OCT) compound (SAKURA 4583, Sakura, Torrance, CA, USA). Blocks of the OCT compound were sectioned at 10 μm on a cryostat (Shandon Cryotome, Thermo Electron Co., Waltham, MA, USA) and stored in a deep freezer until analyzed by immunohistochemistry. Four-micrometer-thick sections were cut from the paraffin blocks, and stained with hematoxylin and eosin. Images of each section were captured with a magnifier digital camera through an Olympus BX40 microscope (Olympus optical Co. Ltd., Tokyo, Japan), and were saved as JPEG files.

Morphometry

The level of alveolarization was determined by measuring the MLI and mean alveolar volume. The mean inter-alveolar distance was measured as MLI, by dividing the total length of the lines drawn across the lung section by the number of intercepts encountered, as described by Thurlbeck [14]. The mean alveolar volume was calculated using the method reported by Snyder et al. [15,16]. Briefly, a grid containing equally spaced crosses was placed on a uniformly enlarged photomicrograph of each lung field. The diameters (ℓ) of the alveoli containing a cross were measured along the horizontal axis of the cross. The cube of the alveolar diameter times π and divided by 3 ($\ell^3 \pi / 3$) was used to estimate the mean alveolar volume. A minimum of two sections per rat and six fields per each section were examined randomly for each analysis.

TUNEL assay

The immunofluorescent TUNEL staining with an in situ cell death detection kit (S7110 ApopTag, Chemicon, Temecula, CA,

USA) was done to measure the extent of apoptosis in the lung. Paraffin section slides were deparaffinized, rehydrated, and digested with Proteinase K (20 µg/ml in PBS) (Sigma Co., St. Louis, MO, USA) at room temperature for 15 minutes and then washed in PBS for 10 minutes. Sections were then incubated with equilibration buffer for 1 minute and immediately incubated with working strength TdT enzyme in a humidified chamber at 37°C for 1 hour. Each section was immersed in a stop/wash buffer and gently rinsed with PBS. Fluorescein isothiocyanate (FITC)-labeled anti-digoxigenin conjugate was applied to the sections which were then incubated at room temperature for 30 minutes in the dark. Nuclear counterstaining was performed with propidium iodide (0.5 µg/ml, Sigma Co., St. Louis, MO, USA). Slides were washed again in PBS, mounted with Vectasheild mounting solution (Vector laboratories, Burlingame, CA, USA), and visualized with a fluorescent microscope (Nikon E600 fluorescence microscope, Tokyo, Japan) using an excitation wavelength of 460–490 nM. Ten non-overlapping fields with a magnifying power of ×200 were examined to count TUNEL positive cells.

Quantification of the PKH26 positive cells

Ten-µm-thick cryosections were mounted with a Vector shield mounting solution containing DAPI (H-1200, Vector, Burlingame, CA, USA). The cell counts for the transplanted or donor-derived cells were measured using PKH26 red fluorescence, as described above after combining the ×20 objective images of the DAPI-stained nuclei signals. Five fields per section were selected randomly, focused, and counted with the naked eye under a fluorescence microscope (Nikon E600, Nikon, Tokyo, Japan) using a filter to detect the PKH26 red fluorescence. The PKH26 red fluorescence was counted manually and averaged per high power field (HPF) in a single animal. Two random sections per animal were evaluated in a blinded manner.

Western blot for p47^{phox}

The upregulation of p47^{phox}, a subunit of NADPH oxidase, both in the cytoplasmic and plasma membrane portion serves as an indicator of NADPH oxidase activation that is responsible for generating reactive oxygen species [17,18]. Tissue slides were incubated for 40 min in PBS containing 0.1% Triton X-100. After blocking with 0.5% BSA, slides were incubated overnight at 4°C with anti-p47^{phox} antibody (1:200) and then exposed for 2 hr at room temperature to FITC-conjugated goat anti mouse immuno-globulin-G (1:200; BD Biosciences, USA). Vectasheld mount medium with DAPI (Vector Laboratories) was used to preserve. Confocal microscopic examination was carried out at 400× magnification using Bio-Rad Radiance 2100 (Bio-Rad Laboratories Inc. Hercules, CA, USA) with krypton/argon laser, and images were achieved using the Laser shop 2000 software (Bio-Rad Laboratories, Inc.). For this purpose, tissue sample from each animal were separated into membrane and cytosolic components for western blot examination. Tissues were homogenized in ice-cold hypertonic solution and centrifuged at 600 g for 10 minutes. The supernatant was ultra-centrifuged at 100,000 g for 1.5 hours. The supernatant contained the cytosolic fraction and the membrane-particulate pellet was resuspended in hypotonic solution containing 1% Triton X-100. Samples were analyzed by western blotting using antibodies against the NADPH oxidase cytosolic subunit, p47^{phox} (1:500, BD Biosciences, San Diego, CA, USA). The bands were recognized by horseradish peroxidase-conjugated anti-mouse secondary antibody (1:1,000, DAKO, Glostrup, Denmark), and then western blots were developed with enhanced chemiluminescence detection reagents (Amersham Pharmacia, Uppsala, Sweden), and exposed to X-ray film (Fuji Photo Film, Tokyo, Japan). The blots were re-probed with antibodies against GAPDH (1:1,000, Santa Cruz Biotechnology Inc., Santa Cruz, CA, USA). To determine the relative degree of membrane purification, the membrane fraction was subjected to immunoblotting for calnexin (1:500 Santa Cruz Biotechnology Inc), a membrane marker.

Protein macroarray

Each lung lysate was analyzed using a rat cytokine array kit (Proteome Profiler™; R&D Systems, Minneapolis, MN, USA). A total of 250 µg of lysate was incubated in the nitrocellulose membrane array overnight at 4°C. After washing away the unbound protein, the array was incubated with a cocktail of phospho-site-specific biotinylated antibodies for 2 h at room temperature, followed by streptavidin–HRP for 30 min. Signals were visualized with chemiluminescent reagents (Amersham Biosciences, Pittsburgh, PA, USA), and recorded on X-ray film. The arrays were scanned, and optical densities were measured using Image J software (NIH) and compared among the experimental groups. The protein macroarray analysis included inflammatory cytokines of interest, including tissue inhibitor of metalloproteinase (TIMP)-1, Chemokine (C-X-C motif) ligand 7 (CXCL7), regulated upon activation normal T-expressed and presumably secreted (RANTES), L-selectin and the soluble form of intercellular adhesion molecule (sICAM)-1.

Myeloperoxidase activity

The activity of MPO, an indicator of neutrophil accumulation, was determined by modification of the method by Gray et al. [19]. The lung tissues were homogenized in a phosphate buffer (pH 7.4) and centrifuged at 30,000 g for 30 min. The pellet was resuspended in another phosphate buffer (50 mM, pH 6.0) containing 0.5% hexadecyltrimethyl ammonium bromide. MPO activity in the resuspended pellet was assayed by measuring absorbance changes spectrophotometrically at 460 nm, using 0.167 mg/mL of O-dianisidine ihydrochloride and 0.0005% hydrogen peroxide. One unit of MPO activity was defined as the quantity of enzyme degrading 1 µM of peroxide/min.

Hepatocyte growth factor (HGF)

Total RNA in the sample was extracted using RNA Trizol according to the manufacturer's protocol (Invitrogen Corporation, Carlsbad, CA, USA). Total RNA concentration was measured by spectrophotometry (Nanodrop Wilmington, DE, USA) at 260 nm. One microgram of RNA was used to produce cDNA with a Protoscript® II RT-PCR kit (New England Biolabs, Ipswich, MA, USA). PCR primers for rat hepatocyte growth factor and rat glyceraldehyde-3-phosphate dehydrogenase (GAPDH) were designed with Primer3 (Whitehead Institute, Cambridge, MA, USA) and synthesized by Bioneer Inc. (Bioneer, Daejeon, Korea). The sequence of primers used was as follows: rat HGF (sense-accctggtgtttcacaagca- antisense-aggggtgtcagggtcaagag-), rat GAPDH (sense- ggccaaaagggtcatcatct-, antisense-gtgatggcatg-gactgtggt-). PCR products were run on a 1.2% agarose gel electrophoresis, visualized by ethidium bromide and scanned by a Gel Doc 2000 analyzer (Bio-Rad, Hercules, CA, USA). The expression levels for each gene were semi-quantified by densitometric analysis using software (Quantity One, Bio-Rad, Hercules, CA, USA). Relative expression levels were estimated by the density ratio of rat GAPDH to rat HGF.

Statistical Analysis

The data are expressed as the mean ± SEM. Survival rates were compared using the Kaplan-Meier analysis followed by a log rank test. For continuous variables with a normal distribution, the groups were compared using a t-test with a Bonferroni correction. Continuous variables that were not normally distributed were analyzed using the Wilcoxon rank test with a Bonferroni correction. All data were analyzed using Stata software (ver. 11.0, StataCorp LP, College Station, TX, USA). Values of $p<0.05$ were considered statistically significant.

Results

Temporal profile of inflammatory responses

In time course experiments of inflammatory responses by measuring TNF-α, IL-1α, IL-1β and IL-6 levels with ELISA at P 1, 3, 5, 7, 10 and 14 in the lung tissue, IL-6 levels after P5 and TNF-α, IL-1α and IL-1β levels after P7 in HC became significantly increased compared to NC up to P 14 (Fig. 1).

Survival rate and body weight gain

Exposure to oxygen (HC) significantly reduced the survival rate to 70.8% ($P<0.05$ vs. NC) at the end of experiment (P21) compared to the 100% survival rate of NC. On the contrary, survival rates of HT3 (91.7%, $P>0.05$ vs. NC) and HT3+10 (87.5%, $P>0.05$ vs. NC) were not different when it compared to NC. However, survival rate of HT10 (75.0%, $P<0.05$ vs. NC) was significantly lower than that of NC (Fig. 2).

Although birth weight was not significantly different between the five experimental groups (7.0±0.13 g, 7.1±0.04 g, 7.1±0.04 g, and 7.1±0.03 in NC, HC, HT3, HT10 and HT3+10, respectively), body weight at P21 in HC (34.3±4.6 g,

$P<0.01$) was significantly lower compared to NC (41.7±2.3 g), and this retarded body weight gain observed in HC was significantly improved in HT3 (39.5±4.7 g, $P<0.01$ vs. HC) and HT3+10 (38.8±4.4 g, $P<0.01$ vs. HC), but not in HT10 (35.7±4.2 g, $P>0.05$ vs. HC, $P<0.05$ vs. HT3, $P<0.05$ vs. HT3+10).

Lung histopathology

Fig. 3A presents typical photomicrographs showing the histopathological differences observed by optical microscopy in each experimental group at P 21. While uniform and small alveoli were observed in NC, impaired alveolar growth, as evidenced by fewer and larger alveoli, focal airspace enlargement and heterogeneous alveolar size were observed in HC compared to NC. After MSCs transplantation, the hyperoxia-induced impairments in alveolar growth and morphological changes were attenuated, particularly in both HT3 and HT3+10 compared to HT10.

In morphometric analyses, the MLI and mean alveolar volume, indicating the size and volume of the alveoli respectively, were significantly higher in HC (67.2±1.2 µm in MLI, $P<0.001$ vs. NC; $19.4\pm1.2\times10^{4}$ µm^3 in mean alveolar volume, $P<0.001$ vs. NC) than in NC (40.8±1.0 µm in MLI and $3.1\pm0.04\times10^{4}$ µm^3 in mean alveolar volume). (Fig. 3B). After MSCs transplantation, these hyperoxia-induced morphometric abnormalities were better attenuated in HT3 (54.0±1.4 µm in MLI, $P<0.001$ vs. HC; $6.7\pm0.9\times10^{4}$ µm^3 in mean alveolar volume $P<0.001$ vs. HC) and HT3+10 (55.3±0.8 µm vs. HC, $P<0.001$; $6.2\pm0.5\times10^{4}$ µm^3 in mean alveolar volume $P<0.001$ vs. HC) compared to those in HT10 (59.4±1.7 µm in MLI, $P<0.001$ vs. HC, $P<0.01$ vs. HT3, , $P<0.05$ vs. HT3+10 ; $10.4\pm1.0\times10^{4}$ µm^3 in mean alveolar volume $P<0.001$ vs. HC, $P<0.01$ vs. HT3, $P<0.01$ vs. HT3+10) (Fig. 3B).

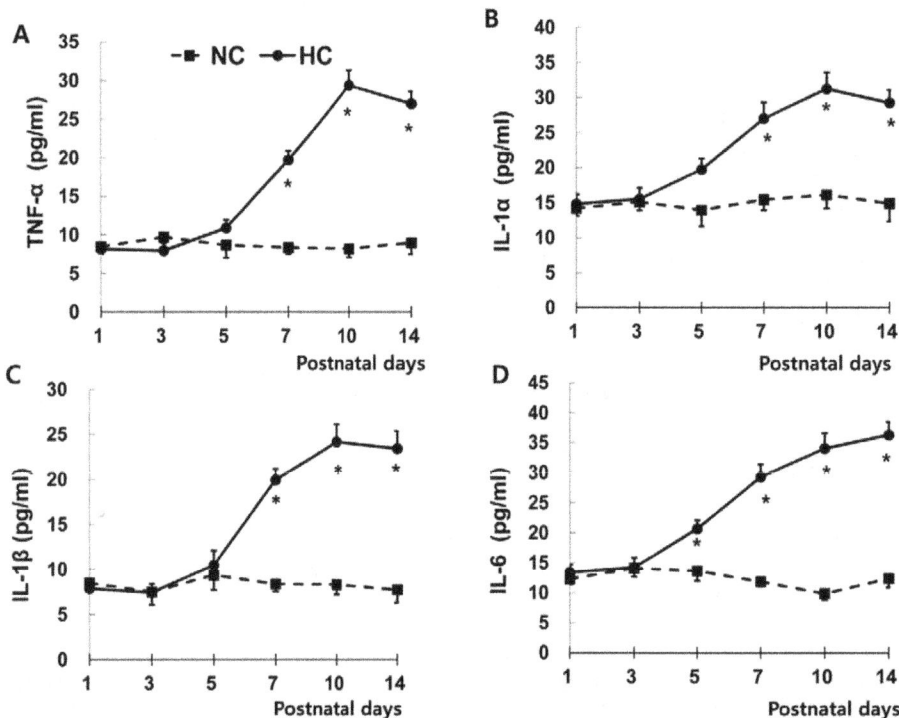

Figure 1. Temporal profiles of inflammatory cytokines. Tumor necrosis factor (TNF)-α, interleukin (IL)-1α, IL-1β, and IL-6 levels measured with ELISA at P 1, 3, 5, 7, 10 and 14 in the rat lung tissue. NC, Normoxia control group; HC, hyperoxia control group. Data; mean±SEM. *$P<0.05$ compared to NC.

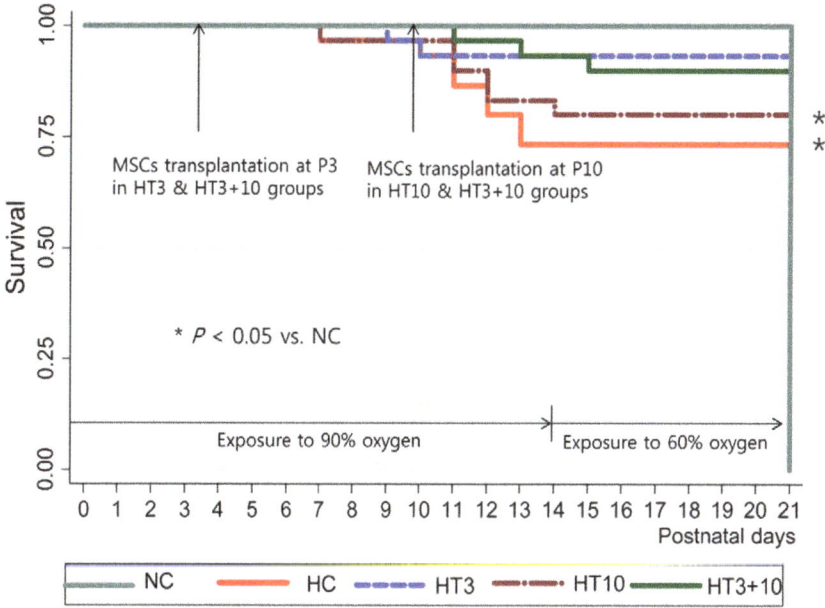

Figure 2. Survival curve. Kaplan-Meier survival curve up to P 21 showing decreased survival. HC compared to NC, and improved survival in both HT3 and HT3+10, but not in HT10. NC, Normoxia control group; HC, hyperoxia control group; HT3, hyperoxia with stem cell transplantation group at P3; HT10, hyperoxia with stem cell treatment group at P10; HT3+10, hyperoxia with stem cell treatment group at P3 and P10. *P<0.05 compared to NC.

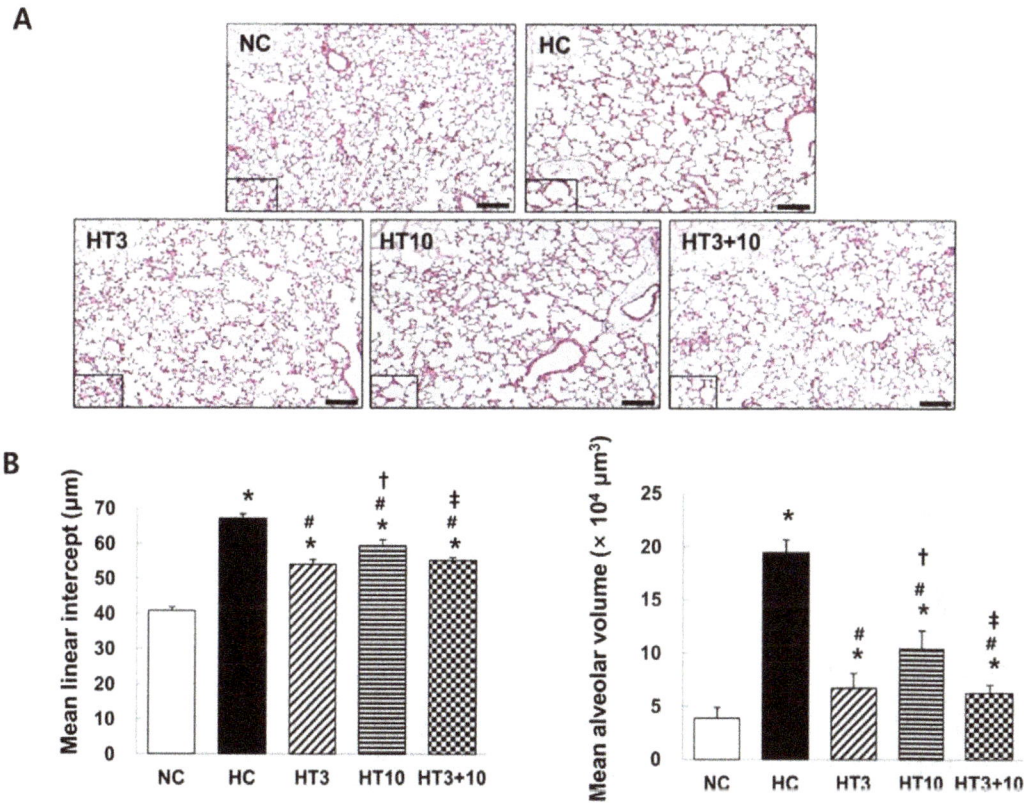

Figure 3. Histology and morphometric analysis of the surviving P21 rat lung. (A): Representative optical microscopy photomicrographs of the lungs stained with hematoxylin and eosin (scale bar = 100 μm). (B): Degree of alveolarization measured by the mean linear intercept (*left*) and mean alveolar volume (*right*). NC, Normoxia control group; HC, hyperoxia control group; HT3, hyperoxia with stem cell transplantation group at P3; HT10, hyperoxia with stem cell treatment group at P10; HT3+10, hyperoxia with stem cell treatment group at P3 and P10. Data; mean±SEM. *P<0.05 compared to NC, # P<0.05 compared to HC,† P<0.05 compared to HT3, ‡ P<0.05 compared to HT10.

The number of TUNEL positive cells in the lung of P21 rats per high power field was significantly increased in HC (15.2 ± 1.1, $P<0.001$) compared to NC (1.1 ± 0.2). This hyperoxia-induced increase in the number of TUNEL positive cells was significantly attenuated in both HT3 (7.6 ± 0.8, $P<0.001$ vs. HC) and HT3+10 (6.6 ± 0.3, $P<0.001$ vs. HC), but not in HT10 (17.4 ± 0.6, $P>0.05$ vs. HC, $P<0.001$ vs. HT3, $P<0.001$ vs. HT3+10) (Fig. 4).

The deposition of PKH26 red fluorescence positive donor cells was observed only in the MSCs transplantation groups, but not in NC and HC (Fig. 5A). The number of donor cells identified per lung field was significantly larger in HT10 (21.5 ± 2.9, $P<0.001$ vs. HT3) and HT3+10 (25.4 ± 1.7, $P<0.001$ vs. HT3) than in HT3 (10.6 ± 1.6). However, there were no significant differences in the donor cells between HT10 and HT3+10 (Fig. 5B).

Cytosolic and membrane expressions of p47^{phox}

Since NADPH oxidase produces oxygen free radicals in both phagocytic [20] and nonphagocytic cells [21,22], hyperoxia-induced production of ROS was evaluated by NADPH oxidase activation, as evidenced by increased cytosolic and membrane expression of a cytosolic subunit of NADPH oxidase p47^{phox}. In fluorescent microscopy, increased p47^{phox} was observed in HC compared to NC, indicating the activation of NADPH oxidase. After MSCs transplantation, the hyperoxia-induced increase in p47^{phox} was attenuated, particularly in both HT3 and HT3+10 compared to HT10 (Fig. 6A). In western blot analyses, significantly higher levels of p47^{phox} were observed in HC both in the cytosolic ($P<0.01$) and membrane ($P<0.05$) fractions than in NC. While the hyperoxia-induced increase in the cytosolic expression of p47^{phox} was significantly attenuated in the MSCs transplantation groups ($P<0.05$ vs. HC) the increase in the membrane fraction was attenuated in both HT3 ($P>0.05$ vs. NC) and HT3+10 ($P>0.05$ vs. NC), but not in HT10 ($P<0.05$ vs. NC).

ELISA and Protein array of cytokines

In HC, significantly increased levels of TNF-α ($P<0.001$ vs. NC), IL-1α ($P<0.001$ vs. NC), IL-1β ($P<0.01$ vs. NC), IL-6 ($P<0.001$ vs. NC) and TGF-β ($P<0.01$ vs. NC) measured by ELISA and TIMP-1 ($P<0.001$ vs. NC), CXCL7 ($P<0.001$ vs. NC), RANTES ($P<0.001$ vs. NC), L-selectin ($P<0.001$ vs. NC) and sICAM-1 ($P<0.05$ vs. NC) measured by protein array were observed compared to NC (Fig. 7). The hyperoxia-induced

increase in these cytokine levels was significantly attenuated in both HT3 and HT3+10, but not in HT10, and the attenuation of IL-1α and IL-6 was more profound in HT3 (IL-1α, $P>0.05$ vs. NC, $P<0.01$ vs. HC; IL-6, $P>0.05$ vs. NC, $P<0.001$ vs. HC) and HT3+10 (IL-1α, $P>0.05$ vs. NC, $P<0.01$ vs. HC; IL-6, $P>0.05$ vs. NC, $P<0.001$ vs. HC) than in HT10 (IL-1α, $P<0.05$ vs. NC, $P<0.05$ vs. HC; IL-6, $P<0.01$ vs. NC, $P<0.01$ vs. HC, $P<0.01$ vs. HT3, $P<0.01$ vs. HT3+10).

ED1 positive cells, Myeloperoxidase activity and Collagen levels

The ED1 positive alveolar macrophages were significantly higher in HC (13.6 ± 1.8, $P<0.001$) than in NC (1.0 ± 0.1). This hyperoxia- induced increase in ED1 positive cells was significantly attenuated with MSCs transplantation, and this attenuation was more profound in HT3 (4.9 ± 0.8, $P<0.001$ vs. HC) and HT3+10 (4.9 ± 0.2, $P<0.001$ vs. HC) than in HT10 (7.9 ± 1.1, $P<0.01$ vs. HC, $P<0.05$ vs. HT3, $P<0.05$ vs. HT3+10) (Fig. 8A).

The MPO activity in HC (8.2 ± 0.5 U, $P<0.001$) was significantly higher than in NC (1.5 ± 0.2 U). The hyperoxia-induced increase in MPO activity was significantly attenuated in both HT3 (6.0 ± 0.2 U, $P<0.001$ vs. HC) and HT3+10 (6.0 ± 0.3 U, $P<0.001$ vs. HC), but not in HT10 (8.6 ± 0.8 U, $P>0.05$ vs. HC, $P<0.01$ vs. HT3, $P<0.01$ vs. HT3+10) (Fig. 8B).

The lung collagen levels at P21 were significantly higher in HC (149 ± 5 µg/mg protein, $P<0.001$) than in NC (81 ± 5 µg/mg protein). This hyperoxia-induced increase in the lung collagen levels was significantly attenuated in both HT3 (124 ± 3 µg/mg protein, $P<0.01$ vs. HC) and HT3+10 (126 ± 4 µg/mg protein, $P<0.01$ vs. HC), but not in HT10 (142 ± 4 µg/mg protein, $P>0.05$ vs. HC, $P<0.05$ vs. HT3, $P<0.05$ vs. HT3+10) (Fig. 8C).

HGF and VEGF

The HGF in the rat lung measured by RT-PCR at P21 were significantly lower in HC ($P<0.05$) than NC. The hyperoxia-induced decrease in lung HGF was significantly up-regulated in both HT3 ($P<0.05$ vs. HC) and HT3+10 ($P<0.01$ vs. HC), but not in HT10 ($P>0.05$ vs. HC, $P<0.05$ vs. HT3, $P<0.01$ vs. HT3+10) (Fig. 9A). The VEGF levels in the rat lungs measured by ELISA at P21 were significantly lower in HC (23.5 ± 1.9 pg/ml, $P<0.001$) than in NC (39.5 ± 4.3 pg/ml). This hyperoxia-induced

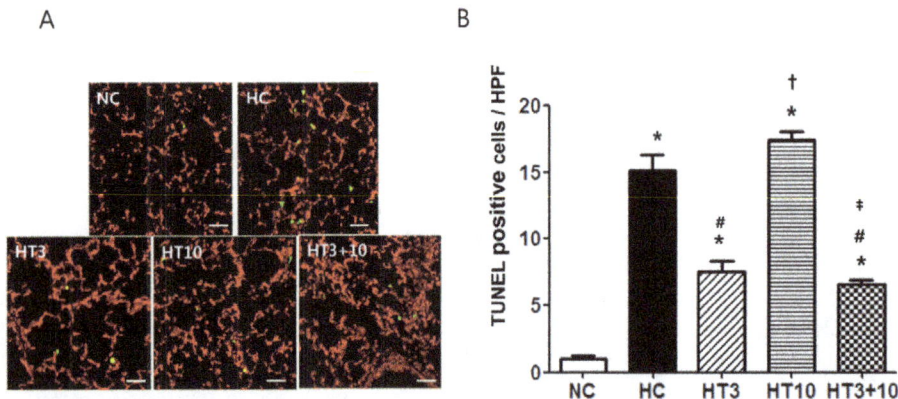

Figure 4. TUNEL positive cells in the distal lungs of the P 21 rat pups. (A): TUNEL positive cells were labeled with FITC (*green*) and the cell nuclei were labeled with propidium iodide (*red*) (Scale bar; 25 µm). (B): Number of observed TUNEL positive cells per high power field. NC, Normoxia control group; HC, hyperoxia control group; HT3, hyperoxia with stem cell transplantation group at P3; HT10, hyperoxia with stem cell treatment group at P10; HT3+10, hyperoxia with stem cell treatment group at P3 and P10. Data; mean±SEM. *$P<0.05$ compared to NC, #$P<0.05$ compared to HC,† $P<0.05$ compared to HT3, ‡ $P<0.05$ compared to HT10.

A

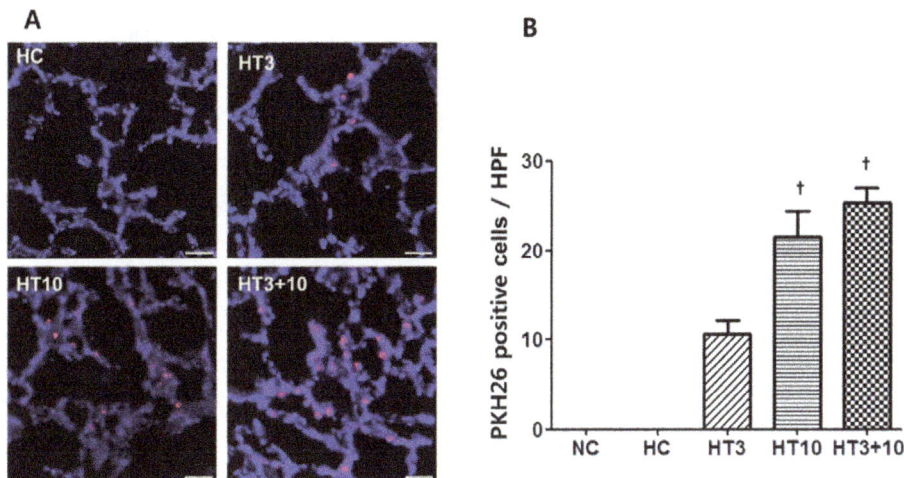

Figure 5. Donor cell localization in the lung of the P 21 rats. (A): Fluorescent microscopic observation of the PKH26 labeled human UCB-derived MSCs (donor cells, *red*) localized in the lungs of the P 21 newborn rats and the nuclei labeled with DAPI (*blue*) (Scale bar; 25 μm). (B): Number of PKH26 positive cells in the lung per high power field. NC, Normoxia control group; HC, hyperoxia control group; HT3, hyperoxia with stem cell transplantation group at P3; HT10, hyperoxia with stem cell treatment group at P10; HT3+10, hyperoxia with stem cell treatment group at P3 and P10. Data; mean±SEM. [†] P<0.05 compared to HT3.

decrease in the lung VEGF level was attenuated in both HT3 (30.6±2.0 pg/ml, P<0.05 vs. HC) and HT10 (33.4±1.6 pg/ml, P<0.01 vs. HC), but not in HT10 (28.1±1.7 pg/ml, P>0.05 vs. HC) (Fig. 9B).

Discussion

In the present study, prolonged exposure of newborn rat pups to hyperoxia for 3 weeks increased mortality, retarded growth, and developed lung injuries similar to those seen in the premature human infants with BPD [23,24], exhibiting decreased alveolarization as evidenced by increased MLI and alveolar volume [25], and significantly increased TUNEL positive cells [26]. Previously, we have shown that the neonatal hyperoxic lung injuries induced by ≥90% oxygen for 2 weeks were significantly attenuated with intratracheal human UCB-derived MSCs transplantation at P5 [7], and these beneficial effects were dose dependent [8]. In the present study, hyperoxic exposure was extended to 3 weeks to guarantee the comparable time span after MSCs transplantation at P10, and the oxygen concentration during the third week was reduced from 90% to 60% because of the concern about increased mortality due to prolonged high oxygen exposure. Only MSCs given at P3 but not at P10 showed protective effects against the hyperoxia-induced lung injuries, and no synergistic effects were observed with combined early+late at P3+10 MSCs transplantation in this study. Overall, these findings suggest that the therapeutic efficacy of human UCB-derived MSCs transplantation is time-dependent, showing protection only during the early but not late phase of inflammation.

In time course experiments of the present study, lung inflammatory cytokine levels such as TNF-α, IL-1α, IL-1β and IL-6 in HC became significantly higher after P5~7 compared to NC. Intratracheal MSCs given at P3 or P5, but not at P10 protected against neonatal hyperoxic lung injuries in our previous [7,8] and present studies. These findings suggest that increased secretion of proinflammatory cytokines and the ensuing full blown host inflammatory milieu might be a strong inhibitor of MSCs protection against neonatal hyperoxic lung injury, and thus the

therapeutic time window of stem cell transplantation in BPD might be limited only to the early phase of inflammation.

In the present study, the number of PKH26 positive cells at P21, indicative of donor cell localization in the lung tissue, was significantly higher in HT10 and HT3+10 than in HT3. These findings suggest that substantial donor cell losses occur early after intratracheal MSCs transplantation [27]. However, significant protective effects against neonatal hyperoxic lung injuries were observed in both HT3 and HT3+10, but not in HT10. Similar results of beneficial effects of MSCs despite low engraftment have also been reported in other disease models such as acute renal failure [28], and cardiac injury [29]. In our previous study [7,8], we also observed only very few donor cells differentiate into type II pneumocytes, Overall, these findings suggest that even a small number of MSCs survived could mediate their therapeutic effects against neonatal hyperoxic lung injuries primarily by secreting key bioactive mediators rather than by direct tissue repair [30], and early timing of MSCs transplantation is critical for their best protective effects. Moreover, although donor cells rapidly faded away after transplantation, the favorable effects of MSCs were persistent up to P21. These findings suggest that the paracrine effects initially induced by stem cells might play a pivotal role in tissue repair, and are sustained later by the intact host tissue protected by MSCs transplantation [31]. However, we cannot exclude the possibility that rejection might have occurred in our study because transplant was performed in a xenograft model; therefore, further studies are needed to clarify this.

Oxidative stress to the immature lung is a well-known risk factor for the development of BPD [32]. NADPH oxidase is a multi-component enzyme complex responsible for production of superoxide anion (O_2^-), which generates other reactive oxygen species such as hydrogen peroxide, hydroxyl radical, and hypochlorous acid [20]. Upon its activation, the cytoplasmic subunits $p47^{phox}$, $p67^{phox}$, $p40^{phox}$ and Rac translocate to membrane bound cytochrome [33]. The membrane translocation of the $p47^{phox}$ can thus be served as an *in vivo* indicator of NADPH oxidase activation in the lung tissue. In our previous study [8], we have observed the dose-dependent anti-oxidative effects of intratracheal MSCs transplantation. In the present study,

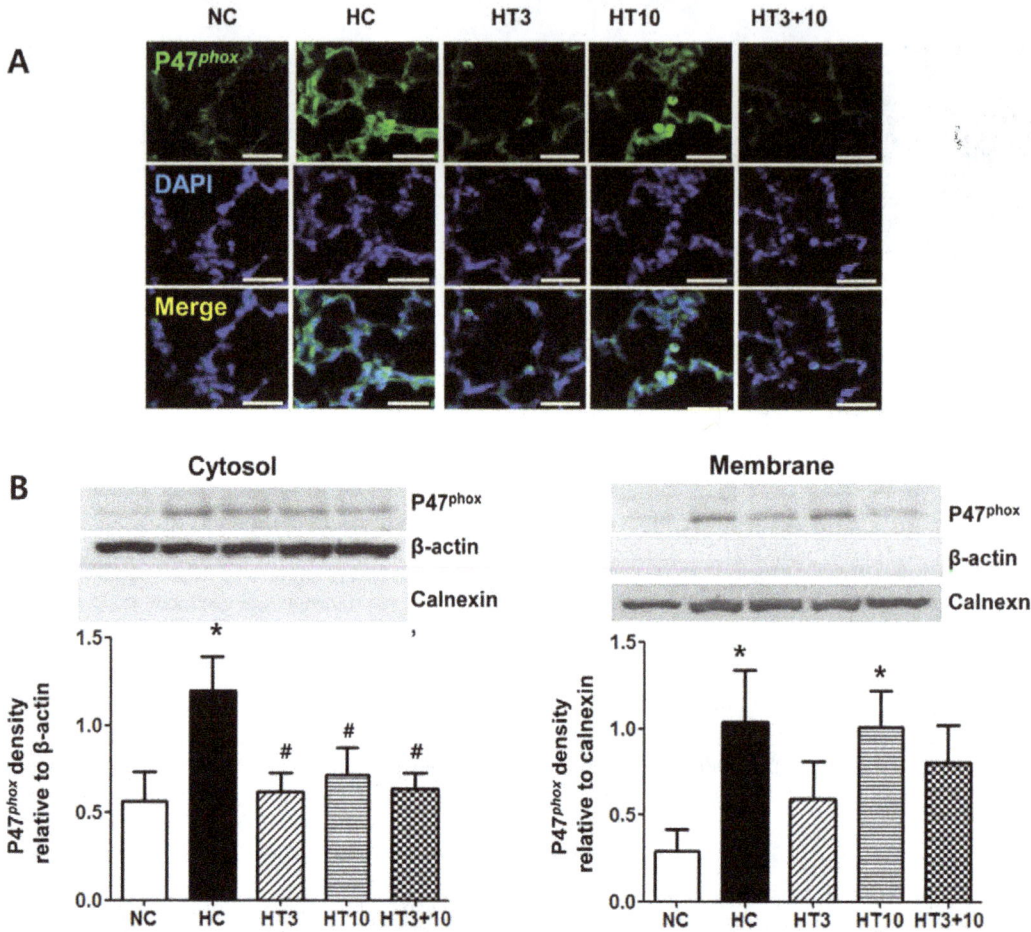

Figure 6. p47^{phox}, cytosolic subunit of nicotinamide adenine dinucleotide phosphate oxidase in the P21 rat lung tissue. (A): Fluorescent microscopic observation of p47^{phox} (green) localized in the lungs of the P21 rats and the nuclei labeled with DAPI (blue) (Scale bar; 25 μm). (B): Representative western blots (top) and densitometric histograms (bottom) in the cytosol (left) and membrane (right) fractions of P21 rat lung homogenates. NC, Normoxia control group; HC, hyperoxia control group; HT3, hyperoxia with stem cell transplantation group at P3; HT10, hyperoxia with stem cell treatment group at P10; HT3+10, hyperoxia with stem cell treatment group at P3 and P10. Data; mean±SEM. *$P<0.05$ compared to NC, # $P<0.05$ compared to HC.

increased expression of the p47^{phox} protein was observed both in the cytosolic and membrane fraction in HC. Although significant attenuation of cytosolic expression of the p47^{phox} was observed after MSCs transplantation, a decrease in membrane translocation of the p47^{phox} was observed in both HT3 and HT3+10, but not in HT10. These findings suggest that MSCs transplantation at the early rather than late phase of inflammation will be the optimal timing for their best anti-oxidative effects.

In our previous studies [7,8], we have shown that inflammatory responses mediated by neutrophils [4] and proinflammatory cytokines [5] play a pivotal role in the development of BPD [6], and that the protective effects of MSCs therapy against hyperoxia-induced lung injuries are mediated primarily by their anti-inflammatory effects rather than by their regenerating capacity. In the present study, hyperoxia-induced increase in ED1 positive alveolar macrophages, lung myeloperoxidase activity and cytokines such as IL-1α, IL-1β, IL-6, TNF-α measured by ELISA, other inflammatory markers such as TIMP-1, CXCL7, RANTES, L-selectin and sICAM-1 measured by protein array were consistently attenuated by MSCs administration at both early (HT3) and combined early+ late (HT3+10), but not at the late (HT10) phase of inflammation. These findings suggest a full-blown

host inflammatory micro-environment might hinder the anti-inflammatory effects of the transplanted MSCs. Further studies will be necessary to elucidate the inhibitory mechanism of endogenous inflammatory factors on transplanted stem cells function.

In our previous studies [7,8], we have shown that the anti-fibrotic effect of transplanted MSCs was associated and probably mediated by their down-modulation of hyperoxia-induced pulmonary inflammatory responses. Significant attenuation of hyperoxia-induced increase in both fibrogenic cytokines such as TGF-β and TIMP-1 [34] along with other inflammatory cytokines, and collagen levels in both HT3 and HT3+10, but not in HT10 support the assumption that the early timing of MSCs transplantation is critical for their best anti-inflammatory and the ensuing anti-fibrotic effects.

In the present study, hyperoxia-induced decrease in growth factors such as VEGF and HGF was significantly up-regulated in both HT3 and HT3+10, but not in HT10 despite higher donor cell localization in the lung tissue at P21 in HT10 than in HT3. These findings suggest that the protective effects of MSCs transplantation such as promotion of angiogenesis, anti-apoptotic effects and reduced inflammation are strongly associated or

A

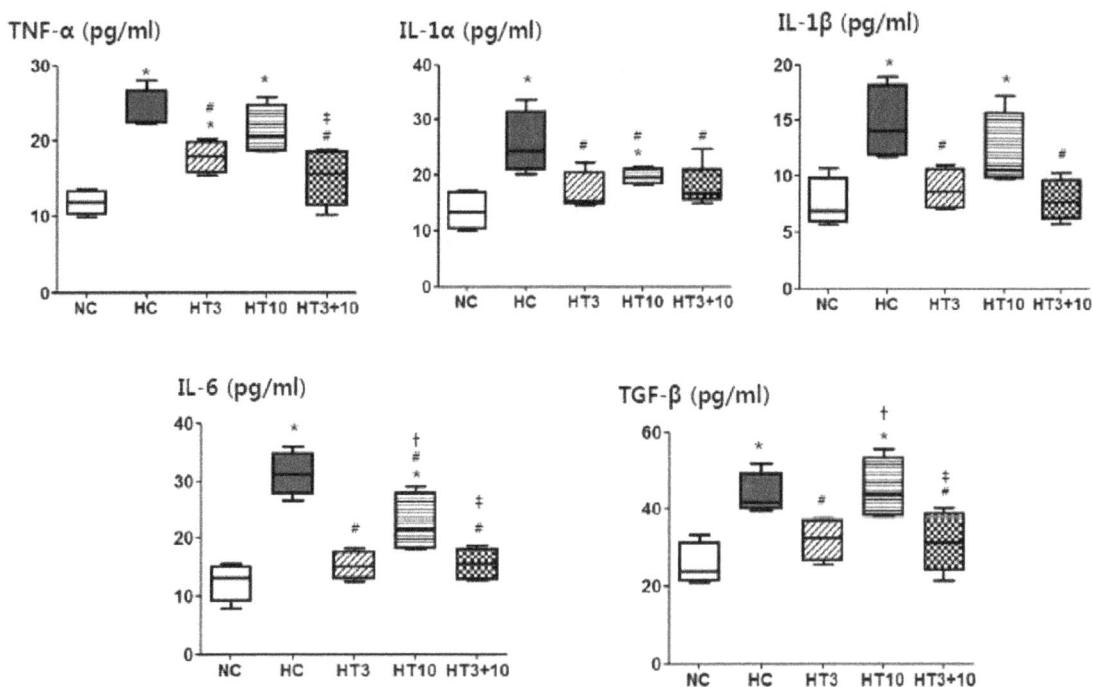

B

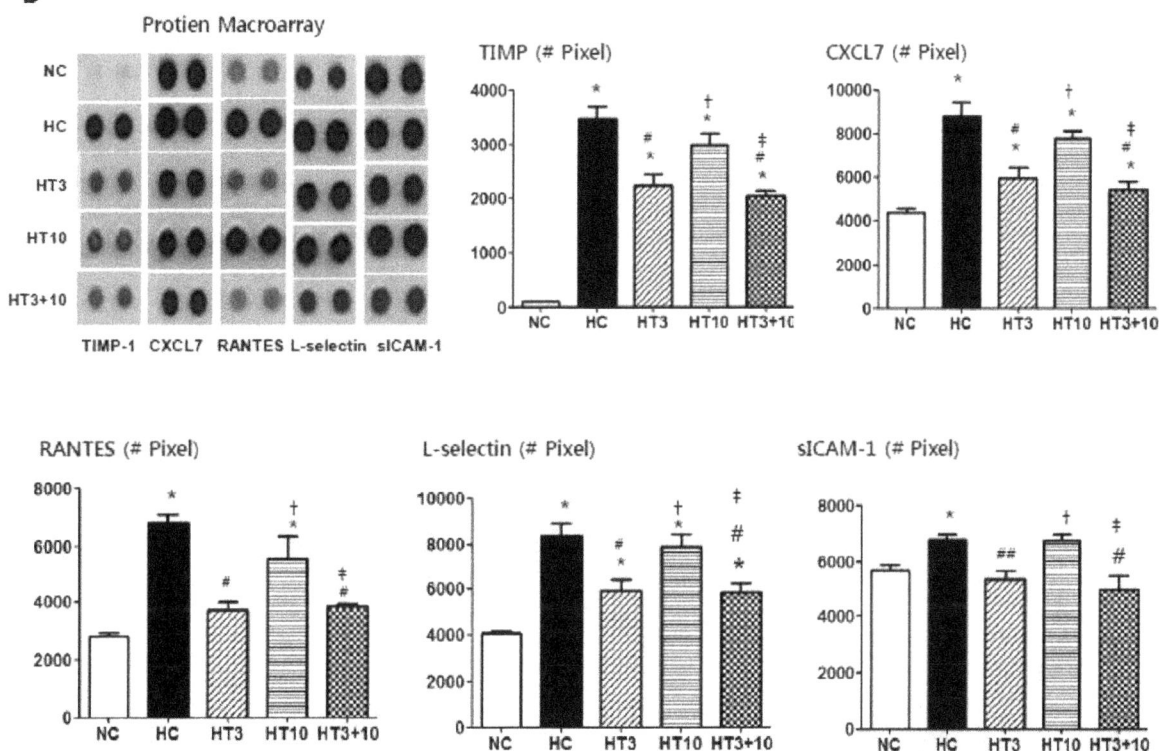

Figure 7. Histograms of inflammatory cytokines and chemokines in the hyperoxic lung injury after MSCs transplantation. TNF-α, IL-1α, IL-1β, IL-6, and TGF-β levels measured by ELISA (A) and TIMP-1, CXCL7, RANTES, L-selectin and sICAM-1 levels measured by protein array at P21 in the rat lung tissue (B,C). NC, Normoxia control group; HC, hyperoxia control group; HT3, hyperoxia with stem cell transplantation group at P3; HT10, hyperoxia with stem cell treatment group at P10; HT3+10, hyperoxia with stem cell treatment group at P3 and P10. Data; mean±SEM. $^{*}P<0.05$ compared to NC, $^{\#}P<0.05$ compared to HC, $^{\dagger}P<0.05$ compared to HT3, $^{\ddagger}P<0.05$ compared to HT10.

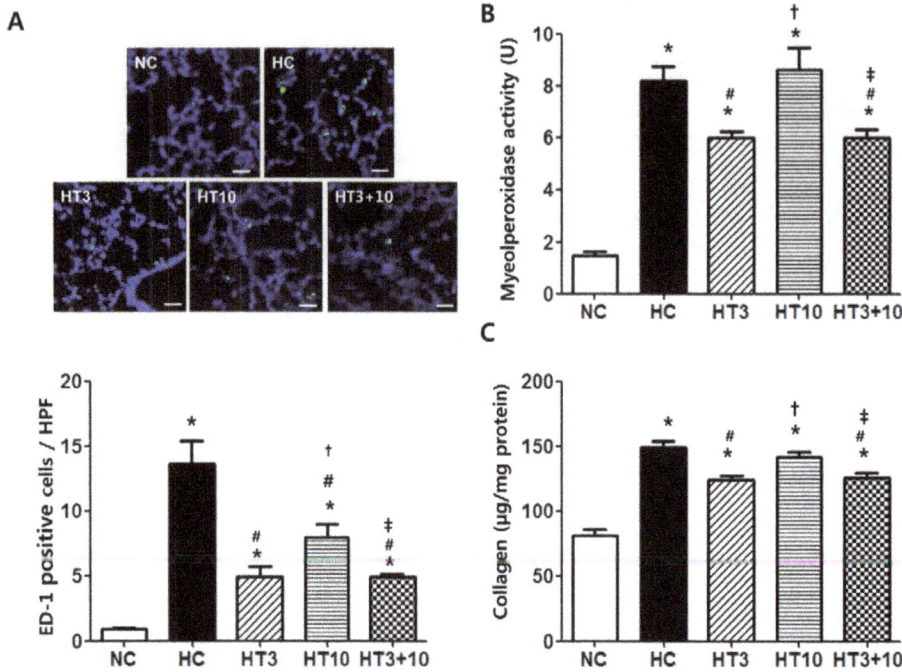

Figure 8. Inflammation with fibrosis in the hyperoxic lung injury after MSCs transplantation. ED1 positive cells indicative of alveolar macrophage were labeled with FITC (*green*) and the nuclei were labeled with DAPI (*blue*) (Scale bar; 25 μm) (*at top*) and number of observed ED1 positive cells per high power field (*below*) (A), myeloperoxidase activity (B), and collagen levels (C) of the rat P21 lung tissues. NC, Normoxia control group; HC, hyperoxia control group; HT3, hyperoxia with stem cell transplantation group at P3; HT10, hyperoxia with stem cell treatment group at P10; HT3+10, hyperoxia with stem cell treatment group at P3 and P10. Data; mean±SEM. *$P<0.05$ compared to NC, # $P<0.05$ compared to HC,[†] $P<0.05$ compared to HT3, ‡ $P<0.05$ compared to HT10.

probably mediated by enhanced secretion of these growth factors [35]. Moreover, as the full blown host inflammatory milieu might hinder the secretion of these growth factors by MSCs [36] the timing of MSCs transplantation early in the inflammation is essential for enhanced expression of these growth factors. Further studies will be necessary to clarify this.

In summary, intratracheal transplantation of human UCB derived MSCs time-dependently attenuated hyperoxia-induced lung pathology such as decreased alveolarization and increased

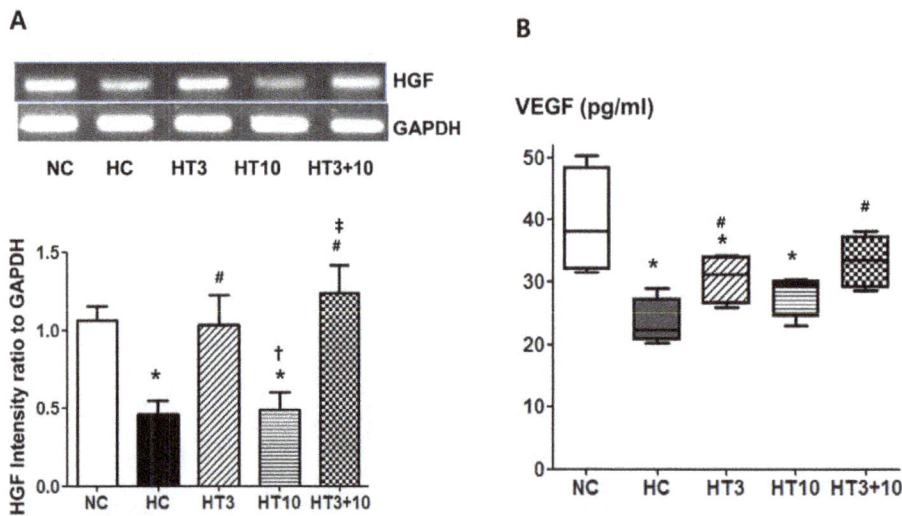

Figure 9. VEGF and HGF in the hyperoxic lung injury after MSCs transplantation. Representative RT-PCR blots (*at top*) and densitometric histograms (*below*) for HGF (A) and VEGF measured with ELISA (B) in the P21 rat lungs. NC, Normoxia control group; HC, hyperoxia control group; HT3, hyperoxia with stem cell transplantation group at P3; HT10, hyperoxia with stem cell treatment group at P10; HT3+10, hyperoxia with stem cell treatment group at P3 and P10. Data; mean±SEM. *$P<0.05$ compared to NC, # $P<0.05$ compared to HC,[†] $P<0.05$ compared to HT3, ‡ $P<0.05$ compared to HT10.

apoptotic cells, oxidative stress, inflammatory responses and the ensuing fibrosis, and up-regulated growth factors such as HGF and VEGF, showing significant protection only in the early at P3 but not in the late at P10 phase of inflammation. There were no synergies with combined early+late MSCs transplantation. These findings are expected to have important implications for future clinical translation to determine the optimal timing of MSCs transplantation for the currently untreatable neonatal hyperoxic lung disease i.e., BPD in premature infants.

Author Contributions

Conceived and designed the experiments: WSP. Performed the experiments: SYA DKS HSY. Analyzed the data: YSC SIS. Contributed reagents/materials/analysis tools: WIO. Wrote the paper: YSC SJC.

References

1. Saigal S, Doyle LW (2008) An overview of mortality and sequelae of preterm birth from infancy to adulthood. Lancet 371: 261–269.
2. Avery ME, Tooley WH, Keller JB, Hurd SS, Bryan MH, et al. (1987) Is chronic lung disease in low birth weight infants preventable? A survey of eight centers. Pediatrics 79: 26–30.
3. Bregman J, Farrell EE (1992) Neurodevelopmental outcome in infants with bronchopulmonary dysplasia. Clin Perinatol 19: 673–694.
4. Fahy JV (2009) Eosinophilic and neutrophilic inflammation in asthma: insights from clinical studies. Proc Am Thorac Soc 6: 256–259.
5. Choo-Wing R, Nedrelow JH, Homer RJ, Elias JA, Bhandari V (2007) Developmental differences in the responses of IL-6 and IL-13 transgenic mice exposed to hyperoxia. Am J Physiol Lung Cell Mol Physiol 293: L142–150.
6. Warner BB, Stuart LA, Papes RA, Wispe JR (1998) Functional and pathological effects of prolonged hyperoxia in neonatal mice. Am J Physiol 275: L110–117.
7. Chang YS, Oh W, Choi SJ, Sung DK, Kim SY, et al. (2009) Human umbilical cord blood-derived mesenchymal stem cells attenuate hyperoxia-induced lung injury in neonatal rats. Cell Transplant 18: 869–886.
8. Chang YS, Choi SJ, Sung DK, Kim SY, Oh W, et al. (2011) Intratracheal transplantation of human umbilical cord blood derived mesenchymal stem cells dose-dependently attenuates hyperoxia-induced lung injury in neonatal rats. Cell Transplant.
9. Jang YK, Jung DH, Jung MH, Kim DH, Yoo KH, et al. (2006) Mesenchymal stem cells feeder layer from human umbilical cord blood for ex vivo expanded growth and proliferation of hematopoietic progenitor cells. Ann Hematol 85: 212–225.
10. Yang SE, Ha CW, Jung M, Jin HJ, Lee M, et al. (2004) Mesenchymal stem/progenitor cells developed in cultures from UC blood. Cytotherapy 6: 476–486.
11. Boiani M, Scholer HR (2005) Regulatory networks in embryo-derived pluripotent stem cells. Nat Rev Mol Cell Biol 6: 872–884.
12. Gang EJ, Bosnakovski D, Figueiredo CA, Visser JW, Perlingeiro RC (2007) SSEA-4 identifies mesenchymal stem cells from bone marrow. Blood 109: 1743–1751.
13. Lee JK, Lee MK, Jin HJ, Kim DS, Yang YS, et al. (2007) Efficient intracytoplasmic labeling of human umbilical cord blood mesenchymal stromal cells with ferumoxides. Cell Transplant 16: 849–857.
14. Thurlbeck WM (1982) Postnatal human lung growth. Thorax 37: 564–571.
15. Cho SJ, George CL, Snyder JM, Acarregui MJ (2005) Retinoic acid and erythropoietin maintain alveolar development in mice treated with an angiogenesis inhibitor. Am J Respir Cell Mol Biol 33: 622–628.
16. Snyder JM, Jenkins-Moore M, Jackson SK, Goss KL, Dai HH, et al. (2005) Alveolarization in retinoic acid receptor-beta-deficient mice. Pediatr Res 57: 384–391.
17. Babior BM (1999) NADPH oxidase: an update. Blood 93: 1464–1476.
18. Cross AR, Segal AW (2004) The NADPH oxidase of professional phagocytes–prototype of the NOX electron transport chain systems. Biochim Biophys Acta 1657: 1–22.
19. Gray KD, Simovic MO, Chapman WC, Blackwell TS, Christman JW, et al. (2003) Endotoxin potentiates lung injury in cerulein-induced pancreatitis. Am J Surg 186: 526–530.
20. Robinson JM, Badwey JA (1995) The NADPH oxidase complex of phagocytic leukocytes: a biochemical and cytochemical view. Histochem Cell Biol 103: 163–180.
21. Hohler B, Holzapfel B, Kummer W (2000) NADPH oxidase subunits and superoxide production in porcine pulmonary artery endothelial cells. Histochem Cell Biol 114: 29–37.
22. Li JM, Shah AM (2002) Intracellular localization and preassembly of the NADPH oxidase complex in cultured endothelial cells. J Biol Chem 277: 19952–19960.
23. Coalson JJ (2003) Pathology of new bronchopulmonary dysplasia. Semin Neonatol 8: 73–81.
24. Jobe AJ (1999) The new BPD: an arrest of lung development. Pediatr Res 46: 641–643.
25. Kunig AM, Balasubramaniam V, Markham NE, Morgan D, Montgomery G, et al. (2005) Recombinant human VEGF treatment enhances alveolarization after hyperoxic lung injury in neonatal rats. Am J Physiol Lung Cell Mol Physiol 289: L529–535.
26. McGrath-Morrow SA, Stahl J (2001) Apoptosis in neonatal murine lung exposed to hyperoxia. Am J Respir Cell Mol Biol 25: 150–155.
27. Reinecke H, Murry CE (2002) Taking the death toll after cardiomyocyte grafting: a reminder of the importance of quantitative biology. J Mol Cell Cardiol 34: 251–253.
28. Togel F, Hu Z, Weiss K, Isaac J, Lange C, et al. (2005) Administered mesenchymal stem cells protect against ischemic acute renal failure through differentiation-independent mechanisms. Am J Physiol Renal Physiol 289: F31–42.
29. Gnecchi M, He H, Noiseux N, Liang OD, Zhang L, et al. (2006) Evidence supporting paracrine hypothesis for Akt-modified mesenchymal stem cell-mediated cardiac protection and functional improvement. FASEB J 20: 661–669.
30. Aslam M, Baveja R, Liang OD, Fernandez-Gonzalez A, Lee C, et al. (2009) Bone marrow stromal cells attenuate lung injury in a murine model of neonatal chronic lung disease. Am J Respir Crit Care Med 180: 1122–1130.
31. Cho HJ, Lee N, Lee JY, Choi YJ, Ii M, et al. (2007) Role of host tissues for sustained humoral effects after endothelial progenitor cell transplantation into the ischemic heart. J Exp Med 204: 3257–3269.
32. Saugstad OD (2003) Bronchopulmonary dysplasia-oxidative stress and antioxidants. Semin Neonatol 8: 39–49.
33. Bastian NR, Hibbs JB, Jr. (1994) Assembly and regulation of NADPH oxidase and nitric oxide synthase. Curr Opin Immunol 6: 131–139.
34. Moodley Y, Atienza D, Manuelpillai U, Samuel CS, Tchongue J, et al. (2009) Human umbilical cord mesenchymal stem cells reduce fibrosis of bleomycin-induced lung injury. Am J Pathol 175: 303–313.
35. Deuse T, Peter C, Fedak PW, Doyle T, Reichenspurner H, et al. (2009) Hepatocyte growth factor or vascular endothelial growth factor gene transfer maximizes mesenchymal stem cell-based myocardial salvage after acute myocardial infarction. Circulation 120: S247–254.
36. Kokaia Z, Martino G, Schwartz M, Lindvall O (2012) Cross-talk between neural stem cells and immune cells: the key to better brain repair? Nat Neurosci 15: 1078–1087.

16

NK Cell Phenotypic Modulation in Lung Cancer Environment

Shi Jin[1,2⑨]**, Yi Deng**[1,3⑨]**, Jun-Wei Hao**[4]**, Yang Li**[1]**, Bin Liu**[1]**, Yan Yu**[2]**, Fu-Dong Shi**[4]**, Qing-Hua Zhou**[1]*

1 Tianjin Key Laboratory of Lung Cancer Metastasis and Tumor Micro-environment, Tianjin Lung Cancer Institute, Tianjin Medical University General Hospital, Tianjin, P.R. China, 2 Department of Medical Oncology, Harbin Medical University Cancer Hospital, Harbin, P.R. China, 3 Cancer Center, Research Institute of Surgery and Daping Hospital, Third Military Medical University, Chongqing, P.R. China, 4 Department of neurology, Tianjin Medical University General Hospital, Tianjin, P.R. China

Abstract

Background: Nature killer (NK) cells play an important role in anti-tumor immunotherapy. But it indicated that tumor cells impacted possibly on NK cell normal functions through some molecules mechanisms in tumor microenvironment.

Materials and methods: Our study analyzed the change about NK cells surface markers (NK cells receptors) through immunofluorescence, flow cytometry and real-time PCR, the killed function from mouse spleen NK cell and human high/low lung cancer cell line by co-culture. Furthermore we certificated the above result on the lung cancer model of SCID mouse.

Results: We showed that the infiltration of NK cells in tumor periphery was related with lung cancer patients' prognosis. And the number of NK cell infiltrating in lung cancer tissue is closely related to the pathological types, size of the primary cancer, smoking history and prognosis of the patients with lung cancer. The expression of NK cells inhibitor receptors increased remarkably in tumor micro-environment, in opposite, the expression of NK cells activated receptors decrease magnificently.

Conclusions: The survival time of lung cancer patient was positively related to NK cell infiltration degree in lung cancer. Thus, the down-regulation of NKG2D, Ly49I and the up-regulation of NKG2A may indicate immune tolerance mechanism and facilitate metastasis in tumor environment. Our research will offer more theory for clinical strategy about tumor immunotherapy.

Editor: Xin-Yuan Guan, The University of Hong Kong, China

Funding: This work was supported by Young People Research Fund from the grants the National Eleventh-Five-Year Key Task Projects of China (No. 2006BAI02A01), the National 973 Program (No. 2010CB529405), Tianjin Scientific Innovation System Program (No. 07SYSYSF05000, 07SYSYJC27900), the China-Sweden Cooperative Foundation (No. 09ZCZDSF04100), the grant National Natural Scientific Foundation of China (No 81201828), Young People Foundation of Heilongjiang Provincial of China (No QC2012C013), Health Department of Heilongjiang Provincial of China (No 2011-124) and Harbin Medical University Cancer Hospital major project Foundation (No: JJZ-2010-01). The funders had no role in study design, data collection and analysis, decision to publish, or preparation of the manuscript.

Competing Interests: The authors have declared that no competing interests exist.

* Email: zhouqh135@163.com

⑨ These authors contributed equally to this work.

Introduction

Lung cancer is one of the most common malignant tumors in the world, which has high morbidity and mortality and accounts for about 25.4% of all tumors. It has been an upward trend of the incidence rate in recent years [1–4]. The American Cancer Society released data show that 222,520 cases of respiratory cancer and 157,300 cases of death in 2010, which is in the first place of morbidity and mortality of all malignant tumors [5]. A clinical statistics of stage IV NSCLC in China showed that the 1-, 2-, 3-, 4- and 5-year survival rate was 44%, 22%, 13%, 9% and 6% respectively [6]. Currently, surgical resection is still the main method to prolong the survival time of lung cancer, but the invasion and metastasis of lung cancer is the biggest obstacle to improve the efficacy of the prognosis of lung cancer. For in-depth study of lung cancer malignant behavior and focus on comprehensive treatment of metastatic lung cancer, it is necessary to establish appropriate animal model to study lung cancer recurrence and metastasis and its comprehensive therapy.

Natural killer (NK) cell, also known as large granular lymphocytes, is an independent and non-specific immune cell. It has no MHC restriction to target cells recognition and destruction, and it can directly kill tumor cells and virus-infected target cells without antigen pre-sensitized [7,8]. It also can produce a large number of immune-active cytokines to enhance or expand its anti-tumor effect, which can be regarded as the first line of the host defense system [9]. Several experimental evidences demonstrated the important role of NK cells in the elimination of tumor cells. Vivier et al report that a low NK cell cytotoxicity in peripheral blood was correlated with an increased cancer risk [10]. Furthermore, NK cells infiltrating in the tumor tissue was associated with good prognosis in colorectal [11], gastric [12], and lung [13] cancers.

Table 1. NK cells phenotype expressed in different pathological type of lung cancer.

Pathological type	NK cellular infiltration extent			Total	χ^2	P value
	Grade1	Grade2	Grade3			
CD56	37(44.0%)	19(22.6%)	28(33.3%)	84(100.0%)	0.126	0.998
CD16	38(45.2%)	19(22.6%)	27(32.1%)	84(100.0%)		
CD56CD16	38(45.2%)	20(23.8%)	26(31.0%)	84(100.0%)		

With the development of tumor formation, malignant tumor cells and infiltrating immune cells interact and composed the tumor micro-environment. Most of studies published showed that a large number of immune cells infiltrating into tumor tissue played an important role in improving tumor prognosis [14,15]. But as we all known, the prognosis of lung-associated malignancies is very terrible, even though there are many immune cells in the lung. We want to know if there is a differential composition of the immune cell infiltrate in malignant and non-malignant lung tissue areas, and even might potentially contribute to this effect. Esendagli G et.al found that in non-small cell lung cancer (NSCLC) patients, NK cells were not almost found in the malignant tissue regions, non-malignant counterparts were selectively populated by NK cells and those NK cells showed strong cytotoxic activity ex vivo [16].

So the impact of NK cell receptor expression and function may be different caused by the interaction between NK cells and tumor in the tumor micro-environment. By exploring NK cells in the body and/or lung cancer micro-environment, discuss its distribution, receptor expression, functional status with lung cancer invasion, metastasis and prognosis, clarify the mechanism of NK cells involved in lung cancer micro-environment from the cellular and molecular levels.

Materials and Methods

Tumor Samples and Ethics Statement

This study was conducted according to the principles expressed in the Declaration of Helsinki. All tumor samples used in this study were obtained from Tianjin Lung Cancer Institute and department of pathology in Tianjin Medical University General Hospital. All patients provided written informed consent for the collection of samples and subsequent analysis. And the study was approved by the Institutional Ethics Committee of Tianjin Medical University General Hospital.

Paraffins Specimen and Frozen tissue origin of Lung cancer

Patients will be eligible for participation in the induction phase of the study if they have: histologic or cytologic diagnosis of NSCLC (including squamous carcinoma, adenocarcinoma and large cell carcinoma); no prior systemic chemotherapy, radiotherapy and biotherapy for lung cancer before surgery; no other cancer history; and ≤80 years of age.

Paraffins Specimen samples were collected from 84 patients diagnosed with lung cancer between January1st 2008 and January 31st 2011 (64 men and 20 women). The median age of patients was 60.7±7.9 years (range 40 to 78 years). There are different pathology types: 37 squamous carcinoma patients, 37 adenocarcinoma patients and 10 large cell carcinoma patients. At the time of diagnosis, patients were assessed according to the AJCC/UICC the sixth classification edition as follows: stage IIA-1 patients, stage IIB- 4 patients, stage IIIA-58 patients, stage IIIB-12 patients, stage IV-9 patients. The samples were applied from Tianjin Medical University Pathology Department.

Frozen tissue samples were generated from 66 surgical samples

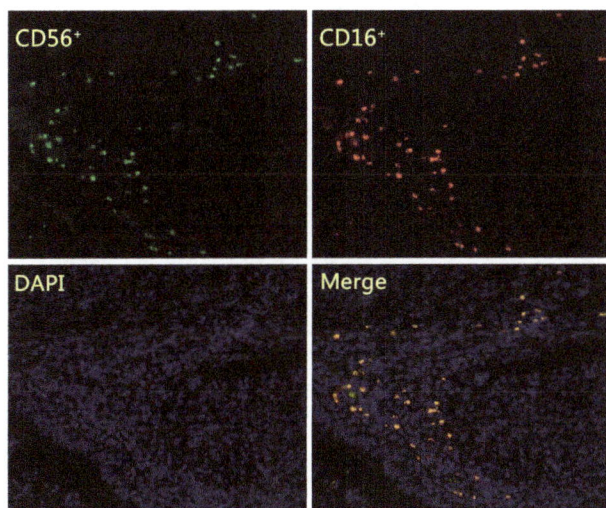

Figure 1. Immune fluorescence detecting the phenotype of NK cells in lung cancer tissues. The infiltrated NK cells in the lung cancer tissue were mainly concentrated in the tumor stroma. NK cells shows with CD56 single positive (green fluorescence), CD16 single positive (red fluorescence) and CD56CD16 double positive (yellow fluorescence) in the lung cancer stroma tissue.

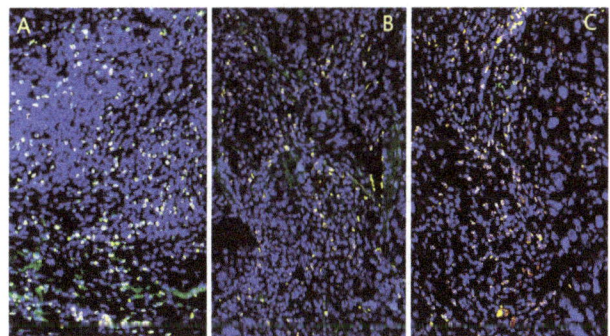

Figure 2. CD56⁺CD16⁺ NK cell infiltration extent in different pathological type of lung cancer. A. Lung squamous carcinoma; B. Lung adenocarcinoma; C. Large cell lung cancer. The expression of NK cells in squamous cell carcinoma was significantly higher than in adenocarcinoma and large cell carcinoma.

Table 2. CD56$^+$CD16$^+$NK cells infiltration extent in different pathological type of lung cancer.

Pathological type	CD56$^+$CD16$^+$NK cellular infiltration extent			Total	χ^2	p value
	Grade1	Grade2	Grade3			
squamous cell carcinoma	9(24.3%)	12(32.4%)	16(43.2%)	37(100.0%)	11.800	0.019*
adenocarcinoma	23(62.2%)	6(16.2%)	8(21.6%)	37(100.0%)		
Large cell cancer	5(50.0%)	1(10.0%)	4(40.0%)	10(100.0%)		
Total	37(44%)	19(22.6%)	28(33.3%)	84(100.0%)		

*p<0.05, Difference have statistical significance.

with lung cancer between January1st 2008 and January1st 2011. There are including 52 men and 14 women. The median age of patients was 60.5±8.4 years (range 40 to 78 years). There were including different pathology types: 28 squamous carcinoma patients, 28 adenocarcinoma patients and 10 large cell carcinoma patients. The patients were assessed according to the AJCC/UICC the sixth classification edition as follows: stage IIA-1 patients, stage IIB-4 patients, stage IIIA-45 patients, stage IIIB-9 patients, stage IV-7 patients. The samples were applied from Tianjin Lung Cancer Research Institute.

Immunofluorescence

Immunophenotypes analysis of CD56 and CD16 were done as follow. In brief, the formalin-fixed, paraffin-embedded sections (4 μm) were warmed by ovenware for 45 min, then deparaffinized in xylene and rehydrated in a graded series of ethanol solutions. The sections were subsequently submerged in citric-sodium citrate buffer solution (pH 7) and microwave at high fire for 5 min, low fire for 15 min, and natural cooling to room temperature to retrieve the antigenicity. Endogenous peroxidase was quenched with 3% H$_2$O$_2$ for 30 min. After washing with PBS, the sections were incubated with 2% BSA for 2 hours in room temperature and then incubated with CD56 and CD16 antibody (Santa Cruz, diluted at 1:100) overnight at 4°C. The sections were incubated with mouse anti-goat and goat anti-mouse fluorescence antibody (Santa Cruz, diluted at 1:200) for 35 min and the DAPI for 5 min. After washing with PBS fourth times, the sections were mounting by glycerol (PH 9.0). The red fluorescence expressed CD56$^+$, the green fluorescence expressed CD16$^+$, the blue fluorescence expressed cell nucleus. We can find the CD56$^+$ and/or CD16$^+$ expressing in the NK cell. The SPOT image analysis software was used in the analysis process. The percentage of CD56 and/or CD16 positive cells was determined by counting per section. The NK cell count of per view field was scored according to the

Table 3. The clinical features of lung cancer patients and NK cell infiltration extent.

Clinical features	Cases	CD56$^+$CD16$^+$NK cellular infiltration extent			χ^2	p value
		Grade1	Grade2	Grade3		
Sex						
Male	64	29(45.3%)	16(25.0%)	19(29.7%)	1.843	0.398
Female	20	8(40.0%)	3(15.0%)	9(45.0%)		
Age						
≤60	39	18(46.2%)	7(17.9%)	14(35.9%)	0.919	0.632
>60	45	19(42.2%)	12(26.7%)	14(31.1%)		
Smoking history						
no	27	13(48.1%)	1(3.7%)	13(48.1%)	9.066	0.011*
have	57	24(42.1%)	18(31.7%)	15(26.3%)		
Primary tumor(T1-4)						
T1-T2	38	23(60.5%)	7(18.4%)	8(21.1%)	7.958	0.019*
T3-T4	46	14(30.4%)	12(26.1%)	20(43.5%)		
Regional lymph node (N0-3)						
N0-N1	17	4(23.5%)	7(41.2%)	6(35.5%)	5.307	0.070
N2-N3	67	33(49.3%)	12(17.9%)	22(32.8%)		
Metastasis (M0-1)						
M0	75	34(45.3%)	18(24.0%)	23(30.7%)	2.346	0.309
M1	9	3(33.3%)	1(11.1%)	5(55.6%)		
Total	84	37(44%)	19(22.6%)	28(33.3%)		

*p<0.05, Difference have statistical significance.

Survival Functions

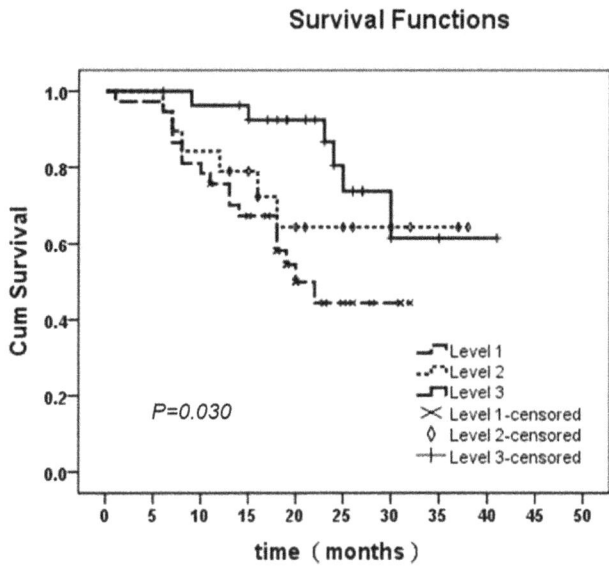

Figure 3. The survival time of different NK cell infiltration extent in the lung cancer. The survival time of lung cancer patient was positively related to NK cell infiltration degree in lung cancer. The more infiltration of NK cells were existed, the longer the survival time of patients did. The patients in level 3 group have the longest survival time. Among three groups statistical significance are exit. (p = 0.030)

following criteria: +, the NK cell counts of per view field<10; ++, the NK cell counts of per view field>10, <20; +++, the NK cell counts of per view field>20. All fields in per section in three independent experiments were calculated.

RNA extraction, cDNA synthesis, and DNA isolation

The total RNA was extracted with the Trizol reagent (Invitrogen, Carlsbad, CA) according to the manufacturer's protocol. The total RNA was digested with R Nase-free D Nase-I (Promega, Madison, USA) and used for cDNA synthesis with the reverse transcriptase system (Takara Biotech, Dalian, China).

Quantitative real-time PCR

The cDNA synthesis was performed as described above. The specific primer of RT experiment were as follow: NK1.1:5'-TCTCTTGAATAAACACACAGCAT -3', NKG2A: 5'- CTGA-GAAGGATTTTG -3', NKG2D: 5'- TTCTCACAGTTCCTCT -3', LY49I: 5'- TTCTATTCTTGCTTTAG -3'. The primer pairs and GAPDH primer pairs were used for Q-PCR with the SYBR Premix Ex Taq RT-PCR Kit (TaKaRa, Dalian, China) in

a ABI PRISM 7900 Real-time System (Bio-Rad) with the following conditions: 95°C for 30 s, 40 amplification cycles (95°C for 5 s and 60°C for 30 s) and a melting cycle from 60°C to 95°C. The data was analyzed using the ABI PRISM 7900 Manager software. All reactions were performed with three technical replicates.

Cell

The high and low metastasis large cell lung cancer cell lines L9981-Luc and NL9980-Luc from Tianjin Lung Cancer Institute [17,18] were maintained in RPMI 1640 medium (Hyclone, America) containing 10% fetal bovine serum (FBS), 100 U/ml penicillin and 100 µg/ml streptomycin (Hyclone, America) in a fully humidified incubator (Nuaire, US Autoflow) at 37°C with 5% CO_2. The cells were kept in an exponential growth phase during experiments.

SCID model

SCID (severe combined immune deficiency) mice purchased from Chinese academy of medical sciences animal institutions were housed in pathogen-free animal facilities. Female mice used were 5–7 wk of age at the experiment's inception. Female SCID mice (16 animals for each experimental group) were inoculated subcutaneously into the right inguen with $2*10^6$ cells suspended in 150 ul of PBS. Nine animals in control group had no inoculation. Tumor sizes were measured every 7 days and their fluorescence intensity were measured with America's true essence of living imaging system (XENOGEN IVIS200). After 6 weeks of observation, dissection was performed and explanted tumors, lungs and spleen were removed for the further analysis. These experiments were repeated at least twice to confirm the results. The animal experimental protocols were approved by the Committee for Ethics of Animal Experimentation and the experiments were conducted in accordance with the Guidelines for Animal Experiments in Tianjin Medical University Cancer Research Center.

Lymphocyte collect and Flow Cytometry detect

The lungs and spleens were polished into pieces. Then the lymphocytes collect were extracted with the Lymphocyte Separation Medium (Shenzhen, China) according to the manufacturer's protocol. Percentages of NK cells were evaluated and separated with flow cytometry using monoclonal antibodies (MoAbs) anti-CD3$^-$ FITC/NK1.1$^+$ PE (BD Phamingen, San Di ego, CA). During analysis, the CD3$^-$/NK1.1$^+$ Population was determined. To determine the surface expression of the NK cell ligands on NK cells, the cells were then stained with the goat anti-mouse NK1.1-FITC, CD3- Alexa Fluor 647, NKG2A-FITC, NKG2D-PE, Ly49I-PE (BD Phamingen, San Di ego, CA) for 30 min at 37°C in

Table 4. NK cells infiltrating extent in the lung cancer and overall survival time.

NK cell	Survival Time(months)				Chi-Square	p value
	<12 (m)	13~24(m)	>25 (m)	Overall		
Level 1	10(27.0%)	21(56.8%)	6(16.2%)	37	7.017	0.030*
Level 2	4(21.1%)	9(47.4%)	6(31.6%)	19		
Level 3	2(7.1%)	14(50.0%)	12(42.9%)	28		
Overall	16(19.0%)	44(52.4%)	24(28.6%)	84		

*p<0.05, Difference have statistical significance.

the dark. The analysis was performed on the FACS Sort (Becton Dickinson, Mountain View, CA) using Cell Quest software (Becton Dickinson) and the cell surface expression was quantified by the value of the mean fluorescence intensities obtained with the specific mAbs.

Co-culture

Purified NK1.1$^+$/CD3$^-$ NK cells (activated with 100U/ml IL-2 during 2 h) from mouse spleen were co-cultured with lung cancer cell line L9981-Luc/NL9980-Luc as (A)0.25:1, (B)0.5:1, (C)1:1 and (D)2:1 for 24, 48, 72 hours. After co-culture, the fluorescence intensity of NK cells was measured with America's true essence of living imaging system.

Quantitative real-time PCR

RNA was isolated from explanted tumors via Trizol and reverse-transcribed using special priming (Invitrogen). Quantitative RT-PCR was performed on an ABI PRISM 7900 instrument, using SYBR green assays. The specific primers are listed in the following (Table 1). The amplification was performed as follows. After initial denaturation step at 95°C for 30 seconds, templates were denatured at 95°C for 5 seconds, primers were annealed and DNA extension was performed at 60°C for 30 seconds (each cycle was repeated 40 times). The expression of target genes was compensated using the expression of GAPDH and presented by the expression ratio between untreated control cells and treated cells.

Statistical analysis

Experiments were performed three times. The Data are presented as mean values ± SD. The statistical evaluation was performed using one-way ANOVA tests or rank-sum test when measurement data is Gaussian distribution with the SPSS Software system, version 17.0. If the data is enumeration data, Chi-square test was used. P values of less than 0.05 were considered statistically significant. Overall survival rate was compared by Kaplan-Meier survivorship curve, Log-rank rank-sum test used among groups.

Results

NK cell localization and morphology characteristic in lung cancer micro-environment

The infiltrated NK cells in the lung cancer tissue were mainly concentrated in the tumor stroma, constituting the tumor micro-environment (Fig.1). In NSCLC tissues, CD56$^+$ NK cells with 1, 2 and 3 degree of infiltration were 44.0%, 22.6%, 33.3%, CD16$^+$ NK cells were 45.2%, 22.6%, 32.1%, and CD56$^+$CD16$^+$ NK cells were 45.2%, 23.8%, 31.0%, respectively. No significant difference was observed ($p>0.05$) among NK cells with CD56 single positive, CD16 single positive and CD56CD16 double positive in the lung cancer tissue (Table 1).

NK cell infiltration and lung cancer patients clinical pathology physiological feature

The 1, 2 and 3 degree with CD56$^+$CD16$^+$ NK cell infiltration were 24.3%, 32.4%, 43.2% in squamous cell carcinomas, and 62.2%, 16.2%, 21.6% in adenocarcinoma and 50.0%, 10.0%, 40.0% in large cell lung cancer, respectively. There was significant difference of CD56$^+$CD16$^+$ NK cell infiltration degree between different pathological types of lung cancer ($p = 0.019$) (Fig.2, Table 2). The expression of NK cells in squamous cell carcinoma was significantly higher than in adenocarcinoma and large cell carcinoma. The 1, 2 and 3 degree with NK cell infiltration were 48.1%, 3.7%, 48.1% in lung cancer patients with no history of smoking, were 42.1%, 31.7% and 26.3% in patients with smoking history. Smoking history of lung cancer patient is related to NK cell infiltration degree ($p = 0.011$). The 1, 2 and 3 degree with NK cell infiltration were 60.6%, 18.4%, 21.1% in the T1-T2 cancer, and 42.1%, 31.7%, 43.5% in the T3-T4 cancer, respectively. A significant difference of NK cell infiltration degree was found between different size of the tumor ($p = 0.019$) (Table 3).

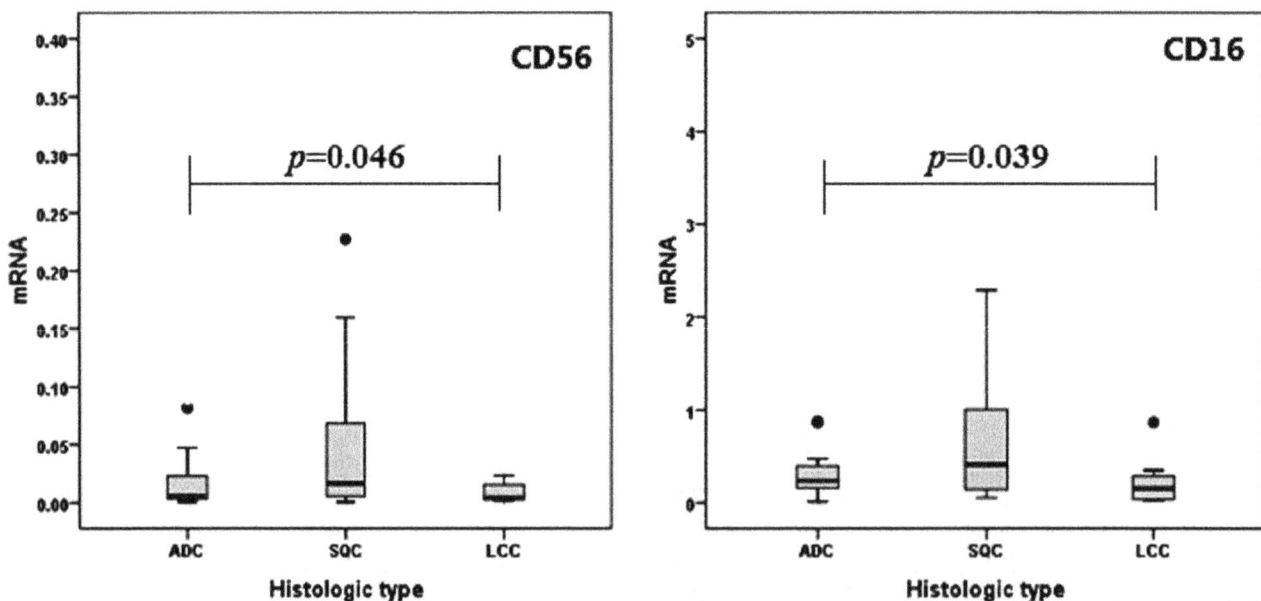

Figure 4. NK cells phenotype mRNA expression levels in different histologic type of lung cancer. NK cells receptors CD56 and CD16 phenotype mRNA in different histologic types of lung cancer have statistical significance.

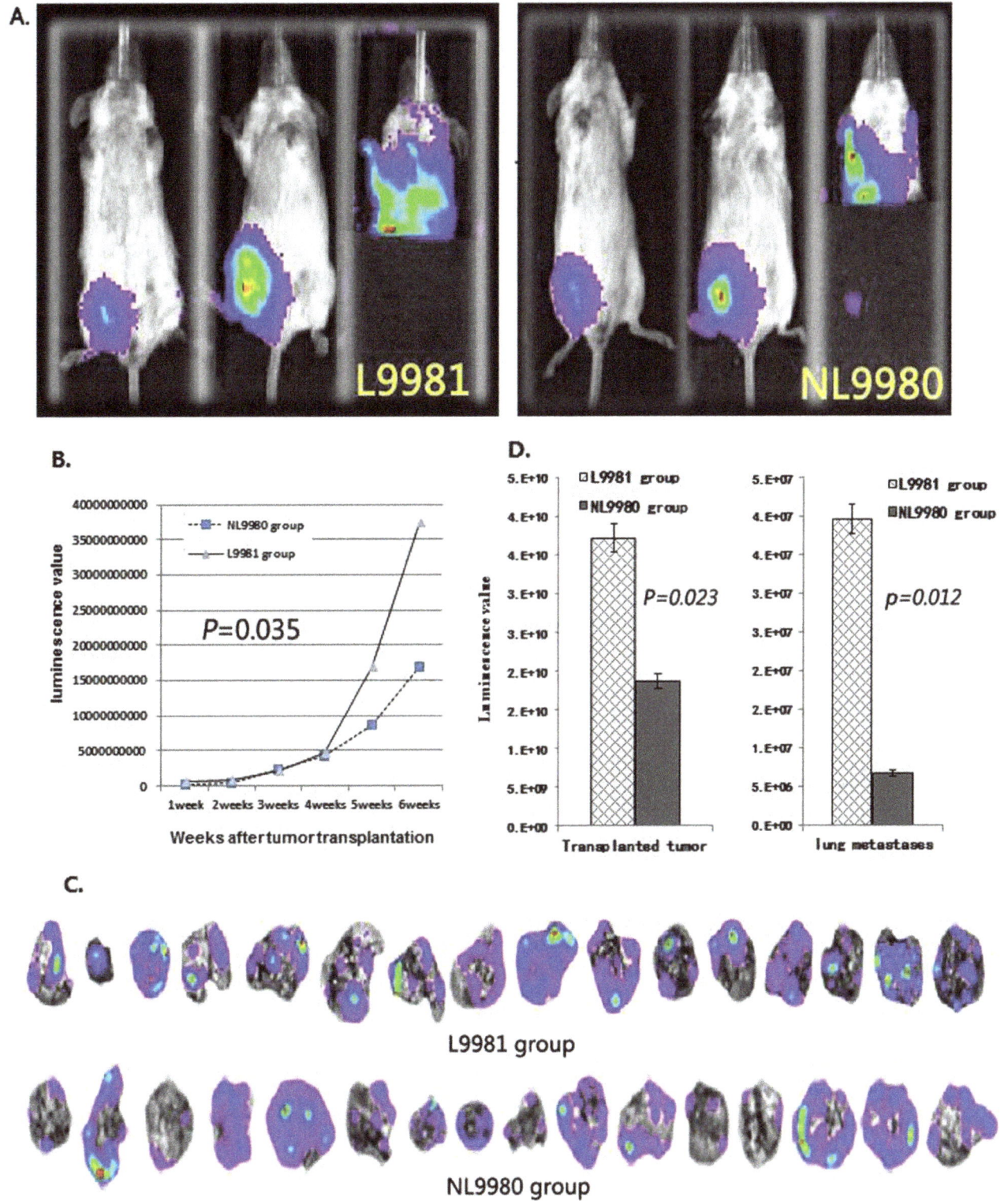

Figure 5. Transplanted tumors-lung metastasis models of high (L9981)/low (NL9980) metastatic human large cell lung cancer cell lines. A: Living fluorescence imaging detect mouse model (the left is the right inguen subcutaneously tumor for 1 week and the middle is for 6 weeks after injection, the right is the lung metastases tumors in six weeks after inoculation.), B: Growth curve of subcutaneously transplant tumor in SCID mouse, C: lung metastases luminescence imaging of tumor-bearing mouse in vitro, D: The comparison of luminescence value between transplanted tumor and lung metastases of high (L9981)/low (NL9980) metastatic human large cell lung cancer cell lines.

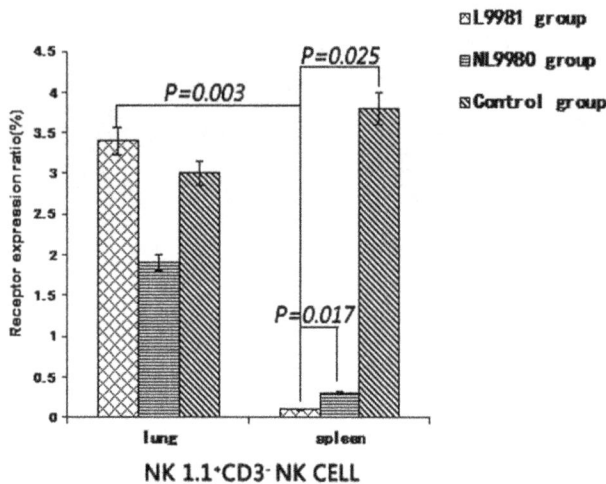

Figure 6. NK1.1$^+$ CD3$^-$ NK cell receptor expression in lung and spleen of different groups. NK1.1$^+$CD3$^-$ NK cells in lungs of high-metastatic group were significantly higher than that in spleen ($p = 0.003$). NK1.1$^+$CD3$^-$ NK cells in spleen of high-metastasis group (0.10±.06) were significantly lower than that in low-metastasis group ($p = 0.017$) and control group ($p = 0.025$).

NK cell infiltration and lung cancer patients prognosis

The survival time of lung cancer patient was positively related to NK cell infiltration degree in lung cancer. The more infiltration of NK cells were existed, the longer the survival time of patients did ($p = 0.030$) (Fig.3, Table 4).

Real-time PCR confirm NK cell infiltration extent in lung cancer

The differences of NK cell receptors CD56 and CD16 mRNA expression between different pathological types of lung cancer was detected and verified by Real-time PCR. We found that NK cells phenotype mRNA in different histologic type of lung cancer have statistical significance (Fig.4). This is in according with the result of the histology.

Transplanted tumors-lung metastasis models established

Transplanted tumors-lung metastasis models were successful established in SCID mouse with high (L9981)/low (NL9980) metastatic human large cell lung cancer cell lines. The distant metastasis of the xenograft tumor was detected by fluorescence imaging in vitro (Fig.5A). Compared with low-metastatic group ($6.84\times10^6\pm3.26\times10^6$), the lung metastases fluorescence value of mice in the high-metastatic group ($30.97\times10^6\pm14.3\times10^6$) was remarkably higher than that in low-metastatic group ($p = 0.035$) (Fig.5B, C, D).

NK cell phenotypic modulation in lung cancer micro-environment

NK1.1$^+$CD3$^-$ NK cells in lungs of high-metastatic group (3.40±0.90) were significantly higher than that in spleen (0.10±0.06) ($p = 0.003$). NK1.1$^+$CD3$^-$ NK cells in spleen of high-metastasis group (0.10±0.06) were significantly lower than that in low-metastasis group (1.66±0.82) and control group (3.80±2.05) ($p = 0.017$, $p = 0.025$) (Fig.6).

NKG2D expression level of NK cells from spleen in high-metastasis group (4.17±0.85) were remarkably lower than that in

control group (7.80±2.67) ($p = 0.034$) and low-metastasis group (6.00±0.96) ($p = 0.040$) (Fig.7B).

NKG2A expression level of NK cells from lung (5.13±2.36) was significantly higher than that from spleen (1.47±0.68) in high-metastatic group ($p = 0.007$) (Fig.7C). NKG2A expression level of NK cells from lung in high-metastatic group (5.13±2.36) were significantly higher than that in low-metastatic group (4.70±1.96) and control group (0.73±0.26) ($p = 0.000$) (Fig.7A).

Ly49I expression level of NK cells from lung in high-metastatic group (4.82±1.78) was remarkably up-regulated than that in spleen (1.50±0.10) ($p = 0.003$) (Fig.7C). The Ly49I expression level of NK cells from the lung (2.79±0.40) was significantly higher than that from the spleen (1.13±0.40) in control group ($p = 0.033$) (Fig.7E). Ly49I expression level of the NK cells from the lung in high-metastatic group (4.82±1.78) and low-metastatic group (6.11±2.23) was significantly higher than that in control group (2.79±0.40) ($p = 0.000$) (Fig.7A). Ly49I expression level of NK cells from the spleen in low-metastatic group (3.40±1.00) was remarkably higher than that in high-metastatic group (1.50±0.10) ($p = 0.010$) and control group (1.13±0.40) ($p = 0.004$) (Fig.7B).

NK cell lethal effect in lung cancer micro-environment

NK1.1$^+$CD3$^-$ NK cells activated by IL-2 in vitro have significant cytotoxic activity to high/low metastatic lung cancer large cells. A significant difference was observed between different effector-target ratio ($p = 0.005$, $p = 0.017$). NK cells had higher cytotoxic activity to NL9980 than that to L9981 in the same effector-target ratio ($p = 0.035$) (Table 5).

NK cell receptor mRNA expressing in subcutaneously transplanted tumor of mouse

In the transplanted tumors of tumor-bearing group, NKG2D expression level of NK cells in high-metastasis group was significantly higher than that in low-metastasis group ($p = 0.018$), and the Ly49I expression level of NK cells in high-metastasis group was also remarkably higher than low-metastasis group ($p = 0.001$). However, no significant difference of the NK1.1 and NKG2A expression level of NK cells was existed between high and low metastasis group ($p > 0.05$) (Fig.8).

Discussion

This study revealed that NK cells infiltration and NK cells receptor expression change in NSCLC tumor environment. From our research, we found that the NK cells infiltrated mainly in the tumor stroma, constituting the tumor micro-environment. These observations are in agreement with previous observations demonstrating that lung tumor micro-environment [16]. In addition, we got the surprise that the number of NK cell infiltrating in lung cancer tissue is closely related to the pathological types, size of the primary cancer, smoking history and prognosis of the patients with lung cancer.

Previous literature implied that some molecules expressing in the tumor and some mediums released from tumor commonly led to tumor escape mechanisms from NK cell immunological surveillance [19,20]. There are high levels of non-classical MHC I molecular HLA - E and HLA - G in the tumor cell surface. They were NK cell activation CD94/receptor NKG2A and cell surface immune globulin sample transcription molecular 2 (ILT2) inhibitory ligand, which can restrain NK cell damage function [21-23]. At the same time, tumor cells can secrete some tumor suppressor factors inhibition of NK cell function, such as IL-10 [24] and TGF-β [25]. Surrounding the tumor infiltrating NK cell, some special changes in some other human tumors had been

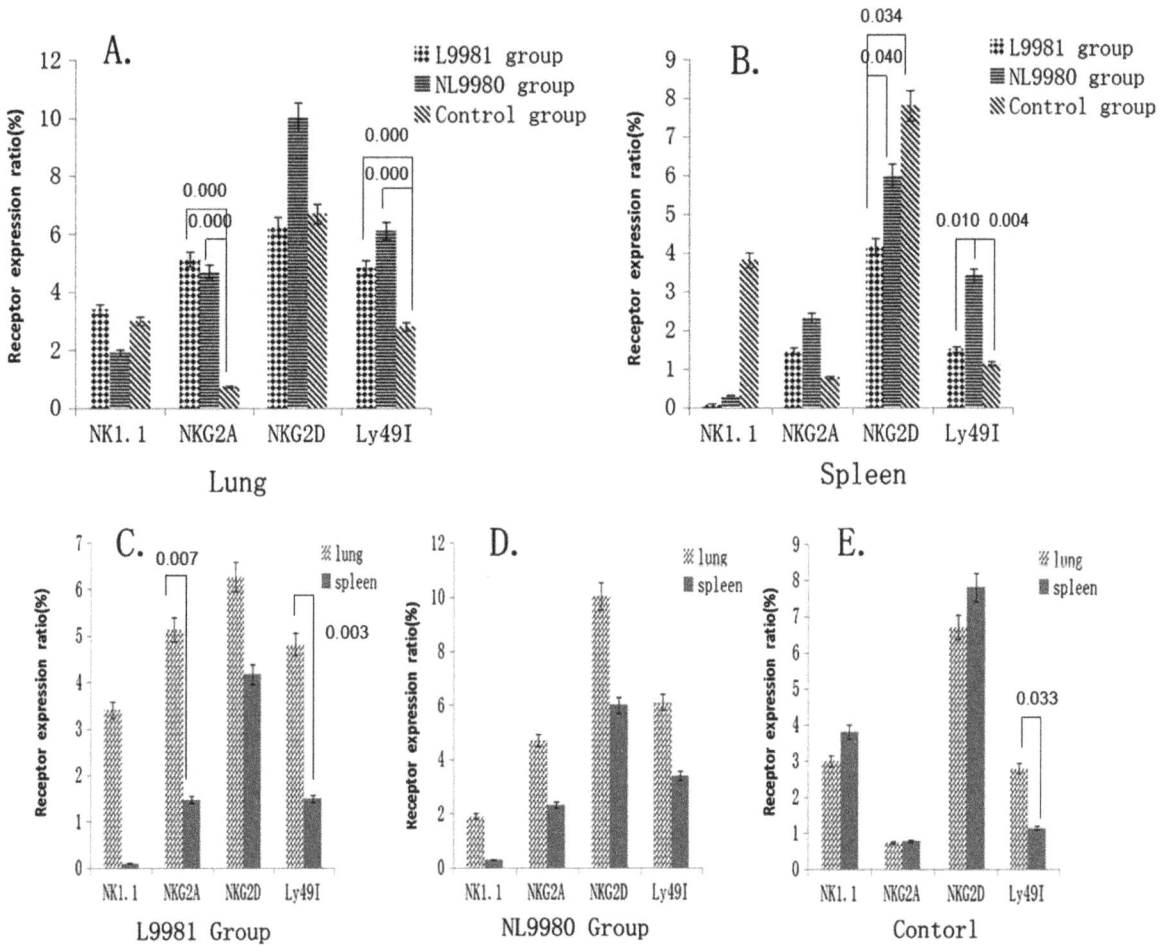

Figure 7. NK cell phenotypic modulation in lung cancer micro-environment. A: NKG2A expression level of NK cells from lung in high-metastatic L9981 group were significantly higher than that in low-metastatic NL9980 group and control group ($p = 0.000$). Ly49I expression level from the lung in L9981 group and NL9980 group was significantly higher than that in control group ($p = 0.000$) **B**: NKG2D expression level of NK cells from spleen in L9981 group (4.17±0.85) were remarkably lower than that in control group ($p = 0.034$) and NL9980 group ($p = 0.040$). Ly49I expression level in NL9980 group was remarkably higher than that in L9981 group ($p = 0.010$) and control group ($p = 0.004$). **C**: NKG2A expression level of NK cells from lung was significantly higher than that from spleen in high-metastatic L9981 group ($p = 0.007$) and Ly49I expression level from lung was remarkably up-regulated than that in spleen ($p = 0.003$) **D**: No significant difference of all the receptors expression level of NK cells was existed in low metastasis NL9980 group. **E**: The Ly49I expression level of NK cells from the lung was significantly higher than that from the spleen in control group ($p = 0.033$).

Table 5. Detection of NK cell cytotoxicity by luminescence *in vitro*.

Group	Time (h)	Luminescence value(E+05)					*p* value	
		0.25:1**	0.5:1**	1:1**	2:1**	Control		
L9981 group	24	181±49.7	160±20.3	123±11.7	99±7.2	221±18.7	0.005*	0.035*
	48	174±19.0	150±35.4	105±10.7	67±7.6	224±26.7		
	72	185±18.9	149±35.2	102±11.2	64±12.6	246±26.9		
NL9980 group	24	131±46.7	122±19.0	113±5.4	11±2.9	123±10.7	0.017*	
	48	124±14.1	119±11.4	113±8.4	18±5.6	125±15.9		
	72	132±14.0	123±10.7	102±8.9	14±5.8	142±17.0		

*$p < 0.05$, Difference have statistical significance.
**NK cell: lung cancer cell.

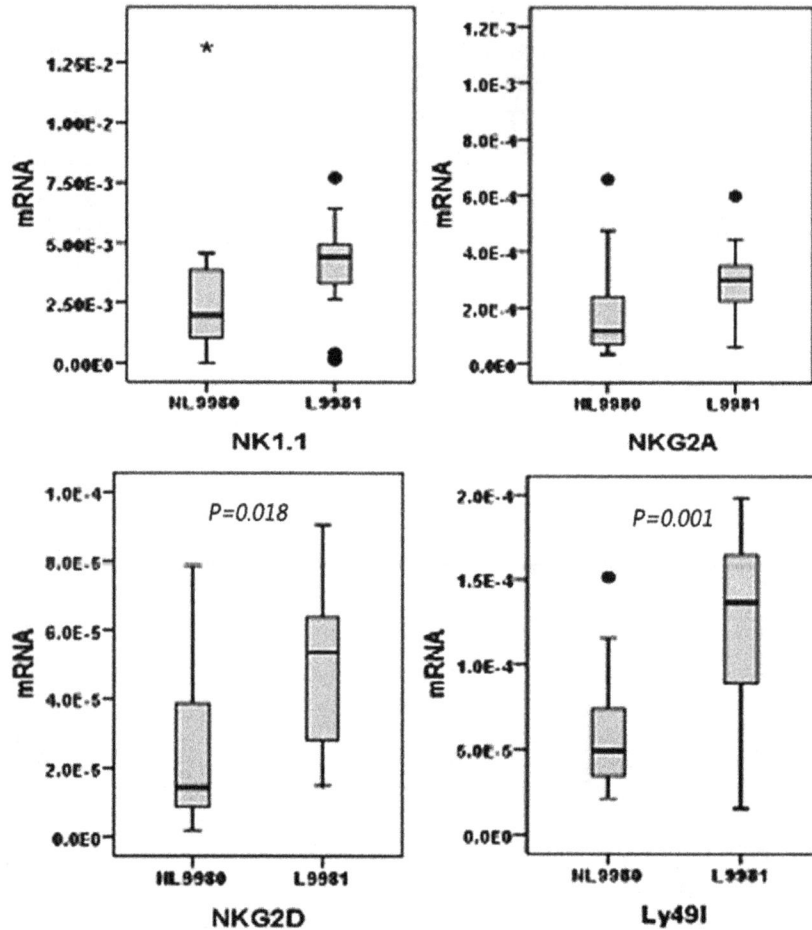

Figure 8. NK cell different receptors mRNA expressing in subcutaneously transplanted tumor of mouse. NKG2D expression level of NK cells in high-metastasis L9981 group was significantly higher than that in low-metastasis NL9980 group ($p = 0.018$), and the Ly49I expression level of NK cells in L9981 group was also remarkably higher than NL9980 group ($p = 0.001$). No significant difference of the NK1.1 and NKG2A expression level of NK cells was existed between high and low metastasis group.

researched. In kidney cancer, the NK cell within tumor only was activated by IL-2 stimulation could have the target cell solution function. And to the same patients there were significant differences between the peripheral blood NK cell phenotype with in tumor [26–28]. The NK cell surface receptor DNAM-1, 2B4, CD16 expression reduced in ovarian cancer, which can result in the NK cell activation function were badly damaged [29].

Our research result prompt that the activated receptor of NK cells is down-regulated and inhibitory receptor of NK cells is up-regulated in the transplanted tumor and the distant metastatic lesions of human large cell lung cancer cell lines, which might be the main reason leading to NK cell killing ability decreased.

NKG2D is a receptor for MHC class I chain-related A and B molecules, which are frequently expressed by epithelial cancers. Ligation of NKG2D induces anti-tumoral effector functions in both NK and T cells. NKG2D recognition plays an important role in tumor immune surveillance [30] and that NKG2D primarily acts to trigger perforin-mediated apoptosis [31]. Our research verified that NKG2D expression level of NK cells from spleen in high-metastasis group were remarkably lower than that in control group ($p = 0.034$) and low-metastasis group ($p = 0.040$). In the transplanted tumors of tumor-bearing group, NKG2D mRNA expression level of NK cells in high-metastasis group was significantly higher than that in low-metastasis group ($p = 0.018$).

NKG2A is an inhibitory NK receptor that has been reported to form disulfide-linked heterodimers with invariant CD94. The NKG2A ligand has been identified as HLA-E, a non-classical MHC class-I b molecule that is widely distributed among various tissues, exhibits relatively low surface expression, and has limited polymorphism [32]. The inhibitory receptor CD94/NKG2A plays a major role in NK cell-mediated lysis of activated CD4$^+$T cells [33]. NKG2A expression level of NK cell from lung was significantly higher than that from spleen in high-metastatic group ($p = 0.007$). NKG2A expression level of NK cells from lung in high-metastatic group were significantly higher than that in low-metastatic group and control group ($p = 0.000$). Thus, the down-regulation of NKG2D and the up-regulation of NKG2A may indicate immune tolerance mechanism and facilitate metastasis in tumor environment.

Interaction of MHC class I with the Ly49 receptors prevent the activation of NK cells and thereby the lysis of the target cell. Thus, NK cells utilize the Ly49 receptors to differentiate 'self' from 'missing-self '. Loss of MHC class I molecules on target cells relieves the NK cell of Ly49-mediated inhibition, thus allowing the NK cells to mediate cytotoxicity [34]. The Ly49I expression level of NK cells from the lung was significantly higher than that from the spleen in control group ($p = 0.033$). Ly49I expression level of the NK cells from the lung in high-metastatic group and low-metastatic group was significantly higher than that in control group ($p = 0.000$). In the transplanted tumors of tumor-bearing group, the Ly49I mRNA expression level of NK cells in high-metastasis group was also remarkably higher than low-metastasis group ($p = 0.001$).

Furthermore, a higher resistant to cytotoxic activity of NK cell exist in the human high-metastatic large cell lung cancer cell line L9981, which is much higher than that in the low-metastatic large cell lung cancer cell line NL9980. In addition, it is possible that other receptors of NK cells changed in tumor environment. In melanoma, NK cells could significantly increase the expression of CD86, and ligation of CD86 with CTLA4Ig significantly increased the ability of NK cells to kill tumor cells [35]. In two spontaneous metastasis models, the B16F10.9 melanoma (B16) and the Lewis lung carcinoma (D122) in the NCR1 knockout mouse, NKp46/NCR1 is directly involved in the killing of B16 and D122 cells in vitro and plays an important role in controlling B16 and D122 metastasis in vivo [36].

So, the variation of NK cell receptors might be useful in the prediction of tumor cell invasion and metastasis capacity, and further studies are needed to figure out the exact mechanism.

Author Contributions

Conceived and designed the experiments: SJ JWH FDS QHZ. Performed the experiments: SJ YD BL YL YY. Analyzed the data: SJ YD. Contributed reagents/materials/analysis tools: JWH FDS QHZ. Wrote the paper: SJ YD QHZ.

References

1. Jemal A, Murray T, Ward E, Samuels A, Tiwari RC, et al. (2005) Cancer statistics, 2005. CA Cancer J Clin 55: 10–30.
2. Yoshimi I, Sobue T (2004) International comparison in cancer statistics: Eastern Asia. Jpn J Clin Oncol 34: 759–763.
3. Parkin DM, Bray F, Ferlay J, Pisani P (2005) Global cancer statistics, 2002. CA Cancer J Clin 55: 74–108.
4. Yang L, Parkin DM, Whelan S, Zhang S, Chen Y, et al. (2005) Statistics on cancer in China: cancer registration in 2002. Eur J Cancer Prev 14: 329–35.
5. Jemal A, Siegel R, Xu J, Ward E (2010) Cancer Statistics, 2010. CA Cancer J Clin 60; 277–300.
6. Peng H, Ma M, Han B (2011) Survival Analysis of 1,742 Patients with Stage IV Non-small Cell Lung Cancer. Zhongguo Fei Ai Za Zhi 14: 362–366.
7. Kiessling R, Klein E, Pross H, Wigzell H (1975) 'Natural' killer cells in the mouse. II. Cytotoxic cells with specificity for mouse Moloney leukemia cells. Characteristics of the killer cell. Eur J Immunol 5: 117–121.
8. Kiessling R, Klein E, Wigzell H (1975) 'Natural' killer cells in the mouse. I. Cytotoxic cells with specificity for mouse Moloney leukemia cells. Specificity and distribution according to genotype. Eur J Immunol 5: 112–117.
9. Kim R, Emi M, Tanabe K (2007) Cancer immunoediting from immune surveilance to immune escape. Immunology 121: 1–14.
10. Vivier E, Ugolini S, Blaise D, Chabannon C, Brossay L (2012) Targeting natural killer cells and nat-ural killer T cells in cancer. Nat Rev Immunol 12; 239–252.
11. Coca S, Perez-Piqueras J, Martinez D, Colmenarejo A, Saez MA, et al. (1997) The prognostic significance of intratumoral natural killer cells in patients with colorectal carcinoma. Cancer 79: 2320–2328.
12. Ishigami S, Natsugoe S, Tokuda K, Nakajo A, Xiangming C, et al. (2000) Clinical impact of intratumoral natural killer cell and dendritic cell infiltration in gastric cancer. Cancer Lett 159: 103–108.
13. Villegas FR, Coca S, Villarrubia VG, Jiménez R, Chillón MJ, et al. (2002) Prognostic significance of tumor infiltrating natural killer cells subset CD57 in patients with squamous cell lung cancer. Lung Cancer 35: 23–28.
14. Farag SS, Caligiuri MA. (2006) Human natural killer cell development and biology. Blood Rev 20: 123–137.
15. Cooper MA, Fehniger TA, Turner SC, Chen KS, Ghaheri BA, et al. (2001) Human natural killer cells: a unique innate immunoregulatory role for the CD56 (bright) subset. Blood 97: 3146–3151.
16. Esendagli G, Bruderek K, Goldmann T, Busche A, Branscheid D, et al. (2008) Malignant and non-malignant lung tissue areas are differentially populated by natural killer cells and regulatory T cells in non-small cell lung cancer. Lung Cancer 59: 32–40.
17. Zhou Q, Wang Y, Che G, Zhu W, Chen X, et al. (2003) Establishment and their biological characteristics of clonal cell subpopulations (NL9980 and L9981) from a human lung large cell carcinoma cell line (WCQH-9801). Zhongguo Fei Ai Za Zhi 6: 464–468.
18. Ren Y, Chen J, Liu H, Yan H, Wang Y, et al. (2008) The study of the tumorigenicity and metastasis ability in human lung cancer cell line L9981 using in vivo imaging. Zhongguo Fei Ai Za Zhi 11: 321–326.
19. Campoli M, Ferrone S (2008) Tumor escape mechanisms: potential role of soluble HLA antigens and NK cells activating ligands. Tissue Antigens 72: 321–334.
20. Zitvogel L, Tesniere A, Kroemer G (2006) Cancer despite immunosurveillance: immunoselection and immunosubversion. Nat Rev Immunol 6: 715–727.
21. LeMaoult J, Zafaranloo K, Le Danff C, Carosella ED (2005) HLA-G up-regulates ILT2, ILT3, ILT4, and KIR2DL4 in antigen presenting cells, NK cells, and T cells. Faseb J 19: 662–664.
22. Levy EM, Bianchini M, Von Euw EM, Barrio MM, Bravo AI, et al. (2008) Human leukocyte antigen-E protein is overexpressed in primary human colorectal cancer. Int J Oncol 32: 633–641.
23. Urosevic M, Dummer R (2008) Human leukocyte antigen-G and cancer immunoediting. Cancer Res 68: 627–630.
24. Salazar-Onfray F, Lopez MN, Mendoza-Naranjo A (2007) Paradoxical effects of cytokines in tumor immune surveillance and tumor immune escape. Cytokine Growth Factor Rev 18: 171–182.
25. Castriconi R, Cantoni C, Della Chiesa M, Vitale M, Marcenaro E, et al. (2003) Transforming growth factor beta 1 inhibits expression of NKp30 and NKG2D receptors: consequences for the NK-mediated killing of dendritic cells. Proc Natl Acad Sci U S A 100: 4120–4125.
26. Richards JO, Chang X, Blaser BW, Caligiuri MA, Zheng P, et al. (2006) Tumor growth impedes natural-killer-cell maturation in the bone marrow. Blood 108: 246–252.
27. Schleypen JS, Baur N, Kammerer R, Nelson PJ, Rohrmann K, et al. (2006) Cytotoxic markers and frequency predict functional capacity of natural killer cells infiltrating renal cell carcinoma. Clin Cancer Res 12: 718–725.
28. Schleypen JS, Von Geldern M, Weiss EH, Kotzias N, Rohrmann K, et al. (2003) Renal cell carcinoma infiltrating natural killer cells express differential repertoires of activating and inhibitory receptors and are inhibited by specific HLA class I allotypes. Int J Cancer 106: 905–912.
29. Carlsten M, Norell H, Bryceson YT, Poschke I, Schedvins K, et al. (2009) Primary human tumor cells expressing CD155 impair tumor targeting by down-regulating DNAM-1 on NK cells. J Immunol 183: 4921–4930.
30. Dasgupta S, Bhattacharya-Chatterjee M, O'Malley BW Jr, Chatterjee SK (2005) Inhibition of NK Cell Activity through TGF-beta 1 by down-regulation of NKG2D in a murine model of head and neck cancer. J Immunol 175: 5541–5550.
31. Hayakawa Y, Kelly JM, Westwood JA, Darcy PK, Diefenbach A, et al. (2002) Cutting edge: tumor rejection mediated by NKG2D receptor-ligand interaction is dependent upon perforin. J Immunol 169: 5377–5381.
32. Sullivan LC, Clements CS, Rossjohn J, Brooks AG (2008) The major histocompatibility complex class Ib molecule HLA-E at the interface between innate and adaptive immunity. Tissue Antigens 72: 415–424.
33. Ljunggren HG, Kärre K (1990) In search of the 'missing self': MHC molecules and NK cell recognition. Immunol Today 11: 237–244.
34. Kärre K (2002) NK cells, MHC class I molecules and the missing self. Scand J Immunol 55: 221–228.
35. Peng Y, Luo G, Zhou J, Wang X, Hu J, et al. (2013) CD86 is an activation receptor for NK cell cytotoxicity against tumor cells. PLoS One 8: e83913.
36. Glasner A, Ghadially H, Gur C, Stanietsky N, Tsukerman P, et al. (2012) Recognition and prevention of tumor metastasis by the NK receptor NKp46/NCR1. J Immunol 188: 2509–2515.

17

LRRC6 Mutation Causes Primary Ciliary Dyskinesia with Dynein Arm Defects

Amjad Horani[1]*, **Thomas W. Ferkol**[1,2], **David Shoseyov**[3], **Mollie G. Wasserman**[4], **Yifat S. Oren**[5], **Batsheva Kerem**[5], **Israel Amirav**[6], **Malena Cohen-Cymberknoh**[3], **Susan K. Dutcher**[7], **Steven L. Brody**[4], **Orly Elpeleg**[8], **Eitan Kerem**[3]

1 Department of Pediatrics, Washington University School of Medicine, St. Louis, Missouri, United States of America, 2 Department of Cell Biology and Physiology, Washington University School of Medicine, St. Louis, Missouri, United States of America, 3 Department of Pediatrics, Hadassah Hebrew University Medical Center, Jerusalem, Israel, 4 Department of Medicine, Washington University School of Medicine, St. Louis, Missouri, United States of America, 5 Department of Genetics, The Hebrew University, Jerusalem, Israel, 6 Department of Pediatrics, Ziv Medical Center, Safed, Israel, 7 Department of Genetics, Washington University School of Medicine, St. Louis, Missouri, United States of America, 8 Monique and Jacques Roboh Department of Genetic Research, Hadassah Hebrew University Medical Center, Jerusalem, Israel

Abstract

Despite recent progress in defining the ciliome, the genetic basis for many cases of primary ciliary dyskinesia (PCD) remains elusive. We evaluated five children from two unrelated, consanguineous Palestinian families who had PCD with typical clinical features, reduced nasal nitric oxide concentrations, and absent dynein arms. Linkage analyses revealed a single common homozygous region on chromosome 8 and one candidate was conserved in organisms with motile cilia. Sequencing revealed a single novel mutation in *LRRC6* (Leucine-rich repeat containing protein 6) that fit the model of autosomal recessive genetic transmission, leading to a change of a highly conserved amino acid from aspartic acid to histidine (Asp146His). LRRC6 was localized to the cytoplasm and was up-regulated during ciliogenesis in human airway epithelial cells in a Foxj1-dependent fashion. Nasal epithelial cells isolated from affected individuals and shRNA-mediated silencing in human airway epithelial cells, showed reduced LRRC6 expression, absent dynein arms, and slowed cilia beat frequency. Dynein arm proteins were either absent or mislocalized to the cytoplasm in airway epithelial cells from a primary ciliary dyskinesia subject. These findings suggest that LRRC6 plays a role in dynein arm assembly or trafficking and when mutated leads to primary ciliary dyskinesia with laterality defects.

Editor: Struan Frederick Airth Grant, The Children's Hospital of Philadelphia, United States of America

Funding: The authors were funded by the Children's Discovery Institute (SLB, SKD, TWF) and National Institutes of Health (NIH) awards HL082657 (TWF), HL056244 (SLB), GM32843 (SKD). The funders had no role in study design, data collection and analysis, decision to publish, or preparation of the manuscript.

Competing Interests: The authors have declared that no competing interests exist.

* E-mail: horani_a@kids.wustl.edu

Introduction

Motile cilia and flagella are essential, highly conserved organelles that extend from the cell to perform specialized functions, including motility and propulsion, and are present in the upper and lower respiratory tract, brain ventricles, and reproductive organs. A motile cilium is composed of an axoneme containing nine outer microtubule doublets and an inner central pair. The outer doublets are associated with dynein motor proteins, organized as outer dynein arms (ODA) and inner dynein arms (IDA). These proteins allow adjacent outer doublets to slide against one other and thus provide movement. Nexin links tether and limit the motion of microtubular doublets, and radial spokes control dynein arm activity relaying signals from the central microtubular pair to the dynein arms [1]. As a vital component of the mucociliary apparatus, cilia are critical for respiratory tract host defense [2], and when dysfunctional, may lead to primary ciliary dyskinesia (PCD) (CILD1: MIM 244400). PCD is a rare, genetically heterogeneous disorder, which is usually inherited as an autosomal recessive trait, and is caused by mutations in genes that code for the dynein proteins or regulatory factors affecting those proteins [1–3]. These genetic defects can render the cilia immotile

or lead to an abnormal beating pattern [4]. Impaired mucociliary clearance in affected individuals may result in acute and chronic infections of the lung, middle ear, and paranasal sinuses [1–3]. Furthermore, cilia defects in the embryonic node during development cause laterality defects, such as *situs inversus totalis* or heterotaxy, in approximately half of PCD cases [5]. Ciliary dysmotility can also cause infertility and has been linked to prenatal hydrocephalus [6,7].

Our understanding of the link between genetic defects and ultrastructural changes of cilia has greatly advanced over the past decade. Owing to conservation of cilia and flagellar structures, studies of these organelles in model organisms, from algae (*Chlamydomonas reinhardtii*) to zebrafish (*Danio rerio*) to mammals, have provided insights into structure, function, and genetics of the human cilium. Thus far, studies using these organisms and others have led to the identification of sixteen different genes that when mutated produce unambiguous clinical phenotypes of PCD in humans. These genes include *DNAH5* (MIM 603335), *DNAI1* (MIM 604366), *DNAI2* (MIM 605483), *TXNDC3* (MIM 607421), *DNAL1* (MIM 610062), *DNAH11* (MIM 603339), *HEATR2* (MIM 614864), *DNAAF1* (MIM 612517), *DNAAF2* (MIM 613190), *DNAAF3* (MIM 614566), *RSPH4A* (MIM 612647), *RSPH9* (MIM

612648), *CCDC39* (MIM 613798), *CCDC40* (MIM 613799), *CCDC103* (MIM 614677) and *HYDIN* (MIM 610812) [8–25]. Several genes, *DNAAF1, DNAAF2, DNAAF3* and *HEATR2*, encode proteins that are involved in dynein arm assembly while the others are essential structural components of the ciliary axoneme. Nonetheless, mutations in these genes still account for less than half of all PCD cases, and our understanding of the critical components of cilia assembly is incomplete [1,6].

Here, we describe a single non-synonymous mutation in *LRRC6* that causes PCD in several members of two unrelated, consanguineous Palestinian families. *LRRC6* is evolutionarily conserved across the phylogenetic tree, and is found in mammals, zebrafish (*D. rerio*), flies (*Drosophila melanogaster*), protozoa (*Trypanosoma brucei*), algae (*C. reinhardtii*), but not in worms (*Caenorhabditis elegans*). There are fourteen other proteins with leucine-rich repeats (LRR) in the cilia proteome [26]. The LRR region in LRRC6 most closely resembles that of the SDS22-like subfamily of LRR proteins [27], a set of proteins with diverse functions, including splicing factors and nuclear export proteins [28]. Airway epithelial cells isolated from affected individuals had reduced LRRC6 expression, axonemal defects with mislocalized dynein proteins, and markedly slowed cilia beat frequency, effects that were all recapitulated by shRNA-mediated knockdown of *LRRC6* in normal airway epithelial cells.

Methods

Patients

Subjects with clinical features consistent with PCD from two unrelated, endogamous families were studied (**Figure 1A and Table 1**).

Ethics Statement

All individuals or their parents provided written informed consent for diagnostic evaluation and genetic characterization. The study protocol was approved by the Hadassah-Hebrew University Human Subjects Committee. Institutional approval was obtained to conduct both human and animal research. Anonymized human airway epithelial cells from surgical excess of large airways that were trimmed during the transplant procedure, of lung donated for transplantation at Washington University in St. Louis were also used in these studies. Research using cells originating from deidentified cadaver specimen (surgical excess of large airways of lung) is exempt from regulation and is not governed by NIH regulation 45 CFR Part 46.

Genetic Analyses and Sequencing

Genetic linkage analysis was performed on three affected members (III-1, III-2 and III-4 in **Figure 1A**) using the GeneChip Human Mapping 250 K Nsp Affymetrix Array as previously described [29]. The sequence of LRRC6 twelve exons and their flanking intronic regions were analyzed by forward and reverse Sanger dideoxy sequencing using the appropriate primers.

Airway Epithelial Cells

Nasal epithelial cells from subjects were obtained from the inferior turbinate by cytology brush [30]. Human airway epithelial cells were isolated from surgical excess of large airways (tracheobronchial segments) that were trimmed during the transplant procedure, of lungs donated for transplantation. Cells were expanded in culture, seeded on supported membranes (Transwell, Corning Inc., Corning, NY), and re-differentiated using air-liquid interface conditions [31]. Cell preparations were maintained in culture for four to ten weeks.

Gene Silencing of Airway Epithelial Cells

shRNA targeted sequences generated by the Children's Discovery Institute shRNA Library Core, were inserted into pLKO.1 lentivirus vectors that includes a U3 promoter and a puromycin resistant cassette. The shRNA sequences used were: GCCCAAGGTAGGAGAAGTAAT (shRNA#1), GAACACAACGACTGT GTCATT (shRNA#2), GATCTCAGACAACGGGTCATT (shRNA#3), CCTGTTTGTTTACTCCT GAAT (shRNA#4) and CCTAAATGTGAATGAGCCCAA (shRNA#5). A non-targeted sequence with a yellow fluorescent protein (YFP) reporter (a gift from Y. Feng and G.D. Longmore), was used as control [32]. Undifferentiated airway epithelial cells were transfected and selected using established protocols [33,34]. Briefly, vesicular stomatitis virus envelope glycoprotein (VSV-G)-pseudotyped vectors were generated by three-plasmid cotransfection of HEK 293T cells using Fugene 6 (Roche, WI). The generated viral supernatant was collected, filtered and used to infect airway epithelial cells. These cells were then selected by adding puromycin to the culture media. Once confluent, airway epithelial cells were grown at an air-liquid interface.

Epithelial Cell Immunofluorescent Staining and Immunoblot Analyses

Normal human lung obtained from excess tissue donated for lung transplantation was fixed, immunostained and imaged as previously described [31,35]. Human tracheobronchial epithelial cells (hTEC) collected from non-PCD subjects and differentiated at an air-liquid interface [31] were similarly examined for protein expression using primary antibodies against LRRC6 (1:100, HPA028058/SAB2103053, Sigma Aldrich, MO), acetylated α-tubulin (1:5000, clone 6-11-B1, Sigma Aldrich), LAMP2 (1:200, Abcam, Cambridge, MA), EEA1 (1:100, BD Biosciences, San Jose, CA), χ-tubulin (1:500, Clone Gtu-88, Sigma-Aldrich), DNAH7 (1:50, Novus Biologicals, Littleton, CO), and DNAI1 (1:5000, gift from Dr. Lawrence Ostrowski, University of North Carolina, Chapel Hill, NC [36]) which were detected using secondary antibodies conjugated to Alexa Fluor dyes (A-21202, A-21206, A-31570 and A-31572; Life Technology, Grand Island, NY). Nuclei were stained using 4′, 6-diamidino-2-phenylindole 1.5 µg/mL. Images were acquired using epifluorescent microscopy and adjusted globally using Photoshop (Adobe Systems, San Jose, CA). Cells were imaged and recorded as previously described [31,35]. For immunoblot analyses, cell supernatants were resolved by SDS-PAGE (7.5%) then transferred to PVDF membranes. The immunoblots were blocked, incubated with anti-LRRC6 (1:100 dilution, SAB1407241, Sigma-Aldrich) or anti-Foxj1 antibody (1:300), and detected with enhanced chemiluminescence using established protocols [35].

RT-PCR Analyses

RNA expression was assessed by RT-PCR amplification using the following oligonucleotide primer sets: human *LRRC6*, 5′-GCAGGCTTTGATGGACGTTG and 5′-GCCTGTAGGTGGTCTTTGCT; murine *LRRC6*, 5′-AAGTTGACCCCAG-CAAGCAT and 5′-CTCACTGGGTTCATCTCGGG; *Foxj1*, 5′-CCCGACGACGTGGACTAC and 5′-GGCGGAA GTAGCAGAAGTTG; *DNAI1*, 5′-AACGACGGCTGTCCCTAAAG and 5′-AGCCTACAAAACGC TCCCTC; and DNAH7, 5′-ACTTGCAGAATCGCATCCCA and 5′-CTCCTCTCCGCTC ACTTGTC, and detected using SYBR green in Lightcycler 480 (Roche, Indianapolis, IN) [37]. Briefly, RNA was isolated from

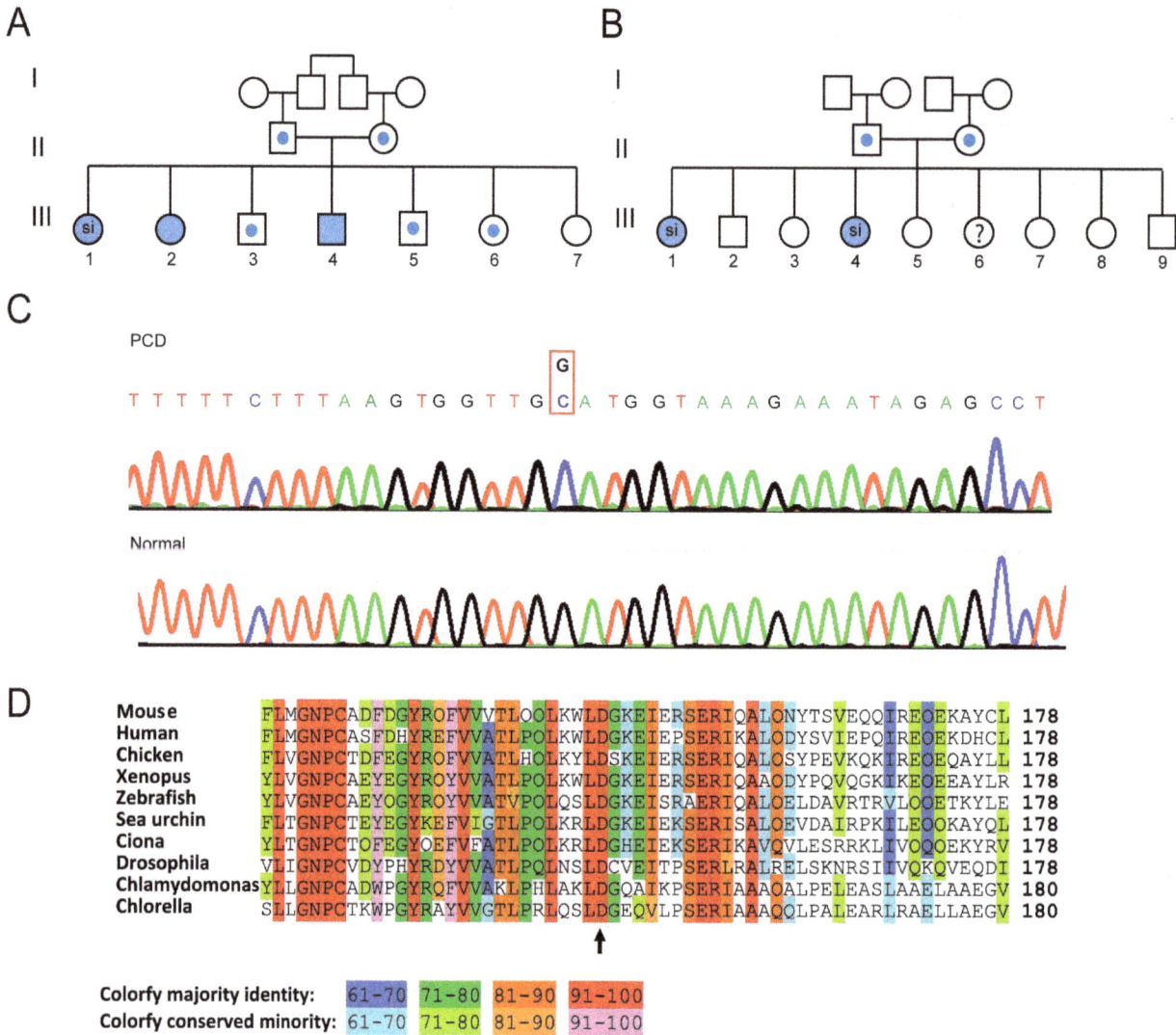

Figure 1. Family pedigree and genetic analyses. Pedigree of consanguineous kindred from two unrelated families in Palestinian communities (**A and B**). Solid symbols: affected individuals; central dots represent heterozygous individuals; Abbreviations: **si**, *situs inversus totalis*. Chromatogram showing the nucleotide sequence (**C**) of the *LRRC6* Exon 5 adjacent to the mutation site, which resulted in G-to-C change at base position, c.436 (Chr8:133645203). Amino acid sequence of the LRRC6 protein around the mutated residue. Note the high degree of conservation in diverse organisms that have motile cilia or flagella (**D**).

cells using an Illustra RNAspin kit (GE Healthcare, Buckinghamshire, UK). RNA was reverse transcribed using a cDNA Reverse Transcription Kit, and then amplified using the TaqMan Fast Universal PCR Master Mix (both from Applied Biosystems, Carlsbad, CA). Gene expression was normalized to glyceraldehyde 3-phosphate dehydrogenase expression.

Table 1. Clinical characteristics of PCD subjects with *LRRC6* mutant alleles.

Patient	Age (years)	Gender	Clinical manifestations	Laterality	Ultrastructural defects	Nasal NO (ppb)
A III-1	28	F	OM, RS, BR	SI	ODA – IDA	46.7
A III-2	25	F	OM, BR, RS	SS	ODA – IDA	10.1
A III-4	15	M	OM, RS, BR	SS	ODA – IDA	31.4
B III 1	21	F	OM, BR	DC	ODA – IDA	26.4
B III 4	13	F	OM, BR	DC	ODA – IDA	ND

Abbreviations: BR, bronchiectasis; DC: dextrocardia; OM, chronic or recurrent otitis media; RS, rhinosinusitis; SI, *situs inversus totalis*; SS, *situs solitus*; ODA, outer dynein arm; IDA, inner dynein arm; ND, not done.

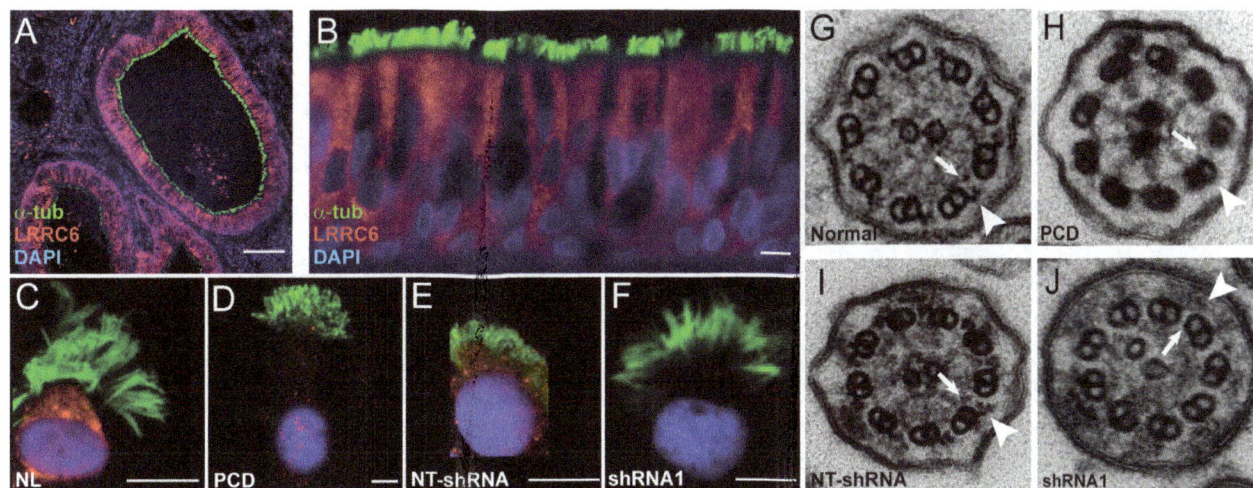

Figure 2. LRRC6 expression in ciliated airway epithelial cells. Photomicrographs of normal human lung section (**A**) (scale bar = 100 µm) and bronchial epithelium (**B**) following immunofluorescent staining for LRRC6, which reveals the cytoplasmic localization of the protein (LRRC6, red) only in ciliated cells (acetylated α-tubulin, a cilia marker, green; DAPI: blue) (scale bar = 10 µm). Immunofluorescent staining of nasal epithelial cells cultured at an air-liquid interface from a healthy subject demonstrating cytoplasmic localization of LRRC6 (**C**) as compared to decreased expression in a cell from a PCD subject (**D**). LRRC6 was similarly present in a non-targeted shRNA (NT) treated airway epithelial cells (**E**) but absent in *LRRC6-specific shRNA* transfected cells (**F**) (scale bar = 10 µm). Ultrastructural appearance of cilia from a normal control (**G**), PCD subject (**H**), and airway epithelial cells following transfection with non-targeted (**I**) and *LRRC6-targeted* (**J**) shRNA sequences. Arrow and arrow-head indicate inner and outer dynein arms, respectively.

Airway Epithelial Cell Videomicroscopy and Electron Microscopy

Nasal epithelial cells collected from subjects with PCD were examined using previously published protocols [38]. Videomicroscopy of ciliated epithelial cells was performed using an inverted microscope with a 20X phase contrast objective (Eclipse Ti-U; Nikon, Melville, NY) enclosed in a customized environmental chamber maintained at 37°C. Images were captured by a high-speed video camera and processed with the Sisson-Ammons Video Analysis system (Ammons Engineering, Mt. Morris, MI, USA) and analyzed using established methodologies [13,39]. Cilia beat frequency was analyzed in at least five fields obtained from each cell preparation. Patient samples were prepared for electron microscopy using previously published protocols; a minimum of 10 ciliary axoneme cross-sections were reviewed and examined in a blinded fashion to define ultrastructure using established criteria [17]. For shRNA treated samples, more than 100 axonemes were blindly reviewed by investigators and scored for ultrastructural defects [13].

Statistical Analyses

Data are expressed as mean ± standard deviation (SD). Statistical comparisons between groups were made using single factor analysis of variance (ANOVA) with Bonferroni correction for multiple comparisons. Individual comparisons were made using Student Two-tail test.

Results and Discussion

Five subjects with clinical features consistent with PCD, including chronic sinusitis, bronchiectasis, recurrent otitis media and laterality defects, from two unrelated, consanguineous Palestinian families were studied (**Figure 1A and Table 1**). Subjects had reduced nasal nitric oxide concentrations; a finding associated with PCD and is suggested as a screening tool [38,40,41]. No ciliary motion compared to healthy controls (**Supplementary video S1 and**

S2) and absent dynein arms (mean ODA and IDA numbers: 0.3±0.4 and 0.4±0.6 per axoneme, respectively; n = 30 axonemal cross sections) were found in at least one of the affected siblings from each family. Analysis of single-nucleotide polymorphism (SNP) haplotype on three affected members in one family (III-1, III-2 and III-4 in **Figure 1A**) revealed multiple regions of homozygosity in each individual, but all three shared a single homozygous genomic region on chromosome 8 (125.70–142.16 Mb, based on Human Genome build 19). Shared haplotype of STR markers that span the region (D8S1720, D8S256 and D8S1743) were noted in two affected siblings from a second family (III-1 and III-4 in **Figure 1B**). Within this common 16.45 Mb genomic region, 43 protein coding genes were present, and seven candidates [*LRRC6*, *KIAA0196* (MIM 610657), *EIF2C2* (MIM 606229), *NDRG1* (MIM 605262), *EFR3A* (MIM 611798), *EIF2C2* (606229), and *DDEF1* (MIM 605953)] were annotated in the ciliary proteome [26]. Only one gene was conserved across all organisms with motile cilia, and DNA sequencing revealed a single, novel, missense mutation that created a G-to-C change at base position c.436 (Chr8:133645203) in exon 5 of *LRRC6* (leucine-rich repeat containing protein 6), which resulted in substitution of aspartic acid to histidine (Asp146His) (**Figure 1C**), an amino acid that is highly conserved in organisms with motile cilia and flagella (**Figure 1D**). The mutation segregated with disease in an autosomal recessive transmission. The five affected individuals were homozygous for the mutated allele whereas the parents and three unaffected siblings from the index family were heterozygous for the mutation. The mutation was not listed in dbSNP135, but was found on 3 of 13006 alleles from 6503 healthy individuals reported in the Exome Variant Server (http://evs.gs.washington.edu/EVS; Exome Variant Server, NHLBI Exome Sequencing Project (ESP), Seattle, WA).

LRRC6 was originally identified as *LRTP* and expressed during spermatogenesis in mice and humans [42]. LRRC6 contains 6 N-terminal LRR repeats, an LRRcap domain and a CS-like domain near the C-terminus [43]. The (Asp146His) falls in the LRRcap domain, a sequence important for protein-protein interaction,

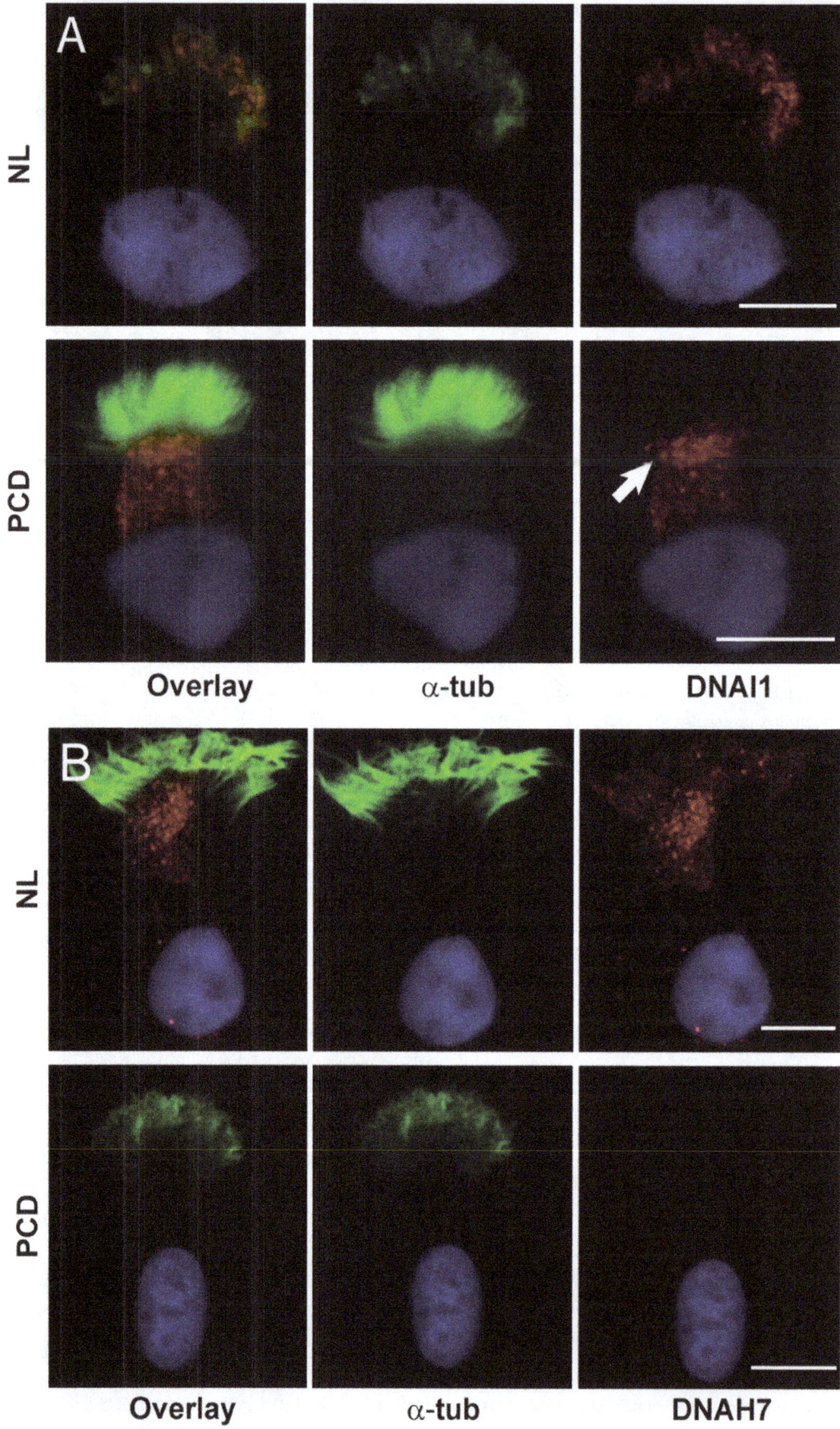

Figure 3. Inner and outer dynein protein mislocalization. Immunofluorescent staining of airway epithelial cells cultured at an air-liquid interface from normal (NL) and PCD subjects (PCD) for DNAI1 (red) (**A**), showing that outer dynein arm marker was localized to cilia of normal cells, but not in PCD cells. DNAI1 was present in the cytoplasm and most prominent beneath the ciliary axoneme in the PCD subject, suggesting mislocalization. The inner dynein arm marker, DNAH7 (red) (**B**), was localized to cilia of normal airway epithelial cells (NL) but absent in cells collected from PCD subjects (PCD). Immunofluorescent staining for DNAI1 or DNHA7 (red), α-tubulin (green) and DAPI (blue) (Scale bar = 10 μm).

regulation of RNA-binding specificity, and RNA nuclear export [44]. Expression of the *C. reinhardtii* orthologue was increased following deflagellation when compared to pretreatment values, consistent with transcriptional up-regulation of flagellar genes during ciliogenesis [45]. The homologous gene in *D. rerio* (*Lrrc6l*), when mutated, results in ciliary motility defects ranging from immotility to disorganized beating in the pronephros and neural tube, but normal axonemal ultrastructure [27]. *D. melanogaster tilB* mutants have defective sperm flagella motility and dysfunctional ciliated dendrites of the chordotonal organs. Furthermore, these mutant sperm axoneme lacked dynein arms [46]. The LRRC6 orthologue, TbLRTP, of the *T. brucei* localizes to basal bodies and is critical for basal body duplication, flagellum assembly, and cytokinesis [47]. Altogether, these data indicate that the LRRC6

protein has conserved functions central to ciliary and flagellar processes.

To better elucidate the function of LRRC6 in cilia assembly, we examined its expression in human airway epithelial cells. LRRC6 was not found in the ciliary axoneme, but was distributed throughout the cytoplasm of ciliated airway epithelial cells (**Figure 2A and 2B**), and localized proximally to basal bodies (**Supplementary Figure S1**), suggesting its involvement in assembly or trafficking during cilia biogenesis.

LRRC6 expression was silenced using an RNAi approach in primary airway epithelial cells obtained from excess tracheal and bronchial tissue from healthy lung transplant donors to define its role in differentiation, cilia assembly, and function. *LRRC6* was reproducibly inhibited by each of the *LRRC6* specific shRNA sequences when compared to cells transfected with non-targeted shRNA sequences as determined using both RT-PCR and immunoblot analyses (**Supplementary Figure S2A and S2B**). Cilia were present on the apical surface of cells treated with shRNA sequences and affected individuals, which showed that LRRC6 was not required for ciliogenesis (**Supplementary Figure S2C**). When compared to non-PCD or non-targeted shRNA transfected cells (**Figures 2C and 2E**, respectively), LRRC6 was markedly reduced in the cytoplasm of nasal epithelial cells from PCD subjects and *LRRC6*-specific shRNA transfected cells (**Figures 2D and 2F**). Furthermore, consistent with the axonemal defect observed in affected subjects (**Figure 2H**), ultrastructural analyses of cilia from silenced airway epithelial cells had truncated or absent dynein arms (**Figure 2J**) compared to normal and non-targeted shRNA transfected cells (**Figure 2G and 2I, respectively**).

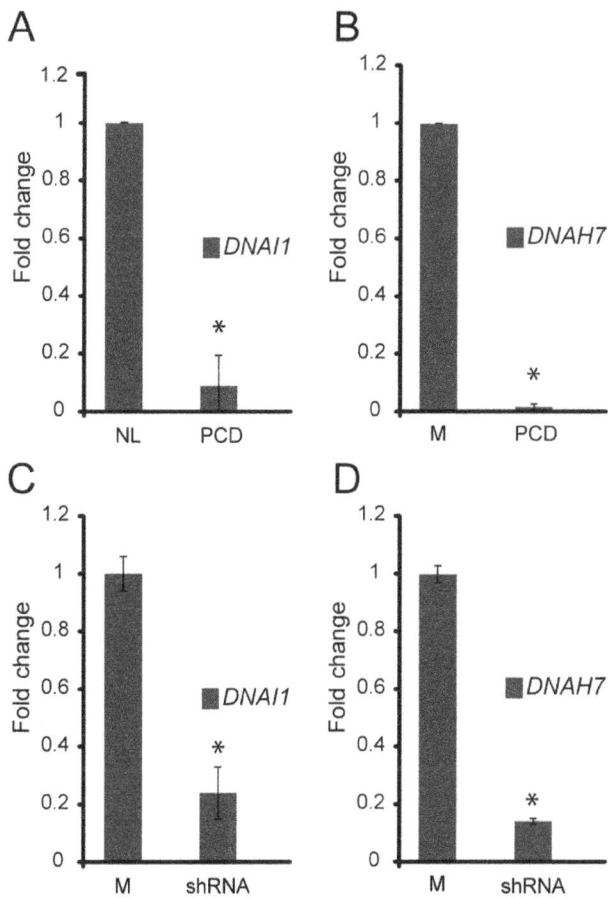

Figure 4. RT PCR analysis of *DNAI1* and *DNAH7* expression in PCD and RNAi silenced cells. *DNAI1* and *DNAH7* expression in nasal cells from PCD subjects (**A and B**) was markedly reduced as compared to cells from a healthy subject (NL) (n = 3 subjects, student t-test, p<0.001). Similarly, *DNAI1 and DNAH7* expression was decreased in *LRRC6*-specific shRNA transfected cells (**C and D**) compared to non-transfected control cells (M) (student t-test, p<0.001). (*) indicates a significant difference compared to control samples.

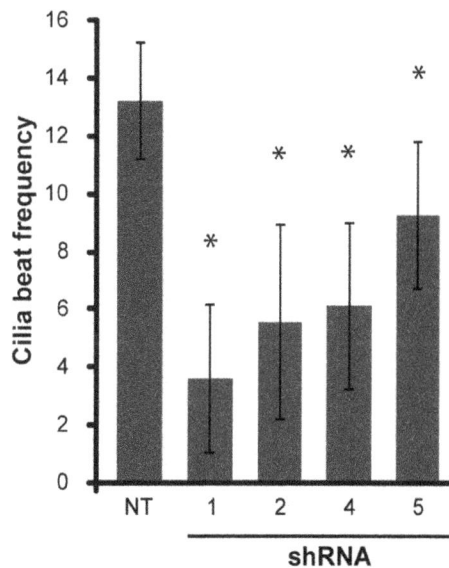

Figure 5. Cilia beat frequency. Mean cilia beat frequency in cells transfected with different shRNA targeted *LRRC6* sequences (n = 50 fields, ANOVA with Bonferroni correction, p<0.005). (*) indicates a significant difference compared to control samples.

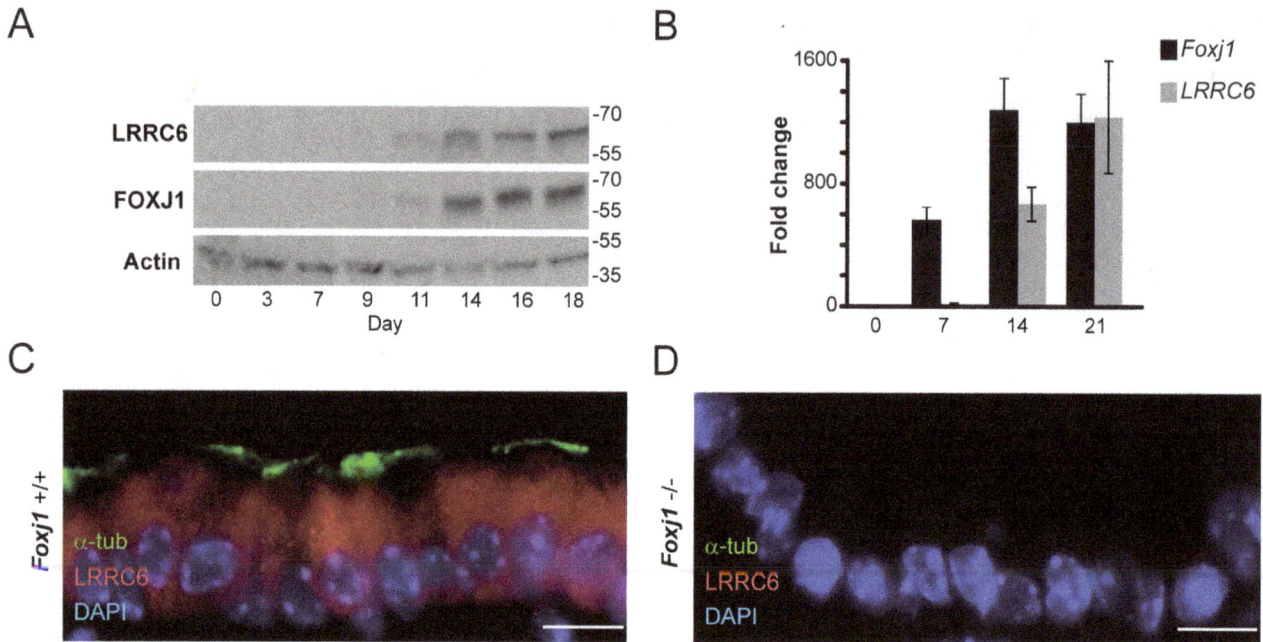

Figure 6. *LRRC6* **relation to** *Foxj1.* Immunoblot analysis of differentiating human tracheal epithelial cells collected from healthy subjects and grown at an air-liquid interface (**A**) showing LRRC6 paralleling Foxj1 expression. *LRRC6* expression measured using RT-PCR (**B**), increased significantly after the onset of ciliogenesis (ANOVA, p = 0.0004; individual student two-tail t-test, p = 0.003 and p = 0.001, comparing expression between day 0 and day 7, and between day 7 and day 14, respectively). *LRRC6* expression in tracheal airway epithelial cells isolated from wild-type mice (*Foxj1*$^{+/+}$) (**C**), compared to cells from Foxj1-deficient littermates (*Foxj1*$^{-/-}$) (**D**), showing that virtually no LRRC6 was detected in the cytoplasm of *Foxj1*$^{-/-}$ cells. Immunofluorescent staining for LRRC6 (red) and α-tubulin (green). (scale bar = 10 μm).

To examine the role of LRRC6 in dynein arm assembly, we immunostained ciliated cells with antibodies against DNAI1, an outer dynein arm polypeptide, and DNAH7, an inner dynein arm polypeptide. Neither DNAI1 nor DNAH7 were detected in cilia from PCD subjects, but DNAI1 was found in the apical cytoplasm of the epithelial cell (**Figure 3A**) suggesting mislocalization of the protein and failure of axonemal transport. In contrast, DNAH7 was not detected in the PCD cells, which may be related to protein degradation or suppressed expression. The latter was further evaluated by examining the expression of *DNAI1* and *DNAH7* in nasal cells for PCD subjects. *DNAI1* and *DNAH7* transcription was markedly reduced in nasal cells from three PCD subjects (III-1, III-2 and III-4 in **Figure 1A**) compared to a healthy control; findings that were also recapitulated in *Lrrc6*-specific shRNA targeted cells, suggesting that mutations in LRRC6 alters the expression of genes encoding some ODA and IDA proteins (**Figure 4**). While these findings indicate that LRRC6 is important for expression, trafficking, or assembly of normal dyneins, the pattern was also reminiscent of mislocalization of the ODA dynein DNAH5, previously described in PCD subjects with certain DNAH5 mutations [48], where mutations in DNAH5, hindered proper trafficking of ODA proteins into the ciliary axoneme and led to their accumulation in the cytoplasm. These findings further support the notion that ODA and possibly IDA proteins are assembled in the cytoplasm and are transported into the cilia axoneme as precursors. Furthermore, airway epithelial cells transfected with *LRRC6*-specific shRNA had markedly slower ciliary motion when compared to controls, as assessed using high-speed videomicroscopy (**Figure 5**). Nasal cells collected from subjects with PCD had no cilia motion when examined using high speed videomicroscopy (**Supplementary Videos S2**) [38].

The relationship between *LRRC6* expression and ciliogenesis, was examined using primary culture of hTEC as previously described [31]. *LRRC6* was initially detected during early ciliary differentiation, which coincided with the expression of the master ciliogenesis gene, *Foxj1* (**Figure 6A and 6B**) [31]. This relationship was further established by assessing *Lrrc6* expression in airway epithelial cells isolated from syngeneic wild-type (*Foxj1*$^{+/+}$) and *Foxj1*-deficient (*Foxj1*$^{-/-}$) mice [49]. *Lrrc6* levels were markedly reduced in *Foxj1*$^{-/-}$ airway epithelial cells when compared to *Foxj1*$^{+/+}$ cells (**Figure 6C and 6D**), indicating that Foxj1 regulated *Lrrc6* expression.

In summary, we show that a mutation in *LRRC6*, Asp146His, caused PCD in affected individuals from two unrelated families, which resulted in axonemal defects of the dynein arms and ciliary dysmotility. The association between LRRC6 and PCD was also recently reported in European subjects, thus confirming the importance of LRRC6 in cilia structure and function [50]. The ultrastructural and functional phenotypes observed in our cohort were recapitulated in *LRRC6*-silenced human airway epithelial cells. Regulated by Foxj1, LRRC6 is expressed in the cytoplasm of normal ciliated airway epithelial cells and absent from the ciliary axoneme, indicating that it is not a structural protein, findings that are consistent with published proteomic analyses that did not detect LRRC6 in cilia [51,52]. The absence of LRRC6 in cilia from these studies, and mislocalization of outer dynein, DNAI1, suggests a role in the preassembly of the dynein arms, like DNAAF1, DNAAF2, and DNAAF3, or their transport to the basal bodies, similar to ODA16 [14,20,25]. The novel finding of reduced expression of the outer and inner arm markers, DNAI1 and DNAH7, may also indicate that LRRC6 is involved in transcriptional regulation of some dynein proteins. Our findings are consistent with observations in other experimental models that conclusively show LRRC6 and its orthologues are involved in cilia assembly and function [50]. Thus, *LRRC6* can be added to the rapidly growing list of genes that when mutated cause PCD.

Supporting Information

Figure S1 Co-localization of LRRC6 with different organelles. Immunofluorescent staining of tracheobronchial epithelial cells from healthy subject showing no co-localization of LRRC6 (red) with markers of endosomes (green), and lysosomes (green). However, LRRC6 localized with χ-tubulin, a marker for basal bodies (green). Nuclei were stained using DAPI (blue). acetylated α-tubulin, a cilia marker, is shown in turquoise (scale bar = 10 μm).

Figure S2 RT PCR analysis of *LRRC6* expression in RNAi silenced cells. (A) *LRRC6* expression in LRRC6-specific shRNA transfected airway epithelial cells **(B)** Immunoblot analyses of airway epithelial cells transfected with three different *LRRC6*-specific shRNA or non-targeted shRNA (NT) sequences and nontransfected control cells (M). **(C)** En face images of LRRC6 in cultured preparations of ciliated airway epithelial cells from a normal donor, transfected with either non-targeted, control shRNA (NT) or different *LRRC6* targeted shRNA sequences. LRRC6 (red), acetylated α-tubulin (green), a ciliated cell marker, and co-stained with DAPI (blue). (scale bar = 20 μm).

Video S1 Healthy human nasal epithelial cells. Nasal epithelial cells from a healthy non-PCD subject showing normal cilia motion.

Video S2 Nasal epithelial cells from a subject with PCD. Nasal epithelial cells from a PCD subject with the *LRRC6* mutation showing no cilia motion.

Acknowledgments

The authors wish to acknowledge Marilyn Levy for assistance with the electron microscopy, Kathryn Akers for technical assistance, and Cassie Mikols and Jian Xu from the Children's Discovery Institute Airway Epithelial Cell Core at Washington University School of Medicine for assistance with cell culture. Drs. Feng and Longmore provided a non-targeted shRNA sequence with yellow fluorescent protein (YFP) reporter, and murine anti-DNAI1 antibody was a generous gift from Dr. Lawrence Ostrowski (University of North Carolina at Chapel Hill).

Author Contributions

Collected patient samples: DS MC IA. Performed initial patient assessment: DS MC. Conceived and designed the experiments: AH TF SB OE EK. Performed the experiments: AH SD MW OE YO YA. Analyzed the data: AH TF DS MW MC SD SB OE BK EK. Contributed reagents/materials/analysis tools: SB SD OE BK EK. Wrote the paper: AH TF SB OE EK.

References

1. Ferkol TW, Leigh MW (2012) Ciliopathies: the central role of cilia in a spectrum of pediatric disorders. J Pediatr 160: 366–371.
2. Knowles MR, Boucher RC (2002) Mucus clearance as a primary innate defense mechanism for mammalian airways. J Clin Invest 109: 571–577.
3. Afzelius BA (1976) A human syndrome caused by immotile cilia. Science 193: 317–319.
4. Chilvers MA, Rutman A, O'Callaghan C (2003) Ciliary beat pattern is associated with specific ultrastructural defects in primary ciliary dyskinesia. J Allergy Clin Immunol 112: 518–524.
5. Kennedy MP, Omran H, Leigh MW, Dell S, Morgan L, et al. (2007) Congenital heart disease and other heterotaxic defects in a large cohort of patients with primary ciliary dyskinesia. Circulation 115: 2814–2821.
6. Leigh MW, Pittman JE, Carson JL, Ferkol TW, Dell SD, et al. (2009) Clinical and genetic aspects of primary ciliary dyskinesia/Kartagener syndrome. Genet Med 11: 473–487.
7. Wessels MW, den Hollander NS, Willems PJ (2003) Mild fetal cerebral ventriculomegaly as a prenatal sonographic marker for Kartagener syndrome. Prenat Diagn 23: 239–242.
8. Olbrich H, Haffner K, Kispert A, Volkel A, Volz A, et al. (2002) Mutations in DNAH5 cause primary ciliary dyskinesia and randomization of left-right asymmetry. Nat Genet 30: 143–144.
9. Guichard C, Harricane MC, Lafitte JJ, Godard P, Zaegel M, et al. (2001) Axonemal dynein intermediate-chain gene (DNAI1) mutations result in situs inversus and primary ciliary dyskinesia (Kartagener syndrome). Am J Hum Genet 68: 1030–1035.
10. Loges NT, Olbrich H, Fenske L, Mussaffi H, Horvath J, et al. (2008) DNAI2 mutations cause primary ciliary dyskinesia with defects in the outer dynein arm. Am J Hum Genet 83: 547–558.
11. Duriez B, Duquesnoy P, Escudier E, Bridoux AM, Escalier D, et al. (2007) A common variant in combination with a nonsense mutation in a member of the thioredoxin family causes primary ciliary dyskinesia. Proc Natl Acad Sci U S A 104: 3336–3341.
12. Horvath J, Fliegauf M, Olbrich H, Kispert A, King SM, et al. (2005) Identification and analysis of axonemal dynein light chain 1 in primary ciliary dyskinesia patients. Am J Respir Cell Mol Biol 33: 41–47.
13. Horani A, Druley TE, Zariwala MA, Patel AC, Levinson BT, et al. (2012) Whole-Exome Capture and Sequencing Identifies HEATR2 Mutation as a Cause of Primary Ciliary Dyskinesia. Am J Hum Genet 91: 685–693.
14. Omran H, Kobayashi D, Olbrich H, Tsukahara T, Loges NT, et al. (2008) Ktu/PF13 is required for cytoplasmic pre-assembly of axonemal dyneins. Nature 456: 611–616.
15. Castleman VH, Romio L, Chodhari R, Hirst RA, de Castro SC, et al. (2009) Mutations in radial spoke head protein genes RSPH9 and RSPH4A cause primary ciliary dyskinesia with central-microtubular-pair abnormalities. Am J Hum Genet 84: 197–209.
16. Blanchon S, Legendre M, Copin B, Duquesnoy P, Montantin G, et al. (2012) Delineation of CCDC39/CCDC40 mutation spectrum and associated phenotypes in primary ciliary dyskinesia. J Med Genet 49: 410–416.
17. Knowles MR, Leigh MW, Carson JL, Davis SD, Dell SD, et al. (2011) Mutations of DNAH11 in patients with primary ciliary dyskinesia with normal ciliary ultrastructure. Thorax 67: 433–441.
18. Pennarun G, Escudier E, Chapelin C, Bridoux AM, Cacheux V, et al. (1999) Loss-of-function mutations in a human gene related to Chlamydomonas reinhardtii dynein IC78 result in primary ciliary dyskinesia. Am J Hum Genet 65: 1508–1519.
19. Bartoloni L, Blouin JL, Pan Y, Gehrig C, Maiti AK, et al. (2002) Mutations in the DNAH11 (axonemal heavy chain dynein type 11) gene cause one form of situs inversus totalis and most likely primary ciliary dyskinesia. Proc Natl Acad Sci U S A 99: 10282–10286.
20. Mitchison HM, Schmidts M, Loges NT, Freshour J, Dritsoula A, et al. (2012) Mutations in axonemal dynein assembly factor DNAAF3 cause primary ciliary dyskinesia. Nat Genet 44: 381–389.
21. Merveille AC, Davis EE, Becker-Heck A, Legendre M, Amirav I, et al. (2011) CCDC39 is required for assembly of inner dynein arms and the dynein regulatory complex and for normal ciliary motility in humans and dogs. Nat Genet 43: 72–78.
22. Becker-Heck A, Zohn IE, Okabe N, Pollock A, Lenhart KB, et al. (2011) The coiled-coil domain containing protein CCDC40 is essential for motile cilia function and left-right axis formation. Nat Genet 43: 79–84.
23. Panizzi JR, Becker-Heck A, Castleman VH, Al-Mutairi DA, Liu Y, et al. (2012) CCDC103 mutations cause primary ciliary dyskinesia by disrupting assembly of ciliary dynein arms. Nat Genet 44: 714–719.
24. Olbrich H, Schmidts M, Werner C, Onoufriadis A, Loges NT, et al. (2012) Recessive HYDIN mutations cause primary ciliary dyskinesia without randomization of left-right body asymmetry. Am J Hum Genet 91: 672–684.
25. Loges NT, Olbrich H, Becker-Heck A, Haffner K, Heer A, et al. (2009) Deletions and point mutations of LRRC50 cause primary ciliary dyskinesia due to dynein arm defects. Am J Hum Genet 85: 883–889.
26. Gherman A, Davis EE, Katsanis N (2006) The ciliary proteome database: an integrated community resource for the genetic and functional dissection of cilia. Nat Genet 38: 961–962.
27. Serluca FC, Xu B, Okabe N, Baker K, Lin SY, et al. (2009) Mutations in zebrafish leucine-rich repeat-containing six-like affect cilia motility and result in pronephric cysts, but have variable effects on left-right patterning. Development 136: 1621–1631.
28. Kobe B, Kajava AV (2001) The leucine-rich repeat as a protein recognition motif. Curr Opin Struct Biol 11: 725–732.
29. Edvardson S, Shaag A, Kolesnikova O, Gomori JM, Tarassov I, et al. (2007) Deleterious mutation in the mitochondrial arginyl-transfer RNA synthetase gene is associated with pontocerebellar hypoplasia. Am J Hum Genet 81: 857–862.

30. Dejima K, Randell SH, Stutts MJ, Senior BA, Boucher RC (2006) Potential role of abnormal ion transport in the pathogenesis of chronic sinusitis. Arch Otolaryngol Head Neck Surg 132: 1352–1362.

31. You Y, Richer EJ, Huang T, Brody SL (2002) Growth and differentiation of mouse tracheal epithelial cells: selection of a proliferative population. Am J Physiol Lung Cell Mol Physiol 283: L1315–1321.

32. Feng Y, Nie L, Thakur MD, Su Q, Chi Z, et al. (2010) A multifunctional lentiviral-based gene knockdown with concurrent rescue that controls for off-target effects of RNAi. Genomics Proteomics Bioinformatics 8: 238–245.

33. Stewart SA, Dykxhoorn DM, Palliser D, Mizuno H, Yu EY, et al. (2003) Lentivirus-delivered stable gene silencing by RNAi in primary cells. RNA 9: 493–501.

34. Lois C, Hong EJ, Pease S, Brown EJ, Baltimore D (2002) Germline transmission and tissue-specific expression of transgenes delivered by lentiviral vectors. Science 295: 868–872.

35. Pan J, You Y, Huang T, Brody SL (2007) RhoA-mediated apical actin enrichment is required for ciliogenesis and promoted by Foxj1. J Cell Sci 120: 1868–1876.

36. Ostrowski LE, Yin W, Rogers TD, Busalacchi KB, Chua M, et al. (2010) Conditional deletion of dnaic1 in a murine model of primary ciliary dyskinesia causes chronic rhinosinusitis. Am J Respir Cell Mol Biol 43: 55–63.

37. Jain R, Ray JM, Pan JH, Brody SL (2012) Sex hormone-dependent regulation of cilia beat frequency in airway epithelium. Am J Respir Cell Mol Biol 46: 446–453.

38. Barbato A, Frischer T, Kuehni CE, Snijders D, Azevedo I, et al. (2009) Primary ciliary dyskinesia: a consensus statement on diagnostic and treatment approaches in children. Eur Respir J 34: 1264–1276.

39. Sisson JH, Stoner JA, Ammons BA, Wyatt TA (2003) All-digital image capture and whole-field analysis of ciliary beat frequency. J Microsc 211: 103–111.

40. Walker WT, Jackson CL, Lackie PM, Hogg C, Lucas JS (2012) Nitric oxide in primary ciliary dyskinesia. Eur Respir J 40: 1024–1032.

41. Noone PG, Leigh MW, Sannuti A, Minnix SL, Carson JL, et al. (2004) Primary ciliary dyskinesia: diagnostic and phenotypic features. Am J Respir Crit Care Med 169: 459–467.

42. Xue JC, Goldberg E (2000) Identification of a novel testis-specific leucine-rich protein in humans and mice. Biol Reprod 62: 1278–1284.

43. UniProt Consortium (2012) Reorganizing the protein space at the Universal Protein Resource (UniProt). Nucleic Acids Res 40: D71–75.

44. Price SR, Evans PR, Nagai K (1998) Crystal structure of the spliceosomal U2B"-U2A' protein complex bound to a fragment of U2 small nuclear RNA. Nature 394: 645–650.

45. Dutcher SK (1995) Flagellar assembly in two hundred and fifty easy-to-follow steps. Trends Genet 11: 398–404.

46. Kavlie RG, Kernan MJ, Eberl DF Hearing in Drosophila requires TilB, a conserved protein associated with ciliary motility. Genetics 185: 177–188.

47. Morgan GW, Denny PW, Vaughan S, Goulding D, Jeffries TR, et al. (2005) An evolutionarily conserved coiled-coil protein implicated in polycystic kidney disease is involved in basal body duplication and flagellar biogenesis in Trypanosoma brucei. Mol Cell Biol 25: 3774–3783.

48. Fliegauf M, Olbrich H, Horvath J, Wildhaber JH, Zariwala MA, et al. (2005) Mislocalization of DNAH5 and DNAH9 in respiratory cells from patients with primary ciliary dyskinesia. Am J Respir Crit Care Med 171: 1343–1349.

49. Brody SL, Yan XH, Wuerffel MK, Song SK, Shapiro SD (2000) Ciliogenesis and left-right axis defects in forkhead factor HFH-4-null mice. Am J Respir Cell Mol Biol 23: 45–51.

50. Kott E, Duquesnoy P, Copin B, Legendre M, Dastot-Le Moal F, et al. (2012) Loss-of-Function Mutations in LRRC6, a Gene Essential for Proper Axonemal Assembly of Inner and Outer Dynein Arms, Cause Primary Ciliary Dyskinesia. Am J Hum Genet 91: 958–964.

51. Pazour GJ, Agrin N, Leszyk J, Witman GB (2005) Proteomic analysis of a eukaryotic cilium. J Cell Biol 170: 103–113.

52. Ostrowski LE, Blackburn K, Radde KM, Moyer MB, Schlatzer DM, et al. (2002) A proteomic analysis of human cilia: identification of novel components. Mol Cell Proteomics 1: 451–465.

18

Bronchial Wall Measurements in Patients after Lung Transplantation: Evaluation of the Diagnostic Value for the Diagnosis of Bronchiolitis Obliterans Syndrome

Sabine Dettmer[1]*, Lars Peters[1], Claudia de Wall[2], Cornelia Schaefer-Prokop[3,4], Michael Schmidt[5], Gregor Warnecke[6], Jens Gottlieb[2], Frank Wacker[1], Hoen-oh Shin[1]

1 Hannover Medical School, Department of Radiology, Hannover, Germany, 2 Hannover Medical School, Department of Respiratory Medicine, Hannover, Germany, 3 Radiologie, Meander Medisch Centrum, Amersfoort, the Netherlands, 4 Radiologie – DIAG, UMC St Radboud, Nijmegen, the Netherlands, 5 Fraunhofer MEVIS, Bremen, Germany, 6 Hannover Medical School, Department of Thoracic and Cardiovascular Surgery, Hannover, Germany

Abstract

Objectives: To prospectively evaluate quantitative airway wall measurements of thin-section CT for the diagnosis of Bronchiolitis Obliterans Syndrome (BOS) following lung transplantation.

Materials and Methods: In 141 CT examinations, bronchial wall thickness (WT), the wall area percentage (WA%) calculated as the ratio of the bronchial wall area and the total area (sum of bronchial wall area and bronchial lumen area) and the difference of the WT on inspiration and expiration (WTdiff) were automatically measured in different bronchial generations. The measurements were correlated with the lung function parameters. WT and WA% in CT examinations of patients with (n = 25) and without (n = 116) BOS, were compared using the unpaired t-test and univariate analysis of variance, while also considering the differing lung volumes.

Results: Measurements could be performed in 2,978 bronchial generations. WT, WA%, and WTdiff did not correlate with the lung function parameters (r<0.5). The WA% on inspiration was significantly greater in patients with BOS than in patients without BOS, even when considering the dependency of the lung volume on the measurements. WT on inspiration and expiration and WA% on expiration did not show significant differences between the groups.

Conclusion: WA% on inspiration was significantly greater in patients with than in those without BOS. However, WA% measurements were significantly dependent on lung volume and showed a high variability, thus not allowing the sole use of bronchial wall measurements to differentiate patients with from those without BOS.

Editor: Nades Palaniyar, The Hospital for Sick Children and The University of Toronto, Canada

Funding: This work (Dettmer and de Wall) was supported by a grant from the German Federal Ministry of Education and Research (reference number: 01EO0802). The funders had no role in study design, data collection and analysis, decision to publish, or preparation of the manuscript.

Competing Interests: The authors have declared that no competing interests exist.

* E-mail: dettmer.sabine@mh-hannover.de

Introduction

Bronchiolitis obliterans syndrome (BOS) is the primary long-term complication following lung transplantation and it considerably influences the prognosis of transplant patients [1]. BOS affects up to 60% of lung transplant recipients during the five years following surgery [2]. Histopathologically, bronchiolitis obliterans (BO) is a fibroproliferative process of the small airways and results in multifocal obliteration of the terminal bronchioli [3]. Characteristic histopathology features are a patchy, submucosal fibrosis in the respiratory bronchioles resulting in nearly total or total occlusion of the small airways. The mechanisms by which BO is mediated are manifold and are not yet completely understood. Alloimmune reactivity appears to have a role as well as antibody-mediated rejection, including activation of innate immune cells and response to enviromental and endogenous factors such as infection and aspiration [4].

BO is difficult to quantify histologically due to the nonuniform distribution of fibrosis. Therefore in 1993, a committee of the International Society for Heart and Lung Transplantation (ISHLT) proposed a clinical description of BO, termed bronchiolitis obliterans syndrome (BOS), with a decrease of FEV_1 (forced expiratory volume in one second) of at least 20% of the postoperative baseline value [5,6] and unexplained by acute rejection, infection or other complications. The severity of BOS is graded according to the degree of obstruction found in pulmonary function tests (PFT): BOS 1 describes a 20–34% decrease in FEV_1 from baseline; BOS 2 a 35–49% decrease in FEV_1; and BOS 3 at least a 50% decrease in FEV_1 from baseline [6]. Although transbronchial biopsy can be used to establish the diagnosis, it is rarely used because of its low sensitivity [7].

The standard workup for the diagnosis of BOS at our lung transplant center initially includes routine lung function tests, bronchoscopy and CT of the chest. If there are decreased values,

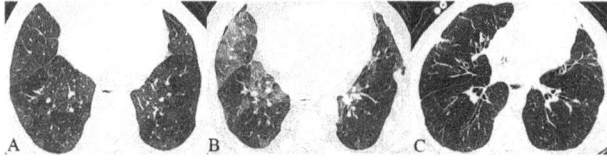

Figure 1. Typical CT findings of BOS include bronchial wall thickening (A), mosaic attenuation (A), air trapping (B) and bronchiectasis (C).

especially for FEV_1, other causes, such as infection, asthma or chronic obstructive disease, are excluded. BOS is diagnosed if no other reason for an obstruction is found and if the impairment persists.

The histopathological changes of the airways seen in BOS result in distinct CT morphological findings such as air trapping [8] and bronchial wall thickening [9] (Figure 1). Other CT findings frequently seen in patients with BOS are bronchiectasis, mucus plugging, and consolidations [9,10,11]. However, it has been shown that none of these findings could predict the development of BOS [12]. There have been repeated efforts to use CT findings to diagnose BOS before it results in clinically apparent functional impairment [10,13]. However, to date these findings have not produced convincing evidence.

During the past 10 years, efforts have been made to measure bronchial wall thickness and bronchial lumen [14]. Contemporary software allows automatic segmentation of the bronchial tree and quantification of the bronchial wall and bronchial lumen [15]. Different mathematical models have been applied with variable accuracy, especially for the smaller and more peripheral airways. The most frequently described method is based on the Full-width-at-half-maximum-principle (FWHM) [16]. However, it has been shown that this method systematically overestimates the wall thickness for small airways [17,18]. The algorithm used in our study is based on the mathematical integration of Hounsfield intensities (intensity integration) across wall regions [19] as this was found to reduce overestimation of WT in small airways and, therefore, seems especially suited for this particular patient group [20].

Previous studies have shown that bronchial wall thickness quantified on CT data is correlated with the lung function parameters in patients with various airway diseases such as COPD [21,22], CF [23], and asthma [24,25].

The purpose of our feasability study is to evaluate whether there is any correlation between the lung function parameters and the CT dimensions of airways and if the airway wall parameters may help to distinguish between lung transplant patients with and those without BOS.

Materials and Methods

Prospective Study Design

Written consent was obtained from all of the patients participating in this study. The consent procedure and study were approved by the Ethics Committee of Hannover Medical School (number 5108).

This prospective study was conducted in a single medical center with a large lung transplant program and more than 100 annual lung transplantations [26]. The study is part of a larger research project to develop imaging tools in recipients who develop BOS after lung transplantation so as to allow an earlier diagnosis and more accurate monitoring of the disease process. Our clinical workup in patients following lung transplantation includes routine

CT scans performed at six, 12 and 24 months after transplantation. We included all individuals who had undergone double or heart and lung transplantation at our clinic when they were between 18 and 68 years of age and with stable graft function ($FEV_1 > 90\%$). Exclusion criteria were severe airway complications after surgery and necessitating intervention, oxygen desaturation during exercise to less than 89% without supplemental oxygen, cardiovascular complications that limited exercise tolerance, single lung and living lobar recipients, and patients with an established diagnosis of BOS at the time of their inclusion and the inability to undergo body plethysmography which may have been due to persistent infection caused by multi-drug-resistant bacteria. Because of the limited number of study patients with clinically manifested BOS during the time between baseline CT and the data inclusion endpoint, we included n = 8, randomly chosen, additional examinations of patients with a clinical diagnosis of BOS for data analysis that fulfilled all of the inclusion criteria stated above with the exception of the availability of a baseline CT with normal PFT.

Study Participants

Our study patient group consisted of 90 lung-transplant patients. The demographic data are presented in Table 1. There were 53 male patients and 37 female patients with a mean age of 45 years (range 18–65 years) at the time of their examination. For 85 patients it was the first transplantation, and five patients underwent a re-transplantation. Eighty-four patients had a double-lung transplantation, and six patients underwent a heart-lung transplantation; however, none of the patients underwent single-lung transplantation.

Of these 90 patients, 45 had one examination, 40 had two examinations, four had three examinations, and one patient had four examinations, resulting in a total of 141 paired CT examinations and lung function tests. One hundred and seventeen examinations were performed in lung transplant patients without BOS and 24 in patients with a clinical diagnosis of BOS (15 were BOS stage 3, two were BOS stage 2, and seven were BOS stage 1). The BOS stages were classified by a pneumologist (CdW) based on FEV_1 and according to the guidelines of the International Society for Heart and Lung Transplantation (ISHLT) [5]. Other reasons for a reduction of FEV_1, such as infection, asthma or chronic obstructive pulmonary disease, were excluded. No patient had clinical signs of an infection at the time of their examination. The mean interval between transplantation and the CT examination was 11 months (range 5–65 months). CT examinations and lung function tests were performed within 24 hours of each other.

CT Data Acquisition

CT examinations were performed at full inspiration (insp) and full expiration (exp) using a 64-row MDCT scanner (Lightspeed VCT, GE Healthcare, Milwaukee, WI, USA), and no intravenous contrast medium was used.

The CT data were aquired using 120 kV, 100 mAs, a rotation time of 0.8 s, and a pitch of 0.984; the slice collimation during acquisition was 1.25 mm. Data reconstruction yielded 1.25-mm slices with an interval of 1 mm using a "standard" reconstruction kernel (soft-tissue). The field of view (FOV) was adapted according to the size of the patient's lung. No separate reconstructions of the right or left lung were performed.

Patients were instructed to hold their breath during full inspiration and expiration, respectively, during the CT data acquisition. CT data were acquired under spirometric control in order to gain information regarding the vital capacity at the time

Table 1. Demographic data of all patients with/without BOS.

		All	Without BOS	With BOS
Number	Patients	90		
	Examinations	141	117 (83%)	24 (17%)
Age (Years)	At timepoint of CT	45 (18–65)	46 (22–65)	45 (18–66)
Gender	Male	53 (59%)	45 (60%)	8 (53%)
	Female	37 (41%)	30 (40%)	7 (47%)
Transplantation	Double lung	84 (93%)	70 (93%)	14 (93%)
	Heart-lung	6 (7%)	5 (7%)	1 (7%)
	First transplantation	85 (94%)	72 (96%)	13 (87%)
	Re-transplantation	5 (6%)	3 (4%)	2 (13%)
Number of CT-examinations	1	45 (50%)		
	2	40 (44%)		
	3	4 (4%)		
	4	1 (1%)		
Underlying disease	Cystic fibrosis	18 (20%)	16 (21%)	2 (13%)
	Emphysema	30 (33%)	26 (35%)	4 (27%)
	Pulmonary fibrosis	20 (22%)	17 (23%)	3 (20%)
	Pulmonary hypertension	5 (6%)	4 (5%)	1 (7%)
	BOS	5 (6%)	3 patients (4%)	2 patients (13%)
	Other	6 (12%)	9 patients (12%)	3 patients (20%)

of the examination and a stable breathhold phase during data acquisition after deep inspiration and expiration, respectively.

Inspiratory and expiratory scans were performed using the same scan protocol. The mean CTDI was 10.1 mGy for both the inspiratory and expiratory CT (range: 3.36–21.9 mGy, SD: 5.08 mGy) and the mean DLPw amounted to 384.3 mGy×cm for the inspiratory and 385.8 mGy×cm for the expiratory scan (range: 117.0–890.5 mGy×cm, SD: 199.5 mGy×cm).

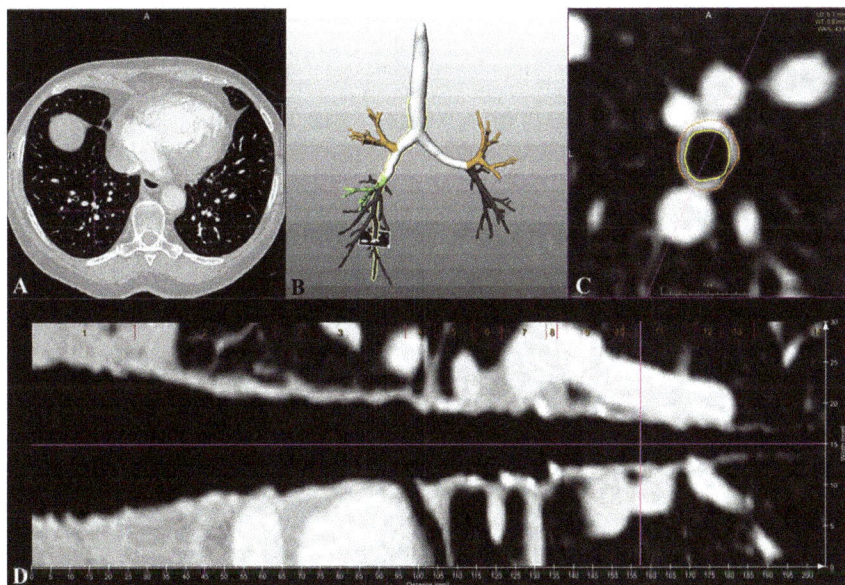

Figure 2. Bronchial wall measurements using the MeVis Airway Examiner. A three-dimensional display of the tracheobronchial tree (B) allowed the selection of the bronchus that should be evaluated (yellow border). For visualization, curved mulitplanar reformation (D) and cross-sectional images perpendicular to the central path, were used (C) and with the viewing direction along the bronchial path. The original dataset is shown in (A) and the selected bronchus is tagged with a cross-line. The location for measurements of the bronchial wall was visualized with a yellow line for the inner and a red line for the outer borderline of the bronchial wall (C).

Table 2. Mean airway wall parameters during inspiration (insp) and expiration (exp) according to the bronchial generation (1 is central, 8 is peripheral).

Generation	WT insp	WT exp	p	WA% insp	WA% exp	p	WTdiff
1	1.76 (0.32)	1.82 (0.38)	0.166	36.53 (5.83)	41.22 (9.52)	<0.001	0.12
2	1.49 (0.33)	1.70 (0.34)	<0.001	39.27 (8.02)	47.07 (10.57)	<0.001	0.25
3	1.38 (0.34)	1.62 (0.40)	<0.001	41.87 (8.68)	50.72 (11.13)	<0.001	0.33
4	1.27 (0.40)	1.49 (0.43)	<0.001	43.69 (8.27)	52.85 (11.54)	<0.001	0.26
5	1.14 (0.43)	1.37 (0.44)	<0.001	42.86 (8.18)	52.39 (11.59)	<0.001	0.22
6	1.09 (0.42)	1.32 (0.41)	<0.001	42.12 (8.65)	53.98 (10.19)	<0.001	0.24
7	1.00 (0.31)	1.26 (0.34)	<0.001	41.47 (6.91)	56.03 (10.04)	<0.001	0.27
8	0.81 (0.20)	1.11 (0.31)	<0.001	36.91 (7.10)	53.66 (8.76)	<0.001	0.30

The WT (mm) and WA% (%) were significantly different between inspiration and expiration (the standard deviation values are in parentheses).

Lung Function Tests

Pulmonary function tests (PFT) were performed using body plethysmography (BodyScope N, Ganshorn Medizin Electronic GmbH, Münnerstadt/Niderlauer, Germany) and the measured values were related to the predicted values calculated according to Quanjier et al. [27]. Spirometry was performed according to the guidelines provided by the American Thoracic Society and the European Respiratory Society [28].

Quantification of the Airway Wall Parameters

For automatic quantification of the airway wall thickness (WT), the lumen diameter (LD), and the wall area percentage (WA%), dedicated software (MEVIS airway examiner, Fraunhofer MEVIS Bremen, Germany) was used [20]. The WA% was calculated as the ratio of the bronchial wall area and the total area (sum of the bronchial wall area and the bronchial lumen area). The difference of the WT between expiration and inspiration (WTdiff) was then calculated separately for each bronchial generation. After fully automatic segmentation of the bronchial tree, a central pathway through the bronchial structures was calculated. The WT and WA% were automatically measured for each cross-sectional image perpendicular to the central pathway after segmentation of the wall contours. Areas not appropriate for measurement, i.e. branching points or areas of adherence of the bronchial wall and vascular structures, were automatically excluded from the measurements. The software highlighted the automatic delineation of the bronchial wall (Figure 2), thus allowing for visual control of the computed segmentation. In cases of incorrect identification of the bronchial wall, the corresponding slice could be manually excluded from the quantitative analysis as a manual segmentation correction was not possible. For the quantitative analysis, two bronchial branches were chosen, the posterior basal segmental bronchus (B10) of the right lung and the apicoposterior segmental bronchus (B01) of the left lung as, therefore, considered data from the upper and lower parts of the lung and from both lungs, could thus be included. We chose the right lower lobe to avoid potential interference of the measurements with the motion artifacts caused by cardiac pulsation in the left lower lobe.

The path of a bronchus was divided in anatomical generations following the anatomic branching from lobar, segmental to subsegmental, and sub-sub-segmental generations and with each ramification defining the beginning of a new generation. Bronchi up to the 7th generation were consistently identified in all scans. More peripheral bronchi up to the 10th generation could not be identified in all scans and were thus only considered if automatic segmentation was successful on both inspiration and expiration. Only bronchial generations with at least 10 valid measurements were included in the analysis. To ensure that the measurement positions were in identical bronchial generations during inspiration and expiration, all images and measurement locations were visually controlled by L.P. und S.D. The WT difference during inspiration and expiration was then calculated. The mean WT of each bronchial generation of inspiration and expiration scans was thereby assessed.

Measurement of Lung Volumes

Lung volumes on inspiration and expiration were measured using MEVIS Pulmo (Fraunhofer MEVIS Bremen, Germany) [29].

Statistical Analysis

Statistical tests were performed using PASW statistics (ver. 18.0, SPSS Inc., Chicago, IL, USA, 2006). The Kolmogorov-Smirnov-

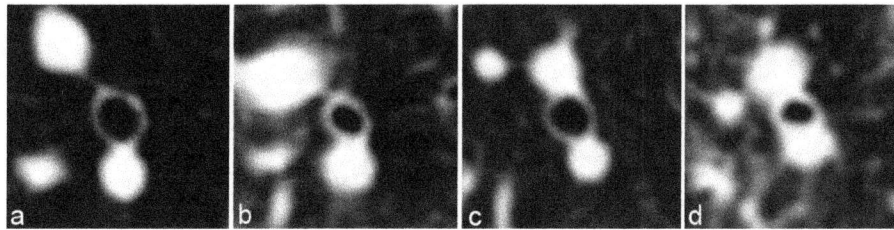

Figure 3. Cross-sectional images perpendicular to the central path of a segmental bronchus (B10) in a patient without (a+b) and one with BOS (c+d) during inspiration (a+c) and expiration (b+d). Differences in the WT between inspiration and expiration are visually apparent in both patients.

test was used to test normal data distribution. The correlation of PFT with the CT measurements obtained bronchus-wise for WT and WA% on inspiration and expiration CT scans, was tested using Pearson's rank correlation coefficient.

The airway wall parameters of stable lung transplant recipients were compared with those of patients with manifested BOS using the independent samples t-test. The WA% and WT measured on inspiration were compared to the expiratory values using the paired samples t-test. To further evaluate the influence of lung volume on bronchial wall measurements, we performed a univariate analysis of variance for The WT and WA% on inspiration and expiration with the lung volume as a covariate comparing patients with and without BOS. This test compares both patient groups considering the depency of the lung volume on measurements.

Results

Airway Dimensions

In the entire study group (without and with BOS), the WT was measured in 2,978 bronchial generations (1,784 on inspiratory scans and 1,194 on expiratory scans) and the WA% in 2,975 bronchial generations (1,786 on inspiratory scans and 1,189 on expiratory scans). The WT difference on inspiration and expiration could be calculated for 1,079 bronchial generations.

The WT continuously decreased when moving from the central (mean WT insp 1st generation: 1.76 mm) to the peripheral bronchial generations (mean WT insp 8th generation: 0.81 mm) (table 2). For all generations the mean WT and mean WA% were significantly greater (paired t-test) on expiration than on inspiration (p<0.001, Table 2, Figure 3) except for the WT in the 1st generation (main bronchus).

Pulmonary Function Tests

The pulmonary function test values are shown in Table 3.

Correlation of the Airway Wall Parameters and the Lung Function Parameters

The Kolmogorov-Smirnov-test showed that the datasets for bronchial wall measurement for each bronchial generation were distributed normally. Pearson's rank correlation coefficient was used to test the correlation between the CT morphologic and lung function parameters.

The analysis did not find any correlation of the overall WT, WA%, and WTdiff with lung function parameters determined on inspiration and expiration (Tables 4 and 5).

For the airway parameters no statistically significant correlation with the lung function parameters could be found except for Peak expiratory flow (PEF) and the ratio of PEF/PEF$_{predicted}$ with WT

insp in the 10th generation, which we regard as coincidential (Tables 4 and 5).

Comparison of the Airway Wall Parameters in Patients with and without BOS

Twenty-five examinations were performed in patients with clinically identified BOS, of which 15 were BOS stage 3. In these 25 examinations, the WT and WA% were measured in 469 bronchial generations. These were compared with the WT and WA% measurements of 2,509 and 2,506 bronchial generations, respectively, in patients without clinical evidence of BOS.

The mean WT on inspiration was slightly higher in patients with BOS than in those without BOS (Table 6), although the difference was not statistically significant. The WT on expiration did not differ significantly with and without BOS, and in the peripheral bronchial generations the WT was slightly higher in patients without BOS. The WA% on inspiration in patients with BOS differed significantly from the measurements seen in stable lung transplant recipients in most bronchial generations (Table 6). The LD is increased in the peripheral bronchial generations in patients with BOS compared to patients without BOS, and thus indicating the development of bronchiectasis (Table 7) although without statistical sgnificance.

The WT and WA% on expiration as well as the WTdiff did not differ significantly in the two patient groups. The WT and WA% were significantly larger on expiration than on inspiration in patients with and without BOS (table 2).

Lung volumes could be measured on 140 of 141 CT examinations. The lung volumes on inspiration in patients with BOS (mean: 4,903 ml) were lower than in patients without BOS (mean: 5,302 ml), although the difference was not significant (p = 0.173). The lung volumes on expiration in patients with BOS (mean: 3,178 ml) were significantly larger than those seen in patients without BOS (mean: 2,495 ml, p = 0.001). The lung volume difference between inspiration and expiration was significantly less in patients with BOS (mean: 1,840 ml) than in patients without BOS (mean: 2,815 ml, p<0.001) (table 8).

The univariate analysis of variance for the WA% revealed a significant influence of lung volume for the WA%. The univariate analysis of variance for the WT and WA%, comparing patients with and without the lung volume as a covariate, revealed a significant difference of the WA% on inspiration in either case (Table 9). Both the presence of BOS and the different lung volume had significant influence on measurements of the WA% on inspiration. The WT on inspiration and expiration and the WA% on expiration did not show a significant difference in either group with and without using the lung volume as a cofactor.

However, the variability of bronchial wall measurements was high and the values for the WA% on inspiration in patients with and without BOS, overlapped considerably (Figure 4).

Table 3. Results (mean values) of the pulmonary function tests for the entire study population and subdivided according to male/female patients and those with/without BOS.

	Mean total	Min total	Max total	standard deviation	Mean male	Mean female	Mean without BOS	Mean with BOS
VC (ml)	3390	1030	5780	1107	3791	2829	3575	2610
VC/pred	0.81	0.22	1.24	0.22	0.79	0.85	0.87	0.57
PEF (l/min)	6.42	1.01	11.7	2.1	7.08	5.48	1.61	3.96
PEF/pred	0.8	0.14	1.19	0.23	0.79	0.81	0.87	0.46
MEF25 (l/min)	1.39	0.12	6.01	0.97	1.57	1.14	1.61	0.42
MEF25/pred	0.73	0.05	2.79	0.49	0.78	0.68	0.85	0.21
MEF50 (l/min)	3.12	0.16	9.55	1.75	3.52	2.57	3.58	1.07
MEF50/pred	0.68	0.03	1.61	0.36	0.73	0.63	0.78	0.22
MEF25–75 (l/min)	2.74	0.15	8.7	1.55	3.08	2.27	3.17	0.85
MEF25–75/pred	0.71	0.04	0.83	0.39	0.76	0.66	0.83	0.21
FEV1 (ml)	2481	330	4690	930	2754	2115	2754	1298
FEV1/pred	0.74	0.09	1.33	0.25	0.74	0.74	0.82	0.36
% of best FEV1	84	23	102	19	84	85	92	45
Tiffeneau	0.73	0.26	1	0.16	0.72	0.74	0.78	0.48

Table 4. Pearson's rank correlation coefficient for the WT and WA% on inspiration for all bronchial generations ($1^{st}-10^{th}$).

	VC	VC/pred	PEF	PEF/pred	MEF25	MEF25/pred	MEF50	MEF50/pred	MEF25-75	MEF25-75/pred	FEV1	FEV1/pred	% best FEV1	Tiffeneau
WT generation 1	0.117	0.048	0.075	0.034	-0.021	-0.023	-0.001	-0.016	0.002	<-0.001	0.081	0.048	0.061	-0.039
WT generation 2	-0.041	-0.166	-0.086	-0.176	-0.173	-0.159	-0.110	-0.117	-0.151	-0.141	-0.121	-0.180	0.103	-0.148
WT generation 3	-0.028	-0.207	-0.071	-0.206	-0.174	-0.187	-0.150	-0.150	-0.152	-0.184	-0.125	-0.213	0.103	-0.159
WT generation 4	0.009	-0.135	0.004	-0.099	-0.148	-0.157	-0.018	-0.044	-0.066	-0.091	-0.052	-0.143	0.126	-0.072
WT generation 5	0.040	-0.069	<-0.001	-0.086	-0.093	-0.084	-0.006	-0.018	-0.025	-0.027	-0.003	-0.054	0.151	-0.085
WT generation 6	0.112	-0.073	0.016	-0.127	-0.098	-0.116	-0.051	-0.092	-0.062	-0.082	0.026	-0.091	0.024	-0.150
WT generation 7	0.196	-0.059	0.098	-0.129	-0.044	-0.109	0.009	-0.070	0.010	-0.055	0.135	-0.060	0.282	-0.102
WT generation 8	-0.353	-0.358	-0.348	-0.348	-0.223	-0.147	-0.102	-0.061	-0.165	-0.084	-0.331	-0.276	0.288	-0.060
WA% generation 1	-0.061	0.062	<-0.001	0.105	-0.036	0.001	-0.011	0.022	-0.029	0.004	-0.009	0.084	0.052	0.106
WA% generation 2	-0.162	-0.170	-0.209	-0.213	-0.235	-0.205	-0.205	-0.191	-0.233	-0.203	-0.230	-0.214	0.072	-0.178
WA% generation 3	-0.256	-0.281	-0.289	-0.320	-0.246	-0.220	-0.241	-0.231	-0.257	-0.251	-0.320	-0.318	0.091	-0.192
WA% generation 4	-0.276	-0.347	-0.263	-0.314	-0.287	-0.276	-0.229	-0.229	-0.260	-0.267	-0.345	-0.378	0.205	-0.189
WA% generation 5	-0.224	-0.291	-0.260	-0.322	-0.252	-0.236	-0.216	-0.214	-0.226	-0.226	-0.280	-0.300	0.191	-0.195
WA% generation 6	-0.221	-0.336	-0.309	-0.406	-0.254	-0.243	-0.270	-0.275	-0.270	-0.267	-0.298	-0.350	0.095	-0.259
WA% generation 7	-0.073	-0.277	-0.051	-0.225	-0.162	-0.199	-0.110	-0.154	-0.117	-0.169	-0.087	-0.214	0.318	-0.008
WA% generation 8	-0.509	-0.487	-0.321	-0.319	-0.190	-0.116	-0.147	-0.101	-0.145	-0.086	-0.404	-0.327	0.480	0.111

For the airway parameters no statistically significant correlation with the lung function parameters was found (all r<0.5 except PEF and the ratio of PEF/PEF$_{predicted}$ with WT insp in generation 10).

Table 5. Pearson's rank correlation coefficient for the WT and WA% on expiration for all bronchial generations and subdivided into bronchial generations (1st–8th).

	VC	VC/pred	PEF	PEF/pred	MEF25	MEF25/pred	MEF50	MEF50/pred	MEF25-75	MEF25-75/pred	FEV1	FEV1/pred	% best FEV1	Tiffeneau
WT generation 1	0.005	−0.115	−0.005	−0.079	0.099	0.073	0.069	0.039	0.062	0.037	0.016	−0.044	0.011	−0.044
WT generation 2	0.043	−0.056	−0.301	−0.110	−0.112	−0.154	−0.050	−0.078	−0.057	−0.087	−0.022	−0.092	−0.019	−0.135
WT generation 3	0.068	−0.018	0.039	−0.019	−0.031	−0.048	0.026	0.016	0.001	−0.019	0.008	−0.043	0.049	−0.075
WT generation 4	0.105	0.009	0.097	0.027	−0.118	−0.144	−0.015	−0.040	−0.046	0.097	0.022	−0.049	0.081	−0.102
WT generation 5	0.018	−0.032	−0.087	−0.137	−0.216	−0.219	−0.120	−0.126	−0.150	−0.150	−0.086	−0.127	−0.051	−0.201
WT generation 6	0.076	−0.011	0.051	−0.007	−0.039	−0.075	0.054	0.028	0.027	0.052	0.034	−0.032	−0.076	−0.027
WT generation 7	0.187	0.082	0.076	−0.011	−0.011	−0.072	0.080	0.031	0.062	0.023	0.126	0.028	0.065	−0.087
WT generation 8	0.209	0.255	0.021	0.052	−0.069	−0.097	0.009	−0.007	−0.022	−0.025	0.100	0.121	−0.215	−0.053
WA% generation 1	−0.068	−0.029	−0.118	−0.076	−0.149	−0.111	−0.153	−0.123	−0.180	−0.143	−0.126	−0.065	0.020	−0.043
WA% generation 2	−0.116	−0.052	−0.143	−0.102	−0.302	−0.304	−0.284	−0.282	−0.302	−0.290	−0.199	−0.171	−0.015	−0.165
WA% generation 3	−0.113	−0.073	−0.146	−0.131	−0.220	−0.200	−0.183	−0.167	−0.216	−0.197	−0.172	−0.140	0.004	−0.127
WA% generation 4	−0.092	−0.073	−0.169	−0.164	−0.325	−0.320	−0.329	−0.321	−0.347	−0.336	−0.189	−0.181	0.079	−0.178
WA% generation 5	−0.112	−0.047	−0.241	−0.213	−0.381	−0.371	−0.371	−0.361	−0.400	−0.383	−0.235	−0.199	−0.045	−0.229
WA% generation 6	−0.120	−0.079	−0.192	−0.173	−0.289	−0.286	−0.266	−0.254	−0.287	−0.279	−0.208	−0.182	−0.100	−0.165
WA% generation 7	0.029	0.067	−0.113	−0.115	−0.238	−0.235	−0.205	−0.205	−0.225	−0.206	−0.061	−0.035	−0.008	−0.121
WA% generation 8	0.011	0.075	−0.076	−0.035	−0.227	−0.235	0.121	−0.120	−0.159	−0.153	−0.084	−0.029	−0.176	−0.061

No statistically significant correlation with the lung function parameters was found between morphometric analysis of the airway parameters on expiration and PFT.

Table 6. Mean WT (mm) and WA% (%) in patients without and with BOS (the standard deviation values are in parentheses).

Generation	WT insp	WT insp BOS	p	WT exsp	WT exsp BOS	p	WA% insp	WA% insp BOS	p	WA% exsp	WA% exsp BOS	p
1	1.86 (0.42)	1.79 (0.39)	0.356	1.8 (0.34)	1.82 (0.46)	0.808	40.03 (8.41)	35.71 (7.08)	0.003	41.23 (8.56)	41.98 (12.04)	0.751
2	1.53 (0.37)	1.62 (0.30)	0.167	1.69 (0.33)	1.67 (0.46)	0.793	40.58 (8.32)	44.32 (9.14)	0.024	47.43 (10.51)	47.67 (11.47)	0.916
3	1.39 (0.39)	1.52 (0.42)	0.056	1.63 (0.37)	1.66 (0.53)	0.756	42.57 (8.78)	45.27 (11.67)	0.182	51.29 (10.65)	52.65 (12.38)	0.529
4	1.25 (0.41)	1.37 (0.44)	0.089	1.51 (0.41)	1.47 (0.54)	0.620	43.64 (8.02)	48.35 (10.32)	0.008	52.85 (11.76)	54 (9.80)	0.627
5	1.11 (0.43)	1.25 (0.49)	0.074	1.36 (0.43)	1.44 (0.48)	0.380	42.83 (8.00)	47.13 (10.53)	0.018	51.84 (11.76)	56.22 (10.94)	0.092
6	0.98 (0.45)	1.04 (0.44)	0.496	1.31 (0.41)	1.3 (0.35)	0.947	40.95 (8.70)	45.34 (12.39)	0.064	53.58 (10.28)	56.76 (9.46)	0.236
7	0.87 (0.31)	1 (0.34)	0.107	1.26 (0.34)	1.21 (0.36)	0.719	39.33 (7.85)	43.96 (7.08)	0.015	56.24 (10.12)	53.91 (8.81)	0.561
8	0.72 (0.22)	0.9 (0.44)	0.122	1.13 (0.31)	0.95 (0.26)	0.261	35.57 (7.25)	42.49 (13.01)	0.063	54.24 (9.12)	49.46 (3.86)	0.313

Significant differences were found for the WA% on inspiration.

Table 7. The mean lumen diameter (LD) in millimeter in patients with and without BOS.

Generation	LD insp	LD insp BOS	LD insp p
1	12.9	12.7	0.799
	(2.82)	(1.97)	
2	10.1	9.9	0.848
	(2.08)	(2.32)	
3	8.8	8.9	0.929
	(2.30)	(2.31)	
4	7.5	7.3	0.719
	(1.98)	(2.53)	
5	6.7	6.2	0.440
	(1.85	(2.51)	
6	6.2	6.5	0.750
	(1.89)	(2.12)	
7	5.8	7.6	0.017
	(1.37)	(1.20)	
8	5.6	6.4	0.265
	(1.15)	(1.60)	

The LD is increased in the peripheral bronchial generations in patients with BOS indicating the development of bronchiectasis. although it failed to demonstrate statistical significance with the exception of 7th generation which we regard as an accidental occurrence (the standard deviation values are in parentheses).

Discussion

In our study, only the WA% on inspiration differed significantly in patients with and without BOS. Therefore, WA% seems to be more suitable for diagnosing BOS than the WT. However, there was a high variability of the measurements due primarily to variable underlying lung volumes which minimize the value of WA% for establishing a diagnosis of BOS based on the imaging findings in individual patients.

CT morphologic parameters and lung function parameters have been found to have statistically significant correlations for a number of airway diseases that differ with respect to the type and anatomic location of their underlying pathology as well as the distribution within the lung. For example, a moderate correlation between the CT airway morphology (WA or LA) and lung function (FEV_1) could be found in patients with COPD [19,20], those with CF [21], and in patients with asthma [22,23].

BOS primarily affects the small airways with diameters<2 mm [1] that cannot be resolved on CT. This raises the question whether bronchial wall measurements of CT data are at all a useful tool for the assessment of BOS. However, previous studies have shown that wall thickening of visually discernible bronchi, i.e. more central bronchial segments, is usually found in patients with BOS [9]. It has also been shown that in patients with COPD the bronchial wall dimensions in relatively large airways, as measured on CT, correlate with those of small airways measured histologically [30]. These reports regarding the meaning of airway CT morphology in other airways diseases [19,21,22] and the fact that bronchial wall thickening is also included as a separate criterion in the CT scoring system for BOS [31] motivated us to perform this study. The goals of our prospective study set-up were: a) to assess bronchial wall dimensions in lung transplant patients without clinical symptoms of BOS; and b) to compare those dimensions with the bronchial wall dimensions of patients with BOS.

In our study we used validated software to detect the WT and the WA% [20]. This software is based on the closed-form solution [19] which is optimized to reduce overestimation of the WT in small airways and is, therefore, specifically suited for lung transplant patients with pathologically small airways. We used the standard reconstruction kernel rather than the sharper lung kernel as it has been shown that this kernel provides more robust measurements [32]. All measurements were carried out automat-

Table 8. The mean lung volumes during inspiration (lung vol insp) and expiration (lung vol exp) and the difference between inspiration and expiration (lung vol diff) in patients with and without BOS.

	without BOS (ml)	with BOS (ml)	p-value
lung vol insp	5302 (1340)	4903 (1013)	0.173
lung vol exp	2495 (832)	3178 (968)	0.001
lung vol diff	2815 (964)	1840 (863)	<0.001

The mean lung volume on expiration (lung vol exp) and the difference between the mean lung volume on inspiration and expiration (lung vol diff) differed significantly (the standard deviation values are in parentheses).

Table 9. Level of significance for univariate analysis of variance for the WT (mm) and WA% on inspiration and expiration and corrected for lung volume comparing patients with and without BOS.

Generation	influence of lung volume				corrected for lung volume			
	WA% insp	WA% exp	WT insp	WT exp	WA% insp	WA% exp	WT insp	WT exp
1	0.096	0.554	0.024	0.057	0.002	0.692	0.527	0.841
2	0.045	0.003	0.498	0.271	0.076	0.415	0.177	0.889
3	<0.001	0.002	0.461	0.463	0.361	0.233	0.052	0.633
4	<0.001	0.113	0.370	0.398	0.007	0.636	0.087	0.469
5	0.001	0.136	0.572	0.172	0.035	0.114	0.076	0.377
6	0.013	<0.001	0.231	0.011	0.100	0.073	0.556	0.609
7	0.026	0.165	0.525	0.206	0.018	0.788	0.102	0.933
8	0.007	0.007	0.916	0.263	0.009	0.478	0.015	0.337

There was a significant influence in the lung volume on the WA% (colums 1–4) and also a significant difference in the WA% on inspiration in patients with and without BOS even if considering the differing lung volumes as cofactor (colums 5–8).

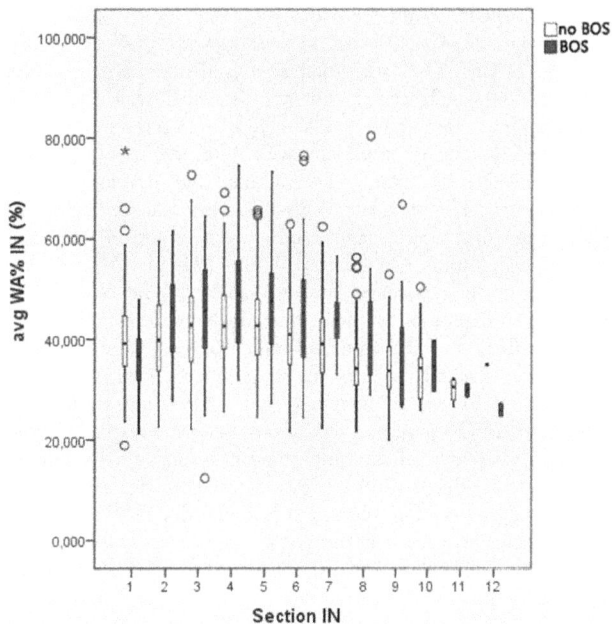

Figure 4. Boxplot showing the average WA% in patients with and without BOS, according to bronchial generations in inspiration. Despite significant differences in the WA% between patients with and those without BOS, there is a substantial overlap in both patient groups.

ically and were thus independent of any user interaction or the CT window settings. Multiple measurements per bronchial generation, in our study at least 10, provided reliable data to also allow for analysis of individual bronchial segments. As there are non-anatomical branching points and smaller branches that might be missed by the program, the measuring points did not necessarily conform to the bronchial generations [19]. To ensure that the measurement locations were identical on inspiration and expiration, all images and measurements were visually checked and "outliers" were eliminated to further increase the accuracy of the quantification.

In our study, there was no correlation of the bronchial wall measurements and the lung function tests performed in lung transplant recipients with and without BOS. The WT on inspiration was slightly higher in patients with BOS than in patients without BOS. This was expected as bronchial wall thickening has been noted in patients with BOS [9], and bronchial wall thickening is used in the CT scoring systems for BOS [31]. However, the difference of the WT on inspiration did not reach statistical significance in those patients with and without BOS. This might be due to the high, dependency of airway measurements on the degree of inspiration, as already shown for the lumen area [33]. This is further supported by the fact that the WT and the WA% were significantly larger on expiration than on inspiration. Regarding the lung volumes that were lower on inspiration and significantly higher on expiration in patients with BOS compared to those without BOS, this might indicate that the influence of the lung volume on measurement of the WT is higher than the presence of BOS. In contrast to the WT, the WA% on inspiration was found to be significantly higher in most bronchial generations in patients with BOS compared to that seen in stable lung transplant patients (Table 5). Therefore, the WA% appears to be a better predictor of BOS than the WT. The WA% is calculated as the ratio of the bronchial wall area and the total area (sum of bronchial wall area and bronchial lumen area). The development of bronchiectasis in patients with BOS leads to a decrease in the WA% (the total area is the denominator and increases in bronchiectasis), whereas bronchial wall thickening results in an increase in the WA% (the wall area is the numerator). As the WA% is higher in patients with BOS, the increase in wall area seems to be more relevant than the development of bronchiectasis. However, the WA% also varied according to the lung volume and showed significantly higher values on expiration than on inspiration. On expiration, the WT increases due to shrinking of the bronchial lumen diameter. The WA% also increases on expiration as the total area (denominator) decreases due to reduction of the bronchial lumen although the wall area (numerator) generally remains the same (the reduced diameter is compensated for by an increased WT). The lung volumes in patients with BOS were non-significantly lower on inspiration and significantly greater on expiration than those in patients without BOS, probably due to obstructive changes. This suggests that the smaller inspiratory lung volumes in patients with BOS contribute to the significant increase of the WA%. This agrees with the study of Zach et al. who showed that the WA% is strongly related to the total lung capacity [34]. In order to be able to eliminate the influence of the lung volume on the difference of the WA% in patients with and those without BOS, we performed a univariate analysis of variance considering the lung volume as a covariate. We could, therefore, confirm the significant influence of the lung volume on the WA%, although we also found significant differences for the WA% on inspiration for the two patient groups after correcting for the influence of the lung volume. These results suggest that the WA% on inspiration is an indicator of both the presence of BOS and the differences in lung volume. However, the inter- and intravariability of the bronchial wall measurements was high in our study. This is not surprising as it is known from pathology studies that BOS shows a very nonuniform anatomic distribution [7]. This makes it necessary to acquire a large number of bronchial wall measurements. Whether bronchial wall measurements alone will be sufficient to diagnose BOS cannot be determined on the basis of our rather small study group. Given the overlap of measurements in patients with and those without BOS, it seems to be more likely at that point that bronchial wall measurements might be a useful adjunct combined with other CT morphologic features such as the presence and amount of air trapping noted on CT. In the future, it will be worthwhile to evaluate whether longitudinal bronchial wall measurements in individuals after lung transplantation are sufficient to document the progression of bronchial wall thickening in patients with

increasing symptoms of BOS and vice versa for those undergoing therapy. Furthermore, it might be interesting to evaluate whether a correcting factor for lung volume can be calculated for bronchial wall measurements as this might help to eliminate the influence of lung volume on measurements. Moreover, it may also be worthwhile to differentiate between patients with the fibrotic and inflammatory phenotypes of BOS.

Our study has a number of limitations. All bronchial wall measurements were performed using one type of software tool. Although the underlying algorithm of this software was thoroughly tested and well-established [19,20], different software tools might yield different results for quantification. Secondly, the number of patients with clinically manifested BOS was much smaller than those without BOS. Also, the number of patients with different severity of BOS stages was too small to allow for a meaningful analysis of the patient subgroups. It is already known that BOS does not occur uniformly or equally affect all bronchi in the lungs. However, in order to provide an objective and standardized method for measurements with high reproducibility we specified the target bronchi prior to the evaluation and did not individually select the target bronchi. In this study we focused on analysis of the bronchial wall measurements and did not include other CT morphological findings such as air trapping. Inclusion of those criteria and the use of airway wall measurements in longitudinal studies will be the foci of future studies.

Conclusion

WA% on inspiration was significantly greater in patients with than in those without BOS. However, WA% measurements were significantly dependent on lung volume and showed a high variability, thus not allowing the sole use of bronchial wall measurements to differentiate patients with from those without BOS.

Acknowledgments

We thank Ms. Mirja Kobbe for her support in post-processing the CT data, Ms. Natalia Flach for providing pulmonary function data, and Bonnie Hami, MA, for assisting with the manuscript editing.

Author Contributions

Conceived and designed the experiments: SD HOS. Performed the experiments: SD LP CdW. Analyzed the data: SD JG HOS CSP. Contributed reagents/materials/analysis tools: MS. Wrote the paper: SD FW GW CSP.

References

1. Al-Githmi I, Batawil N, Shigemura N, Hsin M, Lee TW, et al. (2006) Bronchiolitis obliterans following lung transplantation. Eur J Cardiothorac Surg 30: 846-51.
2. Boehler A, Kesten S, Weder W, Speich R (1998) Bronchiolitis obliterans after lung transplantation: a review. Chest 114: 1411-26.
3. Arcasoy SM, Kotloff RM (1999) Lung transplantation. N Engl J Med 340: 1081-91.
4. Todd JL, Palmer SM (2011) Bronchiolitis obliterans syndrome. Chest 140: 502-8.
5. Cooper JD, Billingham M, Egan T, Hertz MI, Higenbottam T, et al. (1993) A working formulation for the standardization of nomenclature for clinical staging of chronic dysfunction in lung allografts: International Society for Heart and Lung Transplantation. J Heart Lung Transplant 12: 713-6.
6. Estenne M, Maurer JR, Boehler A, Egan JJ, Frost A, et al. (2002) Bronchiolitis obliterans syndrome 2001: an update of the diagnostic criteria. J Heart Lung Transplant 21: 297-310.
7. Chamberlain D, Maurer J, Chaparro C, Idolor L (1994) Evaluation of transbronchial lung biopsy specimens in the diagnosis of bronchiolitis obliterans after lung transplantation. J Heart Lung Transplant 13: 963-71.
8. Bankier AA, Van Muylem A, Knoop C, Estenne M, Gevenois PA (2001) Bronchiolitis obliterans syndrome in heart-lung transplant recipients: diagnosis with expiratory CT. Radiology 218: 533-9.
9. Morrish WF, Herman SJ, Weisbrod GL, Chamberlain DW (1991) Bronchiolitis obliterans after lung transplantation: findings at chest radiography and high-resolution CT. The Toronto Lung Transplant Group. Radiology 179: 487-90.
10. Konen E, Gutierrez C, Chaparro C, Murray CP, Chung T, et al. (2003) Bronchiolitis obliterans syndrome in lung transplant recipients: can thin-section CT findings predict disease before its clinical appearance? Radiology 231: 467-73.
11. Ng YL, Paul N, Patsios D, Walsham A, Chung TB, et al. (2009) Imaging of lung transplantation: review. AJR Am J Roentgenol 192: S1-13.
12. Miller WT Jr, Kotloff RM, Blumenthal NP, Aronchick JM, Gefter WB, et al. (2001) Utility of high resolution computed tomography in predicting bronchiolitis obliterans syndrome following lung transplantation: preliminary findings. J Thorac Imaging Apr;16(2): 76-80.
13. Berstad AE, Aaløkken TM, Kolbenstvedt A, Bjørtuft O (2006) Performance of long-term CT monitoring in diagnosing bronchiolitis obliterans after lung transplantation. Eur J Radiol 58: 124-31.

14. Coxson HO (2008) Quantitative computed tomography assessement of airway wall dimensions: current status and potential applications for phenotyping chronic obstructive pulmonary disease. Proc Am Thorac Soc. 15;5(9): 940–5.

15. Brillet PY, Fetita CI, Beigelman-Aubry C, Saragaglia A, Perchet D, et al. (2007) Quantification of bronchial dimensions at MDCT using dedicated software. Eur Radiol 17(6): 1483–9.

16. Nakano Y, Muller NL, King GG, Niimi A, Kalloger SE, et al. (2002) Quantitative assessment of airway remodeling using high-resolution CT. Chest 122: 271S–5S.

17. Nakano Y, Whittall KP, Kalloger SE, Coxson HO, Flint J, et al. (2002) Development and validation of human airway analysis algorithm using multidetector row CT. Proc SPIE 4683: 460–469.

18. Reinhardt JM, D'Souza ND, Hoffman EA (1997) Accurate measurement of intrathoracic airways. IEEE Trans Med Imaging 16: 820–7.

19. Weinheimer O, Achenbach T, Bletz C, Duber C, Kauczor HU, et al. (2008) About objective 3-d analysis of airway geometry in computerized tomography. IEEE Trans Med Imaging 27: 64–74.

20. Schmidt M, Kuhnigk JM, Krass S, Owsijewitsch M, de Hoop B, et al. (2010) Reproducibility of airway wall thickness measurements. PROC SPIE doi:10.1117/12.844453.

21. Achenbach T, Weinheimer O, Biedermann A, Schmitt S, Freudenstein D, et al. (2008) MDCT assessment of airway wall thickness in COPD patients using a new method: correlations with pulmonary function tests. Eur Radiol 18: 2731–8.

22. Hasegawa M, Nasuhara Y, Onodera Y, Makita H, Nagai K, et al. (2006) Airflow limitation and airway dimensions in chronic obstructive pulmonary disease. Am J Respir Crit Care Med 173(12): 1309–15.

23. Montaudon M, Berger P, Cangini-Sacher A, de Dietrich G, Tunon-de-Lara JM, et al. (2007) Bronchial measurement with three-dimensional quantitative thin-section CT in patients with cystic fibrosis. Radiology 242: 573–81.

24. Montaudon M, Lederlin M, Reich S, Bequeret H, Tunon-de-Lara JM, et al. (2009) Bronchial measurements in patients with asthma: comparison of quantitative thin-section CT findings with those in healthy subjects and correlation with pathologic findings. Radiology 253: 844–53.

25. Chae EJ, Kim TB, Cho YS, Park CS, Seo JB, et al. (2011) Airway Measurement for Airway Remodeling Defined by Post-Bronchodilator FEV1/FVC in Asthma: Investigation Using Inspiration-Expiration Computed Tomography. Allergy Asthma Immunol Res 3: 111–7.

26. Gottlieb J, Szangolies J, Koehnlein T, Golpon H, Simon A, et al. (2008) Long-term azithromycin for bronchiolitis obliterans syndrome after lung transplantation. Transplantation 15;85(1): 36–41.

27. Quanjer PH, Tammeling GJ, Cotes JE, Pedersen OF, Peslin R, et al. (1993) Lung volumes and forced ventilatory flows. Report Working Party Standardization of Lung Function Tests, European Community for Steel and Coal. Official Statement of the European Respiratory Society. Eur Respir J 16: 5–40.

28. Miller MR, Hankinson J, Brusasco V, Burgos F, Casaburi R, et al. (2005) Standardization of spirometry. Eur Respir J 26: 319.

29. Kuhnigk JM, Dicken V, Zidowitz S, Bornemann L, Kuemmerlen B, et al. (2005) New Tools for Computer Assistance in Thoracic CT - Part I: Functional analysis of lungs, lung lobes, and bronchopulmonary segments. RadioGraphics 25: 525–536.

30. Nakano Y, Wong JC, de Jong PA, Buzatu L, Nagao T, et al. (2005) The prediction of small airway dimensions using computed tomography. Am J Respir Crit Care Med 15;171: 142–6.

31. de Jong PA, Dodd JD, Coxson HO, Storness-Bliss C, Paré PD, et al. (2006) Bronchiolitis obliterans following lung transplantation: early detection using computed tomographic scanning. Thorax 61: 799–804.

32. Kim N, Seo JB, Song KS, Chae EJ, Kang SH (2008) Semi-automatic measurement of the airway dimension by computed tomography using the full-width-half-maximum method: a study on the measurement accuracy according to the CT parameters and size of the airway. Korean J Radiol 9: 226–35.

33. Bakker ME, Stolk J, Reiber JH, Stoel BC (2012) Influence of inspiration level on bronchial lumen measurements with computed tomography. Respir Med 106(5): 677–86.

34. Zach JA, Newell JD Jr, Schroeder J, Murphy JR, Curran-Everett D, et al on behalf of the COPDGene Investigators (2012) Quantitative Computed Tomography of the Lungs and Airways in Healthy Nonsmoking Adults. Invest Radiol 47: 596–602.

19

Mononuclear Phagocytes and Airway Epithelial Cells: Novel Sources of Matrix Metalloproteinase-8 (MMP-8) in Patients with Idiopathic Pulmonary Fibrosis

Vanessa J. Craig[1], Francesca Polverino[1,2,3], Maria E. Laucho-Contreras[1], Yuanyuan Shi[1,3], Yushi Liu[1,3], Juan C. Osorio[1], Yohannes Tesfaigzi[4], Victor Pinto-Plata[1], Bernadette R. Gochuico[5], Ivan O. Rosas[1,3], Caroline A. Owen[1,3,4]*

1 Division of Pulmonary and Critical Care Medicine, Brigham and Women's Hospital, Harvard Medical School, Boston, Massachusetts, United States of America, 2 Department of Clinical and Experimental Medicine, University of Parma, Parma, Italy, 3 Pulmonary Fibrosis Program, Lovelace Respiratory Research Institute, Albuquerque, New Mexico, United States of America, 4 Chronic Obstructive Pulmonary Disease Program, Lovelace Respiratory Research Institute, Albuquerque, New Mexico, United States of America, 5 Medical Genetics Branch, National Human Genome Research Institute, National Institutes of Health, Bethesda, Maryland, United States of America

Abstract

Objectives: Matrix metalloproteinase-8 (MMP-8) promotes lung fibrotic responses to bleomycin in mice. Although prior studies reported that MMP-8 levels are increased in plasma and bronchoalveolar lavage fluid (BALF) samples from IPF patients, neither the bioactive forms nor the cellular sources of MMP-8 in idiopathic pulmonary fibrosis (IPF) patients have been identified. It is not known whether MMP-8 expression is dys-regulated in IPF leukocytes or whether MMP-8 plasma levels correlate with IPF outcomes. Our goal was to address these knowledge gaps.

Methods: We measured MMP-8 levels and forms in blood and lung samples from IPF patients versus controls using ELISAs, western blotting, and qPCR, and assessed whether MMP-8 plasma levels in 73 IPF patients correlate with rate of lung function decline and mortality. We used immunostaining to localize MMP-8 expression in IPF lungs. We quantified MMP-8 levels and forms in blood leukocytes from IPF patients versus controls.

Results: IPF patients have increased BALF, whole lung, and plasma levels of soluble MMP-8 protein. Active MMP-8 is the main form elevated in IPF lungs. MMP-8 mRNA levels are increased in monocytes from IPF patients, but IPF patients and controls have similar levels of MMP-8 in PMNs. Surprisingly, macrophages and airway epithelial cells are the main cells expressing MMP-8 in IPF lungs. Plasma and BALF MMP-8 levels do not correlate with decline in lung function and/or mortality in IPF patients.

Conclusion: Blood and lung MMP-8 levels are increased in IPF patients. Active MMP-8 is the main form elevated in IPF lungs. Surprisingly, blood monocytes, lung macrophages, and airway epithelial cells are the main cells in which MMP-8 is upregulated in IPF patients. Plasma and BALF MMP-8 levels are unlikely to serve as a prognostic biomarker for IPF patients. These results provide new information about the expression patterns of MMP-8 in IPF patients.

Editor: Ana Mora, University of Pittsburgh, United States of America

Funding: This work was supported by the Public Health Service, National Heart, Lung, and Blood Institute Grants HL63137, HL086814, HL111835, NIH 2T32 HL007633-26, NIH 5T32 HD007466-15 (www.grants.gov); the American Thoracic Society/Pulmonary Fibrosis Foundation (www.thoracic.org); and the Brigham and Women's Hospital-Lovelace Respiratory Research Institute Consortium (http://brighamandwomens.org and http://www.lrri.org). This work was supported, in part, by the Intramural Research Program of the National Human Genome Research Institute, National Institutes of Health. The funders had no role in study design, data collection and analysis, decision to publish, or preparation of the manuscript.

Competing Interests: The authors have declared that no competing interests exist.

* E-mail: cowen@rics.bwh.harvard.edu

Introduction

IPF is associated with high morbidity and mortality [1] and its incidence is increasing [2,3]. No therapies have been shown to reduce mortality in IPF patients [4–6]. IPF is thought to be caused by an initial (as-yet unidentified) alveolar epithelial injury which is followed by an aberrant wound healing response in the lung [7,8], but the pathways that contribute to this response are not fully understood. An improved understanding of the mechanisms involved in the pathogenesis of IPF may facilitate the development of more efficacious therapeutic approaches for this disease.

One molecule that has recently been linked to fibrotic lung diseases is matrix metalloproteinase-8 (MMP-8 or neutrophil collagenase). MMP-8 degrades type I collagen (the major collagen deposited in IPF lungs) in vitro [9]. However, recent studies have shown that MMP-8 promotes (rather than inhibits) lung fibrosis in bleomycin-treated mice, and this is linked to MMP-8's activities in reducing lung levels of macrophage inflammatory protein 1α

(MIP-1α) and interferon-inducible protein-10 (IP-10) which is an anti-fibrotic cytokine [10–12].

MMP-8 is most highly expressed by neutrophils [13]. However, macrophages stimulated ex vivo with CD40 ligand [14] and activated fibroblasts [10,15,16] also express MMP-8 albeit at lower levels than neutrophils. All MMP-8-expressing cells release a soluble form of MMP-8 as a latent (pro)-proteinase which is then activated in the extracellular space. Activated neutrophils also express another form of MMP-8 on their surface in an inducible fashion [12,17]. Membrane-bound MMP-8 on PMNs is catalytically active but resistant to inhibition by tissue inhibitors of metalloproteinases and could be the key form mediating its activities in vivo [12,17]. However, membrane-bound MMP-8 on PMNs has not been studied in any human disease.

A small number of prior studies have linked MMP-8 to human IPF. One study reported that MMP-8 plasma levels are elevated in IPF patients [18], but this study did not assess whether plasma MMP-8 levels correlate with clinical outcomes or parameters in IPF patients. One study reported that MMP-8 expression was not increased in IPF whole lung samples [19]. Several other studies showed that IPF patients have elevated levels of soluble MMP-8 in bronchoalveolar lavage fluid (BALF) [18,20–22]. One of these studies showed, in a small cohort of IPF subjects, that elevated MMP-8 BALF levels are associated with rapidly declining lung function [21].

Knowledge gaps in the area of MMP-8 and IPF include: 1) which cells in the lung contribute to the elevated BALF MMP-8 levels in IPF patients; 2) whether MMP-8 levels in blood myeloid leukocytes are dysregulated in IPF patients; 3) which is the key form of the proteinase (soluble vs. membrane bound and active vs. latent MMP-8) present in IPF blood and lung samples; and 4) whether substrates that we have identified for MMP-8 in the fibrotic murine lung are also potential substrates for MMP-8 in human IPF lungs. To address these knowledge gaps, we performed a comprehensive analysis of MMP-8 levels and forms in both blood and lung samples from IPF patients versus control subjects. We measured levels of substrates that we have identified for MMP-8 in the fibrotic murine lung (MIP-1α and IP-10) in IPF lung samples to begin to assess whether they might be substrates for MMP-8 in IPF lungs. We also assessed whether plasma MMP-8 levels can serve as a prognostic biomarker for IPF.

Based upon current knowledge of MMP-8 expression patterns, we hypothesized that MMP-8 is mainly expressed by neutrophils and fibroblasts in IPF lungs. As there is evidence that blood neutrophils are activated and undergo degranulation in IPF patients [23], we also hypothesized that MMP-8 levels would be lower in extracts of blood neutrophils and/or higher on the surface of blood neutrophils from IPF patients compared with controls. However, we report for the first time that lung macrophages and airway epithelial cells are the key sources of MMP-8 in IPF lungs. Although we confirmed that plasma MMP-8 levels are increased in IPF patients, surprisingly, MMP-8 levels are not altered in neutrophils from IPF patients. Rather, IPF patients have increased expression of MMP-8 in blood monocytes. Thus, we provide new information about expression and activation patterns of MMP-8 in IPF lung samples which may guide future biomarker studies, and possibly the testing of novel therapeutics targeting MMP-8 for IPF.

Materials and Methods

Human subjects

All research involving human participants was approved by the authors' institutional review board [The Partners Health Care Institutional Review Board (IRB) under protocols #2011P002419

and 2002P000253]. All study subjects signed written informed consent forms that were approved by our IRB. All clinical investigations were conducted according to the principles expressed in the Declaration of Helsinki.

Blood or BALF samples were obtained from healthy volunteers (n = 25 or 12, respectively) and IPF patients (n = 73 or 32, respectively) enrolled in the Brigham and Women's Hospital Interstitial Lung Disease Registry or who signed informed consent and were enrolled in NIH protocols (99-HG-0056 and 04-HG-0211). The diagnosis of IPF was made using ATS/ERS consensus diagnostic criteria [24]. Forced vital capacity (FVC) and diffusing capacity of the lung for carbon monoxide (DLCO)] were recorded on IPF patients for clinical indications. Explanted lung samples from IPF patients undergoing lung transplantation and controls (rejected donor lung transplant tissue) were randomly selected from our IPF bio-repository.

MMP-8, MIP-1α, and IP-10 levels

MMP-8 was quantified in blood and lung samples using an ELISA (R&D Systems, Minneapolis, MN). MMP-8 levels in homogenates of lung samples were corrected for GAPDH levels which were measured in arbitrary units using a commercial kit (eBioscience, San Diego, CA). MMP-8 results were expressed as pg of MMP-8 per arbitrary unit of GAPDH. MIP-1α and IP-10 were quantified in BALF samples using ELISAs (PeproTech, Rocky Hill, NJ). MMP-8 forms were analyzed in BALF (50 microliters/sample) and lung lysates (100 micrograms of protein/sample) using western blotting [12,17] and a polyclonal rabbit anti-human MMP-8 IgG [ab38994; raised against the hinge region of MMP-8 (Abcam, Cambridge, MA)] and quantified using ImageJ software [25].

Leukocyte studies

Neutrophils and monocytes were isolated from blood using density gradient centrifugation [26] and positive selection for CD14 using immuno-magnetic beads (Miltenyi Biotec, San Diego, CA), respectively. Cells were lysed in radio-immunoprecipitation assay (RIPA) buffer containing protease inhibitors (at 5×10^6 cells/ml), and frozen at $-80°C$. Intact neutrophils were immunostained for surface MMP-8 using Alexa 488 and rabbit anti-MMP-8 IgG (ab38994, Abcam) or non-immune rabbit IgG as a control (Dako, Carpinteria, CA) [12,17] and staining quantified using a FACS Canto II flow cytometer (BD, Franklin Lakes, NJ).

Real-time RT-PCR

Real-time RT-PCR was performed on RNA isolated from blood leukocytes and lungs using a MMP-8 gene expression assay (Invitrogen, Eugene, OR), and the comparative cycle threshold method with 18S as an endogenous reference gene [10].

Immunoperoxidase staining

Formalin-fixed lung sections from IPF patients and control subjects were deparaffinized. Antigen retrieval was performed by boiling the sections in 10 mM citrate buffer (pH 6.0) in a microwave for 10 min. Slides were incubated in blocking buffer [1% (w/v) BSA and 10% (v/v) goat serum in Tris buffered saline (TBS; 0.05M Tris containing 0.15 M NaCl and 0.02 M CaCl₂] for 2 h at room temperature. Slides were then incubated with either rabbit anti-MMP-8 IgG or non-immune rabbit IgG for 18 h at 4°C and washed twice in TBS. Slides were incubated in 3% hydrogen peroxide solution for 20 min, washed, incubated again with hydrogen peroxide solution, washed, and incubated for 1 h at room temperature with goat anti-rabbit IgG conjugated to horseradish peroxidase (Bio-Rad, Berkeley, California). Slides were washed, incubated in avidin-biotin complex for 1 h at room temperature, washed again, and developed using 3,3'-diamino-benzidine. Slides were then counterstained with 1% (wt/vol) methyl green solution, dehydrated, and mounted.

Immunofluorescence staining to localize MMP-8 in lung sections

Formalin-fixed lung sections from IPF patients and controls were deparaffinized, and antigen retrieval was performed by heating the slides in a microwave in citrate buffer, as outlined above. The sections were incubated overnight at 4°C with rabbit IgG to human MMP-8 (or non-immune rabbit IgG) and Alexa 546-conjugated goat anti-rabbit F(ab)$_2$. Sections were then washed in PBS and incubated at 37°C for 2 h with either murine anti-CD68 IgG (Dako, Carpinteria, CA), murine anti-vimentin IgG (Abcam), murine anti-surfactant protein C IgG (SP-C, Santa Cruz Biotechnology, Santa Cruz, CA.), murine anti-pancytokeratin IgG (Sigma-Aldrich, St. Louis, MO), or non-immune murine IgG [27]. After washing the lung sections in PBS, Alexa 488-conjugated goat anti-murine F(ab)$_2$ was applied and slides were incubated for additional 1 h at 37°C. Nuclei were then counterstained with 4',6-diamidino-2-phenylindole (DAPI).

Immunostaining to detect apoptosis of alveolar type II epithelial cells in lung sections

To detect the alveolar epithelial type II (ATII) cells undergoing apoptosis, we performed double immunofluorescence staining of lung sections for active (cleaved) caspase-3 and a marker of ATII cells (surfactant protein C; SP-C). Formalin-fixed lung sections from IPF patients and controls were deparaffinized, and antigen retrieval was performed by heating the slides in a microwave in citrate buffer. The sections were incubated overnight at 4°C with murine anti-active caspase-3 IgG (Abcam, Cambridge, MA), or non-immune murine IgG (Sigma-Aldrich, St. Louis MO) followed by Alexa 488-conjugated goat anti-murine F(ab)$_2$. Slides were washed in PBS and incubated with goat anti-SP-C IgG (Santa Cruz Biotechnology, Santa Cruz, CA.) or non-immune goat IgG (Sigma-Aldrich, St. Louis, MO) followed Alexa 546-conjugated rabbit anti-goat F(ab)$_2$. Nuclei were counterstained with DAPI.

Statistics

The results for paired and unpaired data were compared using the Student's t-test for parametric data and the Mann-Whitney rank sum test for non-parametric data; P values less than 0.05 were considered significant. To study associations between MMP-8 plasma levels and FVC or DLCO and, results from patients with ≥2 clinic visits were analyzed and FVC and DLCO results from the second and third visits were expressed as a % of baseline values. Linear regression was performed for each patient and the slope was used to calculate the annual percent change in relative and absolute FVC and DLCO, and Spearman Rank Correlation Coefficients for non-parametric data were calculated. The Cox proportional-hazards regression model was used to determine whether there is a relationship between plasma MMP-8 levels and survival in IPF patients.

Results

MMP-8 levels in IPF lungs

Soluble MMP-8 protein levels are ~5-fold higher in BALF from IPF patients compared with healthy volunteers (Fig. 1A and Table S1 for demographic data on the subjects). Two main forms of MMP-8 are detected in BALF using Western blotting (Fig. 1B): 1) active MMP-8 (M_r~60 kDa) which is the most abundant form; and 2) a ~40 kDa form which likely is a proteolytically processed and inactive form of MMP-8 (containing its hinge region and the hemopexin MMP-8 domains) which we have detected in BALF from mice with acute lung injury [12]. Both forms are increased in IPF BALF (Figs. 1C and 1D). Latent pro-MMP-8 (M_r~80 kDa) is not detected or present at only low levels in BALF samples from IPF cases and controls. MMP-8 protein levels are also strikingly increased in homogenates of lung samples from IPF patients (Fig. 2A), but whole lung MMP-8 steady-state mRNA levels are similar in IPF patients and control subjects (Fig. 2B).

MMP-8 localization in IPF lungs

Based upon current knowledge of MMP-8 expression patterns, we hypothesized that MMP-8 is mainly expressed by PMNs and fibroblasts in IPF lungs. To test this hypothesis, we first performed immunoperoxidase staining of lung sections for MMP-8. There is robust staining for MMP-8 in bronchial epithelial cells in areas of moderately severe and severe fibrosis in IPF lungs. However, there is minimal or no staining for MMP-8 in areas of mild fibrosis in IPF lung and in rejected normal lung transplant donor lungs (Fig. 3A). In addition, positive staining for MMP-8 is present in cells in fibrotic lung tissue but not in control lung tissue (Fig. 3B), and no staining in IPF lung stained with a non-immune control primary antibody (Fig. 3A, right panel).

To confirm these results and identify the cell types in which MMP-8 is regulated in IPF lungs, we double immuno-stained lung sections from explanted IPF lungs and rejected normal lung transplant donor lungs using a green fluorophore for MMP-8 and a red fluorophore for markers of epithelial cells, macrophages, neutrophils, or fibroblasts. Macrophages are strongly stained for MMP-8 in all areas of the lung including areas of mild and severe fibrosis in IPF lung tissue (Fig. 4 upper panel). However, macrophages are not stained for MMP-8 in control lung samples (Fig. 4 lower panel). Bronchial epithelial cells in IPF lung tissue (Fig. 4, upper panel) are positively stained for MMP-8 mainly in areas of severe lung fibrosis (Fig. 4 upper panel). However, in control lung tissue, bronchial epithelial cells stain only weakly for MMP-8 (Fig. 4, lower panel). The few neutrophils present in IPF lungs stain strongly for MMP-8 (Fig. 4 upper panel). Fibroblasts (Fig. 5, upper panel) and fibrobastic foci (not shown) in IPF lung are not stained for MMP-8. Type II alveolar epithelial (ATII) cells stain strongly for MMP-8 in control lung tissue (Fig. 5, lower panel) but there is minimal or no staining for MMP-8 in these cells in areas of moderately severe and severe fibrosis in IPF lungs (Fig. 5). Staining for MMP-8 in ATII cells in areas of mild fibrosis in IPF lung is similar to that in normal lungs (data not shown). There is no staining in lung sections from IPF patients (Fig. 5) or control subjects (data not shown) incubated with isotype-matched non-immune control antibodies, confirming that our staining for MMP-8 and markers of different cell types is specific.

To determine whether the reduced MMP-8 staining in ATII cells in IPF lungs is linked to increased rates of ATII cell apoptosis which has been reported in IPF lungs [28,29], we double immunostained IPF versus normal lungs for a marker of apoptosis (active caspase-3) and a marker of ATII cells (surfactant protein C; SP-C). Positive immunostaining for active caspase-3 is present in areas of moderately severe and severe fibrosis in IPF lung parenchyma but not in normal lung parenchyma (Fig. 6). However, the apoptotic cells in IPF lung parenchyma are not ATII cells as there is minimal or no co-localization of the staining for active caspase-3 and SP-C.

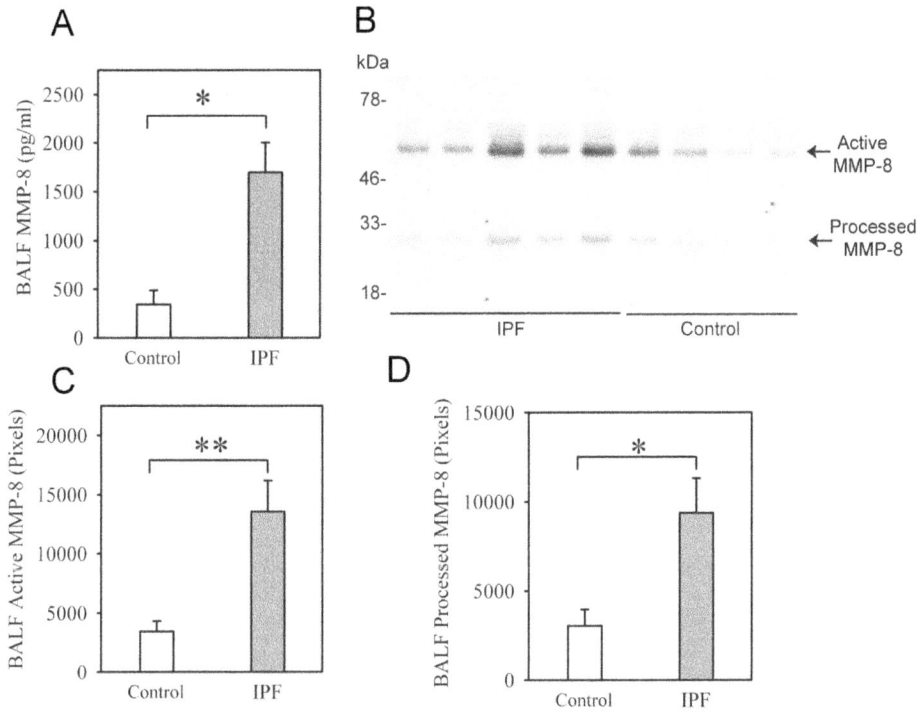

Figure 1. MMP-8 protein levels are increased in IPF BALF samples. In **A**, BAL was performed on IPF patients (n = 32) and healthy volunteers (n = 7), and MMP-8 protein levels were quantified in BAL fluid (BALF) samples using an ELISA. Data are mean + SEM; * indicates p = 0.003. In **B**, we analyzed BALF samples from both groups using Western blotting, and detected both active MMP-8 protein (~60 kDa) and processed MMP-8 (~40 kDa) forms in BALF from IPF patients and healthy volunteers. **B** shows a representative blot of BALF samples from 5 IPF patients and 4 control subjects. In **C–D**, densitometry was used to quantify levels of active MMP-8 (in **C**) and processed MMP-8 (in **D**) in BALF samples. In **C** and **D**, data are mean + SEM; n = 9 control samples and n = 9 IPF samples; asterisk indicates p = 0.022 and ** p = 0.002.

MMP-8 levels in plasma samples

Plasma MMP-8 protein levels are >3–fold higher in IPF patients when compared with levels in healthy volunteers (Fig. 7). Table 1 shows the demographic data on these subjects.

MMP-8 levels in blood neutrophils

As there is evidence that blood neutrophils are activated in IPF patients [23], we hypothesized that MMP-8 protein levels are

lower in extracts of blood neutrophils but higher on the surface of blood neutrophils from IPF patients compared with levels in control subjects. However, we show that MMP-8 protein levels are similar in blood neutrophil extracts from IPF patients and control subjects (Fig. 8A). The percentage of neutrophils that stain positively for surface MMP-8 (which increases when neutrophils are activated [12,17]) is also similar in IPF patients and controls (17.8± SEM 5.6%; n = 32 versus 3.4±1.9%; n = 5, respectively;

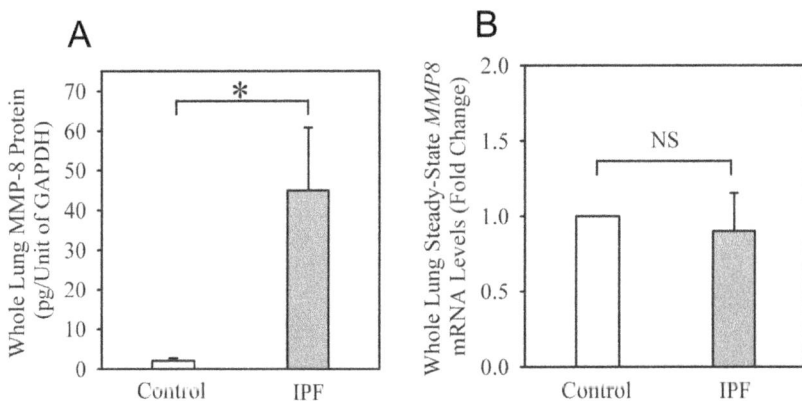

Figure 2. MMP-8 protein levels are increased in IPF whole lung samples. Lung tissue was removed from explanted lungs from IPF patients during lung transplantation (n = 5) or unused transplant donor lungs (control; n = 5). In **A**, MMP-8 protein levels were measured in homogenates of lung samples using an ELISA. Results for MMP-8 were normalized to GAPDH levels (expressed as pg of MMP-8 per arbitrary unit of GAPDH). Data are mean + SEM. Asterisk indicates p<0.03. In **B**, MMP-8 steady-state mRNA levels were measured in RNA isolated from whole lung samples. Data are fold change + SEM; n = 5 control subjects and 4 IPF patients.

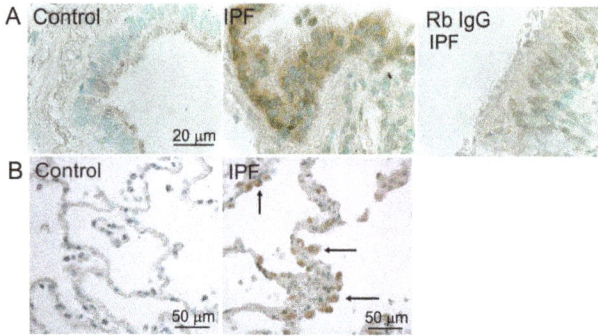

Figure 3. Immunostaining for MMP-8 is increased in IPF lungs.
Lung tissue was obtained from IPF patients undergoing lung transplantation and unused transplant donor lungs (control). Immunoperoxidase staining for MMP-8 was performed on formalin-fixed IPF and control lung sections. In **A**, there is positive (brown) staining for MMP-8 in bronchial epithelial cells in an area of severe fibrosis in the IPF lung but not in bronchial epithelial cells in the control lung section. **B** shows positive (brown) staining for MMP-8 in cells in fibrotic parenchyma in IPF lungs (indicated by the arrows) but not in control lung parenchyma. Lung sections stained with a non-immune rabbit IgG control primary antibody (Rb IgG) showed minimal staining. These results are representative of 3 different lung sections per group. Magnification is X 400.

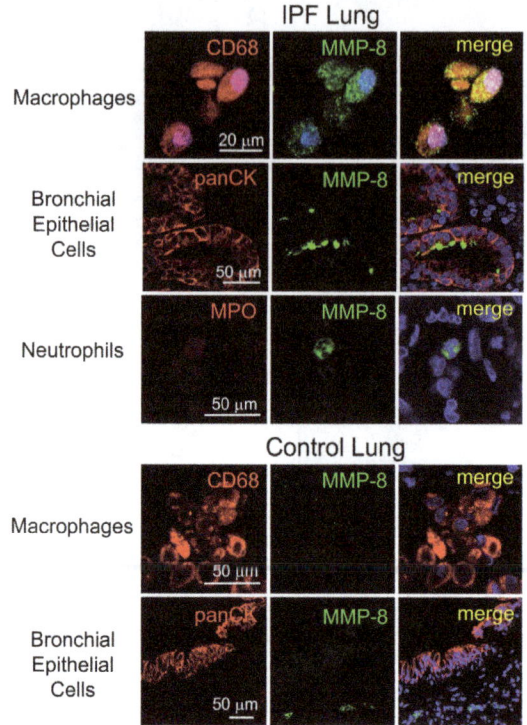

Figure 4. MMP-8 expression is increased in macrophages and bronchial epithelial cells in IPF lungs. Double immunofluorescence staining of an IPF lung section (upper panels) and a control lung section (lower panels) was performed using a red fluorophore (left column) for macrophages (CD68), airway epithelial cells (pancytokeratin; PanCK), or neutrophils (myeloperoxidase; MPO) and with a green fluorophore for MMP-8 (middle column). Lung sections were also stained with isotype-matched non-immune murine and rabbit IgG control antibodies (see Fig. 5). Nuclei were stained with 4',6-diamidino-2-phenylindole (DAPI), and lung sections were examined using a confocal microscope. Merged images (right column) show co-localization of staining for MMP-8 and CD68 and also for MMP-8 and PanCK in the bronchial epithelium of an area of severe fibrosis in the IPF lung (upper panels). The control lung section (lower panels) shows no staining for MMP-8 in macrophages and minimal staining for MMP-8 (middle column) in bronchial epithelial cells. Images are representative of immuno-stained lung sections from 2 controls and 3 patients with IPF. Magnification is X 600 in both panels.

p = 0.79). MMP-8 is not thought to be regulated at the steady state mRNA level in blood PMNs. However, we detected MMP-8 transcripts in PMNs from healthy donors using qRT-RT-PCR. IPF patients and controls have similar low levels of MMP-8 mRNA transcripts in blood neutrophils (Fig. 8B).

MMP-8 levels in blood monocytes

In healthy donors, blood monocyte extracts contain less MMP-8 ($\sim$1 ng/5 million cells) than neutrophil extracts ($\sim$1000 ng/5 million cells) as expected (Figs. 8C and 8A, respectively). MMP-8 protein levels are similar in blood monocyte extracts from IPF patients and control subjects (Fig. 8C). In blood monocytes, MMP-8 mRNA levels are very low or not detectable in normal volunteers (cycle threshold $[C_T]$ >60 cycles for 7 out of 9 healthy volunteers and $\geq$25.3 in 2 healthy volunteers) whereas the C_T for the IPF patients ranges from 5.16 to 22.11. Thus, it is not possible to calculate fold change in monocyte MMP-8 steady state mRNA levels for IPF patents versus healthy subjects using the $\Delta\Delta C_T$ method. Instead, we report MMP-8 steady state mRNA levels using the ΔC_T method for IPF patients versus controls (C_T for MMP-8 - C_T for 18 S as the housekeeping gene). The lower ΔC_T for IPF patients indicates higher MMP-8 mRNA levels in monocytes from IPF patients compared with control subjects (Fig. 8D). We used publicly-available microarray gene expression databases to compare MMP-8 expression in peripheral blood mononuclear cells (PBMCs) from COPD versus healthy control subjects [30] and sarcoidosis patients versus healthy control subjects [31]. Our analysis shows that MMP-8 transcripts are not detected in COPD PBMCs and MMP-8 expression is not significantly increased in PBMCs from patients with sarcoidosis (Table S2).

BALF MIP-1α and IP-10 levels

MMP-8 reduces lung levels of MIP-1α and IP-10 in bleomycin-treated mice to promote pulmonary fibrosis [10–12]. However, BALF levels of MIP-1α and IP-10 are not significantly different in IPF patients and control subjects, and there are trends towards higher (rather than lower) levels of both mediators in IPF patients (Table S3). Among the IPF patients, BALF MMP-8 levels do not correlate significantly with BALF levels of either MIP-1α or IP-10 (Spearman Rank Correlation Coefficients = 0.07 [p = 0.84] and 0.31 [p = 0.29], respectively).

MMP-8 levels in plasma, BALF, and PBMCs and clinical outcomes

MMP-8 plasma levels do not significantly correlate with the annual absolute rate of decline in FVC (Fig. 9A) or DLCO (Fig. 9B) expressed as a percentage of the patients' baseline FVC or DLCO, or absolute FVC and DLCO (data not shown). In addition, plasma MMP-8 levels do not correlate with initial FVC or DLCO at presentation (data not shown). Plasma MMP-8 levels in 66 IPF patients also do not correlate with mortality as assessed using the Cox proportional-hazards model analysis (data not shown).

MMP-8 protein levels in BALF from IPF patients (n = 32) do not correlate with annual absolute rate of decline in FVC or DLCO (data not shown). An analysis of a publicly-available PBMC microarray gene expression dataset on IPF patients [32]

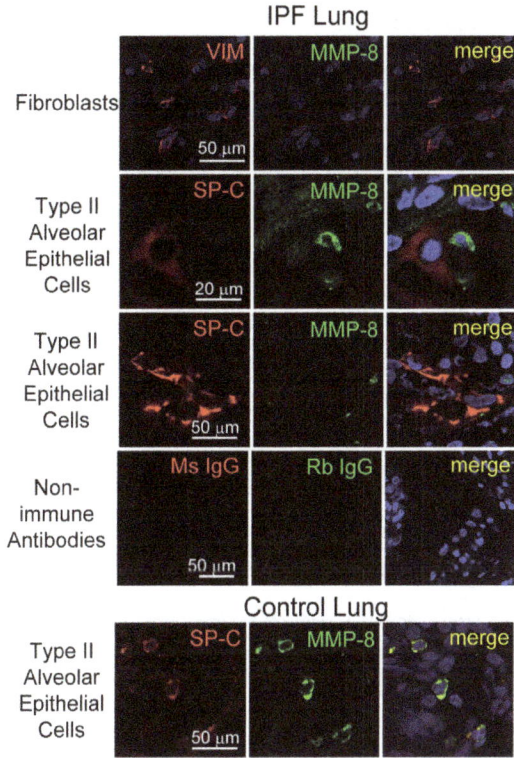

Figure 5. MMP-8 is not expressed in type II alveolar epithelial cells or fibroblasts in IPF lungs. Lung tissue was obtained from IPF patients undergoing lung transplantation (upper panel) or from rejected transplant donor lungs as a control (lower panel). Formalin-fixed lung sections were stained with a red fluorophore (left column) for fibroblasts (vimentin; VIM) or type II alveolar epithelial cells (surfactant protein, SPC) and a green fluorophore for MMP-8 (middle column). Other lung sections were stained with isotype-matched non-immune murine IgG (Ms IgG) or rabbit IgG (Rb IgG). Nuclei were stained with DAPI and lung sections examined using a confocal microscope. Merged images (right column) show no staining for MMP-8 in cells identified as fibroblasts or type II alveolar epithelial (ATII) cells in an area of severe fibrosis in the IPF lung. Control lung sections show positive staining for MMP-8 in type II alveolar epithelial cells (lower panels). Magnification is X 600.

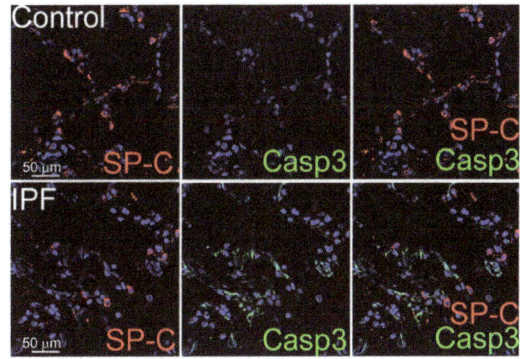

Figure 6. The lack of MMP-8 staining in type II alveolar epithelial cells in IPF lungs is not due to increased rates of apoptosis of these cells. Lung sections from a control and IPF patient were stained with a red fluorophore for a marker of type II alveolar epithelial cells (SP-C, left column) and with a green fluorophore for active caspase-3 (Casp3; middle column as a marker of apoptotic cells). Merged images (right) show apoptotic cells (stained green) in an area of severe fibrosis in the IPF lung, but these apoptotic cells are not ATII cells as assessed by the lack of co-localization of active caspase-3 and SP-C staining. There is no apoptosis in alveolar epithelial cells in the control lung, as expected. The images are representative of immuno-stained lung sections from 2 control subjects and 3 patients with IPF. Magnification is X 600.

for PBMC MMP-8 steady state mRNA levels shows that these levels do not correlate with mortality (personal communication, Naftali Kaminski, MD, Yale University School of Medicine).

Discussion

MMP-8 has been identified as a pro-fibrotic proteinase in the lungs of bleomycin-treated mice [10,11] but much less is known about its roles in human IPF. Herein, we report that MMP-8 plasma levels are higher in IPF patients compared with control subjects in agreement with results reported in one prior study [18]. However, we add to this literature by showing that MMP-8 plasma levels do not correlate with annual rate of decline in lung function or mortality in IPF patients. We hypothesized that MMP-8 levels in blood neutrophils would be altered in IPF patients, as MMP-8 is most highly expressed by neutrophils, and another study reported that blood neutrophils are activated in IPF patients as indicated by increased plasma neutrophil elastase levels in IPF patients [23]. Surprisingly, we found no differences in total cellular or surface levels of MMP-8 in/on blood neutrophils from IPF patients when compared with cellular levels in control subjects. We report for the

first time that MMP-8 gene expression levels are robustly upregulated in blood monocytes in IPF patients, but MMP-8 gene expression in PBMCs does not correlate with mortality in IPF patients when a publicly-available microarray dataset is analyzed.

Consistent with results from prior studies [18,20,21], MMP-8 protein levels are increased in BALF samples from our IPF cohort but do not correlate with pulmonary function. Thus, BALF MMP-8 levels are unlikely to serve as a useful prognostic biomarker for IPF. However, our results add to the literature by showing that the main form of MMP-8 that is increased in IPF BALF is active MMP-8. Although we expected that neutrophils and fibroblasts would express MMP-8 in IPF lungs, our study shows for the first time that lung macrophages and bronchial epithelial cells are the main sources of MMP-8 in IPF lungs. MMP-8 expressed by macrophages and bronchial epithelial cells may contribute to the fibrotic process in IPF lungs.

Until now, MMP-8 has not been well studied in blood samples,

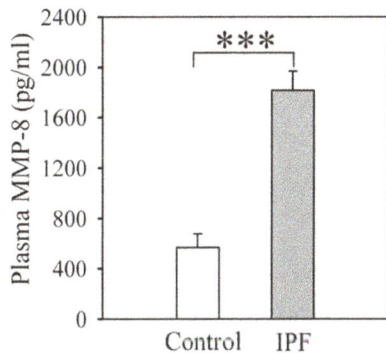

Figure 7. MMP-8 levels are increased in IPF plasma samples. Plasma samples were obtained from patients with IPF and healthy volunteers (control). MMP-8 protein levels were measured using an ELISA. Data are mean + SEM; n = 21 healthy volunteers and n = 73 patients with IPF; asterisks indicate p<0.001.

Table 1. Demographic data on subjects recruited to measure MMP-8 levels in blood samples.

	IPF patients	Control subjects[¶]	P value
Number of subjects	73	25	
Age (years)	68.7 (7.9)[†]	62.9 (10.4)	0.006
Gender (% male)	69.2	80.0	0.446
Caucasian (%)	96.8	96.0	0.642
Hispanic (%)	3.2	12.0	0.276
FVC (L)	2.65 (0.8)	N/A[††]	
FVC (% predicted)	69.8 (18.3)	N/A	
TLC (L)	4.0 (1.1)	N/A	
TLC (% predicted)	67.5 (21.0)	N/A	
DLCO (mL/min/mmHg)	13.3 (6.1)	N/A	
DLCO (% predicted)	49.9 (18.7)	N/A	
Smoking (pack years)	23.3 (14.1)	2.08 (8.2)	<0.001

[†]Data shown are mean results (with SD in parentheses) in both groups for age, gender, forced vital capacity (FVC), FVC % predicted (% pred), total lung capacity (TLC), TLC % predicted, diffusing capacity of the lung for carbon monoxide (DLCO), DLCO % predicted, and smoking pack years.
[††]N/A: not available.
[¶]MMP-8 levels were measured in plasma samples from 21 of the 25 control subjects, MMP-8 levels were measured in leukocytes isolated from up to 7 of the 25 control subjects, and MMP-8 levels were measured in both plasma and leukocyte samples obtained from 3 of the 25 control subjects.

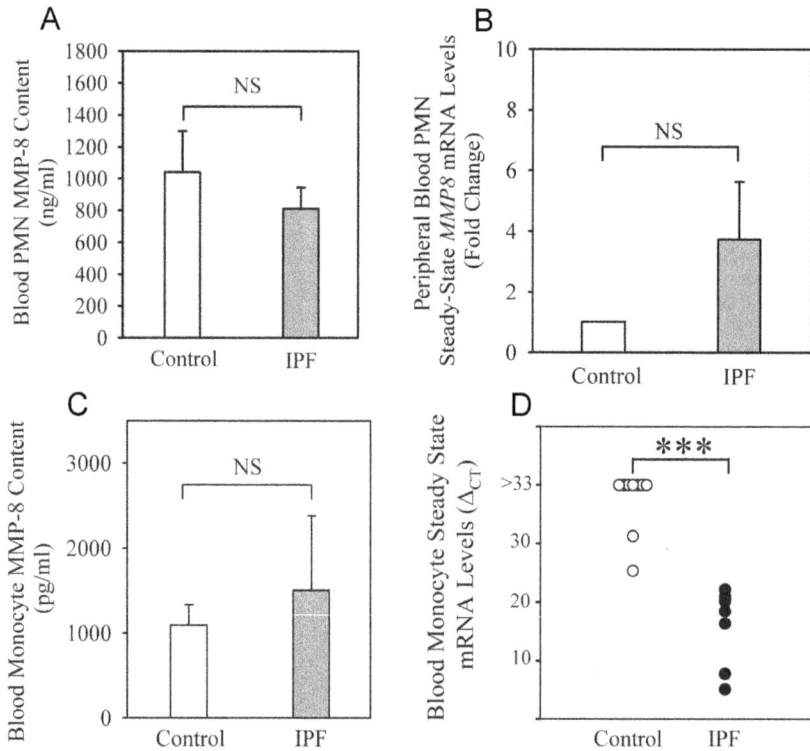

Figure 8. MMP-8 expression is increased in peripheral blood monocytes but not in peripheral blood neutrophils. Neutrophils and monocytes were isolated from blood samples obtained from IPF patients being evaluated for lung transplantation and healthy volunteers. MMP-8 protein levels were measured in neutrophil lysates (**A**) and monocyte lysates (**C**) (all prepared at 5×10^6 cells/ml) using an ELISA. In **A** and **C**, data are mean + SEM, n = 6–7 healthy volunteers and n = 4–22 IPF patients. MMP-8 steady-state mRNA levels were measured in RNA isolated from neutrophils (**B**) and monocytes (**D**) obtained from 7–9 control subjects and 6–9 IPF patients using a commercial gene expression assay for MMP-8 and 18 S as an endogenous reference. Data are expressed as fold change + SEM in **B** and as ΔC_T in **D** (C_T for MMP-8 - C_T for 18 S as MMP-8 transcripts were not detected in 7 out of 9 controls [$C_T > 60$ for MMP-8 and plotted as $\Delta C_T > 33$] or expressed at low levels in monocytes from 2 of the control subjects). Asterisks indicate $p < 0.001$.

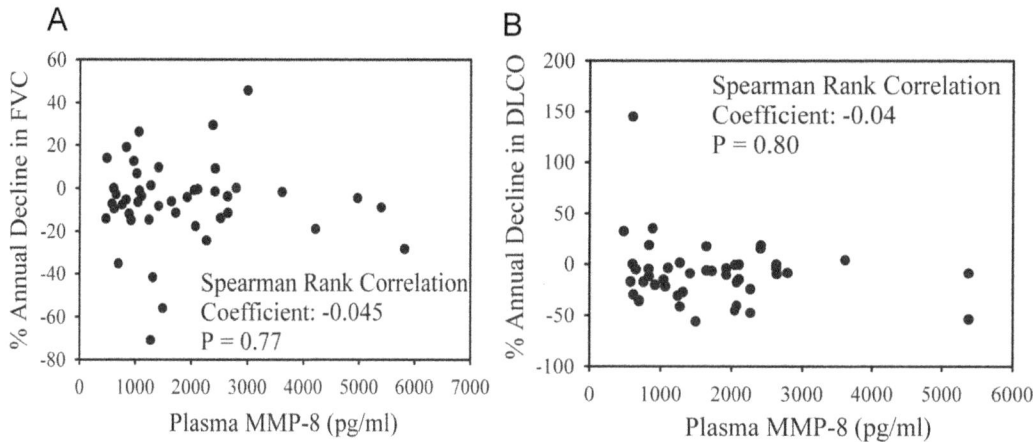

Figure 9. MMP-8 levels in plasma do not correlate with decline in pulmonary function in IPF patients. Serial FVC and DLCO measurements of lung function were performed on IPF patients being evaluated for lung transplantation. Annual rates of decline in both measures were calculated as described in Methods and plotted against plasma MMP-8 levels measured using an ELISA. Correlations between MMP-8 plasma levels and absolute annual rate of decline in FVC (**A**) or DLCO (**B**) were calculated using the Spearman Rank Correlation Coefficient; 45 IPF patients were studied in **A** and **B**.

which are easier to obtain than lung samples for measuring biomarkers. Although mean plasma MMP-8 levels are >3-fold higher in IPF patients compared with controls, our results indicate plasma MMP-8 levels are unlikely to serve as a useful prognostic biomarker for IPF patients as they do not correlate with rate of decline in lung function or mortality in IPF patients. Additionally, plasma MMP-8 levels are not specific for IPF as increased plasma MMP-8 levels occur in patients with active coronary artery disease [33] and breast cancer [34]. However, additional studies are needed to determine whether plasma MMP-8 levels correlate with other clinical outcomes and parameters in IPF patients including disease exacerbations.

Blood neutrophil MMP-8 protein and steady state mRNA levels are similar in IPF patients and control subjects. Until now, it has been thought that MMP-8 is not synthesized de novo by circulating mature neutrophils. Rather, MMP-8 is synthesized by bone marrow precursors of neutrophils and pre-formed MMP-8 protein is stored in neutrophil specific granules and released from these granules into the extracellular space when the cells degranulate [35]. However, in the current study, we detected MMP-8 mRNA transcripts in neutrophils from both IPF patients and healthy control subjects and this likely reflects the more sensitive qRT-RT-PCR method used herein when compared with methods used previously [36]. Membrane-bound MMP-8 on murine PMNs contributes significantly to MMP-8's anti-inflammatory activities in mice with ALI [12,17]. However, we found no differences in the expression of membrane-bound MMP-8 on PMNs from IPF patients versus controls indicating that this form of the proteinase is unlikely to contribute to lung fibrosis in human IPF patients.

MMP-8 is not thought to be a monocyte product. However, we detected MMP-8 mRNA transcripts in monocytes from some healthy subjects, and MMP-8 gene expression is significantly increased in monocytes from IPF patients. The reasons for this finding are not clear, but as MMP-8 gene expression increases in macrophages activated in vitro, mediators released in IPF lungs may induce MMP-8 expression in monocytes. Although MMP-8 gene expression is increased in IPF monocytes, we detected similar low levels of MMP-8 protein in extracts of blood monocyte from both healthy subjects and IPF patients. Likely, monocytes

synthesize and rapidly release (rather than store) MMP-8 protein. It is noteworthy that gene expression profiles of PBMCs (lymphocytes and monocytes) have recently been shown to predict poor outcomes in IPF patients [32]. However, MMP-8 gene expression levels in PBMCs do not correlate with mortality in IPF patients in this publicly-available dataset (personal communication, Naftali Kaminski, MD). Other studies report that patients with COPD and sarcoidosis have increased MMP-8 gene expression in PBMCs [30,31], but we were not able to confirm these findings when we analyzed other publicly-available microarray gene expression datasets of PBMCs from patients with sarcoidosis or COPD versus healthy control subjects (see Table S2). However, increased MMP-8 gene expression in blood monocytes is unlikely to be a predictive or prognostic biomarker for IPF.

Although BALF levels of MMP-8 have been reported to be elevated in IPF patients previously [18,20,21], until now the crucial cellular sources of pro-fibrotic MMP-8 in the lung have not been identified. We report for the first time that macrophages are one key cell type contributing to the elevated MMP-8 levels in IPF lungs, and macrophages in areas of mild as well as severe fibrosis robustly express MMP-8. While bronchial epithelial cells in control lungs do not express MMP-8, robust staining for MMP-8 is detected in bronchial epithelial cells in moderately severe and severe areas of fibrosis in IPF lungs. MMP-8 is also expressed by bronchial epithelium and macrophages in patients with bronchiectasis [37]. Thus, under pathologic conditions, mediators released in the lung may induce MMP-8 expression by bronchial epithelial cells and lung macrophages. Whether MMP-8 expressed by bronchial airway epithelium contributes to the fibrotic process in IPF lungs is not clear. However, MMP-8 expressed by distal airway epithelium could contribute to epithelial to mesenchymal transition.

We detected MMP-8 staining in ATII cells in our control lungs, which has not been reported previously. However, AT II cells have minimal or no MMP-8 expression in areas of moderately severe and severe fibrosis in IPF lungs. Although other studies report that ATII cells have increased apoptosis rates [28,29], our immunostaining results demonstrate apoptosis in cells other than ATII cells in IPF lungs (possibly ATI cells). Thus, it is unlikely that the reduced MMP-8 staining in ATII cells in IPF lungs is due to reduced viability of these cells. While activated murine lung fibroblasts express MMP-8 [10], we did not detect expression of MMP-8 by IPF lung fibroblasts. This underscores the importance of confirming findings obtained in animal models in samples from humans with the disease.

A recent study reported that MMP-8 protein levels are not increased in IPF lung tissue when compared with donor lungs that were not used for lung transplantation as assessed by western blotting [19]. In contrast, we found that MMP-8 protein levels are increased in homogenates of lung samples. The reasons for these different results are not clear but could be related to the status of the donor lung tissue studied. If the discarded donor lung tissue was obtained from donors having lung inflammation or injury due to mechanical ventilation, infection, or other inflammatory responses in the study of Nkyimbeng et al. [19], this could have elevated MMP-8 protein levels in the donor lung and contributed to the lack of a difference in MMP-8 levels between IPF and donor lungs in this study. It is noteworthy that Nkyimbeng et al. detected strong positive staining for MMP-8 in alveolar septae of their control lungs whereas we detected MMP-8 staining only in ATII cells in control lung sections. In addition, different antibodies were used in our study versus that of Nkyimbeng et al. which could recognize different epitopes in MMP-8 leading to differences in the results if these epitopes undergo different proteolytic processing in tissues.

MMP-8 promotes lung fibrosis in mice by decreasing lung levels of MIP-1α and IP-10 [10]. However, in our study, MMP-8 BALF levels do not correlate indirectly with BALF levels of MIP-1α or IP-10 in IPF patients, suggesting that these chemokines may not be MMP-8 substrates and/or MMP-8 has other pro-fibrotic activities in IPF lungs. Also, measuring levels of MMP-8 and chemokines in BALF may not reflect proteolytic events occurring in lung microenvironments other than the alveolar space. It is also noteworthy that delivering a truncated form of MMP-8 to the livers of rats with hepatic cirrhosis reduces hepatic fibrosis [38]. Furthermore, MMP-8 has protective anti-inflammatory activities in mice with acute lung injury [12] and allergen-induced airway inflammation [39], but pro-inflammatory activities during acute hepatic injury in mice [40]. Thus, more studies are needed on human cells and samples to determine whether MMP-8 has pro-fibrotic or beneficial activities in the human lung.

Our study has some limitations including the relatively small number of subjects studied. Also, our healthy subjects are modestly but significantly younger than our IPF patients. MMP-8 levels increase in tissues in mice as they age [41]. However, our analysis of MMP-8 plasma levels in older healthy controls (≥60 years of age; n = 14) versus younger health controls (<60 years of age; n = 11) revealed similar median MMP-8 plasma levels (364 vs. 645 pg/ml, respectively; p = 0.119). Thus, it is unlikely that the higher MMP-8 plasma levels in IPF patients are due to their greater age, but this needs to be confirmed in future studies.

Most of our IPF patients have a history of smoking cigarettes while most of our control subjects are non-smokers. Smoking status could affect MMP-8 levels in blood and lung samples as human PMNs incubated with cigarette smoke extract release increased amounts of MMP-8 and MMP-9 [42]. Additionally, plasma MMP-8 levels correlate with smoking status [43]. Therefore, the greater cigarette smoking history in our IPF cohort compared with that in our control subjects could potentially

contribute to the higher plasma MMP-8 levels observed in the IPF patients.

In conclusion, we confirm that MMP-8 levels are robustly increased in plasma samples from IPF patients. However, we report for the first time that MMP-8 plasma levels do not correlate with mortality or decline in lung function in IPF patients. We identify novel cellular culprits expressing increased levels of MMP-8 in IPF patients (blood monocytes, lung macrophages, and bronchial epithelial cells). We also provide new insights into the form of MMP-8 that is increased in IPF lungs (active MMP-8). Additional studies are needed to determine whether plasma MMP-8 levels correlate with other clinical parameters not studied herein. If MMP-8 is found to have pro-fibrotic activities in human as well as murine lungs, our results may help guide future studies testing the efficacy of novel therapies targeting MMP-8 in halting the progression of lung fibrosis in IPF patients.

Supporting Information

Table S1 Demographic data on subjects recruited to measure MMP-8 protein levels or forms in BALF samples. [†]Data are expressed as mean values for both groups (with SD in parentheses) for age, gender, total lung capacity (TLC), and diffusing capacity of the lung for carbon monoxide (DLCO). [††]BALF from 7 of the 12 control subjects was used to measure MMP-8 protein levels using an ELISA and BALF from 9 of the 12 control subjects was subjected to Western blotting to quantify MMP-8 forms.

Table S2 Results of analysis of Gene Expression Omnibus (GEO) publicly-available microarray gene expression databases for PBMCs in the National Center for Biotechnology Information (NCBI). [†]Gene expression datasets on peripheral blood mononuclear cells that are publicly-available (http://www.ncbi.nlm.nih.gov/geo/) were analyzed using the GEO2R interactive web tool and the GEO query and limma R packages [44] from the Bioconductor project. [††]P-value after adjustment for multiple testing using the Benjamin and Hochberg test [45].

Table S3 MIP-1α and IP-10 levels in BALF samples from IPF cases and control subjects. [†]MIP-1α and IP-10 were measured in BALF samples from 8 IPF cases and 5 control subjects using ELISA kits. [‡]Results are expressed as mean (SEM) values.

Acknowledgments

We thank Bartolome Celli, MD, for critical reading of the manuscript and helpful suggestions.

Author Contributions

Conceived and designed the experiments: VJC FP MLC YL YS YT VPP IOR CAO. Performed the experiments: VJC FP MLC YS JCO CAO. Analyzed the data: VJC FP YS JCO YT BRG IOR CAO. Contributed reagents/materials/analysis tools: YT JOC VPP BRG IOR CAO. Wrote the paper: VJC FP CAO.

References

1. Collard HR, King TE Jr., Bartelson BB, Vourlekis JS, Schwarz MI, et al. (2003) Changes in clinical and physiologic variables predict survival in idiopathic pulmonary fibrosis. Am J Respir Crit Care Med 168: 538–542. 10.1164/rccm.200211-1311OC [doi];200211-1311OC [pii].

2. Gribbin J, Hubbard RB, Le JI, Smith CJ, West J, et al. (2006) Incidence and mortality of idiopathic pulmonary fibrosis and sarcoidosis in the UK. Thorax 61: 980–985. thx.2006.062836 [pii];10.1136/thx.2006.062836 [doi].

3. Navaratnam V, Fleming KM, West J, Smith CJ, Jenkins RG, et al. (2011) The rising incidence of idiopathic pulmonary fibrosis in the U.K. Thorax 66: 462–467. thx.2010.148031 [pii];10.1136/thx.2010.148031 [doi].

4. National Heart Lung and Blood Institute (2012) Evaluating the effectiveness of prednisolone, azathioprine, and N-acetylcysteine in people with Idiopathic Pulmonary Fibrosis (PANTHER-IPF).

5. Noble PW, Albera C, Bradford WZ, Costabel U, Glassberg MK, et al. (2011) Pirfenidone in patients with idiopathic pulmonary fibrosis (CAPACITY): two randomised trials. Lancet 377: 1760–1769. S0140-6736(11)60405-4 [pii];10.1016/S0140-6736(11)60405-4 [doi].

6. Richeldi L, Costabel U, Selman M, Kim DS, Hansell DM, et al. (2011) Efficacy of a tyrosine kinase inhibitor in idiopathic pulmonary fibrosis. N Engl J Med 365: 1079–1087. 10.1056/NEJMoa1103690 [doi].

7. King TE Jr., Pardo A, Selman M (2011) Idiopathic pulmonary fibrosis. Lancet 378: 1949–1961. S0140-6736(11)60052-4 [pii];10.1016/S0140-6736(11)60052-4 [doi].

8. Gunther A, Korfei M, Mahavadi P, von der Beck D, Ruppert C, et al. (2012) Unravelling the progressive pathophysiology of idiopathic pulmonary fibrosis. Eur Respir Rev 21: 152–160. 21/124/152 [pii];10.1183/09059180.00001012 [doi].

9. Hasty KA, Jeffrey JJ, Hibbs MS, Welgus HG (1987) The collagen substrate specificity of human neutrophil collagenase. J Biol Chem 262: 10048–10052.

10. Craig VJ, Quintero PA, Fyfe SE, Patel AS, Knolle MD, et al. (2013) Profibrotic activities for matrix metalloproteinase-8 during bleomycin-mediated lung injury. J Immunol 190: 4283–4296. jimmunol.1201043 [pii];10.4049/jimmunol.1201043 [doi].

11. Garcia-Prieto E, Gonzalez-Lopez A, Cabrera S, Astudillo A, Gutierrez-Fernandez A, et al. (2010) Resistance to bleomycin-induced lung fibrosis in MMP-8 deficient mice is mediated by interleukin-10. PLoS ONE 5: e13242. 10.1371/journal.pone.0013242 [doi].

12. Quintero PA, Knolle MD, Cala LF, Zhuang Y, Owen CA (2010) Matrix metalloproteinase-8 inactivates macrophage inflammatory protein-1 alpha to reduce acute lung inflammation and injury in mice. J Immunol 184: 1575–1588. jimmunol.0900290 [pii];10.4049/jimmunol.0900290 [doi].

13. Hasty KA, Hibbs MS, Kang AH, Mainardi CL (1986) Secreted forms of human neutrophil collagenase. J Biol Chem 261: 5645–5650.

14. Herman MP, Sukhova GK, Libby P, Gerdes N, Tang N, et al. (2001) Expression of neutrophil collagenase (matrix metalloproteinase-8) in human atheroma: a novel collagenolytic pathway suggested by transcriptional profiling. Circulation 104: 1899–1904. 10.1161/hc4101.097419 [doi].

15. Cox SW, Eley BM, Kiili M, Asikainen A, Tervahartiala T, et al. (2006) Collagen degradation by interleukin-1beta-stimulated gingival fibroblasts is accompanied by release and activation of multiple matrix metalloproteinases and cysteine proteinases. Oral Dis 12: 34–40. ODI1153 [pii];10.1111/j.1601-0825.2005.01153.x [doi].

16. Hanemaaijer R, Sorsa T, Konttinen YT, Ding Y, Sutinen M, et al. (1997) Matrix metalloproteinase-8 is expressed in rheumatoid synovial fibroblasts and endothelial cells. Regulation by tumor necrosis factor-α and doxycycline. J Biol Chem 272: 31504–31509.

17. Owen CA, Hu Z, Lopez-Otin C, Shapiro SD (2004) Membrane-bound matrix metalloproteinase-8 on activated polymorphonuclear cells is a potent, tissue inhibitor of metalloproteinase-resistant collagenase and serpinase. J Immunol 172: 7791–7803. 10.4049/jimmunol.172.12.7791 [doi].

18. Rosas IO, Richards TJ, Konishi K, Zhang Y, Gibson K, et al. (2008) MMP1 and MMP7 as potential peripheral blood biomarkers in idiopathic pulmonary fibrosis. PLoS Med 5: e93. 10.1371/journal.pmed.0050093 [doi].

19. Nkyimbeng T, Ruppert C, Shiomi T, Dahal B, Lang G, et al. (2013) Pivotal role of matrix metalloproteinase 13 in extracellular matrix turnover in idiopathic pulmonary fibrosis. PLoS ONE 8: e73279. 10.1371/journal.pone.0073279 [doi];PONE-D-13-14194 [pii].

20. Henry MT, McMahon K, Mackarel AJ, Prikk K, Sorsa T, et al. (2002) Matrix metalloproteinases and tissue inhibitor of metalloproteinase-1 in sarcoidosis and IPF. Eur Respir J 20: 1220–1227. 10.1183/09031936.02.00022302 [doi].

21. McKeown S, Richter AG, O'Kane C, McAuley DF, Thickett DR (2009) MMP expression and abnormal lung permeability are important determinants of outcome in IPF. Eur Respir J 33: 77–84. 09031936.00060708 [pii];10.1183/09031936.00060708 [doi].

22. Willems S, Verleden SE, Vanaudenaerde BM, Wynants M, Dooms C, et al. (2013) Multiplex protein profiling of bronchoalveolar lavage in idiopathic pulmonary fibrosis and hypersensitivity pneumonitis. Ann Thorac Med 8: 38–45. 10.4103/1817-1737.105718 [doi];ATM-8-38 [pii].

23. Obayashi Y, Yamadori I, Fujita J, Yoshinouchi T, Ueda N, et al. (1997) The role of neutrophils in the pathogenesis of idiopathic pulmonary fibrosis. Chest 112: 1338–1343. 10.1378/chest.112.5.1338 [doi].

24. Raghu G, Collard HR, Egan JJ, Martinez FJ, Behr J, et al. (2011) An official ATS/ERS/JRS/ALAT statement: idiopathic pulmonary fibrosis: evidence-based guidelines for diagnosis and management. Am J Respir Crit Care Med 183: 788–824. 183/6/788 [pii];10.1164/rccm.2009-040GL [doi].

25. Schneider CA, Rasband WS, Eliceiri KW (2012) NIH Image to ImageJ: 25 years of image analysis. Nat Methods 9: 671–675.

26. Owen CA, Hu Z, Barrick B, Shapiro SD (2003) Inducible expression of tissue inhibitor of metalloproteinases-resistant matrix metalloproteinase-9 on the cell surface of neutrophils. Am J Resp Cell Mol Biol 29: 283–294. 10.1165/rcmb.2003-0034OC [doi].

27. Knolle MD, Nakajima T, Hergrueter A, Gupta K, Polverino F, et al. (2013) Adam8 limits the development of allergic airway inflammation in mice. J Immunol 190: 6434–6449. jimmunol.1202329 [pii];10.4049/jimmunol.1202329 [doi].

28. Korfei M, Ruppert C, Mahavadi P, Henneke I, Markart P, et al. (2008) Epithelial endoplasmic reticulum stress and apoptosis in sporadic idiopathic pulmonary fibrosis. Am J Respir Crit Care Med 178: 838–846. 200802-313OC [pii];10.1164/rccm.200802-313OC [doi].

29. Maher TM, Evans IC, Bottoms SE, Mercer PF, Thorley AJ, et al. (2010) Diminished prostaglandin E2 contributes to the apoptosis paradox in idiopathic pulmonary fibrosis. Am J Respir Crit Care Med 182: 73–82. 200905-0674OC [pii];10.1164/rccm.200905-0674OC [doi].

30. Bahr TM, Hughes GJ, Armstrong M, Reisdorph R, Coldren CD, et al. (2013) Peripheral blood mononuclear cell gene expression in chronic obstructive pulmonary disease. Am J Respir Cell Mol Biol 49: 316–323. 10.1165/rcmb.2012-0230OC [doi].

31. Zhou T, Zhang W, Sweiss NJ, Chen ES, Moller DR, et al. (2012) Peripheral blood gene expression as a novel genomic biomarker in complicated sarcoidosis. PLoS ONE 7: e44818. 10.1371/journal.pone.0044818 [doi];PONE-D-12-04039 [pii].

32. Herazo-Maya JD, Noth I, Duncan SR, Kim S, Ma SF, et al. (2013) Peripheral blood mononuclear cell gene expression profiles predict poor outcome in idiopathic pulmonary fibrosis. Sci Transl Med 5: 205ra136. 5/205/205ra136 [pii];10.1126/scitranslmed.3005964 [doi].

33. Kato R, Momiyama Y, Ohmori R, Taniguchi H, Nakamura H, et al. (2005) Plasma matrix metalloproteinase-8 concentrations are associated with the presence and severity of coronary artery disease. Circ J 69: 1035–1040. JST.JSTAGE/circj/69.1035 [pii].

34. Decock J, Hendrickx W, Vanleeuw U, Van Belle V, Van Huffel S, et al. (2008) Plasma MMP1 and MMP8 expression in breast cancer: protective role of MMP8 against lymph node metastasis. BMC Cancer 8: 77. 1471-2407-8-77 [pii];10.1186/1471-2407-8-77 [doi].

35. Murphy G, Reynolds JJ, Bretz U, Baggiolini M (1977) Collagenase is a component of the specific granules of human neutrophil leukocytes. Biochem J 162: 195-197.

36. Harris ED Jr., Welgus HG, Krane SM (1984) Regulation of the mammalian collagenases. Coll Relat Res 4: 493–512.

37. Prikk K, Maisi P, Pirila E, Sepper R, Salo T, et al. (2001) In vivo collagenase-2 (MMP-8) expression by human bronchial epithelial cells and monocytes/macrophages in bronchiectasis. J Pathol 194: 232–238. 10.1002/path.849 [pii];10.1002/path.849 [doi].

38. Liu J, Cheng X, Guo Z, Wang Z, Li D, et al. (2013) Truncated active human matrix metalloproteinase-8 delivered by a chimeric adenovirus-hepatitis B virus vector ameliorates rat liver cirrhosis. PLoS ONE 8: e53392. 10.1371/journal.pone.0053392 [doi];PONE-D-12-25745 [pii].

39. Gueders MM, Balbin M, Rocks N, Foidart JM, Gosset P, et al. (2005) Matrix metalloproteinase-8 deficiency promotes granulocytic allergen-induced airway inflammation. J Immunol 175: 2589–2597. 10.4049/jimmunol.175.4.2589 [doi].

40. Van Lint P, Wielockx B, Puimege L, Noel A, Lopez-Otin C, et al. (2005) Resistance of collagenase-2 (matrix metalloproteinase-8)-deficient mice to TNF-induced lethal hepatitis. J Immunol 175: 7642–7649. 175/11/7642 [doi].

41. Salminen HJ, Saamanen AM, Vankemmelbeke MN, Auho PK, Perala MP, et al. (2002) Differential expression patterns of matrix metalloproteinases and their inhibitors during development of osteoarthritis in a transgenic mouse model. Ann Rheum Dis 61: 591–597. 10.1136/ard.61.7.591 [doi].

42. Overbeek SA, Braber S, Koelink PJ, Henricks PA, Mortaz E, et al. (2013) Cigarette smoke-induced collagen destruction; key to chronic neutrophilic airway inflammation? PLoS ONE 8: e55612. 10.1371/journal.pone.0055612 [doi];PONE-D-12-14093 [pii].

43. Aquilante CL, Beitelshees AL, Zineh I (2007) Correlates of serum matrix metalloproteinase-8 (MMP-8) concentrations in nondiabetic subjects without cardiovascular disease. Clin Chim Acta 379: 48–52. S0009-8981(06)00799-6 [pii];10.1016/j.cca.2006.12.006 [doi].

44. Smythe G (2005) Limma: linear models for microarray data. In: Gentleman R, Dudoit S, Irizarry RHW, editors. Bioinformatics and Computational Biology Solutions Using R and Bioconductor. New York, NY: Springer.

45. Benjamini Y, Hochberg Y (1995) Controlling the false discovery rate: a practical and powerful approach to multiple testing. Journal of the Royal Statistical Society Series B 57: 289–300.

20

Intravenous Immunoglobulin for Hypogammaglobulinemia after Lung Transplantation: A Randomized Crossover Trial

David J. Lederer[1,2], Nisha Philip[1], Debbie Rybak[1], Selim M. Arcasoy[1], Steven M. Kawut[3,4]*

1 Department of Medicine, College of Physicians and Surgeons, Columbia University, New York City, New York, United States of America, 2 Department of Epidemiology, Mailman School of Public Health, Columbia University, New York City, New York, United States of America, 3 Department of Medicine, Perelman School of Medicine, University of Pennsylvania, Philadelphia, Pennsylvania, United States of America, 4 Center for Clinical Epidemiology and Biostatistics, Perelman School of Medicine, University of Pennsylvania, Philadelphia, Pennsylvania, United States of America

Abstract

Background: We aimed to determine the effects of treatment with intravenous immunoglobulin on bacterial infections in patients with hypogammaglobulinemia (HGG) after lung transplantation.

Methods: We performed a randomized, double-blind, placebo-controlled two-period crossover trial of immune globulin intravenous (IVIG), 10% Purified (Gamunex, Bayer, Elkhart, IN) monthly in eleven adults who had undergone lung transplantation more than three months previously. We randomized study participants to three doses of IVIG (or 0.1% albumin solution (placebo)) given four weeks apart followed by a twelve week washout and then three doses of placebo (or IVIG). The primary outcome was the number of bacterial infections within each treatment period.

Results: IVIG had no effect on the number of bacterial infections during the treatment period (3 during IVIG and 1 during placebo; odds ratio 3.5, 95% confidence interval 0.4 to 27.6, p = 0.24). There were no effects on other infections, use of antibiotics, or lung function. IVIG significantly increased trough IgG levels at all time points (least square means, 765.3 mg/dl during IVIG and 486.3 mg/dl during placebo, p<0.001). Four serious adverse events (resulting in hospitalization) occurred during the treatment periods (3 during active treatment and 1 during the placebo period, p = 0.37). Chills, flushing, and nausea occurred during one infusion of IVIG.

Conclusions: Treatment with IVIG did not reduce the short-term risk of bacterial infection in patients with HGG after lung transplantation. The clinical efficacy of immunoglobulin supplementation in HGG related to lung transplantation over the long term or with recurrent infections is unknown.

Trial Registration: Clinicaltrials.gov NCT00115778

Editor: Aric Gregson, University of California Los Angeles, United States of America

Funding: This study was funded by an investigator-initiated grant from Bayer Healthcare (now Talecris Pharmaceuticals). The manuscript was written by the authors, and the decision to submit the manuscript for publication was made solely by the authors. This manuscript was sent to the sponsor before submission for publication, however the sponsor had no right to delay or require any revisions to this manuscript. The sponsor had no role in the design of the study, data collection, analysis, interpretation of the data, or the decision to submit the manuscript.

Competing Interests: This study was funded by Bayer Healthcare (now Talecris Pharmaceuticals).

* Email: kawut@upenn.edu

Introduction

Potent immunosuppressive regimens, consisting of a calcineurin inhibitor, an anti-metabolite, and corticosteroids, predominantly target cell-mediated immunity to prevent lung allograft rejection after lung transplantation. Not surprisingly, lung transplant recipients suffer from an increased risk of infection by pathogens such as *Pseudomonas aeruginosa, Staphylococcus aureus,* and cytomegalovirus despite intensive antimicrobial prophylaxis [1,2,3,4,5].

Immunosuppressive therapy after solid organ transplantation may also contribute to humoral immunodeficiency due to hypogammaglobulinemia (HGG). [6,7,8,9] A recent meta-analysis

suggested that severe HGG after solid organ transplantation is associated with an increased risk of early infection and all-cause mortality. [10] In one study of lung transplant recipients, HGG was identified in 70% of lung transplant recipients, of whom 50% had very low immunoglobulin G (IgG) levels (<400 mg/dL). [9] Bacterial, fungal, and viral infections were significantly more common and survival significantly worse among those with HGG. We previously found that 58% of lung transplant recipients had mild incident HGG and 15% had severe HGG, with most episodes occurring within the first year of transplantation. [7] In that study, use of mycophenolate mofetil was an independent risk factor for HGG. We have also shown that the presence of HGG is associated with an increased risk of pneumonia, supporting the clinical importance of HGG in our lung transplant recipients. [8] Moreover, HGG has been reported in recipients of other solid organ transplants, such as heart and kidney, with significant clinical implications [11,12,13].

Intravenous immunoglobulin (IVIG) therapy is the current standard of care for patients with primary and certain secondary immunodeficiency states. Presently, IVIG is FDA-approved for treatment of primary humoral immunodeficiency, Kawasaki syndrome, B-cell chronic lymphocytic leukemia, and bone marrow transplant recipients with recurrent infections, pediatric HIV infection, and idiopathic thrombocytopenic purpura. It is well-established that augmentation of immunoglobulin levels in these immunodeficiency states results in decreases in bacterial infections [14].

IVIG therapy could significantly decrease the incidence and/or severity of infections in lung transplant recipients with HGG, however the use of IVIG in HGG after solid organ transplantation has not been well-studied. Despite the potential benefits, IVIG is relatively difficult to administer (requiring monthly intravenous infusion), has potential adverse reactions, and is very expensive. We performed a pilot phase II clinical trial to determine the efficacy and safety of immunoglobulin supplementation for HGG after lung transplantation.

Materials and Methods

The protocol for this trial and supporting CONSORT checklist are available as supporting information; see Checklist S1 and Protocol S1.

Ethics Statement

The protocol was approved by the Columbia University Medical Center (CUMC) Institutional Review Board and the medical monitor.

Study Design

This was a single-center, randomized double-blind, placebo-controlled, two-period crossover study to determine the efficacy and safety of IVIG in patients with HGG after lung transplantation. The original protocol called for the recruitment of 10 subjects; we enrolled one additional subject after one dropped out. The first subject was randomized in April 2006 and the last subject by July 2008.

The manuscript was written by the authors, and the decision to submit the manuscript for publication was made solely by the authors. This manuscript was sent to the sponsor before submission for publication, however the sponsor had no right to delay or require any revisions to this manuscript. The sponsor did not participate in data analysis or drafting of the manuscript.

Study Participants

We recruited adult lung transplant recipients at Columbia University Medical Center (CUMC) who were at least 3 months out from lung transplantation and had HGG (IgG levels < 500 mg/dL) on two assessments at least one month apart within three months. Study subjects had to be on a stable medical regimen for at least one month before enrollment. We excluded those with acute rejection (defined histologically) or active infection within one month before enrollment, a contraindication to IVIG (acute renal failure, severe selective IgA deficiency, known hypersensitivity to IVIG), pregnancy, or a history of a thrombotic event within three months. The initial protocol called for IgG levels <400 mg/dL, which was increased to <500 mg/dL due to slow enrollment. All participants provided written informed

consent. This study was registered at clinicaltrials.gov before the initiation of enrollment (NCT00115778) (http://clinicaltrials.gov/show/NCT00115778).

Study Procedures

This was a crossover study with two 12 week treatment periods (separated by a 12 week washout period) comparing immune globulin intravenous (Human), 10% Caprylate/Chromatolgraphy Purified (Gamunex) (Bayer, Elkhart, IN) ("IVIG") with 0.1% albumin ("placebo"). The *in vivo* half-life of this form of IVIG is approximately 35 days. The dose of IVIG in this study was 400 mg/kg every 4 weeks, which is a widely used dosage in clinical practice. The initial infusion rate was 0.01 mL/kg/min, titrated to a maximum infusion rate of 0.08 mL/kg/min. Placebo was 0.1% albumin in an equal volume, prepared by the Columbia Research Pharmacy. IVIG and placebo infusion bags had identical color and appearance. All participants were pre-medicated with acetaminophen 650 mg po and diphenhydramine 25 mg po before every study drug infusion.

The Research Pharmacy at Columbia University randomly assigned the treatment order. Investigators, study personnel, and study participants were blinded to the order and identity of the treatments. IGG levels were not performed during the study; samples were banked and then run after the conclusion of the study. Study drug was prepared by an unblinded research pharmacist and delivered to the infusion suite at our medical center where each dose of study drug was administered.

Study participants were evaluated at baseline and at Week 4, 8, 12, 24, 28, 32, and 36. The "Period 1" study drug was administered at baseline and at Week 4 and 8 study visits. The "Period 2" study drug was administered at Week 24, 28, and 32. There was a twelve week washout period between the Period 1 and Period 2. Phlebotomy was performed on the morning of each study visit, before infusion of the study drug. Participants maintained a diary of any new medications or symptoms during the study period.

Outcome Assessments

The primary outcome was the number of bacterial infections during the treatment period. Secondary outcomes included viral, fungal and all non-bacterial infections, hospital admissions, antimicrobial use, serious bacterial infections, trough IgG levels, acute rejection, spirometry, and mortality in each period. The definitions of infectious end points were drawn from an FDA draft document. [15] The necessary criteria were collected prospectively and all infectious events were determined with blinding to the treatment period.

Statistical Analysis

Generalized estimating equations with a compound symmetry covariance structure and logit link were used to estimate odds ratios. Linear mixed effects modeling with an autoregressive covariance structure were used to assess differences in lung function and IgG levels between treatment arms. Models included fixed effects for drug and period. Subject was included as a random effect. Least squares means and 95% confidence intervals for continuous outcomes are reported. Paired sample analysis was performed secondarily.

In order to detect a reduction in the mean number of bacterial infections/patient by one standard deviation over three months with 80% power at an α level of 0.05, we estimated that we would need 10 subjects. This effect estimate was similar to the difference between patients with and without HGG in prior studies. [9] The crossover design of the trial, in which each subject serves as his or

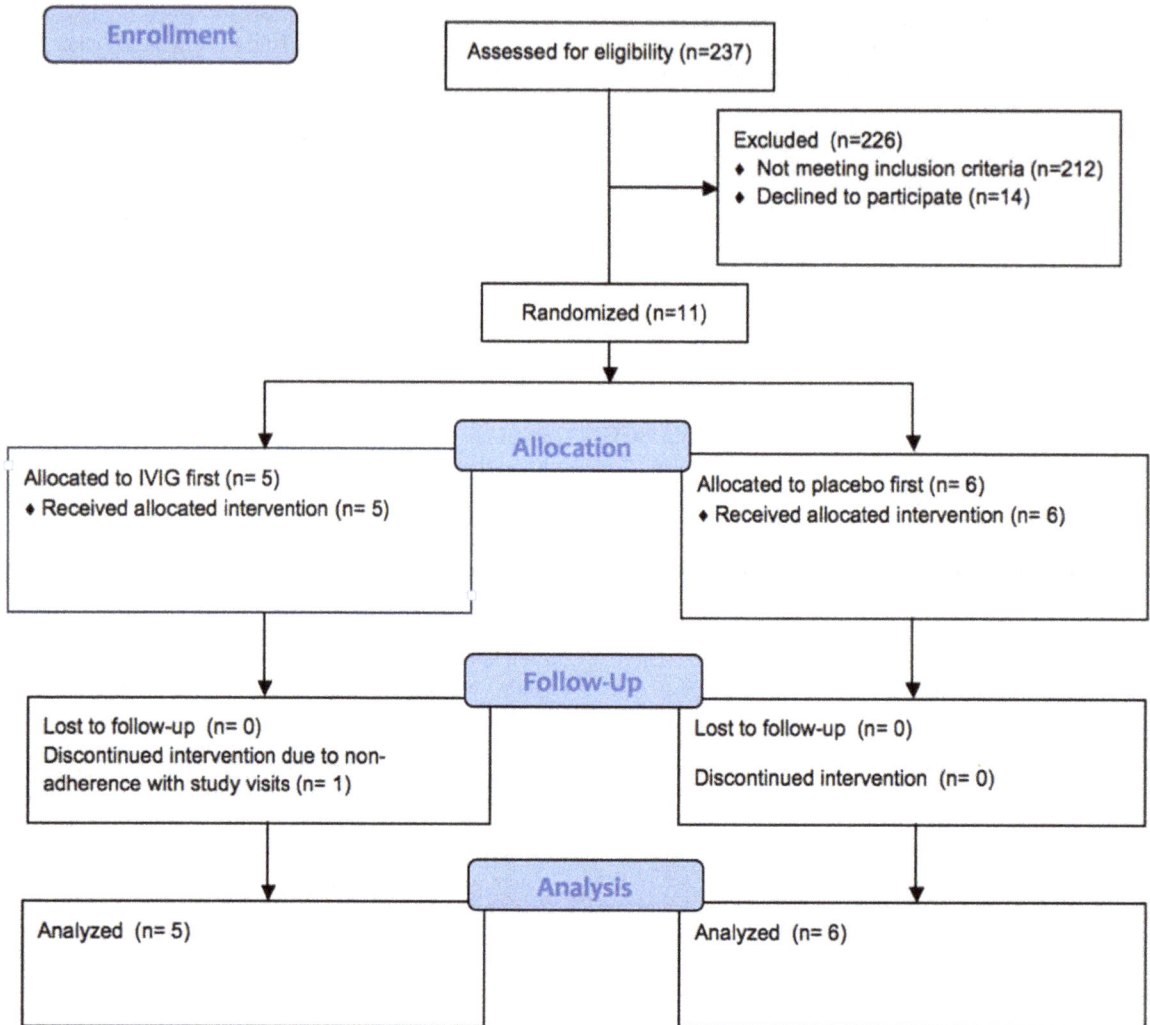

Figure 1. Study flow.

her own control, allows sufficient power for the detection of a clinically significant effect of IVIG with only a small number of patients and is the major strength of this design. For example, a sample size of 10 patients in a crossover trial has more power to detect differences than double the sample size using a parallel group design (i.e., randomizing 10 patients to IVIG and 10 patients to placebo). As we did not have multiple bacterial infections per patient (see below), the power of the study was less than anticipated.

The primary analysis proceeded according to the intent-to-treat principle. All randomized participants were analyzed in their originally assigned group whether or not they discontinued study drug. P values<0.05 were considered significant. Analyses were performed using SAS 9.2 (SAS Institute, Cary, NC). There were no interim analyses or stopping rules planned *a priori* for the trial.

Results

We screened 237 lung transplant recipients between January 2005 and July 2008 (Figure 1). Eleven subjects were eligible and randomized, and 10 completed all study assessments. One subject discontinued the interventions because of inability to comply with the schedule of study visits.

Participant characteristics are shown in Table 1. The mean age was 55 years (range 28 to 66 years) and six (55%) were male. Most were non-Hispanic white. Six underwent lung transplantation for COPD and ten had undergone bilateral transplantation. The median time from transplantation to enrollment was 187 days (interquartile range 153 to 660 days). Five study participants (45%) were taking valganciclovir for prophylaxis against cytomegalovirus. The median baseline IgG level for the study sample at randomization was 487.5 g/dl (IQR 423.5 to 513.8 g/dl), showing the variability over time in IgG levels (as all patients had IgG levels <500 g/dl on two assessments at least one month apart within three months before enrollment).

Subjects received the study treatments in the assigned order. One participant experienced chills, flushing, and nausea during infusion of IVIG. No other infusion-related adverse events occurred. Study drug was discontinued in one subject because of inability to comply with study visits. There were no period or carryover effects.

During the IVIG period, there were three bacterial infections (in three patients) compared to the placebo period, when there was one bacterial infection (in one patient) (odds ratio (OR) 3.5, 95% CI 0.4 to 27.6, p = 0.24; Table 2). Paired sample analyses showed similar results (data not shown). Similarly, there were non-

Table 1. Participant characteristics.

Characteristic	Value
No.	11
Age	60 (28 to 66)
Male	6
Race/ethnicity	
Non-Hispanic white	10
Hispanic white	1
Height, cm	168 (140 to 183)
Weight, kg	68 (52 to 88)
Pre-transplant diagnosis	
Chronic obstructive pulmonary disease	6
Interstitial lung disease	2
Cystic fibrosis	1
Pulmonary arterial hypertension	2
Transplant procedure	
Bilateral	10
Single	1
Days since transplantation	187 (119 to 1330)
Serum creatinine, mg/dl	1.3 (0.9 to 1.8)
Immunosuppressive medications	
Tacrolimus	9
Cyclosporine	2
Azathioprine	5
Mycophenolate mofetil	6
Prednisone	11
Forced vital capacity, % predicted	92 (60 to 112)
Forced expiratory volume in 1 sec, % predicted	109 (65 to 121)
Forced expiratory volume in 1 sec/Forced vital capacity ratio, %	88 (72 to 100)
Forced expiratory flow 25–75, % predicted	128 (50 to 270)

Data are median (range) and frequency.

significant increases in overall infections (IVIG-7 vs. placebo-3, OR 2.7, 95% CI 0.95 to 7.6, p = 0.06), antibiotic initiation (IVIG-9 vs. placebo-8, OR 1.4, 9% CI 0.3 to 6.0, p = 0.61), and hospitalization (IVIG-3 vs. placebo-1, OR 3.5, 95% CI 0.2 to 51.2, p = 0.37; Table 2) during the IVIG period compared to the placebo period. IVIG had no significant effect on lung function over three months (Table 3). As expected, the administration of IVIG significantly increased IgG levels throughout the treatment period compared to placebo (Table 3; Figure 2).

Table 4 shows the adverse events during the IVIG and placebo periods. Five serious adverse- events occurred during the study, and four during a treatment period. Three (pancreatitis, vitreous hemorrhage, and E. coli pneumonia) occurred during the IVIG period and one (hospital admission for thymoglobulin infusion) during the placebo period. There was a hospitalization for a fall during the washout period. The most common adverse events were bronchoscopy (in >50% of participants in both periods). Cough and neck stiffness were more common during IVIG periods.

Discussion

To our knowledge, this is the first randomized, double-blind, placebo-controlled clinical trial of IVIG for HGG after lung transplantation. In a crossover design, we did not find a significant impact of IVIG on bacterial infections or other infectious episodes, despite observing expected increases in IgG levels following IVIG administration. Adverse events were mild and common during both IVIG and placebo periods.

Previous studies have shown associations between the presence of HGG after lung transplant and worse outcomes. We previously demonstrated that lung transplant recipients with severe HGG (IgG<400 mg/dl) had a higher cumulative incidence of pneumonia (63%) compared to that of recipients without HGG (18%), (p = 0.01), but there was no significant increase in the risk of CMV disease. [8] Those with severe HGG also had an increased risk of death. The incidence of severe HGG was about 15% in our prior studies, [7,8] however other investigators have demonstrated even higher prevalences of HGG after lung transplantation. [9] A recent study in pediatric lung transplant recipients found an association between HGG and the risk of infections and hospitalization. [16] More recently, lower post-transplant IgG levels were associated with an increased risk of BOS [6].

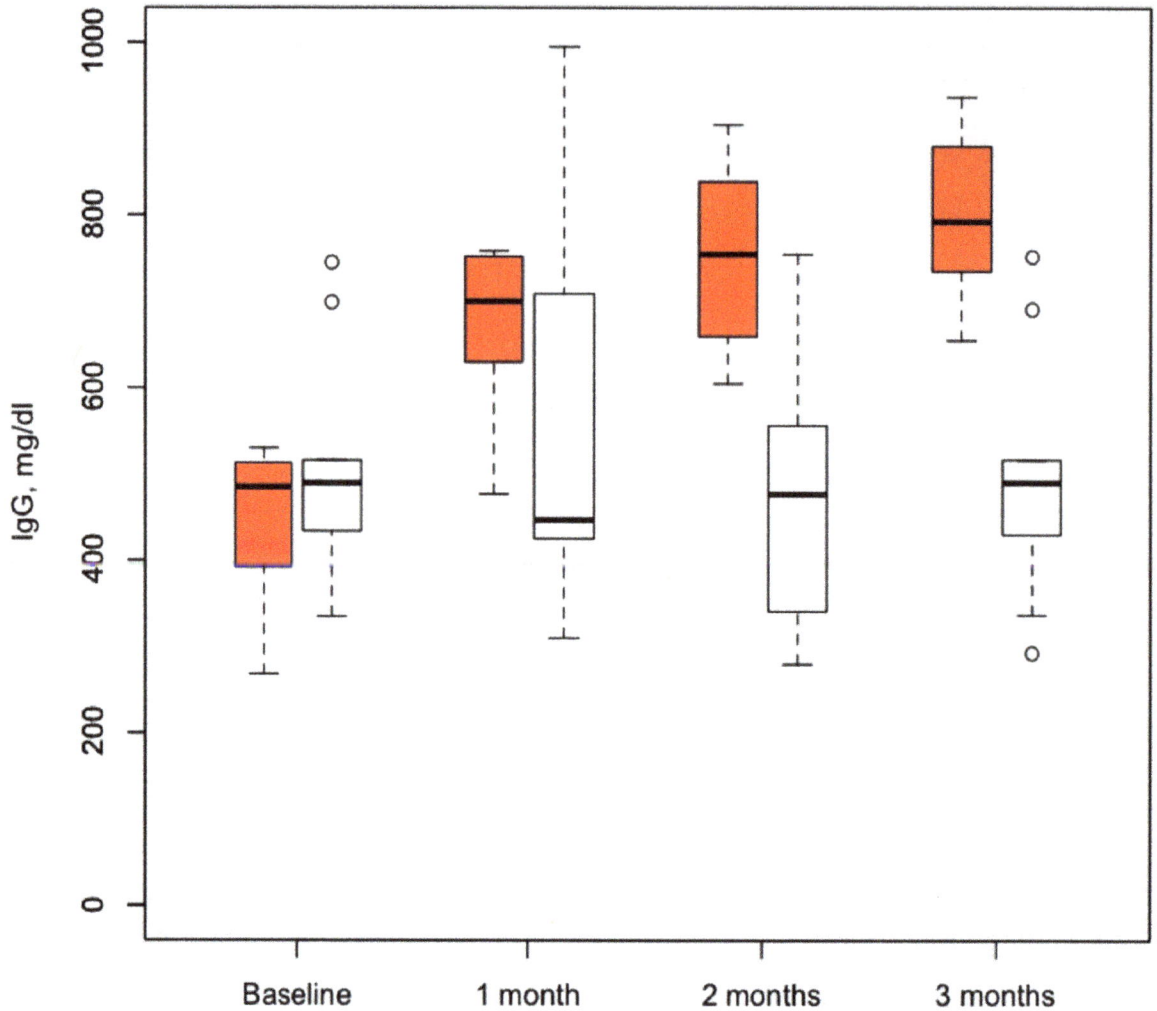

Figure 2. Box (interquartile range) and whisker plots of serum IgG levels during the IVIG period (red) and placebo period (white).

Table 2. Outcomes.

	No. of events occurring during IVIG treatment period	No. of events occurring during placebo treatment period	Odds ratio (IVIG vs. placebo)	95% confidence interval	P value
Bacterial infection	3	1	3.5	0.4 to 27.6	0.24
Viral infection	2	2	0.8	0.1 to 5.9	0.87
Fungal infection	2	0	–	–	
Any infection	7	3	2.7	0.95 to 7.6	0.06
Positive culture	4	2	2.0	0.4 to 9.3	0.37
Antibiotic initiation	9	8	1.4	0.3 to 6.0	0.61
Bronchoscopy	7	6	1.3	0.7 to 2.4	0.47
Hospitalization	3	1	3.5	0.2 to 51.2	0.37
Acute rejection	0	0	–	–	
Lymphocytic bronchiolitis	0	0	–	–	

Table 3. Least square means (95% confidence interval) for spirometry value and serum IgG levels after IVIG and placebo.

	IVIG	Placebo	P value
Forced vital capacity, % predicted	88.8 (86.6–91.1)	89.7 (87.4–92.0)	0.51
Forced expiratory volume in 1 sec, % predicted	95.3 (92.2–98.3)	95.6 (92.5–98.7)	0.84
Forced expiratory volume in 1 sec/forced vital capacity ratio, %	86.9 (84.6–89.1)	85.3 (83.0–87.6)	0.14
Forced expiratory flow 25–75, % predicted	125.0 (114.6–135.4)	119.0 (108.5–129.5)	0.14
IgG, mg/dl	765.3 (720.1–810.6)	486.3 (441.0–531.5)	<0.001

IVIG is the current standard in clinical practice for replacement therapy of patients with primary immunodeficiency states. [17] Currently, IVIG is FDA approved for treatment of primary humoral immunodeficiency, Kawasaki syndrome, chronic lymphocytic leukemia and bone marrow transplant recipients with recurrent infections and idiopathic thrombocytopenic purpura.

Table 4. Adverse events.

Event	IVIG	Placebo	Washout
Any AE	11 (100%)	11 (100%)	11 (100%)
Serious adverse event			
Any SAE	3 (27%)	1 (9%)	1 (9%)
Infusion-related AEs*			
Any infusion-related AE	1 (9%)	0 (0%)	–
Chills	1 (9%)	0 (0%)	–
Flushing	1 (9%)	0 (0%)	–
Nausea	1 (9%)	0 (0%)	–
Infectious			
Fever	2 (18%)	0 (0%)	2 (18%)
Night sweats	0 (0%)	2 (18%)	0 (0%)
Bronchoscopy	7 (64%)	6 (54%)	7 (64%)
Pulmonary			
Dyspnea	1 (9%)	1 (9%)	2 (18%)
Cough	2 (18%)	1 (9%)	1 (9%)
Sputum production	1 (9%)	1 (9%)	1 (9%)
Cardiac			
Palpitations	1 (9%)	1 (9%)	1 (9%)
Pedal edema	0 (0%)	3 (27%)	0 (0%)
Neurological			
Headache	2 (18%)	3 (27%)	0 (0%)
Stiff neck	2 (18%)	0 (0%)	1 (9%)
Genitourinary			
Urinary frequency	1 (9%)	2 (18%)	0 (0%)
Pancreatitis	1 (9%)	0 (0%)	0 (0%)
Gastrointestinal			
Diarrhea	0 (0%)	2 (18%)	1 (9%)
Abdominal discomfort	1 (9%)	2 (18%)	0 (0%)
Heartburn/GER	1 (9%)	1 (9%)	0 (0%)
Other			
Musculoskeletal pain	2 (18%)	2 (18%)	0 (0%)
Acute kidney injury	1 (9%)	0 (0%)	0 (0%)
Vitreous hemorrhage	1 (9%)	0 (0%)	0 (0%)

*AEs with more than 1 occurrence during the study (except for infusion related AEs, acute kidney injury, pancreatitis, and vitreous hemorrhage).

While supplementation using IVIG in HGG after solid organ transplantation would be presumed to be effective, there are several reasons why it may not be. Organ transplant recipients receive a medical regimen that not only reduces B cell function (and antibody production), but also T cell function. HGG might be an epiphenomenon of reduced T cell function and merely replacing antibodies might not improve defenses against infection.

To our knowledge, there is only one other RCT of immunoglobulin replacement for HGG in thoracic organ transplantation. Yamani et al. studied the use of Cytogam in patients with IgG levels between 350 and 500 mg/dl in a randomized, double-blind placebo controlled trial with 13 patients randomized to Cytogam and 10 patients randomized to placebo (5% dextrose). [18] An average of only 1.4 doses were administered per patient, without a standard regimen. The investigators found a decrease in the number of episodes of CMV disease, but no other differences between the groups. These results may not be generalizable as this study 1) used Cytogam in patients who received valganciclovir for CMV prophylaxis for only 4 weeks after transplantation, 2) on average only administered 1–2 doses of study drug for the entire study period, 3) only showed an effect on CMV infection (defined as a positive CMV PCR with fever, malaise, leukopenia, or other evidence of organ disease), and 4) demonstrated no effect on bacterial infections. These data may be difficult to extrapolate to the chronic use of IVIG in lung transplant patients with HGG receiving more prolonged CMV prophylaxis.

Our study had several limitations. While the crossover design provided more power than we would have had with >20 subjects studied in a parallel design, there were few outcomes and our findings could very well be attributable to inadequate power. For the crossover design to be valid, we needed to ensure clinical stability over the time of both treatment periods, necessarily limiting the duration of each. Longer studies with greater numbers of patients would be necessary to detect smaller differences in outcomes. The primary statistical analysis may be anti-conservative in small samples, however no differences in the primary end point were seen and paired sample analyses were similar. We

recruited patients with low IgG levels documented twice over a short period of time. Even so, some of the patients in the study had IgG levels >500 mg/dl at the time of randomization and during the placebo period. This was not attributable to a carryover effect (i.e., the effect of IVIG treatment during the first period continuing into the second period), but likely reflects the variable nature of IgG levels over time. While reflecting the "real world" application of IVIG (i.e., some patients clinically diagnosed with HGG based on two IgG levels in whom IVIG might be prescribed will go on to have IgG levels which are higher), it is possible that IgG levels > 500 mg/dl during the placebo period could have led to bias to the null, even though the study subjects had significantly higher levels of IgG at every time point during treatment with IVIG. Finally, one participant dropped out early in the first period, which could have reduced power as well.

In summary, monthly IVIG therapy did not reduce the incidence of bacterial or other infections compared to placebo over three months in stable adult lung transplant recipients with HGG. Our results do not support the routine clinical use of IVIG in patients with HGG after lung transplant. However, it is unknown whether IVIG may be effective for lung transplant recipients with HGG and repeated or refractory bacterial, fungal, or viral infections.

Author Contributions

Conceived and designed the experiments: DJL SMA SMK NP DR. Performed the experiments: DJL SMA SMK NP DR. Analyzed the data: DJL SMA SMK. Wrote the paper: DJL SMA SMK NP DR.

References

1. Kotloff RM, Thabut G (2011) Lung transplantation. Am J Respir Crit Care Med 184: 159–171.
2. Aguilar-Guisado M, Givalda J, Ussetti P, Ramos A, Morales P, et al. (2007) Pneumonia after lung transplantation in the RESITRA Cohort: a multicenter prospective study. Am J Transplant 7: 1989–1996.
3. de Bruyn G, Whelan TP, Mulligan MS, Raghu G, Limaye AP (2004) Invasive pneumococcal infections in adult lung transplant recipients. Am J Transplant 4: 1366–1371.
4. Husain S, Chan KM, Palmer SM, Hadjiliadis D, Humar A, et al. (2006) Bacteremia in lung transplant recipients in the current era. Am J Transplant 6: 3000–3007.
5. Remund KF, Best M, Egan JJ (2009) Infections relevant to lung transplantation. Proc Am Thorac Soc 6: 94–100.
6. Chambers DC, Davies B, Mathews A, Yerkovich ST, Hopkins PM (2013) Bronchiolitis obliterans syndrome, hypogammaglobulinemia, and infectious complications of lung transplantation. J Heart Lung Transplant 32: 36–43.
7. Yip NH, Lederer DJ, Kawut SM, Wilt JS, D'Ovidio F, et al. (2006) Immunoglobulin G levels before and after lung transplantation. Am J Respir Crit Care Med 173: 917–921.
8. Kawut SM, Shah L, Wilt JS, Dwyer E, Maani PA, et al. (2005) Risk factors and outcomes of hypogammaglobulinemia after lung transplantation. Transplantation 79: 1723–1726.
9. Goldfarb NS, Avery RK, Goormastic M, Mehta AC, Schilz R, et al. (2001) Hypogammaglobulinemia in lung transplant recipients. Transplantation 71: 242–246.
10. Florescu DF, Kalil AC, Qiu F, Schmidt CM, Sandkovsky U (2013) What is the impact of hypogammaglobulinemia on the rate of infections and survival in solid organ transplantation? A meta-analysis. Am J Transplant 13: 2601–2610.
11. Yamani MH, Avery RK, Mawhorter SD, Young JB, Ratliff NB, et al. (2001) Hypogammaglobulinemia following cardiac transplantation: a link between rejection and infection. J Heart Lung Transplant 20: 425–430.
12. Doron S, Ruthazer R, Werner BG, Rabson A, Snydman DR (2006) Hypogammaglobulinemia in liver transplant recipients: incidence, timing, risk factors, and outcomes. Transplantation 81: 697–703.
13. Fernandez-Ruiz M, Lopez-Medrano F, Varela-Pena P, Lora-Pablos D, Garcia-Reyne A, et al. (2012) Monitoring of immunoglobulin levels identifies kidney transplant recipients at high risk of infection. Am J Transplant 12: 2763–2773.
14. Orange JS, Hossny EM, Weiler CR, Ballow M, Berger M, et al. (2006) Use of intravenous immunoglobulin in human disease: a review of evidence by members of the Primary Immunodeficiency Committee of the American Academy of Allergy, Asthma and Immunology. J Allergy Clin Immunol 117: S525–553.
15. Food and Drug Administration. Guidance for Industry: Evaluating Clinical Studies of Antimicrobials in the Division of Anti-Infective Drug Products (draft 02/1997). Center for Drug Evaluation and Research (CDER). Rockville, MD. Available at the FDA website: Available: http://www.fda.gov/Drugs/GuidanceComplianceRegulatoryInformation/Guidances/ucm064980.htm. Accessed 2013 Sep 3.
16. Robertson J, Elidemir O, Saz EU, Gulen F, Schecter M, et al. (2009) Hypogammaglobulinemia: Incidence, risk factors, and outcomes following pediatric lung transplantation. Pediatric transplantation 13: 754–759.
17. Anonymous (1990) NIH consensus conference. Intravenous immunoglobulin. Prevention and treatment of disease. JAMA 264: 3189–3193.
18. Yamani MH, Avery R, Mawhorter SD, McNeill A, Cook D, et al. (2005) The impact of CytoGam on cardiac transplant recipients with moderate hypogammaglobulinemia: a randomized single-center study. J Heart Lung Transplant 24: 1766–1769.

21

Increased Iron Sequestration in Alveolar Macrophages in Chronic Obtructive Pulmonary Disease

Quentin Philippot[1,2], Gaëtan Deslée[2,3], Tracy L. Adair-Kirk[1], Jason C. Woods[4], Derek Byers[1], Susan Conradi[4], Sandra Dury[3,5], Jeanne Marie Perotin[2,3], François Lebargy[3,5], Christelle Cassan[5], Richard Le Naour[5], Michael J. Holtzman[1], Richard A. Pierce[1]*

1 Division of Pulmonary and Critical Care Medicine, Department of Internal Medicine Washington University, St. Louis, Missouri, United States of America, 2 Institut National de la Santé Et de la Recherche Medicale Unit 903, University Hospital, Reims, France, 3 Department of Pulmonary Medicine, University Hospital of Reims, France, 4 Department of Radiology, Washington University, St. Louis, Missouri, United States of America, 5 EA4683, University of Reims, Reims, France

Abstract

Free iron in lung can cause the generation of reactive oxygen species, an important factor in chronic obstructive pulmonary disease (COPD) pathogenesis. Iron accumulation has been implicated in oxidative stress in other diseases, such as Alzheimer's and Parkinson's diseases, but little is known about iron accumulation in COPD. We sought to determine if iron content and the expression of iron transport and/or storage genes in lung differ between controls and COPD subjects, and whether changes in these correlate with airway obstruction. Explanted lung tissue was obtained from transplant donors, GOLD 2–3 COPD subjects, and GOLD 4 lung transplant recipients, and bronchoalveolar lavage (BAL) cells were obtained from non-smokers, healthy smokers, and GOLD 1–3 COPD subjects. Iron-positive cells were quantified histologically, and the expression of iron uptake (transferrin and transferrin receptor), storage (ferritin) and export (ferroportin) genes was examined by real-time RT-PCR assay. Percentage of iron-positive cells and expression levels of iron metabolism genes were examined for correlations with airflow limitation indices (forced expiratory volume in the first second (FEV_1) and the ratio between FEV_1 and forced vital capacity (FEV_1/FVC)). The alveolar macrophage was identified as the predominant iron-positive cell type in lung tissues. Futhermore, the quantity of iron deposit and the percentage of iron positive macrophages were increased with COPD and emphysema severity. The mRNA expression of iron uptake and storage genes transferrin and ferritin were significantly increased in GOLD 4 COPD lungs compared to donors (6.9 and 3.22 fold increase, respectively). In BAL cells, the mRNA expression of transferrin, transferrin receptor and ferritin correlated with airway obstruction. These results support activation of an iron sequestration mechanism by alveolar macrophages in COPD, which we postulate is a protective mechanism against iron induced oxidative stress.

Editor: Rory E. Morty, University of Giessen Lung Center, Germany

Funding: This work was supported by NIH P50HL084922 (J.C.W., D.D., M.J.H., R.A.P.), the Alafi Neuroimaging Laboratory, the Hope Center for Neurological Disorders, and NIH Neuroscience Blueprint Center Core Grant P30 NS057105 to Washington University. The funders had no role in study design, data collection and analysis, decision to publish, or preparation of the manuscript.

Competing Interests: Dr. Holtzman has been the principal investigator for research grants from Hoffman-La Roche and Forest Labs to Washington University.

* E-mail: rpierce@dom.wustl.edu

Introduction

Iron is critical for the maintenance of cell homeostasis, having important roles in respiration, DNA synthesis, energy production, and metabolism. However, excess iron can be detrimental because of its potential to generate harmful free radicals. Because of this, tight regulation of iron metabolism is essential. Perturbation from normal physiologic iron concentrations has been associated with the pathogenesis of aging, neurodegenerative disease,and cancer [1,2], presumably via the generation of excess reactive oxygen species (ROS). The role of iron in other diseases in which oxidative stress has been implicated remains to be determined.

Chronic obstructive pulmonary disease (COPD), comprised of irreversible airways obstruction and alveolar space enlargement or emphysema, is a major cause of mortality and morbidity worldwide [3]. Cigarette smoke is the main etiological factor of COPD [3], which triggers an inflammatory response in the lung. Oxidative stress induced by the free radicals in tobacco smoke and produced by inflammatory cells has been strongly implicated in the pathogenesis of COPD. In addition, excess iron accumulation in the lung has been reported in association with cigarette smoke [4–6] and severe emphysema [7]. Moreover, cigarette smoke can alter lung iron metabolism in animal models [8]. However, it is unknown where iron accumulates in lungs of COPD subjects, if expression of iron uptake and storage genes in the lung differs between controls and subjects with COPD, and whether changes in iron metabolism correlate with disease severity.

This study sought to 1) quantify the iron deposits in the lung tissue of lung transplant donors, GOLD 2–3 (moderate to severe COPD), and GOLD 4 (very severe COPD) subjects, and in bronchoalveolar lavage (BAL) cells from smokers, non-smokers, and GOLD 1–3 COPD subjects, 2) identify the iron-accumulating cell types in the lung parenchyma, 3) determine the expression of transferrin and transferrin receptor (iron uptake), ferritin (iron storage) and ferroportin (iron export), and 4) determine correlations of changes in iron metabolism gene expression with airflow limitation indices (forced expiratory volume in the first second (FEV_1) and the ratio between FEV_1 and forced vital capacity (FEV_1/FVC)) which are indicative of COPD severity.

Materials and Methods

Ethics Statement

The lung parenchyma study was approved by the Human Studies Committee of Washington University and the broncho-alveolar lavage study was approved by the Institutional Review Board of the University Hospital of Reims.

Subjects, Lung Processing, Sampling, and Collection of BAL

Lung samples were obtained from 20 GOLD 4 COPD subjects receiving lung transplant, 9 GOLD 2–3 COPD subjects undergoing resection of lung cancer (avoiding areas affected by tumor), and 8 non-COPD lung donors obtained following size adjustment for transplantation as controls. The lungs were processed as previously described [9]. BAL samples were obtained from a second set of non-cancer, GOLD 1–3 COPD subjects, healthy smokers and healthy non smokers who underwent fiberoptic bronchoscopy according to American Thoracic Society recommendations [10–12]. Briefly, BAL was performed by instilling saline solution in a sub-segmental bronchus, followed by aspiration and discarding of the first 50 ml aliquot. The remaining BAL fluid was centrifuged and cells were used for this study. In both subject sets, COPD diagnosis and GOLD classification was based on spirometric pulmonary function tests according to the Global Initiative for Chronic Obstructive Lung Disease consensus statement[3], and informed, written consent was obtained from each subject.

Histochemical Staining

Ferric iron was detected on serial 5-μm paraformaldehyde-fixed, paraffin-embedded lung sections using Perls DAB staining. Briefly, slides were incubated for 30 min in 5% potassium ferrocyanide (Sigma-Aldrich, St. Louis, MO) and 5% hydrochloric acid, followed by a 15 min incubation in DAB (Peroxidase Substrate Kit; Vector Laboratories, Burlingame, CA). Negative control slides were incubated for 30 min in PBS and 15 min in DAB. Immunohistochemical staining for macrophages, transferrin or ferritin was performed using a Vectastain kit (Vector Laboratories; Burlingame, CA) using mouse anti-CD68 (1:100, KP1; Dako, Kyoto, Japan), rabbit anti-transferrin (1:30 000, A-0061; DakoCytomation, Carpinteria, CA), or anti-H-ferritin (1:2000, F-5012; Sigma) antibodies, respectively. Isotype-matched, nonimmune immunoglobulins served as negative controls.

Quantification and Identification of Iron-positive Cells

Lung sections were stained with Perls-DAB for iron content (brown-black color) and anti-CD68 (red color) to identify macrophages. Dark staining anthracotic material and macrophages with dark-colored content were assessed on a consecutive serial section stained with nuclear fast red only (American Master Tech Scientific Inc., St. Lodi, CA). Slides were scanned using a NanoZoomer 2.0 (Hamamatsu Photonics, K.K., Japan) and the staining was quantified using Image-Pro Plus Software (Media-Cybernetics, Silver Spring, MD). The area of cells positive for iron was calculated using the following formula: *Iron positive cell area = (Area of brown-black color on Perls-DABstained slide − Area of brown-black color on the nuclear fast red slide)/(Area of pink color on the nuclear fast red slide) x 100*. The percentage of iron-positive macrophages was

determined on Perls-DAB-CD68 co-stained slides from 3 randomly selected 10x fields containing ≥ 10 macrophages per field.

RNA Isolation and Quantitative Real-time RT-PCR

Total RNA was isolated from human donor and GOLD 4 COPD lung tissue samples, and BAL cells using TRIzol reagent (Invitrogen, Carlsbad, CA). Quantitative Real-Time RT-PCR was performed as follow: the cDNA was synthesized using SuperScript II reverse transcriptase (Invitrogen). Real-time RT-PCR employed the Fast SYBR Green Master Mix (Applied Biosystems, Foster City, CA) and gene-specific primers (Table S1) on an Eco™ Real-Time PCR System (Illumina, San Diego, CA).Results were standardized using the delta-delta C_T method [13] using the average of the expression GAPDH, HRPT1 (Hypoxanthine phosphoribosyltransferase-1) and PPIA (Peptidylprolyl isomerase-1) for normalization [14,15].

Morphological Analysis

For 14 GOLD 4 COPD and 4 non-COPD subjects, CT-scan of the frozen lungs was performed, and analyzed as previously described [9]. Briefly, the mean radiograph attenuation, expressed in Hounsfield Units (HU), was determined in the CT section corresponding to the lung area of the tissue samples using a separate image processing program (ImageJ; available at: http://rsb.info.nih. gov/ij).

Statistical Analysis

A Student's t test was used to compare between two groups, an Anova analysis with a Tukey-Kramer post-hoc test was used to compare between more than two groups and Spearman rank correlation was used to test for correlations between variables with a $p \leq 0.05$ considered significant.Statistical analysis was performed using Excel 2011 (Microsoft Corporation, Redmond, WA).

Results

Patient Characteristics

Peripheral lung tissue was obtained from 20 GOLD 4 COPD subjects receiving lung transplants for severe emphysema (GOLD 4), 9 GOLD 2–3 COPD subjects undergoing resection of lung cancer (avoiding areas affected by tumor), and 8 non-COPD donor lungs as controls. Their clinical and demographic characteristics are displayed in Table 1. As expected, the donor group consisted of younger, non-smokerssubjects. Pulmonary function tests were not obtained from donors.

In addition to lung tissue samples, BAL cells were obtained from another set of subjects: 8 healthy non-smokers, 8 healthy smokers, and 10 GOLD 1–3 COPD subjects. Their clinical and demographic information are presented in Table 2. As expected, subjects with COPD had increased airflow limitation compared to the healthy non-smokers and the healthy smokers groups. The BAL differentials are also presented in Table 2. The total number of inflammatory cells in the BAL fluid of smokers and COPD subjects were higher than non-smokers. However, in each group the predominant cell type (almost 90%) in the BAL were macrophages.

Increased Iron Deposition in Severe COPD Lungs

Iron accumulation in the lung was examined in 20 GOLD 4 COPD, 9 GOLD 2–3 COPD, and 8 non-COPD lungs by Perls-DAB staining. To distinguish between iron deposits and other dark anthracotic material, consecutive serial sections were stained with nuclear fast red only. To quantify the iron deposits, we calculated

Table 1. Clinical characteristics of subjects included in lung parenchyma study.

Characteristic	Donor	GOLD 2–3 COPD	GOLD 4 COPD
No. of subjects	8	9	20
Age	42±18	62±11*	59±6*
Sex, M/F	4/3 (7/8)	4/5	7/14
Smoking Pack-years	0±0	41±31	55±27
FEV1 (% of predicted)	-	62±17	18±4#
FEV1:FVC	-	57±15	31±9#
BMI (kg/m²)	-	28±5	23±3#

*$p<0.05$ between donor and spirometric GOLD 2–3 or GOLD 4 COPD,
#$p<0.05$ between spirometric GOLD 2–3 and GOLD 4 COPD.

the iron-positive cell area by taking the area of brown-black color on Perls-DAB stained slide minus the area of brown-black color on the nuclear fast red stained slide divided by the area of pink color on the nuclear fast red slide. Iron deposits were rarely found in non-COPD lung parenchyma (Fig. 1A) but were detectable in the parenchyma of GOLD 2–3 COPD lungs and appeared abundant in GOLD 4 COPD lungs (Fig. 1B and 1C, respectively). The iron positive cell area was significantly increased in severe GOLD 4 COPD lungs ($23\pm16\%$) compared to non-COPD ($1.1\pm1.5\%$, $p=1.9\times10^{-5}$) or GOLD 2–3 COPD ($1.6\pm1.5\%$, $p=1.9\times10^{-5}$) lungs (Fig. 1D). Moreover, iron positive cell area was found to correlate with the mean radiograph attenuation at the level of the lung tissue sample which is an index of emphysema severity (Fig. 1E). Our data suggest that excess iron accumulation is also

associated with COPD and emphysema severity, with an increase in lung iron content in GOLD 4 COPD relative to GOLD 2–3 COPD subjects despite similar smoking pack years.

Iron is Localized in Macrophages in COPD Lungs

To quantify the prevalence of iron-positive macrophages, we performed co-staining of Perls-DAB and CD68 in lung sections. As shown in Figure 2B/B' and 2C/C', iron co-localized with macrophages in GOLD 2–3 and GOLD 4 COPD lungs, respectively, but not in non-COPD lungs (Fig. 2A/A'). The percentage of iron-positive macrophages was increased in GOLD 2–3 COPD lungs ($26\% \pm19$, $p=6.1\times10^{-12}$) and GOLD 4 COPD lungs ($68\pm16\%$, $p=6.1\times10^{-12}$) compared to non-COPD lungs ($3.5\pm2.8\%$). Interestingly, the persentage of iron-positive

Table 2. Clinical characteristics of subjects included in BAL study.

Characteristic	Non Smokers	Smokers	GOLD 1–3 COPD
No. of subjects	8	8	10
Age	54±15	45±11	57±7
Sex, M/F	5/3	4/4	8/2
Smoking Pack-years	0±0	39±16*	45±13*
FEV₁ (% of predicted)	96±13	87±5	65±16#
FEV₁/FVC (%)	81±6	78±9	62±9#
BMI (kg/m²)	27±3	27±10	26±5
Treatments (% of patient using the treatment):			
Inhaled LABA	1/8	0/8	5/10
Inhaled SABA	0/8	0/8	1/10
Inhaled LAMA	0/8	0/8	3/10
Inhaled CS	1/8	0/8	4/10
Oral CS	0/8	0/8	1/10
Cellular content of BAL			
Macrophages (%)	87±6	86±9	90±5
Lymphocytes (%)	10±6	7±6	6±3
Neutrophils (%)	2±2	7±8	4±4
Eosinophils (%)	1±2	0±0	0±1
Total cell number per ml	177 571	412 875	237 000

*$p<0.05$ between smokers or COPD and non smokers,
#$p<0.05$ between non smokers or smokers and COPD, LABA = Long-Acting β-Agonists, SABA: Short-Acting β-Agonists., LAMA: Loan-acting muscarinic antagonists, CS: corticosteroids.

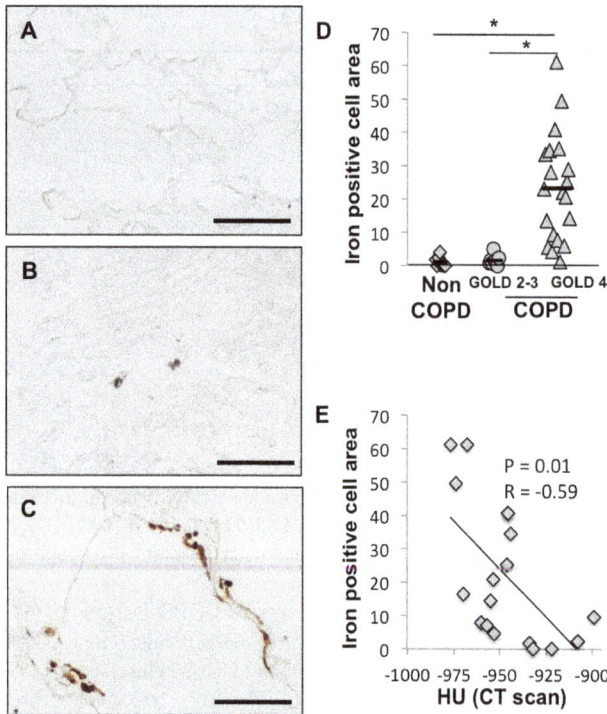

Figure 1. Iron deposits are increased in lungs of COPD subjects. Iron deposits were stained with Perls-DAB staining in lung samples obtained from (A) a patient without COPD, (B) a patient with GOLD 2 COPD and (C) a patient with GOLD 4 COPD. (D) Quantification of iron positive cellular area was performed on lung sections from 8 subjects without COPD, 9 subjects with GOLD 2 or 3 COPD and 20 subjects with GOLD 4 COPD. (E) Correlation between the iron deposits and the mean radiograph attenuation in the same lung area. *p<0.05 (Anova analysis with a Tukey-Kramer post-hoc test); Scale bars = 125 μm.

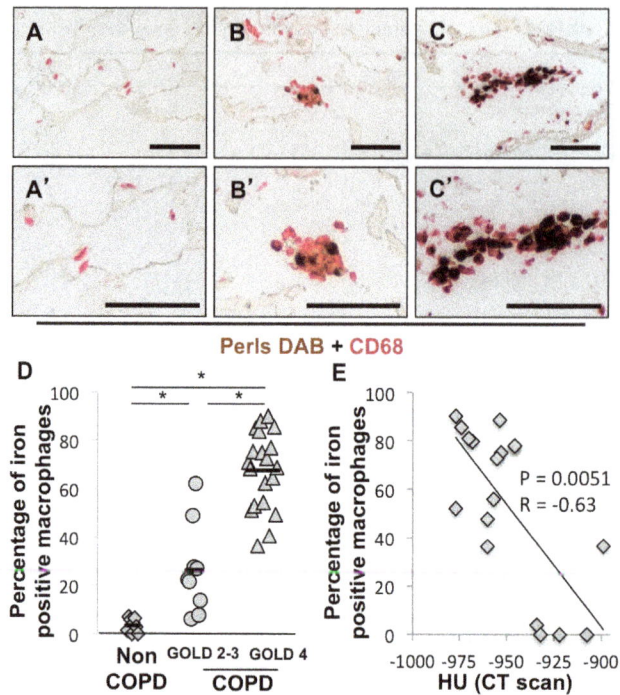

Figure 2. Iron is localized in macrophages in lung of COPD subjects and the percentage of iron positive macrophage increases with severity of disease. Perls-DAB and CD68 costaining was performed in lung samples obtained from (A–A') a patient without COPD, (B–B') a patient with grade 2 COPD and (C–C') a patient with grade 4 COPD. (D) Percentage of iron positive macrophages was assessed in 8 lungs from subjects without COPD, 9 lungs from subjects with GOLD 2 or 3 COPD and lungs from 20 subjects with GOLD 4 COPD. (E) Correlation between the percentage of iron positive macrophages and the mean radiograph attenuation in the same lung area. *p<0.05 (Anova analysis with a Tukey-Kramer post-hoc test); Scale bars = 125 μm.

macrophages correlated with the mean radiograph attenuation of the lung tissue sample (Fig. 2E). These data suggest that the percentage of iron-positive macrophage increases with the severity of COPD and emphysema.

Increased Expression of Iron Uptake Genes in COPD Lungs

Iron metabolism needs to be tightly regulated due to potential harmful effects of excess free iron. Free iron is bound by transferrin, taken into cells by the transferrin receptor, and is stored in cells bound to ferritin. Iron can be exported from cells via ferroportin. The expression of these genes is tightly regulated via the iron-responsive proteins (IREBs), which are able to interact with 5′ or 3′ untranslated region of their mRNA [16]. Among the two orthologous, IREB 2 has been associated with airflow limitation in GWA studies [17–19].

To determine wether the increased iron accumulation in COPD alveolar macrophages was a result of an increase in the expression of mRNAs encoding iron uptake proteins, we assessed the expression of transferrin and the transferrin receptor by real-time RT-PCR using RNA from 8 non-COPD lungsamples and 16 GOLD 4 COPD lungsamples. Transferrin expression was significantly increased in GOLD 4 COPD lungs compared to non-COPD lungs (fold increase = 6.9, p = 5.4×10^{-6}, Fig. 3A). There was no significant difference in the expression of transferrin

receptor between GOLD 4 COPD lungs and non-COPD lungs (Fig. 3B).

To determine which cells in the lungs expressed transferrin and whether the expression of transferrin was associated with iron deposition, lung sections of non-COPD and GOLD 4 COPD subjects were co-stained for Perls-DAB and transferrin. Non-COPD lungs showed scant staining for transferrin, localized mainly to alveolar macrophages based on location and cell morphology (Fig. 3C). However, in GOLD 4 COPD lungs, the majority of the transferrin-positive cells were parenchymal cells, and not the iron-positive alveolar macrophages (Fig. 3D).

Together, these data suggest that iron-uptake gene expression is increased in severe COPD lungs compared to non-COPD lungs, but the iron-binding protein transferrin is not expressed by the macrophages which accumulate the iron.

Expression of Iron Retention and Homeostasis Genes in COPD Lungs

Net iron accumulation could also be caused by an increase in cellular iron retention and/or a decrease in iron export. Accordingly, we examined the expression of genes related to iron retention and export, ferritin and ferroportin, respectively, by real-time RT-PCR using RNA from 8 non-COPD lung samples and 16 GOLD 4 COPD lung samples. Ferritin mRNA expression was significantly increased in GOLD 4 COPD lungs compared to non-

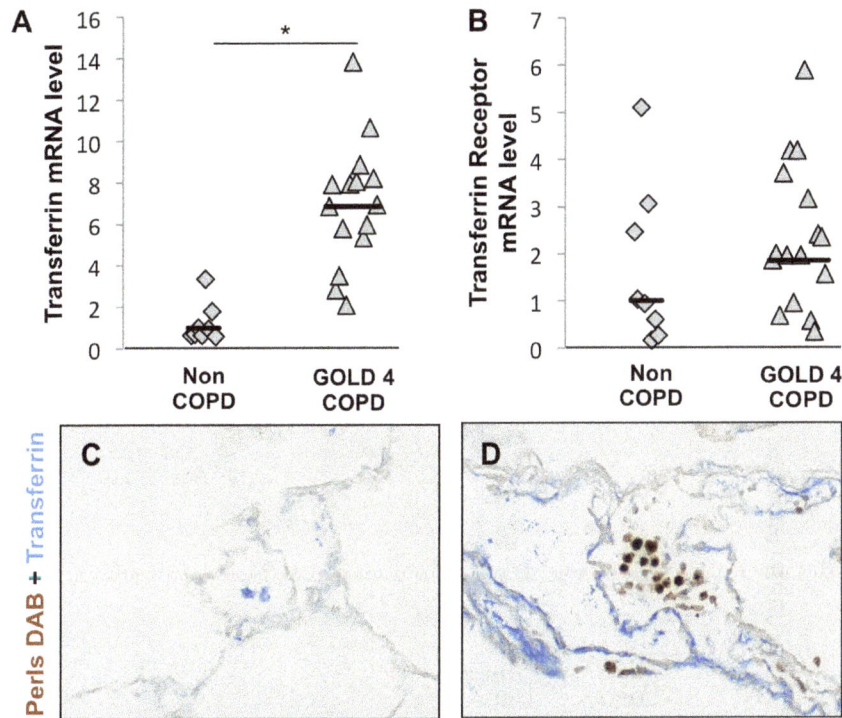

Figure 3. Iron uptake capacities are altered in lungs of COPD subjects. mRNA expression of (A) transferrin and (B) transferrin receptor was investigated in whole-lung total RNA samples obtained from 8 subjects without COPD and 16 subjects with GOLD 4 COPD. Three reference genes (GAPDH, HPRT1 and PPIA) were used for normalization. Costaining for transferrin and iron deposits, by Perls-DAB staining, was performed on lung samples obtained from (C) a subject without COPD and (D) a subject with GOLD 4 COPD. *p<0.05 (Student's t test), Scale bars = 125 μm.

COPD lungs (fold increase = 3.22, p = 0.031, Fig. 4A), while the expression of ferroportin mRNA was unchanged (Fig. 4D). Consistent with the increased intracellular retention of iron in macrophages in COPD lungs, increased ferritin staining in COPD lungs (Fig. 4B) compared to non-COPD lungs (Fig. 4C) localized to alveolar macrophages. IREB2 mRNA expression was signifcantly higher in GOLD4-COPD than in non-COPD (fold increase = 1.6, p = 0.045, Fig. 4E).

We also looked for a correlation between the expression of these iron metabolism related genes and the emphysema severity. We did not find any statistically signficant correlation betwen the expression of these genes and the mean radiograph attenuation of the lung tissue (Table S2).

To determine whether iron deposits and ferritin were present in the same macrophages in COPD lungs, we performed CD68/Perls-DAB and CD68/ferritin co-staining on consecutive GOLD 4 COPD lung sections (Fig. 5). Iron-positive macrophages exhibited strong ferritin staining (arrows). Inversely, iron-negative macrophages did not have any ferritin staining (within circle).

These data suggest that the iron accumulation in alveolar macrophages in severe COPD lungs may, at least in part, be due to an increase in cellular iron retention mechanisms.

Expression of Iron Metabolism Genes in GOLD 1–3 COPD BAL Cells

The data presented in Figures 3 and 4 were obtained using mRNA from whole lung tissue samples. To better understand iron accumulationin alveolar macrophages of severe COPD lungs, we investigated the expression of iron metabolism genes in BAL cells (Fig. 6). By cytological analysis, nearly 90% of cells in the BAL fluid were macrophages (Table 2). Therefore, the data obtained

from these studies may largely reflect gene expression by macrophages.

Compared to non-smokers, transferrin expression by BAL cells from non-COPD smokers and COPD subjects was significantly decreased (fold increase = 0.52 and 0.13 repectively, $p = 5.7 \times 10^{-4}$, Fig. 6A). In contrast, the transferrin receptor was more highly expressed in BAL cells from COPD subjects compared to non-smokers or non-COPD smokers (fold increase = 11 or 14 respectively, $p = 6.7 \times 10^{-3}$, Fig. 6B). When investigating mechanisms of iron retention, we found a significantly higher expression of ferritin by BAL cells from COPD subjects compared to non-smokers (fold increase = 23, p = 0.028, Fig. 6C). Interestingly, whereas ferroportin expression appeared to be similar between BAL cells from non-smokers and COPD subjects, its expression was significantly higher in BAL cells from non-COPD smokers than in the COPDsubjects (fold increase = 7.5, p = 0.028, Fig. 6D). IREB2 expression did not differ between the COPD and the other groups (Fig. 6E). These data support those presented above and show that the expression of iron metabolism genes is altered in alveolar macrophages from COPD patients compared to non-COPD patients which could result in the increased iron accumulation.

Iron Metabolism Gene Expression in BAL Cells Correlates with Airflow Limitation

Next, we investigated correlations between expression of genes related to iron metabolism by BAL cells and airflow limitation indices (Fig. 7). Expression of transferrin positively correlated with both $FEV_1$and the ratio FEV_1/FVC (Fig. 7 A and F). Inversely, expression of the transferrin receptor and ferritin negatively correlated with airflow limitation (Fig. 7 B–G and C–H). Finally,

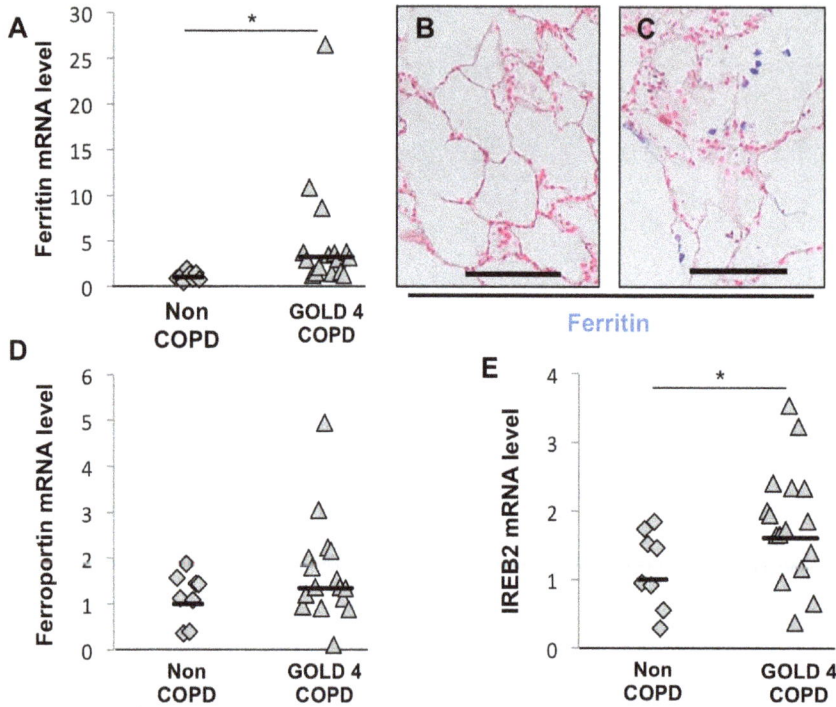

Figure 4. Iron storage capacities are altered in lungs of COPD subjects. mRNA expression of (A) ferritin, (D) ferroportin and (E) IREB2 was investigated in whole-lung total RNA samples obtained from 8 subjects without COPD and 16 subjects with GOLD 4 COPD.Three reference genes (GAPDH, HPRT1 and PPIA) were used for normalization. Immunohistochemistry study of ferritin, with nuclear fast red counterstaining, in lung samples obtained from (B) a subject without COPD and (C) a subject with GOLD 4 COPD. *p<0.05 (Student's t test), Scale bars = 125 µm.

the expression of ferroportin and IREB2 did not significantly correlate with the airflow limitation. Interestingly, expression of these iron related genes did not correlate with hemoglobin or CRP serum concentration. IREB2 expression only correlated with subject age (Table S3). Similarly, expression of studied iron related

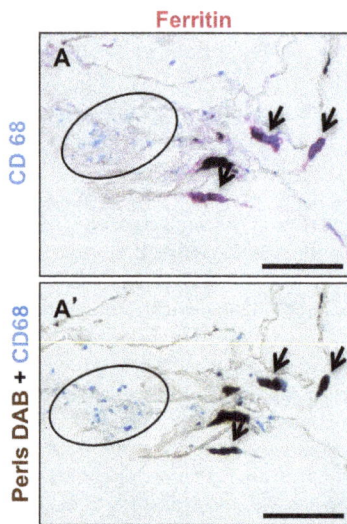

Figure 5. Iron deposits and ferritin staining are colocalized in the same subset of macrophages (A) Costaining for ferritin and CD68 and (A') with Perls-DAB and CD68 in two adjacent lung sections from a GOLD 4 COPD patient. The arrows show iron and ferritin positive macrophages, inside circles are iron and ferritin negative macrophages. Scale bars = 125 µm.

genes was not influenced by the subject sex or the presence of chronic bronchitis (Table S4). The expression of some iron metabolism related genes were associated with dyspnea severity (transferrin), exacerbation rate (transferrin and ferritin) (Table S4) and smoking history including smoking pack-year (transferrin and ferritin) (Table S3) and smoking status (transferrin, ferritin and ferroportin) (Table S5). Finally, in the COPD patients, no relation was found between the presence of an inhaled treatment and the expression of iron metabolism related genes (data not shown).

Globally, these data demonstrate that changes in macrophage expression of iron metabolism genes correlate with airflow limitation and COPD severity.

Discussion

The main findings of this study are that: 1) iron deposits are localized in macrophages in COPD lungs; 2) the quantity of lung iron deposits increases with COPD and emphysema severity; 3) expression of transferrin (involved in iron uptake), and of ferritin (involved in iron storage), are increased in severe COPD lungs whereas ferroportin (involved in cellular excretion of iron) is unchanged; 4) in BAL cells from COPD subjects at GOLD stage 1–3, expression of transferrin receptor and ferritin expression are increased, and 5) indices of airflow limitation correlate with expression of transferrin, transferrin receptor and ferritin in BAL cells from healthy non smokers and smokers, and COPD subjects.

Consistent with our results, iron accumulation has been reported in the lungs of cigarette smokers [4–6] and in severe emphysema [7] but the mechanisms sustaining the iron accumulation in lungs from COPD patients have never been explored. Iron uptake, storage and sequestration are of interest in COPD. Indeed in other diseases associated with aging, including

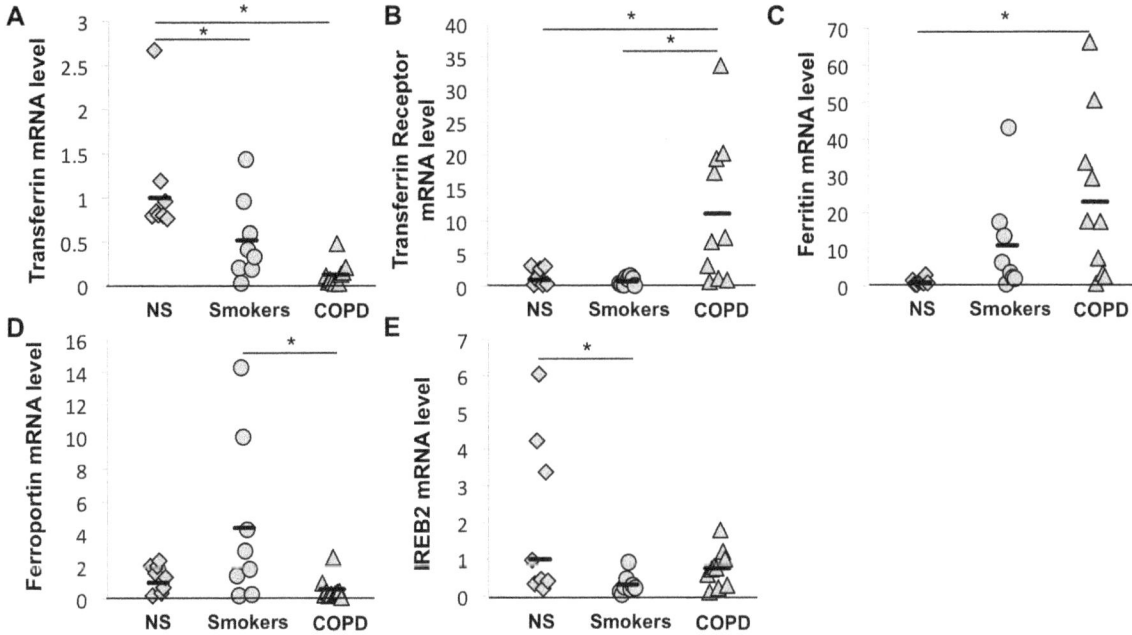

Figure 6. Expression of proteins involved in iron metabolism is altered in BAL cells obtained in subjects with COPD. Expression of proteins involved in iron metabolism in BAL cells collected in 8 non smokers without COPD, 8 smokers without COPD and 10 GOLD 1–3 COPD subjects was examined by RT-PCR.Three reference genes (GAPDH, HPRT1 and PPIA) were used for normalization. *p<0.05 (Anova analysis with a Tukey-Kramer post-hoc test), NS: non smokers.

atherosclerosis, Parkinson's and Alzheimer's, iron depositions are postulated to contribute to excess oxidative stress [2], which is now recognized as important in the pathogenesis of COPD [20,21].

Moreover, free iron acumulation in the lung may promote bacterial growth and influence COPD exacerbation. Therefore,

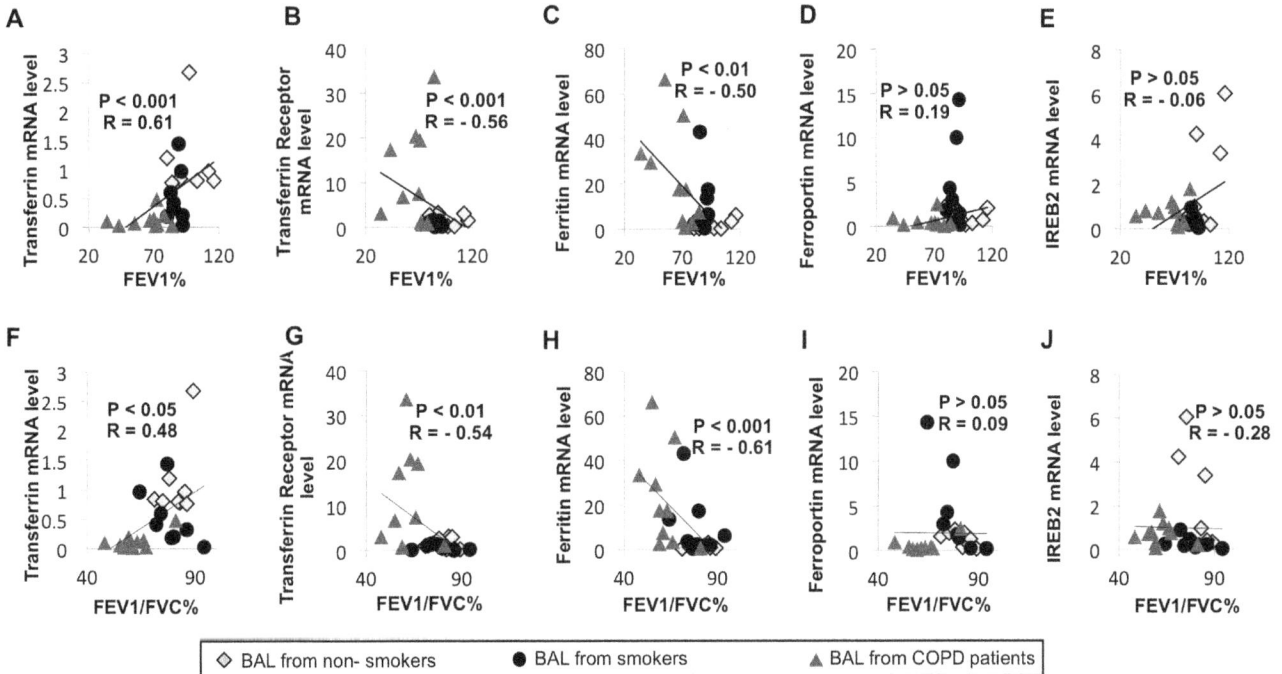

Figure 7. In BAL cells, expression of proteins involved in iron metabolism correlate with airflow limitation. (A–J) Correlation between the expression of genes encoding proteins involved in iron metabolism in BAL cells, as determined by RT-PCR, and airflow limitation was assessed in 8 non smokers without COPD, 8 smokers without COPD and 10 GOLD 1–3 COPD subjects.Three reference genes (GAPDH, HPRT1 and PPIA) were used for normalization. (Spearman rank correlation).

the free iron pool has to be tightly controlled to protect the lung against the harmful properties of iron.

Iron bound by transferrin is taken up into cells by the transferrin receptor, and is stored in cells bound to ferritin. Compared to control lungs, higher transferrin and ferritin expression was found in COPD lungs, and transferrin receptor was higher in BAL from COPD subjects than in healthy subjects. Further, the expression of ferroportin, the only known iron exporter, was unchanged with COPD. These findings support active iron sequestration by alveolar macrophages in COPD lungs, and may represent a protective maneuver intended to control free iron, and therefore, perverse effects of iron. In fact, O. Olakanmi et al have reported that iron sequestration by alveolar macrophages decresease the formation of the highly toxic hydroxyl radical [22] and more recently, it has been shown that iron sequestration by macrophages protects A549 cells against iron toxicity [23]. Consistent with these resluts, we did not find a spatial relationship between the accumulation of 8-hydroxyguanosine, a marker of nucleic acids oxidation, and iron staining in COPD lung specimens in this study (data not shown). While not conclusive, this suggests at least that iron accumulation process in alveolar macrophages does not contribute locally to increased oxidative stress and may even decrease iron induced oxidative stress. Interestingly, current cigarette smoke exposure was not found necessary to alter iron metabolism. Indeed, GOLD 4 COPD subjects in this study had ceased cigarette smoking for at least 6 months prior to transplant and processing of their lung tissue.

The clinical relevance of these findings is supported by the correlations between expression levels of several iron pathway mRNAs in BAL cells and indices of airflow limitation in this study. Ferritin and transferrin receptor expression were increased in COPD subjects and correlated with a decrease in FEV_1 or FEV_1/FVC ratio. IREB2 expression tended to be higher in BAL of COPD subjects and correlated negatively with FEV_1/FVC ratio, supporting a shift in iron metabolism in macrophages in COPD. These studies were limited to smokers, former smokers, and GOLD 2 and -3 COPD subjects, as there is high risk in obtaining BAL from GOLD 4 COPD subjects. Another aspect of the study which may be a limitation is that distinct study sets were employed for the tissue-based and BAL-based experiments. Alternatively, that iron metabolism was altered in separate cohorts of subjects may lend greater weight to the findings. Altering lung iron uptake in macrophages during cigarette smoke exposure in animal model could be employed to test whether this impacts overall lung oxidative stress and the progression of alveolar enlargement. In vitro studies in macrophages could further test the relationships between cigarette smoke exposure, free iron, iron sequestration, ROS generation and oxidative stress.

Overall this study demonstrates that macrophages in the lungs of COPD subjects have increased iron uptake and storage, likely through increased expression of transferrin, transferrin receptor and ferritin, while ferroportin expression is unchanged. This should result in a net gain in iron sequestration in COPD lung macrophages, which we postulate is a protective mechanism intended to reduce free iron and its harmful effects. Similar to the robust anti-oxiodant response reported in COPD lungs [21], it seems likely that iron sequestration may be a mechanism that is intended to limit, but fails to eliminate, progression of COPD. Further investigations are needed to elucidate the contribution of iron sequestration in alveolar macrophages in the complex pathophysiology of COPD.

Supporting Information

Table S1 Sequence of primer pairs used in our RT-PCR reactions.

Table S2 Lack of relationship between subject lung density in CT Hounsfield units and iron metabolism gene expression.

Table S3 Relationships between expression of iron metabolism-related mRNAs age, smoking pack years, and KCO, but not serum variables.

Table S4 Lack of relationship between expression of iron metabolism-related mRNAs and subject gender, dyspnea. Transferrin correlate with the presence of chronic bronchitis. Transferrin and ferritin are correlated with the presence of exacerbations.

Table S5 Expression of transferrin, ferritin and IREB2 are impacted by smoking status.

Acknowledgments

This work was supported by NIH P50HL084922 (J.C.W., D.D., M.J.H., R.A.P.), the Alafi Neuroimaging Laboratory, the Hope Center for Neurological Disorders, and NIH Neuroscience Blueprint Center Core Grant P30 NS057105 to Washington University.

Author Contributions

Performed the experiments: QP TAK. Analyzed the data: QP GD TAK RAP. Contributed reagents/materials/analysis tools: GD JCW DB SC SD FL CC RLN JMP RAP. Wrote the paper: QP GD TAK MJH RAP.

References

1. Jomova K, Valko M (2011) Advances in metal-induced oxidative stress and human disease. Toxicology 283: 65–87. doi:10.1016/j.tox.2011.03.001.

2. Altamura S, Muckenthaler MU (2009) Iron Toxicity in Diseases of Aging: Alzheimer's Disease, Parkinson's Disease and Atherosclerosis. J Alzheimers Dis 16: 879–895. doi:10.3233/JAD-2009-1010.

3. Vestbo J, Hurd SS, Agustí AG, Jones PW, Vogelmeier C, et al. (2013) Global Strategy for the Diagnosis, Management, and Prevention of Chronic Obstructive Pulmonary Disease. Am J Respir Crit Care Med 187: 347–365. doi:10.1164/rccm.201204-0596PP.

4. Thompson AB, Bohling T, Heires A, Linder J, Rennard SI (1991) Lower respiratory tract iron burden is increased in association with cigarette smoking. J Lab Clin Med 117: 493–499.

5. Nelson ME, O'Brien-Ladner AR, Wesselius LJ (1996) Regional variation in iron and iron-binding proteins within the lungs of smokers. Am J Respir Crit Care Med 153: 1353–1358. doi:10.1164/ajrccm.153.4.8616566.

6. Wesselius LJ, Nelson ME, Skikne BS (1994) Increased release of ferritin and iron by iron-loaded alveolar macrophages in cigarette smokers. Am J Respir Crit Care Med 150: 690–695. doi:10.1164/ajrccm.150.3.8087339.

7. Takemoto K, Kawai H, Kuwahara T, Nishina M, Adachi S (1991) Metal concentrations in human lung tissue, with special reference to age, sex, cause of death, emphysema and contamination of lung tissue. Int Arch Occup Environ Health 62: 579–586.

8. Ghio AJ, Hilborn ED, Stonehuerner JG, Dailey LA, Carter JD, et al. (2008) Particulate Matter in Cigarette Smoke Alters Iron Homeostasis to Produce a Biological Effect. Am J Respir Crit Care Med 178: 1130–1138. doi:10.1164/rccm.200802-334OC.

9. Deslee G, Woods JC, Moore C, Conradi SH, Gierada DS, et al. (2009) OXidative damage to nucleic acids in severe emphysema. CHEST J 135: 965–974. doi:10.1378/chest.08-2257.

10. Workshop summary and guidelines: Investigative use of bronchoscopy, lavage, and bronchial biopsies in asthma and other airway diseases (1991). J Allergy Clin Immunol 88: 808–814. doi:10.1016/0091-6749(91)90189-U.

11. Tanino M, Betsuyaku T, Takeyabu K, Tanino Y, Yamaguchi E, et al. (2002) Increased levels of interleukin-8 in BAL fluid from smokers susceptible to pulmonary emphysema. Thorax 57: 405–411. doi:10.1136/thorax.57.5.405.

12. Hattotuwa K, Gamble EA, O'Shaughnessy T, Jeffery PK, Barnes NC (2002) SAfety of bronchoscopy, biopsy, and bal in research patients with copd*. CHEST J 122: 1909–1912. doi:10.1378/chest.122.6.1909.

13. Livak KJ, Schmittgen TD (2001) Analysis of Relative Gene Expression Data Using Real-Time Quantitative PCR and the $2-\Delta\Delta CT$ Method. Methods 25: 402–408. doi:10.1006/meth.2001.1262.

14. Vandesompele J, De Preter K, Pattyn F, Poppe B, Van Roy N, et al. (2002) Accurate normalization of real-time quantitative RT-PCR data by geometric averaging of multiple internal control genes. Genome Biol 3: RESEARCH0034.

15. Glynos C, Dupont LL, Vassilakopoulos T, Papapetropoulos A, Brouckaert P, et al. (2013) The role of soluble guanylyl cyclase in chronic obstructive pulmonary disease. Am J Respir Crit Care Med 188: 789–799. doi:10.1164/rccm.201210-1884OC.

16. Wang J, Pantopoulos K (2011) Regulation of cellular iron metabolism. Biochem J 434: 365–381. doi:10.1042/BJ20101825.

17. Hardin M, Zielinski J, Wan ES, Hersh CP, Castaldi PJ, et al. (2012) CHRNA3/5, IREB2, and ADCY2 Are Associated with Severe Chronic Obstructive Pulmonary Disease in Poland. Am J Respir Cell Mol Biol 47: 203–208. doi:10.1165/rcmb.2012-0011OC.

18. Kim WJ, Wood AM, Barker AF, Brantly ML, Campbell EJ, et al. (2012) Association of IREB2 and CHRNA3 polymorphisms with airflow obstruction in severe alpha-1 antitrypsin deficiency. Respir Res 13: 16. doi:10.1186/1465-9921-13-16.

19. DeMeo DL, Mariani T, Bhattacharya S, Srisuma S, Lange C, et al. (2009) Integration of Genomic and Genetic Approaches Implicates IREB2 as a COPD Susceptibility Gene. Am J Hum Genet 85: 493–502. doi:10.1016/j.ajhg.2009.09.004.

20. Barnes PJ, Shapiro SD, Pauwels RA (2003) Chronic obstructive pulmonary disease: molecular and cellularmechanisms. Eur Respir J 22: 672–688. doi:10.1183/09031936.03.00040703.

21. Rahman I (2005) Oxidative stress in pathogenesis of chronic obstructive pulmonary disease. Cell Biochem Biophys 43: 167–188. doi:10.1385/CBB:43: 1: 167.

22. Olakanmi O, McGowan SE, Hayek MB, Britigan BE (1993) Iron sequestration by macrophages decreases the potential for extracellular hydroxyl radical formation. J Clin Invest 91: 889–899. doi:10.1172/JCI116310.

23. Persson HL, Vainikka LK, Eriksson I, Wennerström U (2013) TNF-α-stimulated macrophages protect A549 lung cells against iron and oxidation. Exp Toxicol Pathol 65: 81–89. doi:10.1016/j.etp.2011.06.004.

22

Expression of Calcineurin Activity after Lung Transplantation: A 2-Year Follow-Up

Sylvia Sanquer[1]*, Catherine Amrein[2], Dominique Grenet[3], Romain Guillemain[2], Bruno Philippe[3], Veronique Boussaud[2], Laurence Herry[1], Celine Lena[1], Alphonsine Diouf[1], Michelle Paunet[4], Eliane M. Billaud[5], Françoise Loriaux[6], Jean-Philippe Jais[7], Robert Barouki[1], Marc Stern[3]

1 Service de Biochimie Métabolomique et Protéomique, Hôpital Universitaire Necker-Enfants Malades Assistance Publique-Hôpitaux de Paris (AP-HP); INSERM UMR-S 747; and Université Paris Descartes, Centre Universitaire des Saints-Pères, Paris, France, 2 Service de Chirurgie Cardio-Vasculaire, Hôpital Européen Georges Pompidou, AP-HP, Paris, France, 3 Service de Pneumologie, Hôpital Foch, Suresnes, France, 4 Laboratoire de Biologie, Hôpital Foch, Suresnes, France, 5 Service de Pharmacologie, Hôpital Européen Georges Pompidou, AP-HP and Université Paris Descartes, Paris, France, 6 Service de Biochimie, Hôpital Européen Georges Pompidou, AP-HP, Paris, France, 7 Service de Biostatistiques, Hôpital Necker-Enfants Malades, AP-HP, Paris, France; Université Paris Descartes, Paris, France

Abstract

The objective of this pharmacodynamic study was to longitudinally assess the activity of calcineurin during the first 2 years after lung transplantation. From March 2004 to October 2008, 107 patients were prospectively enrolled and their follow-up was performed until 2009. Calcineurin activity was measured in peripheral blood mononuclear cells. We report that calcineurin activity was linked to both acute and chronic rejection. An optimal activity for calcineurin with two thresholds was defined, and we found that the risk of rejection was higher when the enzyme activity was above the upper threshold of 102 pmol/mg/min or below the lower threshold of 12 pmol/mg/min. In addition, we report that the occurrence of malignancies and viral infections was significantly higher in patients displaying very low levels of calcineurin activity. Taken together, these findings suggest that the measurement of calcineurin activity may provide useful information for the management of the prevention therapy of patients receiving lung transplantation.

Editor: Aric Gregson, University of California Los Angeles, United States of America

Funding: Funding for this study was provided by the French association Vaincre la Mucoviscidose. The funders had no role in study design, data collection and analysis, decision to publish, or preparation of the manuscript.

Competing Interests: The authors have declared that no competing interests exist.

* E-mail: sylvia.sanquer@gmail.com

Introduction

Organ transplantation is the last alternative therapeutic option for selected patients with end-stage disease of a given organ. The survival of transplanted organs has markedly improved over the past few decades due to the use of immunosuppressive treatments. However, organ survival remains limited by the onset of chronic rejection and devastating adverse drug events. This is particularly true with lung transplantation. Despite increasing improvement in patient care, lung transplantation has the poorest outcomes mainly because of the development of chronic rejection in response to immunologic, ischemic and infectious injury [1–8]. Chronic rejection, which presents as a bronchiolitis obliterans syndrome (BOS), is defined as a progressive airflow obstruction and a deterioration of graft function. It accounts for more than 30% of all mortality after the third year following lung transplantation [8,9]. Moreover, by promoting factor perivascular and peribronchial infiltration of activated lymphocytes into graft tissue, acute rejection remains an important risk factor for the development of BOS [10].

The standard for rejection prevention in lung transplantation consists of an immunosuppressive regimen which includes a calcineurin (CN) inhibitor (CNI) such as cyclosporine (CsA) and tacrolimus [11]. The CNI prophylactic dose is adjusted according to the whole blood concentration of the drug to avoid the occurrence of dose-dependent toxicities. However, the optimal balance of immunosuppression is difficult to achieve following transplantation. Inadequate immunosuppression may lead to transplant rejection and, on the other hand, excessive immunosuppression facilitates the development of severe complications such as infection or malignancy. To date, there are no robust biomarkers that allow the prediction of the extent of immunosuppression afforded by these treatments. This may be a partial explanation for the frequent failure of the immunosuppressive strategy after lung transplantation as illustrated by the facts that 50 to 60% of the patients develop acute rejection and up to 60% of the recipients who survive 5 years after transplantation are affected by BOS [8,9,12].

Different approaches have aimed at reducing the incidence and severity of acute rejection. As a first attempt, we have developed a pharmacodynamic approach for monitoring the extent of immunosuppression following transplantation. This approach is based on the activity of calcineurin, a calcium-calmodulin-dependent phosphatase. Calcineurin activity reflects the combination of the degree of T lymphocyte activation and the inhibitory effect of CNIs [13–17]. Calcineurin is a key factor involved during the early phase of T lymphocyte activation. When CN is activated, it dephosphorylates the nuclear factor of activated T cells (NFAT) which then allows translocation of NFAT into the nucleus. This leads to the synthesis of cytokines that are involved in T lymphocyte proliferation. It has been demonstrated clearly that T cell activation is dependent upon sustained calcium/CN signaling for maximal proliferation and cytokine production [18,19]. Therefore, the CN activity (CN-a) measured in peripheral blood mononuclear cells (PBMCs) issued from allograft recipients receiving CNIs may be considered to be an index of T cell activation and a marker for graft-versus-host disease [20,21].

In this study, we measured CN-a during the first 24 months after lung transplantation and we correlated the activities with the occurrence of acute rejection, BOS and adverse events which are known to be associated with over-immunosuppression, such as malignancies and infections.

Materials and Methods

Ethics Statement

The CALCILUNG study was a prospective observational study of lung transplant recipients. In accordance with French law, the study protocol was approved by the ethics committee of Paris-Broussais-HEGP. Patients enrolled in this study provided informed written consents.

Patients

The study consisted of measuring CN-a during the first 24 months after lung transplantation. Patients were eligible if they were programmed to receive an immunosuppressive treatment consisting of the association of CsA, azathioprine and steroids. Patients followed a typical care regimen for post-lung transplantation patients, including surveillance fiberoptic bronchoscopy and bronchoalveolar lavage, spirometry, systematic transbronchial biopsies for acute rejection monitoring and blood sampling. The first surveillance biopsy was generally scheduled 7 days after transplantation. Subsequently, transbronchial biopsies were performed during the post-transplantation evaluation tests that were scheduled once a month up to the sixth month after lung transplantation and then every three months up to the 24th month after transplantation. Spirometry, generally, was checked once a week up to the third month after lung transplantation, then once a month up to the first year after transplantation and then every three months. In general, the first CN-a assessment was performed before transplantation during the pre-transplantation evaluation tests. Post-transplantation CN-a measurements were performed at least once a month during the first 6 months after transplantation and then every three months. Sampling for CN-a measurements was concomitant to the other monthly scheduled post-transplantation evaluation tests. The transplantation characteristics of the patients enrolled in this study are listed in **Table 1**.

Drug and Pharmacodynamic Monitoring

CsA and CN-a were both determined before the morning dose of CsA, when it was given orally. The clinical outcome of the patients was unknown to the biologist in charge of CN-a analyses and the results of the analyses were not given to the personnel (physicians and nurses) caring for the lung transplant patients. CsA was routinely measured with a locally available immunoassay. Mononuclear cells were isolated from the samples remaining by a Ficoll gradient method and CN-a measurements were made later. Briefly, 25 μg of proteins from mononuclear cells were incubated at 37°C for 30 min in the presence of phosphorylated RII peptide as a substrate of calcineurin. The dephosphorylation of the substrate was quantified by using high-performance liquid chromatography with ultraviolet detection as previously described [20]. Technical validation of this assay showed a correlation coefficient of the linear regression curves (linearity) greater than

Table 1. Basal characteriwstics of patients.

	Total (n = 107)
Age (yr)	36±12
Sex (M/F)	64(60)/43(40)
Initial disease	
cystic fibrosis	64(60)
emphysema	19(18)
others	24(22)
Type of transplantation (single/bilateral)	16(15)/91(85)
CMV mismatch at transplantaion (D+/R-)	26(24)
EBV mismatch at transplantation (D+/R-)	7(7)
Primary graft dysfunction grade III	15±4
Number of CN-a measurements/24 months	6±3
Time of follow-up (months)	41±16
Patients with acute rejection/6 months	77(72)
Patients with BOS grade ≥ I	40(37)
Patients with malignancies	16(15)
Patients with bacterial infections	
≥1 episode	63(59)
≥2 episodes	31(29)
≥3 episodes	15(14)
Patients with viral infections	
≥1 episode	39(36)
≥2 episodes	20(19)
≥3 episodes	7(6.5)
Patients with fungal infections	
≥1 episode	31(29)
≥2 episodes	9(8.4)
≥3 episodes	2(1.9)

Data are summarized as frequencies and percentage for categorical variables and as mean±SD for continuous variables. A total of 670 peripheral blood samples (mean of 6±3 samples per patient, range: 2–14) were obtained during the first 24 months following transplantation. Yr: year; M: male; F: female; EBV: empstein barr virus; CMV: cytomegalovirus; CN-a: calcineurin activity; BOS: bronchiolitis obliterans syndrome.

0.9971 and a variation coefficient (inter-assay variability) less than 10% [20]. The stability of CN-a under our conditions was previously verified by performing pharmacokinetic and pharmacodynamic measurements over a 10-hr time course in stable renal transplant patients treated with CsA. A peak of inhibition of CN-a occurred at approximately the same time as the peak of CsA in whole blood, and the concentrations of both CN-a and CsA gradually returned to baseline levels [20].

Diagnosis of Acute Rejection

Episodes of acute rejection were diagnosed on the basis of pulmonary function tests and histological evaluation of transbronchial biopsies. Acute rejection was graded according to the ISHLT criteria [22]. During the first six months following transplantation, treatment of acute rejection with steroids was initiated in patients with either an alteration or a 3-month stagnation of their pulmonary function and/or in patients for whom a grade A1 or higher was assessed based on their transbronchial biopies. Very few acute rejections of grade higher than A1 were diagnosed in these patients.

Determination of Pulmonary Function

Pulmonary function was estimated from the spirometric data FEV1, representing the forced expiratory volume in one second. To assess the variation of pulmonary function versus time during the first six months after transplantation, FEV1 ratios were calculated from the ratio of the difference between two spirometric values obtained approximately 1 month apart to the number of days between two spirometric measurements. We expressed these ratios in liters per second per day. Because we considered positive FEV1 ratios as a normal evolution of pulmonary function, only null and negative values of FEV1 ratios, which reveal a negative alteration of pulmonary function were taken into account for the study.

Diagnosis of Chronic Rejection/BOS

BOS was diagnosed and graded according to the ISHLT criteria [23]. BOS was defined as a sustained decrease of at least 20 percent in the FEV1 spirometric data as compared to the patient's maximum values in the absence of other causes [23]. Azithromycin therapy was started in patients displaying a strong reduction in FEF_{25-75}. In this study, we took into account the occurrence of BOS of grade I or higher.

Statistical Analysis

The values are expressed as the means$\pm$SD or the medians and percentiles. For the evaluation of the relationship between CN-a and acute rejection, CN-a values were censored when patients received a first IV bolus of steroids. Kernel smoothing curves were generated and the dispersion of extreme CN-a values was determined. For the evaluation of the relationship between CN-a and pulmonary function, we compared the rates of negative altered FEV1 at different CN-a levels. The survival without BOS, overall survival and the occurrence of adverse events were estimated by the Kaplan-Meier method. Other potentially associated risk factors of BOS occurrence were evaluated by using a stepwise logistic regression model.

Analyses were performed by using SAS 9.2 and Graphpad Prism softwares. Two-tailed P<0.05 were deemed significant. In case of multiple group comparisons, p-values were adjusted by the Bonferroni method.

Results

From March 2004 to October 2008, 107 patients who received lung transplants were examined for CN-a monitoring. The initial clinical-biological characteristics of these patients are shown in **Table 1**. Patients were followed until 2009. A total of 670 blood samples (mean of 6 ± 3 samples per patient, range: 2–14) were obtained during the first 24 months following transplantation. We compared the levels of CN-a prior to transplantation in patients with or without cystic fibrosis (CF) since this was the main initial end-stage lung disease that led to lung transplantation in this cohort of patients. There was no difference in the average pre-transplantation CN-a between patients with cystic fibrosis and the other patients (**Fig. 1A**).

Calcineurin Activity and Acute Rejection

The relationship between CN-a and acute rejection was assessed during the first six months after transplantation since acute rejection mainly occurred during that period of time. Of the 107 lung-transplant recipients, 30 (28%) were free of any episode of

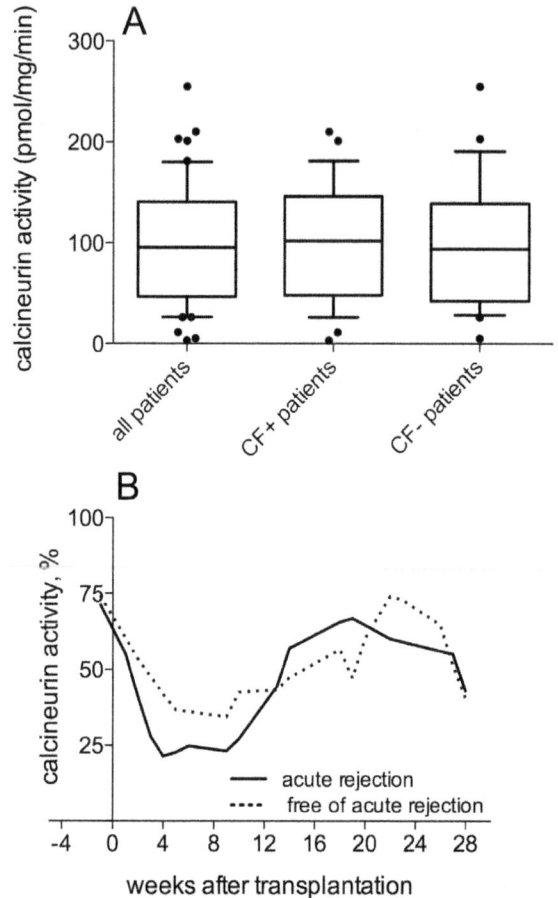

Figure 1. Calcineurin activity and acute rejection. (A) Calcineurin activity (CN-a) was measured before lung transplantation in 52 of the 107 patients enrolled in the participating center. The results are presented as box plots and 10–90 percentile whiskers. We compared CN-a expression prior to transplantation in patients with or without cystic fibrosis (CF) since it is the main initial end-stage lung disease that led to lung transplantation in this cohort of patients and a similar dispersion of the CN-a values was found in CF+ and CF- patients (p = 0.77, Mann-Whitney test). Subsequently, a relationship between extreme values of calcineurin activity and acute rejection was investigated. (B) Comparison across time of the median CN-a levels in patients displaying or not acute rejection: Kernel smoothing curves were generated. The 2 groups of patients displayed similar profiles of CN-a which consist of a phase of enzyme inhibition within the first 10 weeks after transplantation followed by a phase in which enzyme activity is restored. The phase of CN-a inhibition tended to be faster and more marked in patients who had developed acute rejection as compared to patients who were free of acute rejection. Similarly, the increase of enzyme activity to baseline levels tended to be faster and more pronounced in patients who had developed acute rejection.

acute rejection during the first 6 months after transplantation whereas 75 patients (71%) received a first rescue therapy by intravenous bolus (IV) of steroids following a diagnosis of acute rejection based either on their transbronchial biopsies for 68 of them (64%) or on their pulmonary function for 7 of them (7%). Furthermore, 2 patients (2%) were not rescued although an episode of acute rejection was diagnosed. The first episode of acute rejection occurred at a median time of 8 days (extreme values, 5–192 days). A large dispersion of CN-a values was observed, and since no reproducible pattern in CN-a could be discerned, we chose to express the CN-a data using their quartile range. For the patients enrolled in the study, the median of CN-a was 31 pmol/mg/min with values of 9, 12, 14, 17, 62, 84, 102 and 121 pmol/mg/min for the 10th, 15th, 20th, 25th, 75th, 80th, 85th and 90th percentiles, respectively (**Table 2**). We compared the median CN-a levels for the 2 groups of patients (with or without acute rejection) across time, and we generated Kernel smoothing curves (**Fig. 1B**). Although the 2 groups of patients displayed similar profiles of CN-a consisting of a phase of enzyme inhibition within the first 10 weeks after transplantation followed by a phase of restoration of enzyme activity, it appeared that the phase of CN-a inhibition tended to be faster and more marked in patients who developed acute rejection as compared to patients who did not develop acute rejection. Similarly, the increase of enzyme activity, almost to baseline levels, tended to be faster and more pronounced in patients who had developed acute rejection (**Fig. 1B**). We examined the dispersion of CN-a values in the 2 groups of patients by counting the number of values below the 10th to the 25th percentiles and above the 75th to the 90th percentiles (**Table 2**). We found that the number of CN-a values below the 10th–25th percentiles was much higher in the group of patients who had developed acute rejection during the first 10 weeks after transplantation as compared to those that did not develop acute rejection [for example, 7 patients (15%) and 19 patients (40%) with acute rejection vs 2 patients (6%) and 6 patients (17%) free of acute rejection below the 10th and 25th percentiles respectively, **Table 2**]. Similarly, the number of CN-a values above the 75th–90th percentiles was higher in the group of patients who had developed acute rejection during the phase of enzyme activity restoration between 13 to 28 weeks after transplantation [9 patients (35%) and 5 patients (19%) with acute rejection vs 19 patients (30%) and 7 patients (10%) free of acute rejection above the 75th and 90th percentiles respectively, **Table 2**].

Calcineurin Activity and Pulmonary Function

We next examined whether extreme CN-a values were associated with an alteration in pulmonary function during the first 6 months following transplantation. A higher per cent of altered FEV1 ratios was found in patients displaying CN-a values out of the range of 17–62 pmol/mg/min corresponding to the 25th and 75th percentiles as compared to patients displaying values of CN-a within this range [42 (48%) vs 27 (34%), respectively, **Table 3**]. A similar finding was observed for patients having CN-a values out of the range of 12–102 pmol/mg/min corresponding to the 15th and 85th percentiles as compared to patients displaying CN-a values within this range [26 (49%) vs 43 (38%), respectively, **Table 3**]. On the basis of these results, we chose to compare the long-term outcomes of patients who displayed CN-a values within the range of 12–102 pmol/mg/min versus patients who exhibited at least one CN-a value outside this range during the first 24 months after transplantation.

Adverse Events Related to Over-immunosuppression

Because low CN-a levels might reflect an over-immunosuppression, we compared the onset of events known to be associated with over-immunosuppression, such as malignancies and infections, between patients displaying or not CN-a levels below the lower threshold of 12 pmol/mg/min during the first 24 months after transplantation. Of the 107 lung-transplant recipients in this study, 1 patient, who displayed an Epstein-Barr virus-induced lymphoma before any CN-a measurement was made, was not considered for the evaluation of the relationship between CN-a and malignancies. The occurrence of malignancies was significantly higher in patients displaying at least one CN-a value below 12 pmol/mg/min as compared to patients

with higher CN-a values (28% vs 6%, p = 0.0218, Log-rank test, **Fig. 2A**). The assessment of the relationship between CN-a and infections was performed on the 107 patients enrolled in the study by separating the infections of bacterial, viral and fungal origin. The occurrence of bacterial and fungal infections was similar in the 2 groups of patients (**Fig. 2B,C**) whereas that of viral origin was significantly higher in patients displaying at least one CN-a value below 12 pmol/mg/min as compared to patients with higher CN-a levels (15% vs 0%, p = 0.0109, Log-rank test, **Fig. 2D**). This finding was restricted to patients with at least 3 episodes of viral infection (**Fig. 2D**).

Calcineurin Activity and BOS/chronic Rejection

CN-a was monitored the first 24 months after transplantation. We tested for the presence of a relationship between CN-a and the occurrence of BOS. Of the 107 lung-transplant recipients that were studied, 2 patients, who displayed a bronchopulmonary carcinoma and for whom pulmonary function tests were not performed, were not included in this analysis. The median time of follow-up for the patients was of 32.3 months with extreme values of 4–60 months, and that of the occurrence of BOS was of 19 months with a range of 4–53 months. BOS was diagnosed in 14 patients (13%), 35 patients (33%) and 41 patients (38%) 12 months, 36 months and 60 months after transplantation, respectively. Although not statistically significant, the survival without BOS was longer in patients who displayed CN-a levels within the range of 12–102 pmol/mg/min as compared to patients who exhibited at least one CN-a value outside this range (76% vs 43%, p = 0.4717, Log-rank test, **Fig. 3A**). Interestingly, very few patients displayed CN-a values within the range of 12–102 pmol/mg/min throughout the 24-month period of monitoring of CN-a [13 patients (12%) with CN-a values within the range vs 92 patients (88%) with at least one CN-a value out of the range, **Fig. 3A**]. This distribution of values between the two groups of patients (within vs outside of the range 12–102 pmol/mg/min) made it very difficult to determine whether a statistically significant difference in BOS-free survival exists for the groups.

In addition and because BOS was diagnosed mostly after sixth months after transplantation, we restricted the analysis of a relationship between CN-a and BOS to CN-a data obtained between 6 and 24 months after transplantation. Due to the absence of data or the occurrence of BOS before the 6th month after transplantation, 26 patients were not considered in this analysis. With these restrictions, the patients were distributed more evenly between the 2 groups [28 patients (35%) with CN-a values within the range of 12–102 pmol/mg/min vs 51 patients (65%) with at least one CN-a value outside of the range, **Fig. 3B**]. BOS-free survival was found to be significantly higher in patients who displayed CN-a levels within the range of 12–102 pmol/mg/min as compared to patients who exhibited at least one CN-a value outside this range from the 6th month to the 24th month following transplantation (80% vs 40%, p = 0.0118, Log-rank test, **Fig. 3B**). In addition, we have determined whether known risk factors of BOS were involved in the association of CN-a values with BOS during this 18-month period of CN-a monitoring. The association between BOS and CN-a was not significantly accounted for by the following potential risk factors: acute rejection, CMV infection, primary graft dysfunction grade III, anti-HLA antibodies, gastro-oesophageal reflux. In a logistic regression model taking into account the other risk factors, the CN-a range was the only variable significantly associated with BOS (odds ratio 5.7, 95% CI [1.7–19.2], p = 0.045).

Table 2. Dispersion of the values of calcineurin activity.

	1 to 10 weeks after transplantation	13 to 28 weeks after transplantation
Patients free of acute rejection		
number of CN-a determinations	35	68
number of CN-a :		
- ≤10th **percentile** (9 pmol/mg/min)	2(6)	7(10)
- ≤15th **percentile** (12 pmol/mg/min)	2(6)	11(16)
- ≤20th **percentile** (14 pmol/mg/min)	3(9)	14(21)
- ≤25th **percentile** (17 pmol/mg/min)	6(17)	18(26)
- ≥75th **percentile** (62 pmol/mg/min)	6(17)	19(30)
- ≥80th **percentile** (84 pmol/mg/min)	5(14)	14(21)
- ≥85th **percentile** (102 pmol/mg/min)	4(11)	11(16)
- ≥90th **percentile** (121 pmol/mg/min)	2(6)	7(10)
Patients with acute rejection		
number of CN-a determinations	48	26
number of CN-a :		
- ≤10th **percentile** (9 pmol/mg/min)	7(15)	1(4)
- ≤15th **percentile** (12 pmol/mg/min)	10(21)	2(8)
- ≤20th **percentile** (14 pmol/mg/min)	14(29)	2(8)
- ≤25th **percentile** (17 pmol/mg/min)	19(40)	2(8)
- ≥75th **percentile** (62 pmol/mg/min)	5(10)	9(35)
- ≥80th **percentile** (84 pmol/mg/min)	4(8)	8(31)
- ≥85th **percentile** (102 pmol/mg/min)	4(8)	5(19)
- ≥90th **percentile** (121 pmol/mg/min)	2(4)	5(19)

Data are summarized as frequencies and percentage. A total of 103 measurements of calcineurin activity (CN-a) were performed in the group of patients free of acute rejection and of 74 in the group of patients with acute rejection before the occurrence of this event.

Since CN-a levels lower than 12 and higher than 102 pmol/mg/min suggested two putatively different mechanisms by which BOS developed, we next separated these threshold values to determine whether the groups had similar, significant decreases in survival without BOS. A significant reduction in BOS-free survival was found in patients who displayed CN-a levels higher than 102 pmol/mg/min (40% vs 80%, $p = 0.037$, Log-rank test, **Fig. 3C**), whereas a reduction in BOS-free survival in the limit of statistical significance was found in patients who displayed CN-a levels lower than 12 pmol/mg/min (49% vs 80%, $p = 0.0574$, Log-rank test, **Fig. 3C**).

Table 3. Calcineurin activity and pulmonary function.

range of CN-a levels	number of determinations	number of altered FEV1-ratio
25th - 75th percentile (17–62 pmol/mg/min)		
25th–75th in	79	27(34)
25th–75th out	87	42(48)
20th–80th percentile (14–84 pmol/mg/min)		
20th–80th in	96	36(38)
20th–80th out	70	33(47)
15th–85th percentile (12–102 pmol/mg/min)		
15th–85th in	113	43(38)
15th–85th out	53	26(49)
10th–90th percentile (9–121 pmol/mg/min)		
10th–90th in	125	52(42)
10th–90 out	41	17(41)

Data are summarized as frequencies and percentage. The relationship between calcineurin Activity (CN-a) and the forced expiratory volume in one second (FEV1) ratio was studied from A total of 166 values collected from 87 patients (mean of 2±1 data per patient, range : 1–5).

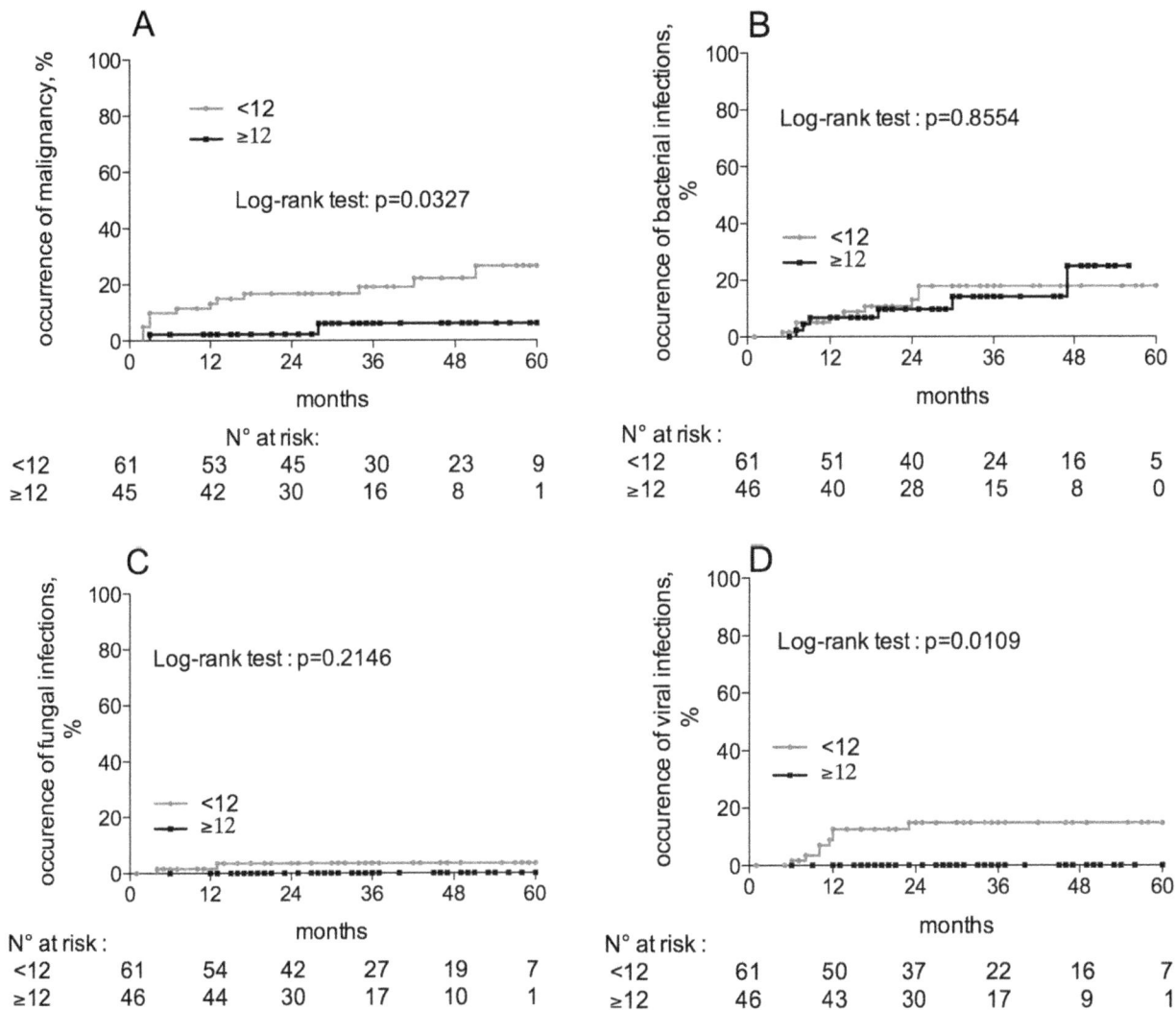

Figure 2. Calcineurin activity and adverse events related to over-immunosuppression. The onset of events known to be related to over-immunosuppression, such as malignancies and infections, was compared between patients displaying or not low CN-a levels by the Kaplan and Meier method. (A) CN-a and malignancies: the occurrence of malignancies was significantly higher in patients displaying at least one CN-a value below 12 pmol/mg/min during the first 24 months after transplantation as compared to patients with higher CN-a values (28% vs 6%, p = 0.0218, Log-rank test). The examination of the relationship between CN-a and infections was performed by separating the infections of bacterial, viral and fungal origin. (B) CN-a and bacterial infections: the occurrence of 3 episodes of bacterial infections was similar in the 2 groups of patients (18% vs 25%, p = 0.85, Log-rank test). (C) CN-a and fungal infections: the occurrence of 3 episodes of fungal infections was similar in the 2 groups of patients (3.5% vs 0%, p = 0.21, Log-rank test). (D) CN-a and viral infections: the occurrence of 3 episodes of viral infections was significantly higher in patients displaying at least one CN-a value below 12 pmol/mg/min during the first 24 months after transplantation compared to patients with higher CN-a values (15% vs 0%, p = 0.01, Log-rank test).

Calcineurin Activity and Overall Survival

Of the 107 patients enrolled in the study, 25 patients (23%) died during follow-up. At this time of the evaluation, no significant difference was found in the overall survival between the 2 groups of patients exhibiting CN-a levels within or outside of the range of 12–102 pmol/mg/min (**Fig. 3D**). This relationship should be re-assessed after a longer period of follow-up.

Calcineurin Activity and Cyclosporine Blood Levels

We next investigated whether CsA blood levels could explain the modification in CN-a that we have observed. However, as shown in **Figure 4**, we did not find any significant correlation between CN-a and CsA blood levels, as also observed in other types of transplantation [20,21,24].

Discussion

The activity of calcineurin measured in the PBMCs of allograft recipients who received inhibitors of calcineurin has been shown to be an index of T cell activation and a marker for graft-versus-host disease [20,21]. It was thought that a high CN-a reflected poor immunosuppression whereas a low CN-a reflected potent immunosuppression. Therefore, our working hypothesis, for the present study, was that the level of CN-a can predict the degree of immunosuppression after lung transplantation, and, thus, be useful for predicting both the occurrence of rejection, related to an inadequate immunosuppression, and the development of severe complications, related to excessively potent immunosuppression. However, we report here that patients who displayed extreme CN-

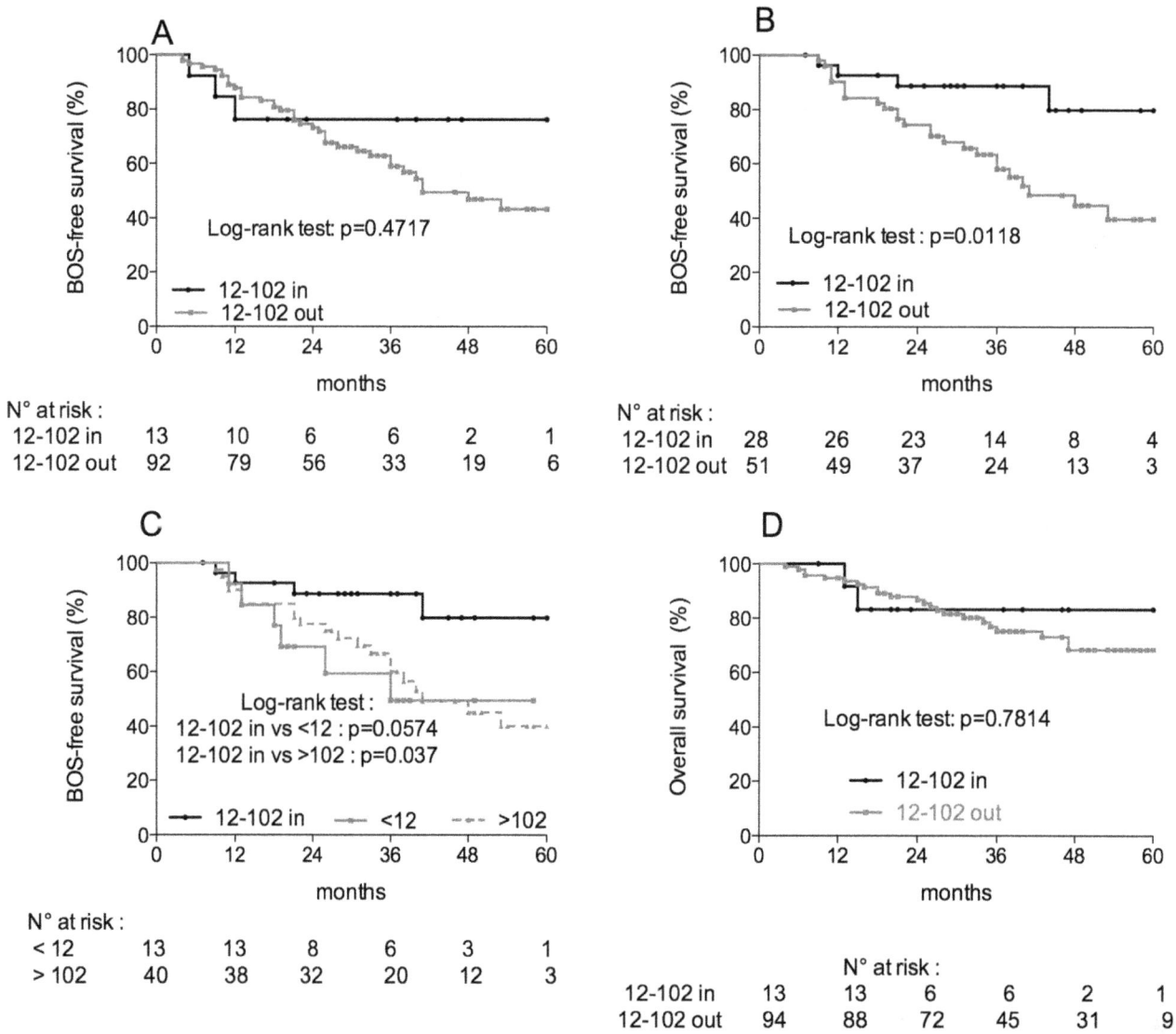

Figure 3. Calcineurin activity, BOS and overall survival. BOS-free survival was estimated at 5 years after transplantation by the Kaplan and Meier method. (A) Calcineurin activity (CN-a) monitoring during the first 24 months after transplantation: although not statistically significant, the survival without BOS was higher in patients who displayed CN-a levels within the range of 12–102 pmol/mg/min as compared to patients who exhibited at least one CN-a value outside this range of 12–102 pmol/mg/min during the first 24 months following transplantation (76% vs 43%, $p = 0.4717$, Log-rank test). (B) CN-a monitoring from the 6th month to the 24th month after transplantation: the survival without BOS was significantly higher in patients who displayed CN-a levels within the range of 12–102 pmol/mg/min as compared to that of patients who exhibited at least one CN-a value outside this range from the 6th month to the 24th months following transplantation (80% vs 40%, $p = 0.0118$, Log-rank test). (C) CN-a monitoring from the 6th to the 24th month after transplantation: the threshold values were further separated in 2 groups : <12 pmol/mg/min, >102 pmol/mg/min. The BOS-free survival in patients from each of these groups was compared to that from patients who displayed CN-a levels within the range of 12–102 pmol/mg/min. A significant reduction of the survival without BOS was found in patients who displayed CN-a levels higher than 102 pmol/mg/min (40% vs 80%, $p = 0.037$, Log-rank test), whereas a reduction in BOS-free survival in the limit of statistical significance was found in patients who displayed CN-a levels lower than 12 pmol/mg/min (49% vs 80%, $p = 0.0574$, Log-rank test). (D) Calcineurin activity and overall survival: no significant difference was found in the overall survival between the 2 groups of patients exhibiting calcineurin activity levels within or outside of the range of 12–102 pmol/mg/min.

a values, either high or low values, were mainly those patients who developed acute rejection and had an altered pulmonary function. These observations led us to define an optimal activity for CN between two thresholds, 12 and 102 pmol/mg/min. Patients who had CN-a values within this range had a significantly higher survival without BOS. Furthermore, the occurrence of malignancies and viral infections was significantly lower in patients who exhibited CN-a values higher than 12 pmol/mg/min.

With the introduction of more potent immunosuppressive agents and newer combinations during the last ten years, patient and graft survivals have dramatically increased following most types of solid organ transplantation. However the incidence of post-transplantation infections and cancer also has increased. It was thought that potent immunosuppression, as reflected by the occurrence of adverse events, was protective against immunogenic stimulation. However, despite a modern immunosuppressive regimen, lung transplantation is characterized by both poor

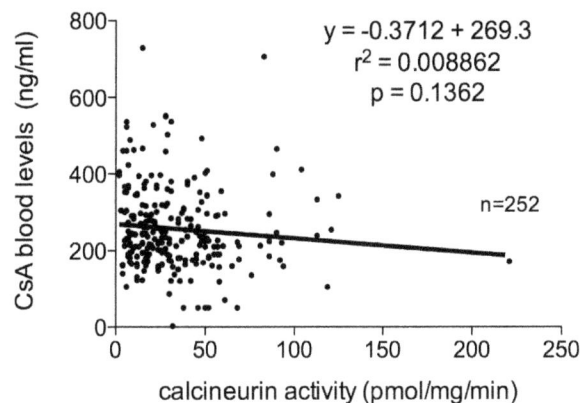

Figure 4. Calcineurin activity and cyclosporine blood levels. The relationship between calcineurin activity (CN-a) and the levels of cyclosporine (CsA) in blood was investigated. No correlation was found between CN-a and the level of CsA in blood.

patient and graft survivals as well as devastating adverse events. The results of the present study may provide a partial explanation for the disappointing long-term outcomes in lung transplant patients. Indeed, we observed extreme CN-a values, below 12 pmol/mg/min or higher than 102 pmol/mg/min, more frequently in the present cohort of lung transplant patients than in other types of transplant patients that we have examined such as hematopoietic stem cell transplant patients [20] or heart transplant patients (unpublished data). In addition, we established a relationship between CN-a and the occurrence of both acute and chronic rejection. This relationship was non-monotonic in that both very low and very high CN-a levels were associated with the onset of acute rejection. As expected, very high CN-a could reflect poor immunosuppression that is not sufficient to counteract the immunogenic activation of T lymphocytes.

On the contrary, the presence of a low threshold was very surprising since very low CN-a levels should have been associated with a strong protection against lymphocyte activation. In fact, the patients with very low CN-a levels were, indeed, strongly immunosuppressed since they developed a higher rate of both malignant diseases and viral infections as compared to patients with higher CN-a levels. Nevertheless, their CN-a levels did not reflect their immunologic potency towards the graft. This finding is consistent with the recently reported activation of a negative feedback loop, via endogenous CN inhibitors, calcipressins, which down-regulate the CN/NFAT signaling pathway when it is activated [25–28]. Although the calcipressin family has been extensively investigated in brain, heart and endothelial cells, a very limited number of studies has been reported concerning the immune system. Additionally, the impact of calcipressins on the effects of immunosuppressive agents in the context of transplantation has never been assessed. Therefore, we anticipate that low CN-a levels displayed by lung transplant patients developing a rejection are associated first with a lymphocyte activation subsequently followed by a strong endogenous down-regulation of the calcineurin/NFAT signaling pathway.

Taken together, these findings on the relationships between CN-a and acute rejection, pulmonary function and the occurrence of adverse events related to over-immunosuppression led us to define an optimal activity for CN between two thresholds, 12 and 102 pmol/mg/min, and to assess, retrospectively, whether patients who displayed CN-a values between these two thresholds had a significantly higher rate of survival without BOS/chronic

rejection. Lung transplantation is the type of organ transplantation that gives the poorest outcomes, with 45% of the recipients dying within 5 years, mainly due to the development of chronic rejection in response to immunologic, ischemic and infectious injury. Unfortunately, once the clinical signs of BOS/chronic rejection appear, it is usually too late to reverse it. We report here that patients who displayed CN-a values within the range of 12–102 pmol/mg/min had a significantly higher rate of survival without BOS/chronic rejection. In addition, this association of BOS/chronic rejection and CN-a values was not explained by the known risk factors of BOS such as acute rejection, CMV infection, primary graft dysfunction grade III, anti-HLA antibodies or gastro-oesophageal reflux. In a logistic regression model taking into account the other risk factors, the CN-a range was the only variable significantly associated with BOS/chronic rejection. Therefore, CN-a may constitute an additional risk factor of BOS. Currently, overall survival is not significantly associated with CN-a values. However, we have to take into account that, in our study, the median time of occurrence of BOS was 19 months and that it has been shown that the median survival after the onset of BOS is 30 months [29]. Therefore, the overall survival according to CN-a values need to be re-assessed after a longer period of follow-up.

The degree of CN inhibition up to 12 hours after treatment with CsA has been shown to vary directly with the blood levels of CsA [30]. However, this relationship might not persist after several months of treatment with CsA because of the potential contribution of lymphocyte stimulation to the drug effect upon the target. Indeed, we report here that blood levels of CsA and trough levels of CN-a are not correlated. This observation is in agreement with previous findings in hematopoietic stem-cell transplant-, in liver transplant- and in kidney transplant-patients [20,21,24,31,32]. However, the absence of correlation between CN-a levels and CsA whole blood concentrations does not mean that the latter is not a predictor of patient outcome.

There are advantages and limitations to using CN-a as a biomarker. First, interpretation by clinicians of CN-a values, which appear to display a considerable dispersion, may prove to be difficult. Second, other markers, such as the degree of T-cell activation in blood [33], in broncho-alveolar fluid [34,35] or increased T-cell pro-inflammatory cytokine production in the graft [36], have been associated with acute rejection. However, as compared to these studies, the main objective of our study was to identify and characterize a rejection marker that is the most directly related to the degree of immunosuppression produced by an anticalcineurin drug such as CsA. Indeed, only this type of marker aids in determining therapeutic options. Consequently, we believe that our observations can help clinicians in their use of CsA. Our findings suggest that CsA should be administered with much more caution during episodes of acute rejection than might have been thought previously. In particular, monitoring of CN-a sequentially after transplantation might be helpful for facilitating the optimization of multidrug immunosuppressant regimens including those employing CsA. The targeting of CN-a levels between the 25th and 75th percentiles, that is between 17 and 62 pmol/mg/min, can be proposed as a desirable therapeutic range in order to avoid values of CN-a outside the range of 12–102 pmol/mg/min that is associated with poor outcome. Indeed, the dose of CsA should be increased for patients with suspected acute rejection and CN-a levels over 62 pmol/mg/min but not for those patients with CN-a levels below 17 pmol/mg/min. In the latter case, a switch to another class of immunosuppressant can be recommended. Recommendations of this type can be made only when the most specific biomarkers are used and not when general biomarkers, only, are available. However, our data are still preliminary and need to be confirmed through a prospective validation cohort. Further investigation of calcineurin levels need to be carried before considering calcineurin levels as a biomarker.

In summary, we have shown that a relationship exists between CN-a and both acute and chronic rejection in lung transplant patients. Further, we have defined an optimal activity for calcineurin between two thresholds : the risk of rejection was higher when the enzyme activity was above the upper threshold of 102 pmol/mg/min or below the lower threshold of 12 pmol/mg/min. In addition, we report that the occurrence of malignancies

and viral infections was significantly higher in patients displaying CN-a below the lower threshold. Based upon these findings, CN-a appears as a potential predictive biomarker that could lead to new guidelines for the management of lung transplant patients.

Author Contributions

Conceived and designed the experiments: SS RB CA RG MS. Performed the experiments: SS CA DG LH RG BP VB RB MS. Analyzed the data: SS CL CA RB JPJ MS. Contributed reagents/materials/analysis tools: SS CL AD MP EMB FL MS. Wrote the paper: SS RB MS.

References

1. American Thoracic Society (1998) International guidelines for the selection of lung transplant candidates. Am J Respir Crit Care Med 158: 335–339.
2. Lin HM, Kauffman HM, McBride MA, Davies DB, Rosendale JD, et al. (1998) Center-specific graft and patient survival rates: 1997 United Network for Organ Sharing (UNOS) report. JAMA 280: 1153–1160.
3. Bando K, Paradis IL, Similo S, Konishi H, Komatsu K, et al. (1995) Obliterative bronchiolitis after lung and heart-lung transplantation: an analysis of risk factors and management. J Thorac Cardiovasc Surg 110: 4–13.
4. Sharples LD, Tamm M, McNeil K, Higenbottam TW, Stewart S, et al. (1996) Development of bronchiolitis obliterans in recipients of heart-lung transplantation – early risk factors. Transplantation 61: 560–566.
5. Trulock EP (1993) Management of lung transplant rejection. Chest 103: 1566–1576.
6. Yousem SA (1993) Lymphocytic bronchitis/bronchiolitis in lung allograft recipients. Am J Surg Pathol 17: 491–496.
7. Yousem SA, Duncan SR, Griffith BP (1992) Intersticial and airspace granulation tissue reactions in lung transplant recipients. Am J Surg Pathol 16: 877–884.
8. Estenne M, Hertz MI (2002) Bronchiolitis obliterans after human lung transplantation. Am J Respir Crit Care Med 166: 440–444.
9. Al-Githmi I, Batawil N, Shigemura N, Hsin M, Lee TW, et al. (2006) Bronchiolitis obliterans following lung transplantation. Eur J Cardiothorac Surg 30: 846–851.
10. Sharples LD, McNeil K, Stewart S, Wallork J (2002) Risk factors for bronchiolitis obliterans: a systematic review of recent publications. J Heart Lung Transplant 21: 271–281.
11. Arcasoy SM, Kotloff RM (1999) Lung transplantation. N E J M 340: 1081–1091.
12. Martinu T, Chan DF, Palmer SM (2009) Acute rejection and humoral sensitization in lung transplant recipients. Proc Am Thorac Soc 6: 54–65.
13. Batiuk TD, Kung L, Halloran PF (1997) Evidence that calcineurin is rate-limiting for primary human lymphocyte activation. J Clin Invest 100: 1894–1901.
14. Graef IA, Chen F, Chen L, Kuo A, Crabtree GR (2001) Signal transduced by Ca(2+)/calcineurin and NFATc3/c4 pattern the developing vasculature. Cell 105: 863–875.
15. Beals CR, Sheridan CM, Turck CW, Gardner P, Crabtree GR (1997) Nuclear export of NF-ATc enhanced by glycogen synthase kinase-3. Science 275: 1930–1934.
16. Okamura H, Aramburu J, Garcia-Rodriguez C, Viola JPB, Raghavan A, et al. (2000) Concerted dephosphorylation of the transcription factor NFAT1 induces a conformational switch that regulates transcriptional activity. Mol Cell 6: 539–550.
17. Timmerman LA, Clipstone NA, Ho SN, Northrop JP, Crabtree GR (1996) Rapid shuttling of NF-AT in discrimination of Ca2+ signals and immunosuppression. Nature 383: 837–840.
18. Huppa JB, Gleimer M, Sumen C, Davis MM (2003) Continuous T cell receptor signaling required for synapse maintenance and full effector potential. Nature Immunol 4: 749–755.
19. Feske S, Okamura H, Hogan PG, Rao A (2003) Ca2+/calcineurin signaling in cells of the immune system. Biochem Biophysic Res Com 31: 1117–1132.
20. Sanquer S, Schwarzinger M, Maury S, Yakouben K, Rafi H, et al. (2004) Calcineurin activity as a functional index of immunosuppression after allogeneic stem-cell transplantation. Transplantation 77: 854–858.

21. Fukudo M, Yano I, Masuda S, Fukatsu S, Katsura T, et al. (2005) Pharmacodynamic analysis of tacrolimus and cyclosporine in living-donor liver transplant patients. Clin Pharmacol Therap 78: 168–181.
22. Yousem SA, Berry GJ, Gagle PT, Chamberlain D, Husain AN, et al. (1996) Revision of the 1990 working formulation for the classification of pulmonary allograft rejection: Lung Rejection Study Group. J Heart Lung Transplant 15: 1–15.
23. Estenne M, Maurer JR, Boehler A, Egan JJ, Frost A, et al. (2002) Bronchiolitis obliterans syndrome 2001: An update of the diagnostic criteria. J Heart Lung Transplant 21: 297–310.
24. Caruso R, Perico N, Cattananeo D, Piccinina G, Bonazzola S, et al. (2001) Whole-blood calcineurin activity is not predicted by cyclosporine blood concentration in renal transplant recipients. Clin Chem 47: 1679–1687.
25. Fuentes JJ, Genesca L, Kingsbury TJ, Cunningham KW, Pérez-Riba M, et al. (2000) DSCR1, overexpressed in Down syndrome, is an inhibitor of calcineurin-mediated signaling pathways. Hum Mol Genet 9: 1681–1690.
26. Kingsbury TJ, Cuningham KW (2000) A conserved family of calcineurin regulators. Genes Dev 14: 1595–1604.
27. Gorlach J, Fox DS, Cutler NS, Cox GM, Perfect JR, et al. (2000) Identification and characterization of a highly conserved calcineurin binding protein, CBP1/calcipressin, in Cryptococcus neoformans. EMBO J 19: 3618–3629.
28. Ryeom S, Greenwald R, Sharpe AH, McKeon F (2003) The threshold pattern of calcineurin-dependent gene expression is altered by loss of the endogenous inhibitor calcipressin. Nature Immunol 9: 874–878.
29. Finlen-Copeland CA, Snyder LD, Zaas DW, Turbyfill WJ, Davies WA, et al. (2010) Survival after bronchiolitis obliterans syndrome among bilateral lung transplant patients. Am J Respir Crit Care Med 182: 784–789.
30. Halloran PF, Helms LMH, Kung L, Noujaim J (1999) The temporal profile of calcineurin inhibition by cyclosporine in vivo. Transplantation 68: 1356–1361.
31. Yano I (2008) Pharmacodynamic monitoring of calcineurin phosphatase activity in transplant patients treated with calcineurin inhibitors. Drug Metab Pharmacokinet 23: 150–157.
32. Yano I, Masuda S, Egawa H, Sugimoto M, Fukudo M, et al. (2012) Significance of trough monitoring for tacrolimus blood concentration and calcineurin activity in adult patients undergoing primary living-donor liver transplantation. Eur J Clin Pharmacol 68: 259–266.
33. Schowengerdt KO, Ficker FJ, Bahjat KS, Kuntz ST (2000) Increased expression of the lymphocyte early activation marker CD69 in peripheral blood correlates with histologic evidence of cardiac allograft rejection. Transplantation 69: 2102–2107.
34. Gregson AL, Hoji A, Saggar R, Ross DJ, Kubak BM, et al. (2008) Bronchoalveolar immunologic profile of acute human lung transplant allograft rejection. Transplantation 85: 1056–1059.
35. Crim C, Keller CA, Dunphy CH, Maluf HM, Ohar JA (1996) Flow cytometric analysis of lung lymphocytes in lung transplant recipients. Am J Respir Crit Care med 153: 1041–1046.
36. Hodge G, Hodge S, Chambers DC, Reynolds PN, Holmes M (2012) Increased expression of graft intraepithelial T-cell pro-inflammatory cytokines compared with native lung during episodes of acute rejection. J Heart Lung Transplant 31: 538–544.

23

Pregnancy Outcomes in Liver and Cardiothoracic Transplant Recipients: A UK National Cohort Study

Olaa Mohamed-Ahmed[1]*, Cathy Nelson-Piercy[2,3], Kate Bramham[2], Haiyan Gao[1], Jennifer J. Kurinczuk[1], Peter Brocklehurst[4], Marian Knight[1]

1 National Perinatal Epidemiology Unit, Nuffield Department of Population Health, University of Oxford, United Kingdom, 2 Division of Women's Health, King's College London, Women's Health Academic Centre, King's Health Partners, United Kingdom, 3 Obstetric Medicine, Guy's and St Thomas' NHS Foundation Trust, London, United Kingdom, 4 Institute for Women's Health, University College London, United Kingdom

Abstract

Introduction: There are an increasing number of reports of pregnancy in transplant recipients but many questions remain regarding the effect of the transplant on pregnancy outcome, the pregnancy on the graft and the medication on the fetus. The majority of studies reporting outcomes in transplant recipients have focused on women with kidney transplants, and have included retrospective, voluntary registries or single centre studies.

Methods: The UK Obstetric Surveillance System (UKOSS) was used to prospectively identify all pregnant women with a liver or cardiothoracic transplant in the United Kingdom, between January 2007 and January 2012. Data were collected on demographics, transplant characteristics, immunosuppression regimens, antenatal care, maternal, graft and neonatal outcomes. In an exploratory analysis, we tested for associations between "poor fetal outcome" and medications used before or during pregnancy.

Results and conclusions: We report 62 pregnancies in 56 liver transplant recipients and 14 pregnancies in 14 cardiothoracic transplant recipients (including 10 heart, three lung and one heart-lung recipient). Liver transplant recipients, in comparison to cardiothoracic, had similar livebirth rates (92% vs. 87%) but better fetal outcomes (median gestational age 38 weeks vs. 35 weeks; median birthweight 2698 g vs. 2365 g), fewer caesarean deliveries (47% vs. 62%), fewer maternal intensive care (ICU) admissions (19% vs. 29%) and fewer neonatal ICU admissions (25% vs. 54%). Nine women (12%) were taking mycophenolate mofetil at conception, which was associated with adverse fetal outcomes. Pregnancy in transplant recipients may have successful outcomes, but complication rates are high, emphasising the role of pre-conception counselling and further research into the long-term effect on maternal and graft survival rates.

Editor: Claire Thorne, UCL Institute of Child Health, University College London, United Kingdom

Funding: This paper reports on an independent study that is funded by the Policy Research Programme in the Department of Health. The views expressed are not necessarily those of the Department. The funders had no role in study design, data collection and analysis, decision to publish, or preparation of the manuscript.

Competing Interests: The authors have declared that no competing interests exist.

* E-mail: olaa.mohamed-ahmed@npeu.ox.ac.uk

Introduction

Over the past 50 years, more than 14,000 women with solid organ transplants have had pregnancies, worldwide [1]. The majority of studies on pregnancy outcomes in women with transplants have included only women with renal transplants, with information obtained from national, retrospective, voluntary registries, with the only currently active registry being the National Transplantation Pregnancy Registry (NTPR), in the United States of America (USA) [2–4].

An international conference on reproduction and transplantation highlighted the need for prospective observational studies [5], and recognised that many unanswered questions remain. For the practicing clinician, further information is required regarding the effect of the transplant on pregnancy, the effect of pregnancy on the graft and the impact of medications on the fetus, particularly in non-renal transplant recipients [6].

The aim of this study was to use the United Kingdom Obstetric Surveillance System (UKOSS), which collects data on rare disorders in pregnancy [7], to conduct a national, prospective cohort study of pregnancy outcomes in liver and cardiothoracic transplant recipients.

Methods

We aimed to identify all pregnant women in the United Kingdom (UK), between January 2007 and January 2012, who had previously undergone liver or cardiothoracic transplantation.

The UKOSS methodology has been described in detail elsewhere [7]. In brief, nominated clinicians in each consultant-led maternity unit in the UK were sent a case notification card each month and asked to report all cases. They were also asked to return cards indicating a "nil report" in order to distinguish no cases of liver and cardiothoracic transplant recipients from a lack

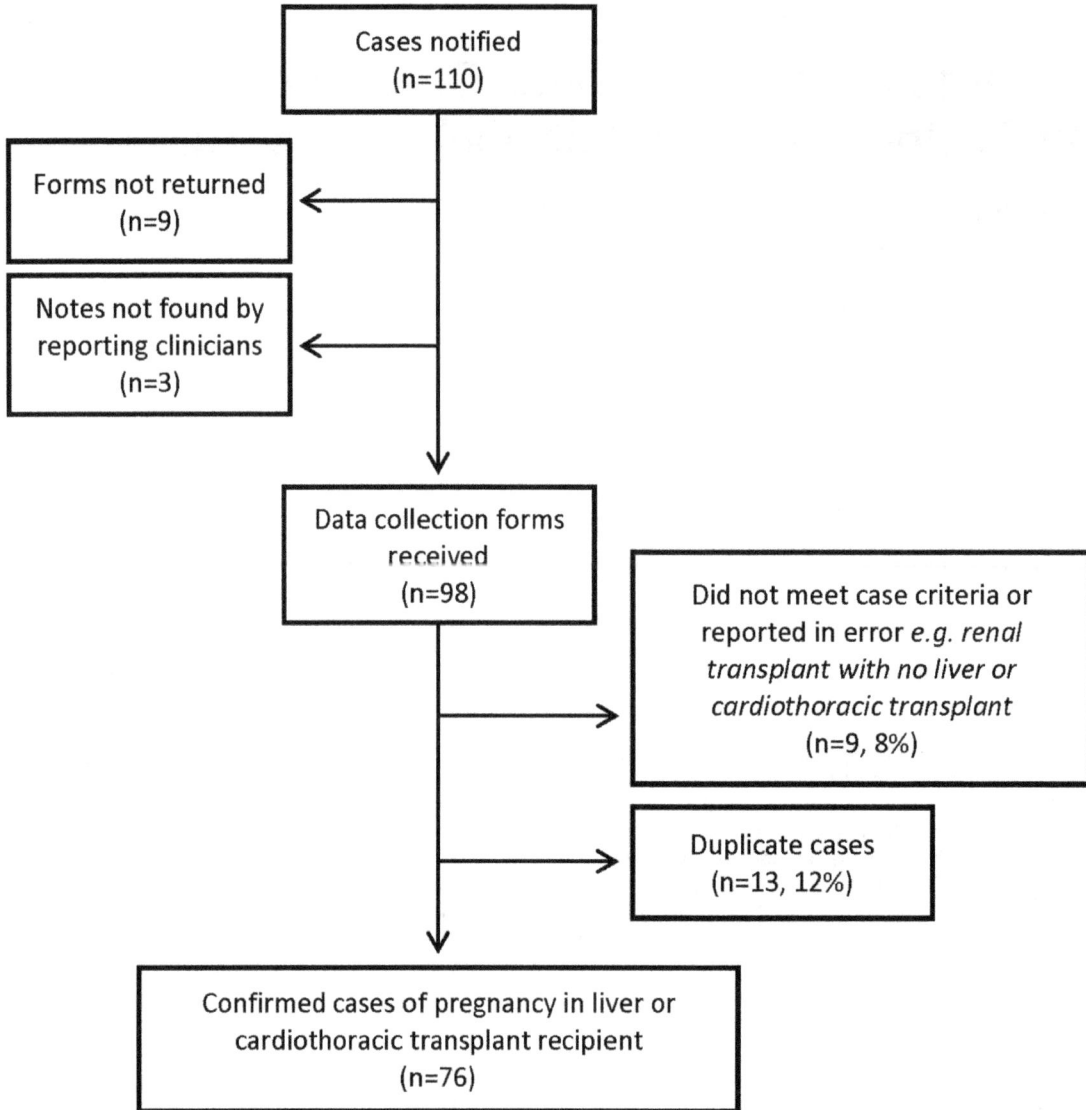

Figure 1. Case reporting and completeness of data collection.

of response. Reporting clinicians were then asked to complete data collection forms to provide information about cases (Figure 1).

We collected data on demographics, transplant characteristics, immunosuppression regimens, antenatal care, and maternal, graft and neonatal outcomes. All data collected were anonymous and the entire cohort of women giving birth in the UK was included. As the study spanned five years, year of birth, height and the organ transplanted were used to identify successive pregnancies in the same recipient.

Continuous variables were summarized as means (standard deviations), or medians (inter-quartile or entire ranges) for skewed data. Categorical variables were summarized as frequencies (percentages).

Small-for-gestational age was calculated by comparing birth-weight to revised British 1990 birth centiles [8], using LMSgrowth software [9]. As data were not collected on the sex of infants born to the transplant recipients, a best-case scenario was generated assuming all infants were female and worst-case scenario assuming

all infants were male. Any infants below the 10th centile were considered to be small-for-gestational age.

Poor fetal outcome was defined as any pregnancy resulting in a stillbirth, miscarriage, very low birthweight (<1500 g), small-for-gestational age (<10th centile, best-case scenario), congenital anomaly, neonatal unit admission and very preterm birth (<32 weeks). This was used to generate a categorical variable which was tested for association with medications used before or during pregnancy. To allow for non-independence of multiple pregnancies from the same women, logistic regression with cluster analysis was used to generate odds ratios, p-values and 95% confidence intervals.

All statistical analyses were carried out using STATA 11 SE software (StataCorp LP, College Station, TX).

Ethics Statement

The UK Obstetric Surveillance System general methodology (ref: 04/MRE02/45) and this study (ref: 06/MRE02/78) were approved by the London Multicentre Research Ethics Committee.

Results

All 228 hospitals in the UK with obstetrician-led maternity units participated in the study (100% of eligible units), with data collection from January 2007 until February 2012. Nineteen hospitals ceased reporting cases during the study period, because the admitting units had closed. Case ascertainment is presented in Figure 1.

Patient Characteristics

We identified 62 pregnancies in 56 liver transplant recipients and 14 pregnancies in 14 cardiothoracic transplant recipients, including 10 heart, three lung and one heart-lung recipient.

The demographic, maternal and transplant characteristics of the population are presented in Table 1.

Women with a liver transplant had a median age of 30 years at pregnancy (range 18–39 years), median age of 21 years at first transplantation (range 2–36 years, 34% below age 18) and a median transplant to conception interval of 6.5 years (range 4

months to 20 years). Seven women conceived within two years of liver transplantation, with two occurring within the first year. The most common indications for transplantation (Table 2) were acute liver failure (secondary to drug toxicity), biliary atresia, metabolic diseases, seronegative and autoimmune hepatitides.

Women with a cardiothoracic transplant had a median age of 26 at delivery (range 20–38 years), median age of 21 at first transplantation (range 4–33 years, 43% below age 18) and a median transplant to conception interval of 8 years (range 2–16 years), reflecting the burden of congenital disease, with almost half (n = 6) transplanted for congenital heart disease and cystic fibrosis (Table 2). No women conceived within two years of receiving a cardiothoracic transplant.

Management

Of the 76 transplant recipients, 45 received antenatal care in the usual hospital for their area of residence (59%). Of those who received care at another hospital, 28 (37%) were referred because of their underlying medical condition.

Table 1. Demographic, maternal and transplant characteristics of liver and cardiothoracic transplant recipients.

Demographic Characteristics	Liver transplant cohort (n = 62)	Cardiothoracic transplant cohort (n = 14)
Maternal age (years)		
<20	3 (5)	0 (0)
20–34	45 (73)	11 (79)
≥35	14 (23)	3 (21)
Ethnic group[1]		
White	44 (80)	12 (92)
Non-White	11 (20)	1 (8)
Socio-economic status		
Managerial/Professional	17 (33)	2 (15)
Non-managerial/Other	26 (51)	6 (46)
Unemployed	8 (16)	5 (38)
Smoking status		
Smoked during pregnancy	16 (27)	3 (21)
Did not smoke during pregnancy	43 (73)	11 (79)
Body mass index		
Normal (<25)	34 (57)	11 (79)
Overweight (25–29)	18 (30)	1 (7)
Obese (≥30)	8 (13)	2 (14)
Multiple pregnancy		
No	62 (100)	13 (93)
Yes	0 (0)	1 (7)
Parity		
0	34 (55)	10 (71)
1	18 (29)	4 (29)
2+	10 (16)	0 (0)
Transplant to conception interval		
Less than 1 year	2 (3)	0 (0)
1–2 years	5 (8)	0 (0)
2–5 years	16 (26)	3 (21)
More than 5 years	39 (63)	11 (79)

Data are shown as n (%), with percentages referring to complete data only.
[1]Reported for 70 transplant women, rather than 76 pregnancies, as this characteristic will not have changed with repeated pregnancies.

Table 2. Indication for transplantation in liver transplant recipients (n = 56) and cardiothoracic transplant recipients (n = 14).

Category	Indication	Number (%)
Liver transplant recipients	**Acute liver failure**	**15 (27)**
	Paracetamol	7 (13)
	Other (ecstasy, sulfasalazine, viral)	8 (14)
	Biliary atresia	**8 (14)**
	Cirrhosis	**13 (23)**
	Seronegative/autoimmune hepatitis	11 (20)
	Other (alcohol, amyloid)	2 (3)
	Metabolic disease	**13 (23)**
	Wilson's disease	8 (14)
	Other (tyrosinaemia, alpha-1 antitrypsin deficiency)	5 (9)
	Other (Budd-Chiari syndrome, primary sclerosing cholangitis, cystic fibrosis, malignancy)	**7 (13)**
Cardiothoracic transplant recipients	**Bronchiectatic disease**	**3 (21)**
	Cystic fibrosis	2 (14)
	Obliterative bronchiectasis	1 (7)
	Cardiomyopathies	**6 (43)**
	Viral	3 (21)
	Dilated	2 (14)
	Non-infective	1 (7)
	Congenital heart disease and primary pulmonary hypertension	**5 (36)**

Immunosuppressants and Medication during Pregnancy

Tacrolimus was the most commonly used immunosuppressant in both groups of recipients (n = 58, 76%), followed by prednisolone (38%) and azathioprine (36%), as shown in Table 3. Nine women were taking mycophenolate mofetil (MMF) at conception, with three continuing MMF throughout the pregnancy (doses ranging from 500 to 2000 mg per day); one woman took sirolimus throughout her pregnancy.

Three women took ACE inhibitors or angiotensin receptor blockers at conception and 11 women took aspirin at conception.

Fetal Outcomes

Fetal outcomes are reported in Table 4 and Table 5. There were 70 live births (91% of all pregnancies), and the live birth proportion was similar between the cardiothoracic and liver

Table 3. Medications taken before or during pregnancy.

Drugs	Liver transplant cohort (n = 62)	Cardiothoracic transplant cohort (n = 14)
Immunosuppressants		
Azathioprine	20 (32)	7 (50)
Cyclosporine	12 (19)	5 (36)
Prednisolone	24 (39)	5 (36)
Mycophenolate mofetil	7 (11)	2 (14)
Tacrolimus	49 (79)	9 (64)
Sirolimus	1 (2)	0 (0)
Antihypertensives		
ACE inhibitors and angiotensin receptor blockers	1 (2)	2 (14)
Calcium-channel blockers	4 (6)	1 (7)
Other antihypertensives	5 (8)	6 (43)
Other		
Aspirin	8 (13)	3 (21)
Dyspepsia drugs e.g. omeprazole, ranitidine	10 (16)	2 (14)
Anticoagulants	3 (5)	1 (7)

Data are shown as n (%), with percentages referring to complete data only.

Table 4. Birth outcomes for 77 fetuses born to liver and cardiothoracic transplant recipients[1].

Birth outcome	Entire cohort (n = 77)
Livebirth[2]	70 (91)
Termination of pregnancy for deteriorating maternal condition	1 (1)
First or second trimester miscarriage	4 (5)
Stillbirth	2 (3)

[1]Data have been grouped for confidentiality purposes, due to small numbers.
[2]Includes 57 livebirths to women with liver transplants and 13 livebirths to women with cardiothoracic transplants.

recipients. There were two stillbirths, five miscarriages/terminations and no neonatal deaths.

The median gestational age for live births to women with liver transplants was 38 weeks, compared to 35 in the cardiothoracic cohort (42% vs. 54% born before 37 weeks' gestation). The median birthweight in the liver cohort was 2698 g (range 1115–3995 g), with 37% classified as low birthweight (<2500 g), compared to 2364 g (range 1480–3420 g) in the cardiothoracic cohort and 54% classified as low birthweight.

Thirty percent of neonates were admitted to a neonatal unit, with 54% (n = 7) of the cardiothoracic cohort compared with 25% of the liver cohort (n = 14). Our "best-case scenario" estimated only one small-for-gestational age infant in the cardiothoracic cohort (8%), compared to 9 (16%) in the liver cohort; "worst-case scenario" estimated three (23%) and 12 (21%), respectively.

In our exploratory analysis, MMF had a statistically significant association with poor fetal outcomes (p = 0.04, data not shown), with seven of nine women, who received it prior to or during pregnancy, experiencing adverse outcomes (odds ratio 5.31, 95% confidence interval 1.05–26.96, Table 6). No other immunosuppressant was associated with adverse fetal outcomes.

Women receiving aspirin appeared less likely to have a poor fetal outcome (p = 0.02, data not shown), with an odds ratio (OR) of 0.21 (95% confidence interval 0.05–0.78).

Sixty-three percent of women were breastfeeding their infants at discharge (n = 44).

Maternal Outcomes and Complications
Maternal outcomes are presented in Table 7. One cardiac transplant recipient was delivered at 30 weeks' gestation for

Table 5. Fetal outcomes[1] in liver (n = 57) and cardiothoracic transplant recipients (n = 13)*.

	Liver transplant cohort n (%)	Cardiothoracic transplant cohort n (%)
Apgar score at 5 minutes		
More than 7	56 (98)	11 (85)
Less than 7	1 (2)	2 (15)
Gestational age at delivery		
Less than 32 weeks	0 (0)	2 (15)
32–37 weeks	24 (42)	5 (38)
More than 37 weeks	33 (58)	6 (46)
Birthweight		
1000–1499 g	1 (2)	1 (8)
1500–1999 g	6 (11)	3 (23)
2000–2499 g	14 (25)	3 (23)
More than 2500 g	36 (63)	6 (46)
Small-for-gestational age		
Best-case scenario	9 (16)	1 (8)
Worst case scenario	12 (21)	3 (23)
Congenital anomaly	0 (0)	0 (0)
Neonatal unit admission	14 (25)	7 (54)
Infant breastfed		
Yes	36 (63)	8 (62)
No	13 (23)	2 (15)
Not known	8 (14)	3 (23)

Data are shown as n (%), with percentages referring to complete data only.
[1]Denominator includes all live births,
*including one multiple pregnancy in cardiothoracic cohort.

Table 6. Association of fetal outcomes with medications taken before or during pregnancy, in liver and cardiothoracic transplant recipients (n = 77)[1].

	Good fetal outcome (n = 43)	Poor fetal outcome[2] (n = 34)	Total (n = 77)	Odds ratio (95% confidence interval)
Immunosuppressants[3]				
Azathioprine	16 (37)	12 (35)	28 (36)	0.92 (0.36–2.23)
Cyclosporine	10 (23)	8 (24)	18 (23)	1.02 (0.37–2.78)
Prednisolone	18 (42)	12 (35)	30 (39)	0.76 (0.30–1.94)
Mycophenolate mofetil	2 (5)	7 (21)	9 (12)	5.31 (1.05–27.0)
Tacrolimus	33 (77)	25 (74)	58 (75)	0.84 (0.31–2.30)
Sirolimus	0 (0)	1 (3)	1 (1)	Insufficient data
Anti-hypertensives[4]				
ACE inhibitors and ARBs	2 (5)	1 (3)	3 (4)	0.62 (0.05–7.27)
Calcium-channel blockers	4 (9)	1 (3)	5 (6)	0.30 (0.03–2.86)
Other	5 (12)	6 (18)	11 (14)	1.63 (0.45–5.91)
Other[4]				
Aspirin	10 (23)	2 (6)	12 (16)	0.21 (0.05–0.78)
Dyspepsia drugs	7 (16)	5 (15)	12 (16)	0.89 (0.27–2.84)
Anticoagulants	3 (7)	2 (6)	5 (6)	0.83 (0.19–3.63)

Data are shown as n (%), with percentages referring to complete data only, except for the last column which gives odds ratios with 95% confidence intervals in parentheses.
[1]Denominator refers to all pregnancies, including one multiple pregnancy, but with cluster analysis for 70 women as six women had repeated pregnancies.
[2]Poor fetal outcome was defined as any pregnancy resulting in a stillbirth, miscarriage, very low birthweight (<1500 g), small-for-gestational age (<10th centile, best-case scenario), congenital anomaly, neonatal unit admission and very preterm birth (<32 weeks).
[3]Refers to medications taken before and/or during pregnancy.
[4]Refers to medications taken before pregnancy.
ACE = Angiotensin-converting enzyme inhibitor; ARB = Angiotensin II receptor antagonist.

deteriorating graft function, was admitted to intensive care and died 12 days later, with post-mortem biopsy confirming acute rejection. Two other women (one liver recipient, one cardiothoracic recipient) were reported to have an episode of rejection, neither underwent biopsy.

Sixteen transplant recipients (21% of total; 12 liver recipients, 19%, four cardiothoracic recipients, 29%) were admitted to an intensive care (ITU) or high dependency unit (HDU), though this tended to be for a short duration (median 2 days, range 1–12 days).

Half of the cohort (n = 35) underwent caesarean section, with the majority classed as Grade 3–4 (59%, n = 20) urgency, where there was no immediate maternal or fetal compromise.

The most common indications for emergency caesarean delivery (urgency grade 1–2, 41%, n = 14) were fetal compromise (n = 9), including reduced fetal movements, cardiotocography abnormality and cord prolapse, and maternal compromise (n = 5), including pre-eclampsia and deteriorating graft function. Four women underwent non-emergency caesarean section solely due to their transplant or transplant surgery and two were at maternal request.

Ten women (13%) were diagnosed with pre-eclampsia during pregnancy and the percentage was similar between liver and cardiothoracic recipients. Six women were diagnosed with gestational diabetes, all of whom were on tacrolimus therapy throughout their pregnancy; four of the six women were also taking prednisolone.

Seventeen women (22%) were reported to have renal dysfunction during pregnancy with a 30% increase in serum creatinine

and seven women (9%) had serum creatinine greater than 150 umol/l during the third trimester.

Cardiothoracic transplant recipients had higher creatinine levels during pregnancy than liver transplant recipients, with mean serum creatinine of 104 during first trimester (vs. 77), and greater increases by the third trimester (see Figure 2). Creatinine did not decrease in the second trimester for liver transplant recipients.

Ten women (16%) in the liver transplant group had a diastolic blood pressure greater than 100 mmHg, whilst seven (11%) had a systolic blood pressure greater than 160 mmHg. Three women (21%) in the cardiothoracic group had a diastolic blood pressure of more than 100 mmHg, though none had a systolic blood pressure greater than 160 mmHg.

Discussion

This study reports national, prospectively-collected pregnancy outcome data for UK liver and cardiothoracic transplant recipients, over a five year period. Similar to other studies [1,10–12], we have found that the majority of pregnancies are successful in transplant recipients, but with a high rate of complications.

Liver transplant recipients, in comparison to cardiothoracic and renal transplant recipients from a separate UKOSS cohort [13], had similar livebirth rates (92% vs. 87% vs. 91%, respectively) but lower prematurity rates (42% vs. 54% vs. 52%), fewer low birthweight babies (37% vs. 54% vs. 48%), lower caesarean delivery rates (47% vs. 62% vs. 64%), similar maternal ICU admissions (19% vs. 29% vs. 21%) and fewer neonatal ICU admissions (25% vs. 54% vs. 38%). This same study found that a comparison cohort, of women from the general maternity

Table 7. Maternal outcomes in liver and cardiothoracic transplant recipients.

Maternal outcomes	Liver transplant cohort (n = 62)	Cardiothoracic cohort (n = 14)
Maternal death	0 (0)	1 (7)
Critical care admission	12 (19)	4 (29)
Duration of stay:		
1–2 days	8 (67)	3 (75)
More than 2 days	4 (33)	1 (25)
Episode of rejection	1 (2)	2 (14)
Caesarean section	27 (47)	8 (62)
Grade of urgency[1]:		
Grade 1–2	12 (46)	2 (25)
Grade 3–4	14 (54)	6 (75)
Renal function during pregnancy		
Highest serum creatinine >150 umol/l	5 (8)	4 (29)
Highest serum creatinine >125 umol/l	10 (16)	5 (36)
Highest serum creatinine >100 umol/l	20 (32)	11 (79)
More than 30% increase in serum creatinine	12 (19)	5 (36)
More than 20% increase in serum creatinine	21 (34)	9 (64)
Blood pressure during pregnancy		
Highest systolic blood pressure >160 mmHg	7 (11)	0 (0)
Highest diastolic blood pressure >100 mmHg	10 (16)	3 (21)
Conditions during pregnancy		
Pre-eclampsia	8 (13)	2 (14)
Gestational diabetes	4 (6)	2 (14)

Data are shown as n (%), with percentages referring to complete data only.
[1]Grade 1 involves an immediate threat to the life of the woman or fetus; Grade 2 involves maternal or fetal compromise which is not immediately life-threatening; Grade 3 involves a need for early delivery but no maternal or fetal compromise; Grade 4 requires delivery at a time to suit the woman and maternity team [36].

population had higher livebirth rates (99%), lower prematurity rates (8%), fewer low birthweight babies (8%) and lower caesarean delivery rates (24%), further supporting the finding of a higher rate of complications in transplant recipients [13]. Thus complication rates in all transplant recipients are higher than in the general UK population, though liver recipients appear to have better rates than cardiothoracic and renal transplant recipients.

This is consistent with existing literature, in which more complications have been found in renal than liver transplant recipients, in both single-centre studies [14] and meta-analyses [10]. However, few studies have compared cardiothoracic transplant to other organ recipients [1,3] and no meta-analyses exist.

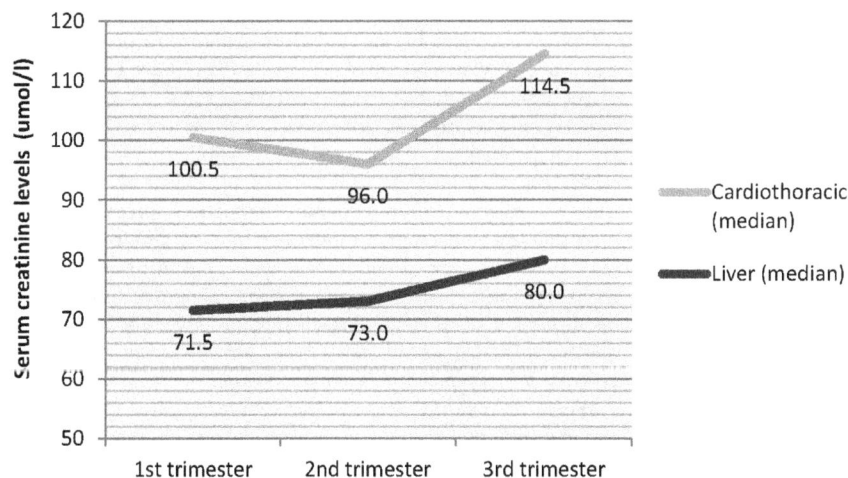

Figure 2. **Highest serum creatinine level during each trimester of pregnancy, for liver and cardiothoracic transplant recipients.**

While our study suggests poorer prognosis in the cardiothoracic group compared to our liver recipients, our cohort also had the lowest mean gestational age (35.5 weeks) and lowest mean birthweight (2441 g) when compared to the other cardiothoracic recipients in the literature (range 36.4–38.3 weeks, range 2600–2143 g) [6,15–17]. As a national, prospective study we would expect our data to be less subject to selection bias and reporting bias inherent in single-centre studies and voluntary registries. Nonetheless, an important caveat to this finding is the comparatively small number of cases analysed, and no external source of case ascertainment was identified for our study period, as the UK Transplant Pregnancy Registry only covered 1994 to 2001.

In a national, retrospective study conducted in Sweden [18], which considered obstetric complications before and after organ transplantation, high rates were found in women who conceived in the years before transplant, particularly in renal compared to liver transplant recipients, suggesting the important role of pre-existing disease in affecting outcomes, particularly chronic kidney disease and hypertension [19]. These factors are likely to be applicable to our cardiothoracic cohort due to the high prevalence of moderately severe, pre-existing renal impairment, as evidenced by high creatinine levels (Figure 2), and congenital disease in this group of women (Table 2). Though our study found 21% (n = 3) of cardiothoracic recipients had diastolic blood pressure over 100 mmHg, other studies of heart transplant recipients and lung transplant recipients, specifically, have found rates of 39% and 52%, respectively [12], though it is not clear which thresholds for blood pressure or definition of "hypertension" they have used.

Another factor to consider is the generally poorer prognosis of cardiothoracic transplant recipients outside of pregnancy. National statistics have shown one-year survival in UK females of reproductive age (15–49 years), transplanted between 2005 and 2007 for kidney, heart, heart-lung, lung and liver was 98–100%, 85%, 71%, 79%, 93% respectively (unpublished data, NHS Blood and Transplant). Five-year survival in UK females of reproductive age, transplanted between 2005 and 2007 for kidney, heart, heart-lung, lung and liver was 92–98%, 80%, 57%, 53% and 80% respectively. Thus, one-year survival and five-year survival are generally lowest in cardiothoracic transplant recipients, and worse in liver than renal transplant recipients, which will be partly related to chronic rejection in the form of bronchiolitis obliterans syndrome [20] and cardiac allograft vasculopathy [21] limiting graft and patient survival after lung or cardiac transplantation, respectively, even in non-pregnant populations.

We cannot comment on whether the reasons women choose to become pregnant vary between regions within the UK or worldwide, and between transplant groups. It is possible that those women who became pregnant represent a healthier cohort than women who did not become pregnant, and this is a limitation that may distort results when making comparisons between groups.

Allograft Function and Rejection in Pregnancy

Our study reports rejection rates of 2% in liver recipients (n = 1) and 14% in cardiothoracic recipients (n = 2). This was biopsy-proven in one of the cardiothoracic recipients, who died as a result of acute rejection. There were no other graft losses or biopsies undertaken. The UKOSS study of renal transplant recipients found 2% (n = 2) had rejection episodes [13].

Other studies have reported higher rates of rejection in liver recipients. For example, in a UK-based study, Christopher et al. [22] found 17% (n = 12) had rejection episodes during pregnancy, with an additional two cases (3%) occurring post-partum. Nagy et al. [23], in the USA, found 10.5% (n = 4) experienced rejection

during pregnancy and a further two (5%) post-partum. In both studies, there were no graft losses or re-transplantations during pregnancy. Both studies were single-centre studies, conducted in transplant units. A survey-based study of female solid organ transplant recipients in British Columbia, Canada, found that 21% (n = 7) experienced a rejection episode [24].

The National Transplantation Pregnancy Registry (NTPR) found rejection rates of 16% in lung transplant recipients (n = 5), 0% in 5 heart-lung transplant recipients and 11% in heart transplant recipients (n = 11), with graft loss within 2 years of pregnancy of 3%, 20% and 14%, respectively [12]. A case series of cystic fibrosis lung transplant recipients found a particularly high rate of rejection (40%, n = 4), with progressive graft dysfunction resulting in death in all four women within 38 months of delivery [25].

Of note, two recent case reports [26,27] document pregnancy-related sensitisation to HLA antigens, leading to rejection and graft failure in cardiac transplant recipients. One of the cases required re-transplantation (five months post-partum) [26], whilst the other died two years later [27]. These case reports highlight that although cardiothoracic recipients are at increased risk of graft loss and have lower survival rates, further research to explore the role of anti-HLA antibodies is needed [6].

Medication at Conception and during Pregnancy

Evidence about the potential effects on pregnancy of the older immunosuppressive drugs is well established [28], however, there is less experience with some of the newer medications in pregnancy. Our study adds to the growing body of evidence that mycophenolate mofetil can lead to adverse fetal outcomes including congenital anomalies and a high probability of fetal loss [29].

Congenital anomalies most commonly associated with "mycophenolate embryopathy" include microtia and orofacial cleft defects [30], though there remain questions regarding the role of complex immunosuppressant regimens and interactions. None of these specific anomalies were reported in our cohort.

Of note, one of two patients to receive mycophenolate, with no adverse fetal outcome, was treated with anticoagulants and anti-platelet agents throughout pregnancy. The group receiving aspirin at conception had a statistically significant lower likelihood of adverse fetal outcomes, which is consistent with a recent meta-analysis considering perinatal death, growth restriction and preterm birth [31].

Only one patient in our study had exposure to sirolimus; she had a poor pregnancy outcome. Though there have been reports of successful pregnancies with sirolimus (16 of 23 pregnancies resulted in livebirths in one report [12]), uncertainty remains regarding potential teratogenic effects [32]. Interestingly, an earlier report from the NTPR found no livebirths in women who had continued on sirolimus throughout pregnancy, but successful fetal outcomes in those discontinuing during pregnancy [33]. It is important to note that most transplant recipients were receiving more than one medication and this may affect interpretation of the role of each medication in contributing to outcomes; a caveat in nearly all obvservational studies of pregnancy in women with complex diseases.

While the majority (60%) of our cohort breastfed their infants and current international consensus suggests it should not be viewed as absolutely contraindicated [5], the topic remains controversial and many centres advocate avoidance to their patients [15,17]. Recent evidence suggests that tacrolimus therapy should not be a contraindication to breast feeding [34,35]. The role of registries, such as the NTPR, will be integral in long-term follow-up of offspring for any adverse events.

Conclusion

In common with most of the literature, our study found the majority of pregnancies in liver and cardiothoracic transplant recipients were successful, although there were high complication rates. Liver transplant recipients appear to have a better prognosis than both renal and cardiothoracic recipients, which may be related to them having a lower incidence of renal dysfunction, hypertension, congenital diseases and graft loss. This study confirmed the impact of renal dysfunction on pregnancy outcomes and the need for ongoing monitoring throughout pregnancy. We found an association between mycophenolate mofetil and poor fetal outcomes. Given the risks of graft rejection on maternal survival, this emphasises the role of pre-conception counselling in addressing these risks. Further research will be needed to investigate the long-term effects of pregnancy on maternal and graft survival rates, for which surveillance systems and national registries will prove invaluable.

Acknowledgments

This study would not have been possible without the contribution and enthusiasm of the UKOSS reporting clinicians who notified cases and completed the data collection forms.

Author Contributions

Conceived and designed the experiments: CNP JJK PB MK. Analyzed the data: OMA. Wrote the paper: OMA. Contributed to writing the manuscript: CNP KB HG JJK PB MK. Contributed to the analysis: JJK MK HG.

References

1. McKay DB, Josephson MA (2006) Pregnancy in recipients of solid organs–effects on mother and child. N Engl J Med 354: 1281 1293.
2. Coscia LA, Constantinescu S, Moritz MJ, Frank AM, Ramirez CB, et al. (2010) Report from the National Transplantation Pregnancy Registry (NTPR): outcomes of pregnancy after transplantation. Clin Transpl: 65–85.
3. Sibanda N, Briggs JD, Davison JM, Johnson RJ, Rudge CJ (2007) Pregnancy after organ transplantation: a report from the UK Transplant pregnancy registry. Transplantation 83: 1301–1307.
4. Rizzoni G, Ehrich JH, Broyer M, Brunner FP, Brynger H, et al. (1992) Successful pregnancies in women on renal replacement therapy: report from the EDTA Registry. Nephrol Dial Transplant 7: 279–287.
5. McKay DB, Josephson MA, Armenti VT, August P, Coscia LA, et al. (2005) Reproduction and transplantation: report on the AST Consensus Conference on Reproductive Issues and Transplantation. Am J Transplant 5: 1592–1599.
6. Cowan SW, Davison JM, Doria C, Moritz MJ, Armenti VT (2012) Pregnancy after cardiac transplantation. Cardiol Clin 30: 441–452.
7. Knight M, Kurinczuk JJ, Tuffnell D, Brocklehurst P (2005) The UK Obstetric Surveillance System for rare disorders of pregnancy. British Journal of Obstetrics and Gynaecology 112: 263–265.
8. Cole TJ, Williams AF, Wright CM (2011) Revised birth centiles for weight, length and head circumference in the UK-WHO growth charts. Ann Hum Biol 38: 7–11.
9. Pan H, Cole TJ (2012) LMSgrowth, a Microsoft Excel add-in to access growth references based on the LMS method. 2.77 ed.
10. Deshpande NA, James NT, Kucirka LM, Boyarsky BJ, Garonzik-Wang JM, et al. (2012) Pregnancy outcomes of liver transplant recipients: a systematic review and meta-analysis. Liver Transpl 18: 621–629.
11. Coffin CS, Shaheen AA, Burak KW, Myers RP (2010) Pregnancy outcomes among liver transplant recipients in the United States: a nationwide case-control analysis. Liver Transpl 16: 56–63.
12. National Transplantation Pregnancy Registry (2012) 2011 Annual Report. Gift of Life Institute, Philadelphia, PA.
13. Bramham K, Nelson-Piercy C, Gao H, Pierce M, Bush N, et al. (2013) Pregnancy in renal transplant recipients: a UK national cohort study. Clin J Am Soc Nephrol 8: 290–298.
14. Blume C, Sensoy A, Gross MM, Guenter HH, Haller H, et al. (2013) A comparison of the outcome of pregnancies after liver and kidney transplantation. Transplantation 95: 222–227.
15. Baron O, Hubaut J, Galetta D, Treilhaud M, Horeau D, et al. (2002) Pregnancy and heart-lung transplantation. J Heart Lung Transplant 21: 914–917.
16. Estensen M, Gude E, Ekmehag B, Lommi J, Bjortuft O, et al. (2011) Pregnancy in heart- and heart/lung recipients can be problematic. Scand Cardiovasc J 45: 349–353.
17. Miniero R, Tardivo I, Centofanti P, Goggi C, Mammana C, et al. (2004) Pregnancy in heart transplant recipients. J Heart Lung Transplant 23: 898–901.
18. Kallen B, Westgren M, Aberg A, Olausson PO (2005) Pregnancy outcome after maternal organ transplantation in Sweden. BJOG 112: 904–909.
19. Flack JM, Ferdinand KC, Nasser SA, Rossi NF (2010) Hypertension in special populations: chronic kidney disease, organ transplant recipients, pregnancy, autonomic dysfunction, racial and ethnic populations. Cardiol Clin 28: 623–638.
20. Weigt SS, DerHovanessian A, Wallace WD, Lynch JP, 3rd, Belperio JA (2013) Bronchiolitis obliterans syndrome: the Achilles' heel of lung transplantation. Semin Respir Crit Care Med 34: 336–351.
21. Valantine H (2004) Cardiac allograft vasculopathy after heart transplantation: risk factors and management. J Heart Lung Transplant 23: S187–193.
22. Christopher V, Al-Chalabi T, Richardson PD, Muiesan P, Rela M, et al. (2006) Pregnancy outcome after liver transplantation: a single-center experience of 71 pregnancies in 45 recipients. Liver Transpl 12: 1138–1143.
23. Nagy S, Bush MC, Berkowitz R, Fishbein TM, Gomez-Lobo V (2003) Pregnancy outcome in liver transplant recipients. Obstet Gynecol 102: 121–128.
24. Humphreys RA, Wong HH, Milner R, Matsuda-Abedini M (2012) Pregnancy outcomes among solid organ transplant recipients in British Columbia. J Obstet Gynaecol Can 34: 416–424.
25. Gyi KM, Hodson ME, Yacoub MY (2006) Pregnancy in cystic fibrosis lung transplant recipients: case series and review. J Cyst Fibros 5: 171–175.
26. Ginwalla M, Pando MJ, Khush KK (2013) Pregnancy-related human leukocyte antigen sensitization leading to cardiac allograft vasculopathy and graft failure in a heart transplant recipient: a case report. Transplant Proc 45: 800–802.
27. O'Boyle PJ, Smith JD, Danskine AJ, Lyster HS, Burke MM, et al. (2010) De novo HLA sensitization and antibody mediated rejection following pregnancy in a heart transplant recipient. Am J Transplant 10: 180–183.
28. Hou S (2013) Pregnancy in renal transplant recipients. Adv Chronic Kidney Dis 20: 253–259.
29. Hoeltzenbein M, Elefant E, Vial T, Finkel-Pekarsky V, Stephens S, et al. (2012) Teratogenicity of mycophenolate confirmed in a prospective study of the European Network of Teratology Information Services. Am J Med Genet A 158A: 588–596.
30. Ang GS, Simpson SA, Reddy AR (2008) Mycophenolate mofetil embryopathy may be dose and timing dependent. Am J Med Genet A 146A: 1963–1966.
31. Roberge S, Nicolaides KH, Demers S, Villa P, Bujold E (2013) Prevention of perinatal death and adverse perinatal outcome using low-dose aspirin: a meta-analysis. Ultrasound Obstet Gynecol 41: 491–499.
32. Armenti VT, Constantinescu S, Moritz MJ, Davison JM (2008) Pregnancy after transplantation. Transplant Rev (Orlando) 22: 223–240.
33. Sifontis NM, Coscia LA, Constantinescu S, Lavelanet AF, Moritz MJ, et al. (2006) Pregnancy outcomes in solid organ transplant recipients with exposure to mycophenolate mofetil or sirolimus. Transplantation 82: 1698–1702.
34. Bramham K, Chusney G, Lee J, Lightstone L, Nelson-Piercy C (2013) Breastfeeding and tacrolimus: serial monitoring in breast-fed and bottle-fed infants. Clin J Am Soc Nephrol 8: 563–567.
35. Sau A, Clarke S, Bass J, Kaiser A, Marinaki A, et al. (2007) Azathioprine and breastfeeding: is it safe? BJOG 114: 498–501.
36. Royal College of Obstetrics and Gynaecology and Royal College of Anaethetists (2010) Classification of urgency of Caesarean section - a continuum of risk. Good Practice No. 11. London: Royal College of Obstetrics and Gynaecology.

Permissions

The contributors of this book come from diverse backgrounds, making this book a truly international effort. This book will bring forth new frontiers with its revolutionizing research information and detailed analysis of the nascent developments around the world.

We would like to thank all the contributing authors for lending their expertise to make the book truly unique. They have played a crucial role in the development of this book. Without their invaluable contributions this book wouldn't have been possible. They have made vital efforts to compile up to date information on the varied aspects of this subject to make this book a valuable addition to the collection of many professionals and students.

This book was conceptualized with the vision of imparting up-to-date information and advanced data in this field. To ensure the same, a matchless editorial board was set up. Every individual on the board went through rigorous rounds of assessment to prove their worth. After which they invested a large part of their time researching and compiling the most relevant data for our readers.

The editorial board has been involved in producing this book since its inception. They have spent rigorous hours researching and exploring the diverse topics which have resulted in the successful publishing of this book. They have passed on their knowledge of decades through this book. To expedite this challenging task, the publisher supported the team at every step. A small team of assistant editors was also appointed to further simplify the editing procedure and attain best results for the readers.

Apart from the editorial board, the designing team has also invested a significant amount of their time in understanding the subject and creating the most relevant covers. They scrutinized every image to scout for the most suitable representation of the subject and create an appropriate cover for the book.

The publishing team has been an ardent support to the editorial, designing and production team. Their endless efforts to recruit the best for this project, has resulted in the accomplishment of this book. They are a veteran in the field of academics and their pool of knowledge is as vast as their experience in printing. Their expertise and guidance has proved useful at every step. Their uncompromising quality standards have made this book an exceptional effort. Their encouragement from time to time has been an inspiration for everyone.

The publisher and the editorial board hope that this book will prove to be a valuable piece of knowledge for researchers, students, practitioners and scholars across the globe.

List of Contributors

Robert P. Dickson, John R. Erb-Downward, Natalie Walker, Fernando J. Martinez and Vibha N. Lama
Division of Pulmonary and Critical Care Medicine, Department of Internal Medicine, University of Michigan Medical School, Ann Arbor, Michigan, United States of America

Christine M. Freeman
Division of Pulmonary and Critical Care Medicine, Department of Internal Medicine, University of Michigan Medical School, Ann Arbor, Michigan, United States of America
Research Service, Department of Veterans Affairs Health Care System, Ann Arbor, Michigan, United States of America

Brittan S. Scales and Gary B. Huffnagle
Division of Pulmonary and Critical Care Medicine, Department of Internal Medicine, University of Michigan Medical School, Ann Arbor, Michigan, United States of America
Department of Microbiology and Immunology, University of Michigan Medical School, Ann Arbor, Michigan, United States of America

James M. Beck
Department of Medicine, University of Colorado Denver, Aurora, Colorado and Medicine Service, Veterans Affairs Eastern Colorado Health Care System, Denver, Colorado, United States of America,

Jeffrey L. Curtis
Division of Pulmonary and Critical Care Medicine, Department of Internal Medicine, University of Michigan Medical School, Ann Arbor, Michigan, United States of America
Pulmonary & Critical Care Medicine Section, Medical Service, VA Ann Arbor Healthcare System, Ann Arbor, Michigan, United States of America

Teng Moua and Tobias Peikert
Division of Pulmonary/Critical Care, Mayo Clinic Rochester, Rochester, Minnesota, United States of America

Ladan Zand, Dingxin Qin and Qi Qian
Division of Nephrology, Mayo Clinic Rochester, Rochester, Minnesota, United States of America

Robert P. Hartman and Thomas E. Hartman
Department of Radiology, Mayo Clinic Rochester, Rochester, Minnesota, United States of America

Thi H. O. Nguyen, Glen P. Westall, Tara E. Bull, Aislin C. Meehan, Nicole A. Mifsud and Tom C. Kotsimbos
Department of Medicine, Monash University, Central Clinical School, The Alfred Centre, Melbourne, Victoria, Australia
Department of Allergy, Immunology and Respiratory Medicine, The Alfred Hospital, Melbourne, Victoria, Australia

Chi-Ping Day and Glenn Merlino
Laboratory of Cancer Biology and Genetics, National Cancer Institute, Bethesda, Maryland, United States of America

John Carter and Carrie Bonomi
In Vivo Evaluation, Leidos Biomedical Research Inc., Frederick National Laboratory for Cancer Research, Frederick, Maryland, United States of America

Zoe Weaver Ohler, Rajaa El Meskini and Philip Martin
Center for Advanced Preclinical Research of Leidos Biomedical Research Inc., Frederick National Laboratory for Cancer Research, Frederick, Maryland, United States of America

Cari Graff-Cherry and Lionel Feigenbaum
Laboratory Animal Science Program, Leidos Biomedical Research Inc., Frederick National Laboratory for Cancer Research, Frederick, Maryland, United States of America

Thomas Tüting
Department of Dermatology and Allergy, University Hospital Bonn, Bonn, Germany

Terry Van Dyke
Center for Advanced Preclinical Research of The Center for Cancer Research, National Cancer Institute, Frederick, Maryland, United States of America

Melinda Hollingshead
Biological Testing Branch, Developmental Therapeutics Program, National Cancer Institute, Frederick, Maryland, United States of America

Matthew D. Stone
Waters Corporation, Milford, Massachusetts, United States of America
Department of Biochemistry, Molecular Biology and Biophysics, University of Minnesota, Minneapolis, Minnesota, United States of America

Stephen B. Harvey and Gary L. Nelsestuen
Department of Biochemistry, Molecular Biology and Biophysics, University of Minnesota, Minneapolis, Minnesota, United States of America

Cavan Reilly
Department of Biostatistics, University of Minnesota, Minneapolis, Minnesota, United States of America

Marshall I. Hertz
Department of Medicine, University of Minnesota, Minneapolis, Minnesota, United States of America

Chris H. Wendt
Department of Medicine, University of Minnesota, Minneapolis, Minnesota, United States of America
Department of Medicine, Veterans Administration Medical Center, University of Minnesota, Minneapolis, Minnesota, United States

Wenteh Chang, Ke Wei, Susan S. Jacobs, Cheryl H. Chang and Glenn D. Rosen
Division of Pulmonary and Critical Care Medicine, Stanford University School of Medicine, Stanford, California, United States of America

Lawrence Ho
Division of Pulmonary and Critical Care Medicine, University of Washington School of Medicine, Seattle, Washington, United States of America

Gerald J. Berry
Department of Pathology, Stanford University School of Medicine, Stanford, California, United States of America

Hendrik Suhling, Jessica Rademacher, Imke Zinowsky, Jan Fuge, Mark Greer, Tobias Welte and Jens Gottlieb
Dept. of Respiratory Medicine, Hannover Medical School, Hannover, Germany

Gregor Warnecke and Axel Haverich
Dept. of Cardiothoracic, Transplantation and Vascular Surgery, Hannover Medical School, Hannover, Germany

Jacqueline M. Smits
Eurotransplant International Foundation, Leiden, The Netherlands

Anna Bertram
Dept. of Nephrology and Hypertension, Hannover Medical School, Hannover, Germany

Steven R. White, Timothy Floreth and Chuanhong Liao
Departments of Medicine and Health Studies, University of Chicago, Chicago, Illinois, United States of America

Sangeeta M. Bhorade
Department of Medicine, Northwestern University, Chicago, Illinois, United States of America

Aislin C. Meehan, Nicole A. Mifsud, Thi H. O. Nguyen, Tom C. Kotsimbos and Glen P. Westall
Department of Medicine, Monash University, Melbourne, Victoria, Australia
Department of Allergy, Immunology and Respiratory Medicine, The Alfred Hospital, Melbourne, Victoria, Australia

Bronwyn J. Levvey and Greg I. Snell
Department of Allergy, Immunology and Respiratory Medicine, The Alfred Hospital, Melbourne, Victoria, Australia

Fiorella Calabrese, Francesca Lunardi, Elisabetta Balestro, Egle Perissinotto, Emanuela Rossi, Nazarena Nannini, Giuseppe Marulli and Federico Rea
Department of Cardiac, Thoracic and Vascular Sciences, University of Padova, Padova, Italy

Anja Kipar
Department of Infection Biology, University of Liverpool, Liverpool, United Kingdom
School of Veterinary Science, University of Liverpool, Liverpool, United Kingdom
Veterinary Pathology, Department of Basic Veterinary Science, Faculty of Veterinary Medicine, University of Helsinki, Helsinki, Finlan

James P. Stewart
Department of Infection Biology, University of Liverpool, Liverpool, United Kingdom
School of Veterinary Science, University of Liverpool, Liverpool, United Kingdom

Yao Liu, Yi Liu, Lili Su and Shu-juan Jiang
Department of Respiratory Medicine, Provincial Hospital Affiliated to Shandong University, Jinan, Shandong, China

Nicole Scheuing, Reinhard W. Holl and Julia M. Hermann
Institute of Epidemiology and Medical Biometry, Central Institute for Biomedical Technology, University of Ulm, Ulm, Germany

Gerd Dockter
Cystic Fibrosis Centre, Saarland University Hospital for Pediatric and Adolescent Medicine, Homburg/Saar, Germany

Sibylle Junge
Clinic for Pediatric Pneumology and Neonatology, Hannover Medical School, Hannover, Germany

Cordula Koerner-Rettberg and Manfred Ballmann
Department of Pediatric Pulmonology, St. Josef Hospital Pediatric Clinic, Ruhr University Bochum, Bochum, Germany

Lutz Naehrlich
Department of Pediatrics, Justus-Liebig University Giessen, Giessen, Germany

Christina Smaczny
Medical Clinic I, Pneumology and Allergology, University Hospital Frankfurt/Main, Goethe University, Frankfurt/Main, Germany

Doris Staab
Division of Pulmonology and Immunology, Department of Pediatrics, Charité Berlin, Berlin, Germany

Gabriela Thalhammer
Department for Pediatric Pulmonology and Allergology, Medical University of Graz, Graz, Austria

Silke van Koningsbruggen-Rietschel
Cystic Fibrosis Centre Cologne, Childrens Hospital, University of Cologne, Cologne, Germany

Bernhard Moser, Anna Megerle, Stefan Janik, Shahrokh Taghavi and Walter Klepetko
Department of Thoracic Surgery, Division of Surgery, Medical University Vienna, Vienna, Austria

Christine Bekos and Hendrik Jan Ankersmit
Department of Thoracic Surgery, Division of Surgery, Medical University Vienna, Vienna, Austria
Christian Doppler Laboratory for the Diagnosis and Regeneration of Cardiac and Thoracic Diseases, Medical University Vienna, Vienna, Austria

Tamás Szerafin
Department of Cardiac Surgery, University of Debrecen, Debrecen, Hungary

Peter Birner and Ana-Iris Schiefer
Department of Pathology, Medical University Vienna, Vienna, Austria

Michael Mildner
Department of Dermatology, Medical University Vienna, Vienna, Austria

Irene Lang, Nika Skoro-Sajer and Roela Sadushi-Kolici
Department of Internal Medicine II, Division of Cardiology, Medical University Vienna, Vienna, Austria

Kashif Raza and Marshall I. Hertz
Pulmonary, Allergy, Critical Care and Sleep Medicine, University of Minnesota, Minneapolis, Minnesota, United States of America

Trevor Larsen and Nath Samaratunga
Breck High School, Edina, Minnesota, United States of America

Andrew P. Price, Carolyn Meyer, Amy Matson, Michael J. Ehrhardt, Samuel Fogas and Jakub Tolar
Pediatric Blood and Bone Marrow Transplant Program, University of Minnesota Cancer Center, Minneapolis, Minnesota, United States of America

Angela Panoskaltsis-Mortari
Pulmonary, Allergy, Critical Care and Sleep Medicine, University of Minnesota, Minneapolis, Minnesota, United States of America
Pediatric Blood and Bone Marrow Transplant Program, University of Minnesota Cancer Center, Minneapolis, Minnesota, United States of America

Yun Sil Chang and Won Soon Park
Department of Pediatrics, Samsung Medical Center, Sungkyunkwan University School of Medicine, Seoul, Korea
Samsung Biomedical Research Institute, Sungkyunkwan University School of Medicine, Seoul, Korea

Soo Jin Choi and Won Il Oh
Biomedical Research Institute, MEDIPOST Co., Ltd., Seoul, Korea

So Yoon Ahn, Se In Sung and Hye Soo Yoo
Department of Pediatrics, Samsung Medical Center, Sungkyunkwan University School of Medicine, Seoul, Korea

Dong Kyung Sung
Samsung Biomedical Research Institute, Sungkyunkwan University School of Medicine, Seoul, Korea

Shi Jin
Tianjin Key Laboratory of Lung Cancer Metastasis and Tumor Micro-environment, Tianjin Lung Cancer Institute, Tianjin Medical University General Hospital, Tianjin, P.R. China
Department of Medical Oncology, Harbin Medical University Cancer Hospital, Harbin, P.R. China

Yi Deng
Tianjin Key Laboratory of Lung Cancer Metastasis and Tumor Micro-environment, Tianjin Lung Cancer Institute, Tianjin Medical University General Hospital, Tianjin, P.R. China
Cancer Center, Research Institute of Surgery and Daping Hospital, Third Military Medical University, Chongqing, P.R. China

Jun-Wei Hao and Fu-Dong Shi
Department of neurology, Tianjin Medical University General Hospital, Tianjin, P.R. China

Yang Li, Bin Liu and Qing-Hua Zhou
Tianjin Key Laboratory of Lung Cancer Metastasis and Tumor Micro-environment, Tianjin Lung Cancer Institute, Tianjin Medical University General Hospital, Tianjin, P.R. China

Yan Yu
Department of Medical Oncology, Harbin Medical University Cancer Hospital, Harbin, P.R. China

Amjad Horani
Department of Pediatrics, Washington University School of Medicine, St. Louis, Missouri, United States of America

Thomas W. Ferkol
Department of Pediatrics, Washington University School of Medicine, St. Louis, Missouri, United States of America
Department of Cell Biology and Physiology, Washington University School of Medicine, St. Louis, Missouri, United States of America

David Shoseyov, Malena Cohen-Cymberknoh and Eitan Kerem
Department of Pediatrics, Hadassah Hebrew University Medical Center, Jerusalem, Israel

Mollie G. Wasserman and Steven L. Brody
Department of Medicine, Washington University School of Medicine, St. Louis, Missouri, United States of America

Yifat S. Oren and Batsheva Kerem
Department of Genetics, The Hebrew University, Jerusalem, Israel

Israel Amirav
Department of Pediatrics, Ziv Medical Center, Safed, Israel

Susan K. Dutcher
Department of Genetics, Washington University School of Medicine, St. Louis, Missouri, United States of America

Orly Elpeleg
Monique and Jacques Roboh Department of Genetic Research, Hadassah Hebrew University Medical Center, Jerusalem, Israel

Sabine Dettmer, Lars Peters, Frank Wacker and Hoen-oh Shin
Hannover Medical School, Department of Radiology, Hannover, Germany

Claudia de Wall and Jens Gottlieb
Hannover Medical School, Department of Respiratory Medicine, Hannover, Germany

Cornelia Schaefer-Prokop
Radiologie, Meander Medisch Centrum, Amersfoort, the Netherlands
Radiologie – DIAG, UMC St Radboud, Nijmegen, the Netherlands

Michael Schmidt
Fraunhofer MEVIS, Bremen, Germany

Gregor Warnecke
Hannover Medical School, Department of Thoracic and Cardiovascular Surgery, Hannover, Germany

Vanessa J. Craig, Maria E. Laucho-Contreras, Juan C. Osorio and Victor Pinto-Plata
Division of Pulmonary and Critical Care Medicine, Brigham and Women's Hospital, Harvard Medical School, Boston, Massachusetts, United States of America,

Francesca Polverino
Division of Pulmonary and Critical Care Medicine, Brigham and Women's Hospital, Harvard Medical School, Boston, Massachusetts, United States of America,
Department of Clinical and Experimental Medicine, University of Parma, Parma, Italy
Pulmonary Fibrosis Program, Lovelace Respiratory Research Institute, Albuquerque, New Mexico, United States of America

Yuanyuan Shi, Ivan O. Rosas and Yushi Liu
Division of Pulmonary and Critical Care Medicine, Brigham and Women's Hospital, Harvard Medical School, Boston, Massachusetts, United States of America,
Pulmonary Fibrosis Program, Lovelace Respiratory Research Institute, Albuquerque, New Mexico, United States of America

Yohannes Tesfaigzi
Chronic Obstructive Pulmonary Disease Program, Lovelace Respiratory Research Institute, Albuquerque, New Mexico, United States of America

Bernadette R. Gochuico
Medical Genetics Branch, National Human Genome Research Institute, National Institutes of Health, Bethesda, Maryland, United States of America

Caroline A. Owen
Division of Pulmonary and Critical Care Medicine, Brigham and Women's Hospital, Harvard Medical School, Boston, Massachusetts, United States of America,
Pulmonary Fibrosis Program, Lovelace Respiratory Research Institute, Albuquerque, New Mexico, United States of America

Chronic Obstructive Pulmonary Disease Program, Lovelace Respiratory Research Institute, Albuquerque, New Mexico, United States of America

David J. Lederer
Department of Medicine, College of Physicians and Surgeons, Columbia University, New York City, New York, United States of America
Department of Epidemiology, Mailman School of Public Health, Columbia University, New York City, New York, United States of America

Nisha Philip, Debbie Rybak and Selim M. Arcasoy
Department of Medicine, College of Physicians and Surgeons, Columbia University, New York City, New York, United States of America

Steven M. Kawut
Department of Medicine, Perelman School of Medicine, University of Pennsylvania, Philadelphia, Pennsylvania, United States of America
Center for Clinical Epidemiology and Biostatistics, Perelman School of Medicine, University of Pennsylvania, Philadelphia, Pennsylvania, United States of America

Quentin Philippot
Division of Pulmonary and Critical Care Medicine, Department of Internal Medicine Washington University, St. Louis, Missouri, United States of America
Institut National de la Santé Et de la Recherche Medicale Unit 903, University Hospital, Reims, France

Gaëtan Deslée and Jeanne Marie Perotin
Institut National de la Santé Et de la Recherche Medicale Unit 903, University Hospital, Reims, France
Department of Pulmonary Medicine, University Hospital of Reims, France

Tracy L. Adair-Kirk, Derek Byers, Michael J. Holtzman and Richard A. Pierce
Division of Pulmonary and Critical Care Medicine, Department of Internal Medicine Washington University, St. Louis, Missouri, United States of America

Jason C. Woods and Susan Conradi
Department of Radiology, Washington University, St. Louis, Missouri, United States of America

Sandra Dury and François Lebargy
Department of Pulmonary Medicine, University Hospital of Reims, France
EA4683, University of Reims, Reims, France

Christelle Cassan and Richard Le Naour
EA4683, University of Reims, Reims, France

Sylvia Sanquer, Laurence Herry, Celine Lena, Alphonsine Diouf and Robert Barouki
Service de Biochimie Métabolomique et Protéomique, Hôpital Universitaire Necker-Enfants Malades Assistance Publique-Hôpitaux de Paris (AP-HP); INSERM UMR-S 747; and Université Paris Descartes, Centre Universitaire des Saints-Pères, Paris, France

Catherine Amrein, Romain Guillemain and Veronique Boussaud
Service de Chirurgie Cardio-Vasculaire, Hôpital Européen Georges Pompidou, AP-HP, Paris, France

Dominique Grenet, Bruno Philippe and Marc Stern
Service de Pneumologie, Hôpital Foch, Suresnes, France

Michelle Paunet
Laboratoire de Biologie, Hôpital Foch, Suresnes, France

Eliane M. Billaud
Service de Pharmacologie, Hôpital Européen Georges Pompidou, AP-HP and Université Paris Descartes, Paris, France

Françoise Loriaux
Service de Biochimie, Hôpital Européen Georges Pompidou, AP-HP, Paris, France,

Jean-Philippe Jai
Service de Biostatistiques, Hôpital Necker-Enfants Malades, AP-HP, Paris, France; Université Paris Descartes, Paris, France

Olaa Mohamed-Ahmed, Haiyan Gao, Jennifer J. Kurinczuk and Marian Knight
National Perinatal Epidemiology Unit, Nuffield Department of Population Health, University of Oxford, United Kingdom

Cathy Nelson-Piercy
Division of Women's Health, King's College London, Women's Health Academic Centre, King's Health Partners, United Kingdom
Obstetric Medicine, Guy's and St Thomas' NHS Foundation Trust, London, United Kingdom

Kate Bramham
Division of Women's Health, King's College London, Women's Health Academic Centre, King's Health Partners, United Kingdom

Peter Brocklehurst
Institute for Women's Health, University College London, United Kingdom

Index